**SECOND EDITION**

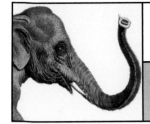

### APPLETON & LANGE

## OUTLINE REVIEW FOR THE

# PHYSICIAN ASSISTANT EXAMINATION

**Albert F. Simon, MEd, PA-C**
Chairman, Department of Physician Assistant Sciences
Saint Francis University
Loretto, Pennsylvania

**Anthony A. Miller, MEd, PA-C**
Associate Professor & Director
Division of Physician Assistant Studies
Shenandoah University
Winchester, Virginia

**Appleton & Lange Reviews/McGraw-Hill**
Medical Publishing Division

New York   Chicago   San Francisco   Lisbon   London   Madrid
Mexico City   Milan   New Delhi   San Juan   Seoul   Singapore   Sydney   Toronto

**Appleton & Lange Outline Review for the Physician Assistant Examination, Second Edition**

5 6 7 8 9 0  CUS/CUS  0 9 8 7

ISBN 0-07-140289-6

---

**Notice**

Medicine is an ever-changing science. As new research and clinical experience broaden our knowledge, changes in treatment and drug therapy are required. The authors and the publisher of this work have checked with sources believed to be reliable in their efforts to provide information that is complete and generally in accord with the standards accepted at the time of publication. However, in view of the possibility of human error or changes in medical sciences, neither the authors nor the publisher nor any other party who has been involved in the preparation or publication of this work warrants that the information contained herein is in every respect accurate or complete, and they disclaim all responsibility for any errors or omissions or for the results obtained from use of the information contained in this work. Readers are encouraged to confirm the information contained herein with other sources. For example and in particular, readers are advised to check the product information sheet included in the package of each drug they plan to administer to be certain that the information contained in this work is accurate and that changes have not been made in the recommended dose or in the contraindications for administration. This recommendation is of particular importance in connection with new or infrequently used drugs.

---

This book was set in New Baskerville by Circle Graphics.
The editors were Michael J. Brown and Christie Naglieri.
The production supervisor was Sherri Souffrance.
Project management was provided by Columbia Publishing Services.
Von Hoffmann Graphics was printer and binder.

This book is printed on acid-free paper.

**Library of Congress Cataloging-in-Publication Data**

Appleton & Lange outline review for the physician assistant examination / [edited by]
    Albert F. Simon, Anthony A. Miller.—2nd ed.
        p. ; cm.
    Includes bibliographical references and index.
    ISBN 0-07-140289-6
    1. Physicians' assistants—Examinations, questions, etc.  I. Title: Outline review for the
physician assistant examination. II. Simon, Albert F. III. Miller, Anthony A.
    [DNLM: 1. Physician Assistants—Examination Questions. 2. Physician
Assistants—Outlines. W 18.2 A6487 2003]
    R697.P45A667 2003
    610.69'53'076—dc21
                                                                            2003053964

Please tell the author and publisher what you think of this book by sending your comments to pa@mcgraw-hill.com. Please put the author and title of the book in the subject line.

# Contributors

**Salah Ayachi, PhD, PA-C**
Associate Professor
Physician Assistant Studies
The University of Texas Medical Branch
Galveston, Texas
*Cardiovascular Diseases*

**J. Dennis Blessing, PhD, PA-C**
Professor and Chairman
Department of Physician Assistant Studies
University of Texas Health Sciences
   Center at San Antonio
*Ophthalmology*

**Kathryn Boyer, MS, PA-C**
Leukemia Department
University of Texas
M.D. Anderson Cancer Center
Houston, Texas
*Hematology and Oncology*

**Dwight M. Deter, PA-C**
Physician Assistant
Southwest Endocrine Consultants
El Paso, Texas
*Endocrinology*

**William R. Duryea, PhD, PA-C**
Master of Medical Science Program
Department of Physician Assistant Sciences
Saint Francis University
Loretto, Pennsylvania
*Infectious Disease*

**Raymond L. Eifel, MS, PA-C**
Assistant Professor
Division of Physician Assistant Studies
Shenandoah University
Winchester, Virginia
*Male Genitourinary Disorders*

**Steve B. Fisher, MHA, PA-C**
Assistant Professor
Department of Clinical Science
College of Health Sciences
Division of Physician Assistant Studies
University of Kentucky, Lexington
Professional Staff, Department of Surgery
Division of Neurosurgery
University of Kentucky Medical Center, Lexington
*Surgery*

**Anita Duhl Glicken, MSW**
Professor
Department of Pediatrics
Child Health Associate/Physician
   Assistant Program
University of Colorado Health Sciences Center
Aurora, Colorado
*Psychiatry*

**Constance Goldgar, MS, PA-C**
Research Associate Professor
Family and Preventive Medicine
University of Utah
Salt Lake City
*Obstetrics and Gynecology*

**Nancy Ivansek, MA, PA-C**
Coordinator, Sarcoidosis Center of Excellence
Cleveland Clinic Foundation
Cleveland, Ohio
*Gastroenterology and Nutrition*

**Brenda L. Jasper, MPAS, PA-C**
Physician Assistant
Renal-Endocrine Associates, P.C.
West Penn Allegheny Health System
Forbes Regional Hospital
Monroeville, Pennsylvania
*Renal Disease*

**P. Eugene Jones, PhD, PA-C**
Professor and Chairman
Department of Physician Assistant Studies
The University of Texas Southwestern
    Medical Center at Dallas
*Dermatology*

**Rebecca Luebke, MSBS, PA-C**
Physician Assistant
Fallen Timbers Family Physicians, Inc.
Maumee, Ohio
*Ear, Nose, and Throat*

**William H. Marquardt, MA, PA-C**
Chair
Physician Assistant Department
Nova Southeastern University
Ft. Lauderdale, Florida
*Neurology*

**Matthew McQuillan, MS, PA-C**
Assistant Professor and Faculty
Physician Assistant Program
University of Medicine and Dentistry of
    New Jersey, Piscataway
Physician Assistant
The Doctor Is In
Clinton, New Jersey
*Pulmonary Diseases*

**Dawn Morton-Rias, PD, RPA-C**
Interim Dean
College of Health Related Professions
Assistant Professor
Physician Assistant Program
State University of New York
Health Sciences Center at Brooklyn-Downstate
    Medical Center
Brooklyn, New York
*Obstetrics and Gynecology*

**Paula Phelps, MHE, PA-C**
Assistant Professor
Physician Assistant Program
Idaho State University, Pocatello, Idaho
*Obstetrics and Gynecology*

**Maura Polansky, MS, PA-C**
Physician Assistant
Division of Cancer Medicine
Gastrointestinal Oncology Center
Program Director
Postgraduate Physician Assistant
    Oncology Program
M.D. Anderson Cancer Center, Houston, Texas
*Hematology and Oncology*

**Richard R. Rahr, EdD, PA-C**
Professor and Chair
Physician Assistant Studies
The University of Texas Medical Branch
Galveston, Texas
*Cardiovascular Diseases*

**Jill Reichman, MPH, PA-C**
Associate Director and Associate Professor
Physician Assistant Program
University of Medicine and Dentistry of
    New Jersey, Piscataway
*Pulmonary Diseases*

**Lisa N. Reyna, MPAS, PA-C**
Clinical Coordinator and Assistant Professor
Department of Physician Assistant Studies
University of Texas Health Sciences Center at
    San Antonio
*Ophthalmology*

**Douglas R. Southard, PhD, MPH, PA-C**
Director
Department of Clinical Research
Carilon Medical Center, Roanoke, Virginia
*Psychiatry*

**Sarah A. Toth, MS, PA-C**
Physician Assistant
Texas Ear, Nose, and Throat Consultants, PLLC
Houston, Texas
*Pediatrics*

**Donna L. Yeisley, MEd, PA-C**
Associate Professor
Department of Physician Assistant Sciences
Saint Francis University, Loretto, Pennsylvania
*Rheumatology and Orthopedics*

# Contents

# Preface

The second edition of *Appleton & Lange Outline Review for the Physician Assistant Examination* has undergone extensive content revision and updating. Once again we have called on content experts throughout the medical disciplines to provide a concise outline to highlight important points and help structure your review of materials for the Physician Assistant National Certifying Examination (PANCE) and Physician Assistant National Recertifying Examination (PANRE) examinations. The content of this edition still is patterned after the examination blueprint of topics from the NCCPA to ensure an adequate coverage of the topics you may encounter on the PANRE and PANCE examinations. Physician assistant students may also find the *Outline Review* helpful as they prepare for end of rotation or summative examinations during their course of study.

The benefit of the *Outline Review* will be enhanced by using it in conjunction with your favorite textbook of medicine and *Appleton & Lange Review for the Physician Assistant* to design an overall comprehensive study plan. We think you will fine the *Outline Review* particularly effective in illustrating the important points about disease processes and conditions you are likely to encounter both in practice and on examinations.

We would like to thank the contributors for their expert assistance in developing and updating the material for this text and their long hours of dedication to assist those who will follow them in this profession. The folks at McGraw-Hill continue to provide sound guidance for us with their suggestions throughout the publication process. Finally, thanks to our families, friends, and colleagues who continue to support us.

*Albert F. Simon, MEd, PA-C*
*Anthony A. Miller, MEd, PA-C*

# Helpful Hints for Taking the Certifying Exam

## CONTENT PREPARATION

✓ Take a refresher course.

✓ Set a weekly schedule for exam preparation: start early, don't try to cram.

✓ If possible, design your review schedule to correlate with your clinical rotation schedule to maximize learning.

✓ Design your reading around the examination content outline. For more information on the content and procedures, go to the NCCPA web site and click on "exams"

  ○ http://www.nccpa.net

✓ Remember the PANCE and PANRE exams are primary care oriented.

✓ Select reference books that are up-to-date and easy to read.

✓ Use this outline review to refresh your memory and determine gaps in knowledge; take notes as you review, mark unfamiliar words or phrases, then look them up.

✓ Use practice tests to diagnose strengths and weaknesses. *Appleton & Lange Review for the Physician Assistant,* 4th edition offers 1,200 exam questions for review and an excellent practice exam on CD. The Association of Physician Assistant Programs (APAP) offers a practice exam called GRADRAT. To order, go to http://www.apap.org and click on "Products and Services."

✓ Practice test-taking to improve speed and proficiency.

✓ Use the practice diskette from NCCPA to familiarize yourself with the test format.

## TEST PREPARATION

✓ Register for the exam on time.

✓ Mark your calendar with the assigned date, time, and test center.

✓ Make sure you know how to get to the test center; allow extra time for travel, and be early the day of the exam.

✓ Get plenty of rest the night before.

✓ Be sure you are well nourished, but don't eat a full meal just before the exam.

✓ Dress comfortably in layers, so you can adjust to the temperature of the test center.

✓ Make sure you have the admission card and identification before you leave for the test center.

✓ Keep a positive attitude. Proper preparation helps provide confidence.

## DURING THE EXAM

✓ Make sure you are comfortable.

✓ Avoid distractions—concentrate (bring ear plugs if necessary).

✓ Read directions carefully.

✓ Pace yourself to avoid rushing at the end.

✓ Avoid "jumping the gun"—consider all possible answers before selecting.

✓ Don't get discouraged over one or two questions. Some items are designed to be more difficult.

✓ Answer items you are sure of first, then go back to the difficult ones.

✓ Don't change answers unless you are sure you marked incorrectly.

✓ Use the process of elimination to narrow your choices.

✓ Answer all questions, generally there are no penalties for guessing.

✓ Go back to finish skipped items before ending exam.

## AFTER THE EXAM

✓ Celebrate!

# Dermatology 1

*P. Eugene Jones, PhD, PA-C*

## I. ECZEMATOUS ERUPTIONS

### A. Dermatitis

#### 1. Atopic

▶ **Scientific Concepts**

Although the exact etiology of atopic dermatitis (atopic eczema) remains uncertain, the implication of an immunologic disorder as the etiology is supported by the presence of elevated serum immunoglobulin E (IgE) levels and a clinical similarity to primary T cell immunodeficiency disorders. Primarily manifesting in infancy and childhood, the diagnosis of atopic dermatitis is based on a combination of historical and clinical findings rather than any specific diagnostic laboratory test.

▶ **History & Physical**

Known as "the itch that rashes," atopic dermatitis presents more often in infancy and childhood as a chronic recurring condition commonly associated with differing combinations of major and associated clinical features. Major features include pruritus, lichenification, flexor and extensor crease involvement, chronicity, and a personal or family history of atopy (specifically allergic rhinitis and/or asthma). Associated features are numerous and include pityriasis alba, xerosis, ichthyosis vulgaris, keratosis pilaris, sensitivity to wool, nonspecific pruritic dermatoses, and hyperlinear palmar creases. Patients present in differing stages of acuity and chronicity with excoriated, erythematous, weeping, crusted, and scaly lesions progressing to lichenified and fibrotic papules and plaques. The constellation of acute, subacute, and chronic features and classic history of atopy, coupled with intense pruritus and skin sensitivity, suggest the diagnosis.

▶ **Diagnostic Studies**

None, based on history and physical examination.

▶ **Diagnosis**

Rule out other disorders of the eczematous eruption category (see Index).

▶ **Clinical Therapeutics**

Skin hydration, avoidance of aggravating flare factors such as environmental elements, emotional stressors, and infection. The cornerstone of medicinal treatment has been topical steroids, but newer therapy for unresponsive or intolerant cases consist of ascomycins and nonsteroidal immunomodulators such as tacrolimus (Protopic®) ointment applied bid and continued for 1 week after lesions are cleared.

▶ **Clinical Intervention**

No surgical or procedural interventions indicated.

▶ **Health Maintenance Issues**

Adequate cutaneous hydration remains a hallmark for preventive therapy. Lukewarm and less frequent bathing with soap- and fragrance-free cleansers, followed by application of occlusive emollients and avoidance of trigger factors is important, particularly in the drying winter months.

## 2. Contact Dermatitis

### ► Scientific Concepts

Contact (allergic, eczematous) dermatitis is a delayed cell-mediated hypersensitivity reaction stimulated by exposure to a sensitizing agent. The exception to this is toxic contact dermatitis occurring after a single exposure to harsh agents such as petroleum byproducts or strongly acidic or basic chemicals.

### ► History & Physical

Lesions may develop within days to weeks or may present after months to years of exposure. Symptoms may include intense pruritus and burning. Contact dermatitis may present as acute, subacute, or chronic lesions, with acute lesions seen as papules and plaques of erythema and edema with crusted and oozing vesicles. Subacute presentations typically include less erythema with scale and superficial desquamation. Lichenified plaques, excoriation, scale, and postinflammatory hyperpigmentation is seen with chronic presentations. Lesion patterns are often linear from contact, and lesion distribution ranges according to contact distribution.

### ► Diagnostic Studies

Following resolution of acute or subacute episodes, patch testing may offer diagnostic confirmation of uncertain causes.

### ► Diagnosis

Rule out other disorders of the eczematous eruption category (see Index).

### ► Clinical Therapeutics

Current therapy includes Burow's solution dressings for weeping vesiculobullous eruptions; high-potency topical steroids where indicated; tapering course of oral steroids for severe cases. Newer therapy with topical anti-inflammatory agents such as the ascomycin group or tacrolimus is gaining popularity.

### ► Clinical Intervention

No surgical or procedural interventions indicated.

### ► Health Maintenance Issues

Avoidance of known precipitating agents.

## 3. Diaper Dermatitis

### ► Scientific Concepts

A superficial cutaneous infection of intertriginous folds typically precipitated by fecal/urine soilage and moisture that may be complicated by the presence of *Candida* organisms.

### ► History & Physical

Skin erythema with papules, pustules, oozing, erosion, marginal scale, peripheral satellite papules, and pustules.

### ► Diagnostic Studies

Potassium hydroxide (KOH) test to rule out dermatophyte etiology; culture and sensitivity if bacterial organisms are suspected.

### ► Diagnosis

Rule out other disorders of the eczematous eruption category (see Index).

► Clinical Therapeutics

Topical anti-*Candida* agents; consider oral if refractory to topical or if widespread. If irritant origin consider hydrocortisone-iodoquinol (Vytone®) cream bid.

► Clinical Intervention

No surgical or procedural interventions indicated.

► Health Maintenance Issues

Keep intertriginous areas clean and dry; daily topical antifungal powder may be indicated.

## 4. Dyshidrotic Eczema

► Scientific Concepts

The origin of dyshidrotic eczema (pomphylox, vesicular palmoplantar eczema) is uncertain but is often regarded to be constitutional. Despite the term *dyshidrotic*, sweat glands are not involved.

► History & Physical

Recurrent episodes of pruritus of lateral fingers, palms or soles with deep-seated "tapioca-like" vesicles followed by papules, painful fissures, scaling, and lichenification.

► Diagnostic Studies

None, based on history and physical examination.

► Diagnosis

Rule out other disorders of the eczematous eruption category (see Index) and possible id reaction from tinea pedis.

► Clinical Therapeutics

High-potency topical steroids under occlusion for 1 to 2 weeks. Consider oral course of prednisone, antibiotics if secondarily infected, PUVA (psoralen plus ultraviolet light therapy) in severe cases.

► Clinical Intervention

No surgical or procedural interventions indicated.

► Health Maintenance Issues

None.

## 5. Nummular Eczema

► Scientific Concepts

The etiology of nummular (discoid) eczema is unknown. It is unrelated to atopy and circulating IgE levels are normal.

► History & Physical

Intensely pruritic coin-shaped papules and plaques with erythema, excoriations, scale, and lichenification typically occurring in regional clusters.

► Diagnostic Studies

Consider culture and sensitivity if secondarily infected.

► Diagnosis

Rule out other disorders of the eczematous eruption category (see Index). Rule out dermatophyte infection.

► **Clinical Therapeutics**

Skin hydration and moisturization, potent topical steroids bid unless contraindicated by location, consider intralesional triamcinolone for isolated papules/plaques.

► **Clinical Intervention**

No surgical or procedural interventions indicated. Consider PUVA or ultraviolet B light (UVB) if unresponsive to topical preparations.

► **Health Maintenance Issues**

Lesions are often secondarily infected; avoid lesion contamination.

## 6. Perioral Dermatitis

► **Scientific Concepts**

Unknown etiology.

► **History & Physical**

Inflammatory papules and pustules with erythema and scale distributed in the perioral area with typical sparing of the vermillion border, seen predominantly in young women.

► **Diagnostic Studies**

None, based on history and physical examination.

► **Diagnosis**

Rule out other disorders of the eczematous eruption category (see Index). Rule out acne and rosacea.

► **Clinical Therapeutics**

Topical steroids can worsen the condition and must be avoided. Commence therapy with oral antibiotics for 1 month then taper over another month (tetracycline, doxycycline, or minocycline). Topical metronidazole, clindamycin, sulfonamides, or erythromycin bid for maintenance therapy.

► **Clinical Intervention**

No surgical or procedural interventions indicated.

► **Health Maintenance Issues**

Inquire about use of possible trigger agents containing cinnamic aldehyde, found in tartar control toothpaste, chewing gum, and breath mints.

## 7. Seborrheic Dermatitis

► **Scientific Concepts**

Thought to be associated with *Pityrosporum ovale* yeast; also influenced by genetic and environmental factors.

► **History & Physical**

Erythematous lesions with yellow-orange scale found in areas with greater concentration of sebaceous glands (scalp, eyebrows, glabella, nasolabial folds, beard area, axillae, external auditory canals, postauricular folds, presternal area, inframammary folds, and groin). In infants, scalp scale referred to as *cradle cap*. Scalp scale alone (seborrhea) is dandruff.

► **Diagnostic Studies**

None.

► Diagnosis

Rule out other disorders of the eczematous eruption category (see Index).

► Clinical Therapeutics

Scalp lesions respond well to over-the-counter shampoos containing selenium sulfide and zinc pyrithione. Ketoconazole shampoo (1% over the counter, 2% prescription) can be applied and lathered to all affected areas. Low potency topical steroids of 1 to 2.5% hydrocortisone or desonide cream qd to bid are effective.

► Clinical Intervention

No surgical or procedural interventions indicated.

► Health Maintenance Issues

Preventive therapy of weekly ketoconazole or tar-based shampoos, intermittent application of topical steroid creams.

## 8. Stasis Dermatitis

► Scientific Concepts

Occurs in the setting of chronic venous insufficiency of the lower extremities secondary to incompetent valves and communicating vein backflow restriction.

► History & Physical

See inflammatory papules, stippled hyperpigmentation, excoriations, dermal sclerosis, scale, and crust in patients with known chronic venous insufficiency. Atrophie blanche and ulcerations may be seen, typically medially and proximal to the ankles.

► Diagnostic Studies

Doppler ultrasound studies to evaluate arterial flow; color-coded duplex sonography or venograms to detect incompetent veins. Diagnosis typically made by combination of history, physical exam, and Doppler sonography.

► Diagnosis

Rule out other disorders of the eczematous eruption category (see Index) as well as congenital arteriovenous fistulas and deep vein phlebitis.

► Clinical Therapeutics

See Clinical Intervention.

► Clinical Intervention

Elevation, fitted compression stockings, management of underlying cardiovascular pathology, sclerotherapy, and possible vascular surgery referral.

► Health Maintenance Issues

Approach underlying factors contributing to cardiovascular pathology.

## B. Lichen Simplex Chronicus

► Scientific Concepts

A localized eczematous eruption possibly related to epidermal nerve proliferation and hyperexcitability resulting in extreme sensitivity and pruritus. A characteristic feature of atopy.

► **History & Physical**

Lesions may be present from weeks to years and present as localized lichenified plaques in characteristic areas of the posterior neck, ankles, dorsal feet, genitalia area, upper thighs, and perianal area.

► **Diagnostic Studies**

None.

► **Diagnosis**

Rule out other disorders of the eczematous eruption category (see Index).

► **Clinical Therapeutics**

High potency topical steroids, antihistamines for pruritus.

► **Clinical Intervention**

Consider occlusive dressings over topical steroids or steroid-impregnated tape, intralesional triamcinolone; consider Unna Boot for distal lower extremity lesions.

► **Health Maintenance Issues**

Reinforce need for patients to stop rubbing and scratching.

## II. PAPULOSQUAMOUS DISEASES

### A. Dermatophyte Infections

► **Scientific Concepts**

Dermatophytes are fungi that typically infect the stratum corneum layer of skin, hair, and nails. Dermatophytes originating from animals and soil may also infect humans. Causal organisms of human predilection includes *Epidermophyton, Microsporum,* and *Trichophyton* spp. Predisposing host factors include immune compromise, age, gender, race, geographic location, warm moist climate, skin occlusion, and trauma.

► **History & Physical**

In the presence of predisposing historical factors, physical examination typically reveals an erythematous, well-marginated, annual plaque or patch with central clearing and a vesicular, scaly border. Pruritus and burning is occasionally present.

► **Diagnostic Studies**

KOH looking for translucent, branching, rod-shaped filaments of uniform width (hyphae) in dermatophyte infections, with spores and nonbranching hyphae seen in superficial *Candida* and tinea versicolor infections. Wood's lamp helpful if fluorescence positive; fungal culture diagnostic.

► **Diagnosis**

The differential diagnosis of papulosquamous lesions is lengthy (see Bibliography). Dermatophytosis complications include deep inflammatory infections from zoophilic fungi, secondary bacterial infections, post-inflammatory hyperpigmentation, kerion, and generalized infection in the immunocompromised.

► Clinical Therapeutics

Topical or oral antifungal agents, depending upon severity and duration of infection.

► Clinical Intervention

No procedural interventions are indicated.

► Health Maintenance Issues

Avoidance of precipitating factors.

## 1. Tinea Versicolor

► Scientific Concepts

Overgrowth of lipophilic normal skin flora *Pityrosporum ovale* and *Pityrosporum orbiculare* found in areas of increased sebaceous activity. Endogenous (pregnancy, immunosuppression, Cushing's disease) or exogenous (topical steroids, heat, humidity) factors lower skin resistance allowing organisms to proliferate. Enzymatic oxidation of fatty acids results in classic hypomelanosis of lesions.

► History & Physical

Blotchy hypopigmented sharply demarcated lesions for weeks to months noted primarily on the upper trunk, arms, neck, and abdomen. May be hyperpigmented in darker skin. Multiple circular macules with fine superficial scale presenting in a range of various colors.

► Diagnostic Studies

KOH revealing filamentous hyphae and globular yeast forms ("spaghetti and meatballs"). Blue-green fluorescence with Wood's lamp.

► Diagnosis

Rule out vitiligo, pityriasis alba, postinflammatory hypopigmentation, tinea corporis, pityriasis rosea, guttate psoriasis, and nummular eczema.

► Clinical Therapeutics

Selenium sulfide 2.5% lotion or shampoo daily for 1 week, ketoconazole 2% shampoo daily for 1 week, azole creams qd-bid for 2 weeks.

► Clinical Intervention

No procedural interventions are indicated.

► Health Maintenance Issues

Prophylactic ketoconazole or selenium sulfide shampoos once to twice a week.

## 2. Tinea Corporis

► Scientific Concepts

A suitable environment on host skin associated with trauma, maceration, occlusion, and increased temperature disrupts the barrier function of the stratum corneum, resulting in overgrowth of dermatophytes. The most common etiologic agents are from the *Trichophyton, Microsporum,* and *Epidermophyton* species.

► History & Physical

Spread by direct contact from person to person, inanimate objects, and pets. Commonly presents as an annular lesion with an active scaly erythematous border.

▶ Diagnostic Studies

KOH, fungal culture, or periodic acid-Schiff (PAS) stain from biopsied material.

▶ Diagnosis

Differentiate from other papulosquamous disorders, erythema migrans, subacute lupus erythematosus, and mycosis fungoides.

▶ Clinical Therapeutics

Topical antifungal agents (imidazoles = clotrimazole, miconazole, ketoconazole, econazole, oxiconizole, sulconizole; allylamines = naftifine, terbinafine; naphthiomates = tolnaftate; substituted pyridone = ciclopirox olamine).

▶ Clinical Intervention

No procedural interventions are indicated.

▶ Health Maintenance Issues

Avoidance of precipitating compromise of stratum corneum.

## 3. Tinea Pedis

▶ Scientific Concepts

Common dermatophyte infection from *Trichophyton* and *Epidermophyton* species in summer or tropical environment, with occlusive footwear, and closed communities (military, athletic teams).

▶ History & Physical

Pruritus and occlusion accompanied by heat manifested as chronic intertriginous lesions with macerated fissures and scale; superficial white scale in a moccasin-type distribution, a vesiculobullous pattern, or an acute ulcerative process.

▶ Diagnostic Studies

KOH, fungal culture, or PAS stain from biopsied material.

▶ Diagnosis

Differentiate from impetigo, psoriasis, dyshidrotic eczema, allergic contact dermatitis.

▶ Clinical Therapeutics

May require oral antifungal agents due to thickness on plantar stratum corneum, otherwise topical antifungal agents as described in tinea corporis.

▶ Clinical Intervention

No procedural interventions are indicated.

▶ Health Maintenance Issues

Avoid walking barefoot on contaminated floors.

## B. Drug Eruptions

▶ Scientific Concepts

Drug eruptions in the papulosquamous category include exanthematous, acneiform, eczematous, and lichenoid reactions. Drug eruptions can mimic all dermatologic morphology and are typically caused by an immunologically mediated hypersensitivity response.

► History & Physical

Exanthematous eruptions may be associated with the administration of amoxicillin or ampicillin in the presence of mononucleosis, the administration of sulfonamides to human immunodeficiency virus (HIV) positive individuals, or a history of prior drug sensitization. Drugs contributing to exanthematous eruptions include antibiotics (specifically penicillin derivatives), nonsteroidal anti-inflammatory drugs (NSAIDs), barbiturates, nitrofurantoin, hydantoin, isoniazid, benzodiazepines, phenothiazines, and sulfonamides. Presentation typically includes disseminated pruritic erythematous macules and/or papules in a symmetrical distribution on the trunk and extremities.

► Diagnostic Studies

Diagnosis based on history and physical examination, confirmed by histologic examination of punch biopsy.

► Diagnosis

Rule out viral exanthem, secondary syphilis, pityriasis rosea, allergic contact dermatitis.

► Clinical Therapeutics

Identify and discontinue offending drug.

► Clinical Intervention

No procedural interventions are indicated.

► Health Maintenance Issues

Following diagnosis inform patient to avoid similar drug exposures due to concern for potential anaphylactic reaction.

## 1. Lichen Planus

► Scientific Concepts

Idiopathic disorder of skin and mucous membranes lasting months to years.

► History & Physical

Classically described by the "five P's" that include pruritic purple (violaceous) planar (flat) polygonal papules seen on the wrists, lumbar area, shins, and penis. May include painful mucous membrane lesions with a reticulated pattern of lacy white hyperkeratosis (Wickham's striae).

► Diagnostic Studies

Confirmed by histologic examination of punch biopsy.

► Diagnosis

Rule out lupus erythematosus, psoriasis, pityriasis rosea, eczema, lichen simplex chronicus.

► Clinical Therapeutics

Topical, intralesional, or oral steroids may be necessary to control symptoms.

► Clinical Intervention

No procedural interventions are indicated.

► Health Maintenance Issues

Increased incidence of oral cancer following oral lichen planus.

## 2. Pityriasis Rosea

▶ **Scientific Concepts**

A common benign papulosquamous disorder of unknown etiology.

▶ **History & Physical**

A single oval/round scaly patch resembling tinea corporis develops followed days to weeks later by crops of smaller lesions on the trunk and proximal extremities. Lesions typically appear along skin lines and can resemble a "Christmas tree" pattern on the trunk. Scale is fine and wrinkled in a collarette around each lesion.

▶ **Diagnostic Studies**

None available; consider rapid plasma reagin (RPR) to rule out secondary syphilis and KOH to rule out tinea corporis.

▶ **Diagnosis**

Rule out secondary syphilis, guttate psoriasis, viral exanthems, tinea corporis, nummular eczema, and drug eruptions.

▶ **Clinical Therapeutics**

Treat symptomatically.

▶ **Clinical Intervention**

No procedural interventions are indicated.

▶ **Health Maintenance Issues**

None; condition is benign.

## 3. Psoriasis

▶ **Scientific Concepts**

A hereditary autoimmune disorder of multiple clinical presentations associated with human leukocyte antigens (HLAs) and activated T cells manifesting as keratinocyte proliferation and a characteristic inflammatory pattern.

▶ **History & Physical**

Bimodal mean onset ages of 8 and 55 with peak onset in early 20s; early onset predicts increased disease severity. Typical salmon-pink papules and plaques with silvery-white micaceous scale in symmetrical distribution. Predominant locations are scalp, elbows, knees, palms, finger, soles, gluteal cleft and lower lumbar area, intertriginous areas, penis, and fingernails. May be generalized, erythrodermic, or arthritic. Köebner's phenomenon (psoriatic papule/plaque arising from area of trauma) common.

▶ **Diagnostic Studies**

Dermatopathology of punch biopsy lesion reveals characteristic diagnostic findings.

▶ **Diagnosis**

Differentiate among chronic plaque type, guttate, erythrodermic, and psoriatic arthritis. Consider seborrheic dermatitis, lichen simplex chronicus, tinea corporis, and mycosis fungoides.

▶ **Clinical Therapeutics**

A range of treatment modalities exists. If body surface area involvement exceeds 20% consider systemic and/or light box therapy. Topical therapy includes steroid preparations, vitamin $D_3$ analogs (Calcipotriol), anthralin, tar compounds, and occlusive tape and dressings. Intralesional steroid therapy considered for localized plaques. Consider narrow-band UVB, PUVA, methotrexate, etretinate, or cyclosporine for extensive involvement.

► **Clinical Intervention**
No procedural interventions are indicated.

► **Health Maintenance Issues**
Stress reduction, carefully monitored sunlight exposure may help reduce severity of lesions.

## III. DESQUAMATION

### A. Erythema Multiforme

► **Scientific Concepts**
An acute inflammatory hypersensitivity syndrome of multifactorial etiology, including pregnancy, drugs, malignancy, infection, and idiopathic. Erythema multiforme (EM) minor (absence of mucous membrane involvement) may be associated with herpes simplex virus (HSV) infection in up to 100% of cases. The more severe presentations of EM major, Stevens-Johnson syndrome (SJS), or toxic epidermal necrolysis (TEN) are thought to be due to drug reactions in the majority of cases.

► **History & Physical**
Dull red urticarial papules with iris/targetoid lesions displaying central vesicles and bullae predisposed to the hands, feet, forearms, face, elbows, knees, and genitalia. May include mucous membrane erosions, but not extensive variant as seen in SJS and TEN. May recur in crops.

► **Diagnostic Studies**
None.

► **Diagnosis**
Differentiate from urticaria, drug eruptions, secondary syphilis. If oral involvement, consider herpes simplex, pemphigus, and acute lupus erythematosus.

► **Clinical Therapeutics**
Observation; symptomatic supportive therapy. Observe for progression to SJS or TEN.

► **Clinical Intervention**
No procedural interventions are indicated.

► **Health Maintenance Issues**
Avoid known precipitating factors such as exposure to etiologic agents.

## B. Stevens-Johnson Syndrome (SJS)

▶ **Scientific Concepts**

A more severe form of EM thought to be secondary to a drug reaction. Common precipitating agents include sulfonamides, phenytoin, barbiturates, phenylbutazone, penicillin, or allopurinol.

▶ **History & Physical**

Upper respiratory infection (URI) prodrome for 1 to 14 days followed by widespread vesicles and bullae on purpuric targetoid macules with often severe mucous membrane involvement with high morbidity and mortality.

▶ **Diagnostic Studies**

Punch biopsy with direct immunofluorescence if lesions are not classic.

▶ **Diagnosis**

Differentiate from TEN and Staph Scalded Skin Syndrome (SSSS).

▶ **Clinical Therapeutics**

Supportive therapy; disease is self-limited if no complications arise; systemic corticosteroid therapy remains controversial.

▶ **Clinical Intervention**

No procedural interventions are indicated unless endotracheal intubation and advanced life support measures are necessary.

▶ **Health Maintenance Issues**

Diligently pursue possible etiology to avoid future recurrence that may be life threatening.

## C. Toxic Epidermal Necrolysis

▶ **Scientific Concepts**

A progression of SJS to diffuse generalized full-thickness epidermal detachment with pathophysiologic similarities to burn injuries resulting in large sheets of epidermal shedding.

▶ **History & Physical**

Fever with URI-like symptoms precedes conjunctivitis and stomatitis by 1 to 2 weeks followed by diffuse painful erythematous skin with epidermal shearing from friction (Nikolsky's sign). Complications include purulent conjunctivitis, bronchopneumonia, septicemia, and fluid and electrolyte loss.

▶ **Diagnostic Studies**

Same as SJS.

▶ **Diagnosis**

Same as SJS.

▶ **Clinical Therapeutics**

Burn center fluid, electrolyte, and skin replacement therapy.

▶ **Clinical Intervention**

Advanced life support measures as necessary.

▶ **Health Maintenance Issues**

Same as SJS.

## IV. VESICULOBULLOUS ERUPTIONS

### A. Bullous Pemphigoid

▶ Scientific Concepts

A rare subepidermal blistering autoimmune disease of unknown etiology.

▶ History & Physical

Large tense bullae arising from an erythematous edematous annular base, more commonly on the lower abdomen and flexor extremity surfaces in the sixth decade and beyond.

▶ Diagnostic Studies

Punch biopsy with direct and indirect immunofluorescence is diagnostic.

▶ Diagnosis

Differentiate from epidermolysis bullosa acquisita, dermatitis herpetiformis, pemphigus, bullous systemic lupus erythematosus (SLE), and bullous drug eruptions.

▶ Clinical Therapeutics

Often self-limited but may last years. May require topical or oral steroids, immunosuppressive agents, sulfones, and antibiotics such as tetracycline or erythromycin.

▶ Clinical Intervention

No procedural interventions are indicated.

▶ Health Maintenance Issues

None.

## V. ACNEIFORM LESIONS

### A. Acne Vulgaris

▶ Scientific Concepts

A disease of the pilosebaceous unit caused by the proliferation and modification of sebum by *Propionibacterium acnes* in predisposed patients with increased sebum production, resulting in cohesive hyperkeratosis and pilosebaceous duct obstruction.

▶ History & Physical

Acne typically affects the face, neck, shoulders, and back, with onset near puberty and lessening as adolescence ends, with varying intensity and duration. Examination of these areas may reveal differing combinations of inflammatory lesions (papules, pustules, and nodules) (Table 1–1) and noninflammatory lesions (open comedons [blackheads] and closed comedons [whiteheads]). Premenstrual flares may occur.

▶ Diagnostic Studies

None.

► table 1-1

**ACNE CLASSIFICATION AND GRADING**

| Lesion Type | Mild | Moderate | Severe |
|---|---|---|---|
| Papules/Pustules | +/++ | ++/+++ | +++/++++ |
| Nodules | 0 | +/++ | +++ |

*Source: Adapted from TP Habif,* Clinical Dermatology: A Color Guide to Diagnosis and Therapy, *3rd ed., St. Louis: Mosby, 1996.*

► **Diagnosis**

Characteristic clinical history and appearance is usually diagnostic; differentiate from steroid acne, occupational acne, acne mechanica, acne cosmetica, and acne rosacea. Complications include treatment failure, potentially severe psychosocial effects, occupational disability, and disfigurement.

► **Clinical Therapeutics**

Depending on severity and response, therapeutics can include adapalene, tretinoin, benzoyl peroxide, drying agents, topical or oral antibiotics, intralesional steroids, acne surgery, and isotretinoin.

► **Clinical Intervention**

Acne surgery expresses comedons and drains pustules; intralesional steroids rapidly control larger lesions.

► **Health Maintenance Issues**

Patient education regarding misconceptions; assessment of psychological factors; appropriate follow-up instructions and continuous treatment for optimal results.

## B. Rosacea

► **Scientific Concepts**

Pathogenesis remains uncertain but may be linked to gastrointestinal (GI) disturbances (including presence of *H. pylori*), *Demodex folliculorum* mites, or psychogenic factors.

► **History & Physical**

Predominantly in 30- to 50-year-old females, with predisposing history of vasomotor lability (flushing and blushing) followed by persistent erythema with telangiectasias, papules, pustules, and rarely nodules in the central facial area, typically worsened by sunlight, temperature extremes, stress, hot or spicy foods, or alcohol.

► **Diagnostic Studies**

Based on history and physical examination.

► **Diagnosis**

Rule out acne, seborrheic dermatitis, folliculitis, and perioral dermatitis.

▶ Clinical Therapeutics

Initially oral agents including tetracycline, doxycycline, or minocycline combined with topical agents including metronidazole, sodium sulfacetamide, or topical antibiotics to achieve control, followed by maintenance therapy with topical agents.

▶ Clinical Intervention

No procedural interventions are indicated.

▶ Health Maintenance Issues

Sunlight and precipitating factor avoidance, sun protective factor (SPF) 15 or greater sunscreen on a daily-use basis.

## C. Folliculitis

▶ Scientific Concepts

Chemical or microbial inflammation of hair follicles characterized by a follicular papule, pustule, erosion, or crust.

▶ History & Physical

Grouped lesions on any body surface, more common on scalp, beard area, and limbs, typically appearing as pustules pierced by individual hairs.

▶ Diagnostic Studies

Consider Gram stain to identify bacteria, KOH to isolate yeast or hyphae, or culture and sensitivity (C&S) of pustule contents.

▶ Diagnosis

Differential includes pseudofolliculitis barbae, keratosis pilaris, contact dermatitis.

▶ Clinical Therapeutics

Appropriate antimicrobials to cover etiologic agent(s).

▶ Clinical Intervention

Topical antibacterial cream, soap, or shampoo, as indicated.

▶ Health Maintenance Issues

Increased personal hygiene, avoid causative factors, suspect immunodeficiency in recalcitrant cases. Risk factors include poor hygiene, hydrocarbon exposure, immunodeficiency, abraded or injured skin.

## VI. VERRUCOUS LESIONS

## A. Seborrheic Keratosis

▶ Scientific Concepts

A common, hereditary (probably autosomal dominant) benign lesion that begins to appear in the third decade and may increase to hundreds/thousands of lesions in the elderly.

▶ History & Physical

Begin as small skin-colored or tan macule, progress to slightly elevated tan to brown lesions that may include a stippled/cobblestoned surface texture with plaque type elevation, horn cysts, and variegated colors of tan, brown, black, and skin-colored. Well-circumscribed and may become erythematous at borders from friction or excoriation.

▶ Diagnostic Studies
Dermatopathology by shave biopsy reveals characteristic keratinocyte proliferation.

▶ Diagnosis
Always differentiate from malignant melanoma and squamous cell carcinoma; consider verruca vulgaris, solar lentigo, pigmented actinic keratosis.

▶ Clinical Therapeutics
None.

▶ Clinical Intervention
Cryosurgery or curettage if indicated in irritated lesions; shave biopsy indicated unless certain of diagnosis.

▶ Health Maintenance Issues
Inform patient of likelihood of new lesion development and possible recurrence of lesions at treated sites.

## B. Actinic (Solar) Keratosis

▶ Scientific Concepts
Etiology is cumulative ultraviolet radiation in susceptible persons; increased incidence in lighter skin color, outdoor workers, and equatorial regions.

▶ History & Physical
Adherent white, yellow-brown, brown, or reddish scale that is rough to palpation ("sandpaper" texture) on sun-exposed surfaces.

▶ Diagnostic Studies
Dermatopathology of shave biopsy reveals characteristic pleomorphic keratinocytes.

▶ Diagnosis
Differentiate from basal cell carcinoma, squamous cell carcinoma, verruca, irritated seborrheic keratoses.

▶ Clinical Therapeutics
Cryosurgery typically effective, consider fluorouracil, retinoids, peels, or laser surgery.

▶ Clinical Intervention
Consider 20% aminolevulinic acid HCl in conjunction with photodynamic therapy for treatment of face or scalp lesions.

▶ Health Maintenance Issues
Liberal use of ultraviolet A (UVA)/UVB sunscreens on a daily application basis. Treat all actinic keratoses because approximately 10% will progress to squamous cell carcinoma if left untreated.

## VII. INSECTS/PARASITES

### A. Lice

▶ Scientific Concepts
*Pediculus humanus, Pediculus corporis,* and *Phthirius pubis* are blood-sucking lice that favor distinct body areas. *P. humanus* (head lice) favor

the scalp; *P. corporis* (body lice) favor the body, and *Phthirius pubis* (pubic or crab lice) favor the pubic region. Antigen, toxin, or enzyme-laden saliva is introduced cutaneously by stylet penetration of the skin, producing varying sensitivity and severity of reaction.

► **History & Physical**

Active infection with head lice presents with visible adult lice or nits on hair shafts. Body lice present with findings of lice and or eggs in seams of clothing. Pubic lice present with marked pruritus and visible lice or nits in the pubic hair area. Examination may reveal hypersensitivity bite reactions (papular urticaria), bites in clusters or groups, or pruritic wheals in exposed areas.

► **Diagnostic Studies**

Microscopy may reveal nits or lice; diagnosis based on history and physical examination.

► **Diagnosis**

Differential includes eczema, scabies, seborrhea, lichen simplex chronicus, impetigo.

► **Clinical Therapeutics**

Varies according to lice type and location, includes topical permethrin/pyrethrin, lindane 1% shampoo, ivermectin lotion, shampoo, or oral.

► **Clinical Intervention**

None.

► **Health Maintenance Issues**

Risk factors are environmental, socioeconomic, and lack of preventive measures.

## B. Scabies

► **Scientific Concepts**

The *Sarcoptes scabiei* mite is responsible for human scabies, a contagious condition arising from skin-to-skin contact with an infected person or from mite-infested bedding or clothing. Fertilized females burrow into the stratum corneum, depositing eggs and fecal pellets (scybala). Hypersensitivity reactions result in characteristic signs and symptoms and may take weeks to develop in first infection.

► **History & Physical**

Onset of minor itching that spreads mites to other areas, resulting in nocturnal pruritus that progresses to intractable generalized pruritus. Clinical appearance varies, but typical distribution includes linear or serpiginous intraepidermal burrows in the finger web spaces, wrists, lateral aspects of hands and feet, axillae, genitalia, and buttocks.

► **Diagnostic Studies**

Scabies prep slide (burrow scrapings covered with mineral oil) to examine for mites, eggs, or scybala.

► **Diagnosis**

Typical clinical findings, confirmed by microscopy. Differential includes drug eruption, eczema, psoriasis, or impetigo. Complicated by continuing pruritus up to several weeks following treatment due to mite antigen hypersensitivity reaction.

▶ **Clinical Therapeutics**
Topical permethrin or lindane; oral ivermectin; antihistamines; topical or oral corticosteroids.

▶ **Clinical Intervention**
No surgical or procedural interventions indicated.

▶ **Health Maintenance Issues**
Institutional facilities (nursing homes, prisons) increase risk. Decontaminate environment; examine and treat sexual and household contacts.

## C. Spiders

▶ **Scientific Concepts**
Black widow (*Lactrodectus mactans*) and brown recluse (*Loxoscelidae recluses*) spiders inflict the most morbidity among U.S. spider bites. The black widow venom is neurotoxic; the brown recluse venom is polyproteinaceous and necrotizing.

▶ **History & Physical**
*Black widow:* Painful or painless envenomation followed by generalized abdominal, back, and leg pain, possibly spreading within minutes to hours to include the entire torso and legs with severe abdominal pain and spasm worsening for 24 hours then gradually subsiding over 2 to 3 days.

*Brown recluse:* Ranges from mild local urticaria to full-thickness skin necrosis. Painless envenomation followed in several hours by central bulla with surrounding gray to purple discoloration surrounded by a zone of erythema, the classic "red, white, and blue" sign of brown recluse envenomation.

▶ **Diagnostic Studies**
Witnessed envenomation is only diagnostic certainty.

▶ **Diagnosis**
Differential includes cellulitis, necrotizing soft tissue infection, drug reaction.

▶ **Clinical Therapeutics**
*Black widow:* Consider antivenin therapy, muscle relaxants, and analgesic/supportive therapy.

*Brown recluse:* Conservative therapy with immobilization, ice, elevation; consider antibiotics and tetanus toxoid if necessary; consider Dapsone 50–100 mg/day; avoid early surgical intervention.

▶ **Clinical Intervention**
As noted previously.

▶ **Health Maintenance Issues**
Avoid spider habitats.

## VIII.  NEOPLASMS

### A.  Basal Cell Carcinoma (BCC)

▶ Scientific Concepts

The most common type of skin cancer, BCC has a limited capacity to metastasize, but can be locally invasive, aggressive, and destructive. Rare in darker-pigmented persons; susceptibility increases with prolonged sun exposure history.

▶ History & Physical

A bleeding or scabbing lesion that heals and recurs is the most common presenting complaint. Typical lesions are round/ovoid smooth papules or nodules with a pearly translucent rolled border containing threadlike telangiectasias and a depressed/umbilicated center, located on sun-exposed skin. However, BCC can occur in many clinical forms with varying presentations.

▶ Diagnostic Studies

Confirmed by histopathologic examination of lesion biopsy.

▶ Diagnosis

Differentiate from keratoacanthoma, squamous cell carcinoma, and malignant melanoma by biopsy.

▶ Clinical Therapeutics

No adequate medicinal treatment currently available.

▶ Clinical Intervention

Depending on clinical presentation, cell type, and tumor size and location, BCC treatment modalities can include electrodessication and curettage, simple surgical excision, or Mohs' micrographic surgery.

▶ Health Maintenance Issues

Because patients with one BCC often develop another, quarterly follow-up is indicated to inspect for new lesions.

### B.  Squamous Cell Carcinoma (SCC)

▶ Scientific Concepts

Commonly occurring in sun-exposed areas, SCCs may arise from normal skin, actinically damaged skin, or from underlying actinic keratoses. Those arising from the lip, apparently normal skin, or sites of chronic inflammation are more aggressive.

▶ History & Physical

Unlike BCCs, SCCs are more commonly found on the scalp, dorsal surface of the hands, and superior aspect of the pinnae. Lower extremity lesions are more common in women. Typical lesions present as indurated erythematous-yellowish papules, plaques, or nodules in a polygonal, ovoid, or round shape. Crusting, erosion, and ulceration may be present, with a firm elevated margin.

▶ Diagnostic Studies

Confirmed by histopathologic examination of lesion biopsy.

▶ Diagnosis

Differentiate from nummular eczema, psoriasis, Paget's disease, BCC.

► **Clinical Therapeutics**

No effective oral therapies available.

► **Clinical Intervention**

Depending on clinical presentation, cell type, and tumor size and location, SCC treatment modalities can include simple surgical excision, Mohs' micrographic surgery, radiation, and chemotherapy.

► **Health Maintenance Issues**

Risk factors include light skin, poor tanning ability, older age, outdoor occupations, exposure to chemical carcinogens, and geographic area of residence. The lifetime probability of developing SCC varies from 1.5 to 11%, depending on risk factors. BCCs are three times more common that SCCs.

## C. Malignant Melanoma

► **Scientific Concepts**

Malignant transformation of epidermal melanocytes presenting as pigmented lesions, more frequently in fair-skinned patients; etiology predominately associated with sun exposure. Melanomas present as superficial spreading melanoma (70%), nodular melanoma (15%), lentigo maligna (4–10%), and acral lentiginous melanoma (2–8%).

► **History & Physical**

Melanomas typically manifest as pigmented lesions that change in color, symmetry, size, symptoms, or shape over weeks to months in 20- to 40-year-olds. Asymmetric lesions greater than 6 mm in diameter with an admixture of colors and an irregular border are highly suspicious.

► **Diagnostic Studies**

Diagnosis and staging require complete excisional biopsy or punch/ incisional biopsy for larger lesions; curettage or shave biopsies are contraindicated due to inability to accurately stage level of involvement.

► **Diagnosis**

Differentiate from melanocytic nevus (a benign proliferation of melanocytes), atypical nevus (a benign acquired precursor to melanoma and a marker for melanoma risk), and blue nevus (a benign acquired nevus). Complications include metastatic disease; prognosis based on Clark's staging.

► **Clinical Therapeutics**

No effective oral or topical treatment available for primary malignant melanoma; metastatic disease may require a combination of chemotherapy/immunotherapy.

► **Clinical Intervention**

Complete surgical excision is the treatment of choice for malignant melanoma.

► **Health Maintenance Issues**

Avoidance of sun exposure (of particular note is blistering sunburn before age of 18), liberal use of sunscreen of greater that SPF 15, frequent total body examinations following diagnosis.

## IX. HAIR AND NAILS

### A. Alopecia Areata

▶ **Scientific Concepts**

A relatively common, localized area of hair loss (typically the scalp) in a well-demarcated round or oval-shaped lesion without evidence of inflammation. Etiology remains unknown but suspected to be an autoimmune phenomenon.

▶ **History & Physical**

Typically occurs under age 25; may occur in patches of varying stages of hair loss and regrowth. No cutaneous symptoms; predilection for scalp, eyebrows, eyelashes, beard, and pubic hair.

▶ **Diagnostic Studies**

None.

▶ **Diagnosis**

Based on typical clinical picture.

▶ **Clinical Therapeutics**

High potency topical steroids may be effective; oral steroids induce regrowth but alopecia may recur upon discontinuation; oral PUVA (photochemotherapy) may be indicated in extensive cases.

▶ **Clinical Intervention**

Intralesional steroids provide effective temporary resolution.

▶ **Health Maintenance Issues**

Prepubescent alopecia has greater incidence of leading to repeated episodes and progression to total alopecia.

### B. Androgenetic Alopecia

▶ **Scientific Concepts**

Predominantly a male condition secondary to effect of androgen on hair follicles and genetic predisposition (polygenic/autosomal dominant in males; autosomal recessive in females).

▶ **History & Physical**

Male pattern begins as bitemporal thinning progressing to increased frontal hair loss and eventual occipital scalp alopecia progressing in some to complete balding of the top with sparing in a band around the sides and lower occiput. Female pattern begins on crown and may extend to frank baldness of crown; characteristically leaves a frontal fringe not present in male pattern.

▶ **Diagnostic Studies**

Diagnosis based on history and physical examination; if menstrual irregularity, infertility, hirsutism, cystic acne, virilism, or galactorrhea present in females, order total testosterone, dehydroepiandrosterone sulfate (DHEAS), prolactin, and thyroid-stimulating hormone (TSH).

▶ **Diagnosis**

Consider hormonal imbalance (increased androgens) and thyroid dysfunction.

▶ Clinical Therapeutics
Oral finasteride 1 mg/day in males only; topical minoxidil (2% and 5%) qd available for men and women.

▶ Clinical Intervention
None. Consider hair transplants if patient desires.

▶ Health Maintenance Issues
None.

## C. Onychomycosis

▶ Scientific Concepts
Onychomycosis is an infectious process of the nails caused by a variety of yeasts, molds, and fungi. The subtype *tinea unguium* is caused by the dermatophyte group of fungi.

▶ History & Physical
Predominately on the toenails (particularly the great toe), onychomycosis typically presents with a history of marginated streaks or plaques on the nails, with eventual dystrophic thickening and hyperkeratotic debris beneath the nail.

▶ Diagnostic Studies
Direct microscopic examination via KOH prep; Sabouraud's agar fungal culture to isolate pathogen.

▶ Diagnosis
Positive KOH or fungal culture is diagnostic. Progressive nail involvement occurs if untreated.

▶ Clinical Therapeutics
Griseofulvin, azoles (itraconazole, ketoconazole, fluconazole), allylamines (terbinafine). Consider topical ciclopirox 8%.

▶ Clinical Intervention
Nail debulking by mechanical means or complete removal may be indicated if thickening precludes ability to wear shoes, etc.

▶ Health Maintenance Issues
Avoidance of occlusive footwear, overcrowding, communal bathing, and circulatory disturbances.

## D. Paronychia

▶ Scientific Concepts
A digital cellulitis/abscess of the proximal or lateral nailfold; causative organisms may include bacterial, viral, and/or fungal.

▶ History & Physical
Repeated exposure to moisture or trauma predisposes individuals to developing a paronychia. Examination reveals tenderness, pain, erythema, and edema of the proximal or lateral digit nail fold.

▶ Diagnostic Studies
Drainage or aspirate from infected digit may be cultured to identify pathogens.

► Diagnosis

Differentiate acute versus chronic digital cellulitis/paronychia by speed of onset and occupational predisposition (medical and dental personnel, dishwashers).

► Clinical Therapeutics

Oral antibiotic therapy for 7–10 days with appropriate antistaphylococcal coverage.

► Clinical Intervention

Paronychia typically requires incision and drainage in addition to antibiotics.

► Health Maintenance Issues

Hand and foot care instructions with goal of dry environment; glove use when appropriate; avoidance of skin breakdown, trauma, and manipulation.

## X. VIRAL DISEASES

### A. Condyloma Accuminatum

► Scientific Concepts

More than 150 human papillomavirus (HPV) types have been identified and associated with various cutaneous lesions. The most common mucosal surface manifestation of HPV is genital warts (condyloma accuminatum). HPV infections are typically self-limited unless presenting in immunocompromised patients.

► History & Physical

Warts may persist for years if untreated. Typically manifesting as verrucous "cauliflower" papules and plaques in the anogenital region.

► Diagnostic Studies

Typically made on clinical findings. Acetowhitening test (applying acetic acid-soaked gauze to suspicious areas for 5 to 10 minutes turns dysplastic/neoplastic tissue white). Dermatopathology to confirm diagnosis and rule out progression to squamous cell carcinoma if indicated.

► Diagnosis

Rule out squamous cell carcinoma.

► Clinical Therapeutics

Imiquimod 5% cream, numerous over-the-counter and prescription topical agents containing acetic acid, trichloracetic acid, salicylic acid, formaldehyde, or podophyllin are available.

► Clinical Intervention

Liquid nitrogen, laser surgery, surgical excision, and electrodessication and curettage are used with varying degrees of success, depending upon the size and location of warts. Condyloma accuminatum warrant more aggressive therapies.

► Health Maintenance Issues

Condyloma accuminatum HPV types have a major role in the pathogenesis of carcinoma of the anogenital epithelium. HPV can be transmitted to the fetus during delivery, resulting in anogenital warts or recurrent respiratory papillomatosis. HPV also has an important etiologic role in carcinoma of the cervix and cervical intraepithelial neoplasia (CIN).

## B. Exanthems

► **Scientific Concepts**

With the advent of widespread pediatric immunizations, the most commonly presenting viral exanthems are from the enteroviruses: echovirus and coxsackievirus.

► **History & Physical**

Typically present as a maculopapular confluent and generalized exanthem that may include urticarial, vesicular, or petechial components. May be accompanied by systemic symptoms such as fever, nausea, vomiting, diarrhea, photophobia, and lymphadenopathy.

► **Diagnostic Studies**

Serum viral titers.

► **Diagnosis**

May be indistinguishable from drug eruptions.

► **Clinical Therapeutics**

Symptomatic therapy.

► **Clinical Intervention**

None.

► **Health Maintenance Issues**

Avoidance of known infected individuals.

## C. Herpes Simplex Virus (Nongenital)

► **Scientific Concepts**

Herpes simplex is a deoxyribonucleic acid (DNA) virus. Herpes labialis ("cold sore," "fever blister") is due to herpes simplex virus type 1 (HSV-1) in 80 to 90% of cases. Transmission is typically skin-to-skin contact.

► **History & Physical**

Symptomatic primary herpes infection typically includes vesicles at inoculation site with regional lymphadenopathy, fever, malaise, and myalgias. In children, primary herpetic gingivostomatitis is more common presentation. In recurrent infection, prodrome of tingling, itching, or burning sensation typically precedes skin changes by 24 hours. Vesicles erode to grouped ulcerations.

► **Diagnostic Studies**

Tzanck smear reveals multinucleated giant cells; viral cultures available.

► **Diagnosis**

Differential includes impetigo, aphthous stomatitis, herpes zoster, syphilitic chancre, herpangina.

► **Clinical Therapeutics**

Consider acyclovir, valacyclovir, famciclovir.

▶ Clinical Intervention
No clinical procedures indicated.

▶ Health Maintenance Issues
Avoid contact with neonates and immunocompromised. Frequent hand washing. Increased HSV-1 transmission is associated with crowded and lower socioeconomic conditions.

## D. Molluscum Contagiosum

▶ Scientific Concepts
A self-limited epidermal viral infection caused by a poxvirus, occurring in children and sexually active adults.

▶ History & Physical
Lesions typically present as small, discrete, solid, skin-colored papules with a central umbilication, occurring on exposed skin sites in children and genital region in sexually active adults.

▶ Diagnostic Studies
Molluscum contagiosum virus has not been successfully cultured.

▶ Diagnosis
Based on distinct clinical appearance of lesions.

▶ Clinical Therapeutics
No oral medications available.

▶ Clinical Intervention
Curettage or cryosurgery; HIV-infected patients with numerous or large lesions may require electrodessication.

▶ Health Maintenance Issues
Lesions will resolve spontaneously unless patient is infected with HIV. Avoid skin-to-skin contact with mollusca-infected individuals.

## E. Verrucae (Human Papillomavirus, HPV)

▶ Scientific Concepts
See Scientific Concepts of condyloma accuminatum. More than 150 HPV types have been identified and associated with various cutaneous lesions, with the most prevalent being common warts (verruca vulgaris), plantar warts (verruca plantaris), and flat warts (verruca plana). HPV infections are typically self-limited unless presenting in immunocompromised patients.

▶ History & Physical
Warts may persist for years if untreated. Typically manifesting as papules and plaques, HPV commonly infects keratinized skin.

▶ Diagnostic Studies
Typically made on clinical findings.

▶ Diagnosis
Although potentially persistent, HPV infections typically resolve spontaneously in immunocompetent patients.

► Clinical Therapeutics

5-fluorouracil (for flat warts) has been used successfully as a topical agent; numerous over-the-counter and prescription topical agents containing acetic acid, trichloracetic acid, salicylic acid, formaldehyde, or podophyllin are available for common warts.

► Clinical Intervention

A variety of therapeutic modalities are used with varying degrees of success, depending upon the type and location of warts. Most common are cryosurgery or electrodessication and curettage. Unless clinically warranted, aggressive therapies are often painful and may be accompanied by scarring. Condyloma accuminatum and plantar warts warrant more aggressive therapies.

► Health Maintenance Issues

See condyloma accuminatum Health Maintenance Issues.

## F. Herpes Zoster (Shingles)

► Scientific Concepts

Recrudescence of latent varicella zoster infection presenting as a cutaneous viral infection generally involving the skin of a single dermatome; classically occurring unilaterally. Following chickenpox, the virus remains latent in the sensory dorsal root ganglion cells. Reactivation of latent varicella zoster has been attributed to age, immunosuppression, lymphoma, fatigue, emotional upset, and radiation therapy.

► History & Physical

Cutaneous eruption preceded by several days of pain, presenting as papules and plaques of erythema in a unilateral dermatomal distribution, with vesicular formation often within hours of plaque development. Vesicles become pustular, crust, and heal, usually without scarring. Duration of eruption correlates with patient age, severity of eruption, and presence of immunosuppression, and ranges from 2 to 6 weeks. Preherpetic neuralgia, dermatomal hyperesthesia, fever, headache, and malaise may precede the eruption by several days.

► Diagnostic Studies

Same as varicella.

► Diagnosis

Characteristic clinical history and appearance is usually diagnostic.

► Clinical Therapeutics

Antiviral therapy with valacyclovir, famciclovir, or acyclovir; nerve blocks; tricyclic antidepressants.

► Clinical Intervention

No clinical procedures indicated. Monitor for complications.

► Health Maintenance Issues

Pain is more severe in elderly; immunocompromised are more likely to have skin necrosis and scarring, postherpetic neuralgia, and disseminated herpes zoster. Herpes zoster ophthalmicus can occur when the ophthalmic division of the trigeminal nerve is involved, with anterior uveitis and keratitis presenting more commonly. Complications include long-term ocular disease and postherpetic neuralgia, reduced by prompt treatment with valacyclovir, famciclovir, or acyclovir.

## G. Varicella (Chickenpox)

▶ **Scientific Concepts**

Extremely communicable varicella zoster virus (VZV) disease (a DNA virus of the herpesvirus family) transmitted by respiratory droplets or direct contact with infected vesicles. Communicable from 1 to 2 days prior to rash onset until all lesions crusted. Average incubation period 14 days. Postinfection immunity is usually lifelong; herpes zoster may later develop by reactivation of latent VZV from sensory ganglia.

▶ **History & Physical**

Pediatric prodromal symptoms include fever, headache, malaise just prior to or at onset of cutaneous eruption. Adult symptoms may include chills, malaise, and backache. Lesions begin on trunk then spread to face and extremities; extent of involvement varies considerably and may be subclinical. New lesions typically appear as "dewdrop-like" vesicles on an erythematous base. Fresh crops occur irregularly for 3 to 5 days, resulting in intermingled papules, vesicles, and crusts. Lesions may also occur on mucous membranes.

▶ **Diagnostic Studies**

Viral culture of vesicular fluid; direct fluorescent antibody; Tzanck smear demonstrating multinucleated giant cells (valuable test but does not differentiate varicella from herpes simplex).

▶ **Diagnosis**

Characteristic clinical history and appearance is usually diagnostic. May be clinically indistinguishable from disseminated herpes zoster or coxsackievirus viral exanthem. Viral cultures are definitive. Lesions may become secondarily infected; complications can include encephalitis and Reye's syndrome, varicella pneumonia in adults, and higher complication rates in immunosuppressed patients.

▶ **Clinical Therapeutics**

*Topical:* Antipruritic lotions, oatmeal baths, cool compresses, Burow's solution soaks (1:40 dilution).

*Systemic:* Antihistamines, acyclovir, acetaminophen (no salicylates in children due to risk of Reye's syndrome).

▶ **Clinical Intervention**

No clinical procedures indicated. Monitor for complications.

▶ **Health Maintenance Issues**

Isolation from seronegative contacts required. Maternal VZV infection during pregnancy can result in congenital varicella syndrome with significant embryopathies, disseminated varicella in newborns, and significant morbidity and mortality. Consider use of zoster immune globulin (ZIG), varicella zoster immune globulin (VZIG), gamma globulin, acyclovir, or vidarabine in selected and appropriate immunocompromised or pregnant candidates. Varicella vaccine (Varivax®) is recommended in healthy children at 12 months or vaccination of susceptible children within 3 days of exposure to prevent or attenuate the infection.

# XI. BACTERIAL INFECTIONS

## A. Cellulitis

▶ **Scientific Concepts**

A skin infection typically caused by group A beta-hemolytic streptococci (GABHS) and/or *Staphylococcus aureus*. Organisms typically enter broken skin then proliferate and spread locally.

▶ **History & Physical**

Examination reveals edema, erythema, tenderness, and heat at the affected area (typically extremities).

▶ **Diagnostic Studies**

Cultures of entry sites or aspirate to identify pathogens have a low yield; blood cultures can confirm bacteremia.

▶ **Diagnosis**

Fever, chills, malaise, and proximally spreading lymphangitis accompanied by lymphadenitis may be seen in erysipelas, a group A strep variant of cellulitis. Differential includes allergic contact dermatitis and urticaria.

▶ **Clinical Therapeutics**

Clinical recognition of distinctive features require empiric treatment with a penicillinase-resistant penicillin, a cephalosporin, or erythromycin.

▶ **Clinical Intervention**

No procedural interventions are indicated. Monitor for hematogenous spread and bacteremia.

▶ **Health Maintenance Issues**

Recurrent episodes require prolonged antimicrobial prophylaxis and careful history to elicit predisposing factors.

## B. Vasculitis

▶ **Scientific Concepts**

A hypersensitivity reaction to circulating immune complexes from antigens ranging from exogenous to endogenous sources including drugs and infectious agents.

▶ **History & Physical**

Previous infection or drug ingestion weeks before onset of pruritus, burning, malaise, and peripheral neuritis manifested in hallmark lesions of nonblanching palpable purpura typically localized to the lower third of the legs, the buttocks, and arms.

▶ **Diagnostic Studies**

No specific tests; diagnosis by history and physical examination.

▶ **Diagnosis**

Differentiate from thrombocytopenic purpura, disseminated intravascular coagulation (DIC), septic vasculitis.

▶ **Clinical Therapeutics**

Antibiotics if secondary to bacterial infection; consider oral steroids and cytotoxic immunosuppressives if indicated.

► Clinical Intervention
None.

► Health Maintenance Issues
Avoidance of precipitating factors.

## C. Erysipelas

► Scientific Concepts
Erysipelas is an uncommon cellulitic presentation that is distinguished by marked dermal lymphatic vessel involvement typically due to GABHS. In contrast, cellulitis may begin as erysipelas but extends deeper into the dermis and subcutaneous tissues.

► History & Physical
See cellulitis.

► Diagnostic Studies
See cellulitis.

► Diagnosis
See cellulitis.

► Clinical Therapeutics
See cellulitis.

► Clinical Intervention
See cellulitis.

► Health Maintenance Issues
See cellulitis.

## D. Impetigo

► Scientific Concepts
A common, contagious superficial skin infection typically found on the face, caused by staphylococci, streptococci, or both. Manifests as bullous and nonbullous versions.

► History & Physical
Higher rates seen in children in close physical contact; may follow minor skin injury; frequently occurs on intact skin. May present with mild itching and soreness. More common in infants and children, presenting with one or more vesicles that ooze and form a honey-colored crust; regional lymphadenopathy likely.

► Diagnostic Studies
Skin lesion and nasopharyngeal cultures may isolate causative agents.

► Diagnosis
Characteristic clinical history and appearance is usually diagnostic. Clinical appearance may resemble rhus dermatitis, atopic dermatitis, varicella zoster or herpes simplex vesicles, or ecthyma. Complications include poststreptococcal glomerulonephritis, cellulitis, bacteremia, septic arthritis, and osteomyelitis.

► Clinical Therapeutics
Requires topical or systemic antimicrobial coverage against GABHS and *S. aureus*.

► **Clinical Intervention**
Lesion debridement with warm water soaks.

► **Health Maintenance Issues**
Monitor infants for life-threatening secondary infections. Predisposing factors include poor hygiene and moist, warm environments. Topical mupirocin bid for 5 days to nares to eliminate carrier state.

## XII. OTHER

### A. Acanthosis Nigricans

► **Scientific Concepts**
A condition with five types of epidermal changes possibly related to heredity, endocrinopathies, obesity, drug administration, and, in type 5, malignancy. Type I is hereditary benign acanthosis nigricans (AN). Type 2 is benign AN associated with insulin resistance. Type 3 is pseudo AN, a complication of obesity. Type 4, drug-induced AN, is associated with nicotinic acid, steroids, or hormones.

► **History & Physical**
Classic lesions appear initially as hyperpigmentation of the intertriginious folds, specifically in the axillae and around the neck, followed by velvety thickening and accentuation of skin lines accompanied by an increase in acrochordons.

► **Diagnostic Studies**
Rule out diabetes mellitus and in malignant AN (type 5) rule out associated carcinoma.

► **Diagnosis**
Differentiate from tinea versicolor.

► **Clinical Therapeutics**
None.

► **Clinical Intervention**
None.

► **Health Maintenance Issues**
Treat underlying disorder, maintain ideal body weight.

### B. Burns

► **Scientific Concepts**
Burns produce thermal skin and tissue injury. Classification by degrees; minor erythema = first degree; blistering = second degree, with pain accompanying first and second degree; third degree = full thickness burn with charring.

► **History & Physical**
Assess burn degree and depth; determine etiology and duration of exposure.

► **Diagnostic Studies**
None; rule of nines estimates extent of burn. Adult values = 18% each leg, 9% each arm, 18% front of trunk, 18% back of trunk, and 9% head.

▶ Diagnosis

Based on history and physical examination.

▶ Clinical Therapeutics

May include fluid and electrolyte resuscitation, burn cleaning and debridement, and grafting.

▶ Clinical Intervention

Appropriate antibiotics and tetanus toxoid may be required.

▶ Health Maintenance Issues

Appropriate physical and occupational therapy and rehabilitation may be indicated.

## C. Decubitus Ulcer (Pressure Ulcer)

▶ Scientific Concepts

Ischemic tissue necrosis caused by skin compression, shear forces, and friction over bony prominences, typically in bedridden patients.

▶ History & Physical

Progressing through stages from localized blanching erythema to nonblanching erythema to ulceration of varying depths, resulting in ulceration over bony prominences following prolonged hospitalization or immobility.

▶ Diagnostic Studies

Based on history and physical examination.

▶ Diagnosis

Differential includes pyoderma gangrenosum, malignant ulcer, thermal burn, vasculitis ulcer, and infectious ulcer. Complications include osteomyelitis, bacteremia, and sepsis.

▶ Clinical Therapeutics

Early lesions may respond to topical antibiotics, hydrogels, or hydrocolloidal dressings.

▶ Clinical Intervention

Surgical management includes debridement, flaps, and skin grafts.

▶ Health Maintenance Issues

Frequent skin inspection, patient repositioning, massage, skin care, nutritional status monitoring, and early mobilization.

## D. Leg Ulcers

▶ Scientific Concepts

Lower-extremity ulcers typically arise from chronic venous or arterial insufficiency or peripheral sensory neuropathy.

▶ History & Physical

Ulcers secondary to venous insufficiency historically have lower-extremity aching and swelling exacerbated by dependency and alleviated by elevation. One typically sees ischemic blue-red patch followed by punched-out, irregular-edged ulceration over the malleoli or distal medial calf, often accompanied by lymphedema. If secondary to arterial insufficiency, one may see shiny, atrophic skin with alopecia of lower legs and feet.

► **Diagnostic Studies**

May require differing studies to determine underlying pathology/comorbid factors such as sickle cell anemia, diabetes, collagen vascular disease, syphilis.

► **Diagnosis**

Differential includes vasculitis, infection, trauma, pressure ulcer, pyoderma gangrenosum, sickle cell anemia.

► **Clinical Therapeutics**

May require systemic antibiotics for secondary infection; treatment of underlying disease states.

► **Clinical Intervention**

May include corrective surgical debridement, wound therapy, elastic support stockings, systemic antibiotics for secondary infection, and skin grafting.

► **Health Maintenance Issues**

Avoidance of smoking and control of systemic diseases such as hypertension and diabetes mellitus, correction of anemias or malnourished state, exercise, weight reduction in obese.

## E. Hidradenitis Suppurativa

► **Scientific Concepts**

Pathogenesis is unknown but condition is associated with inflammatory changes to apocrine glands with infection, suppuration, fibrosis, and sinus tract formation. Associated with genetic predisposition for acne.

► **History & Physical**

Typically onset is in puberty, females > males. One sees inflammatory nodules/abscesses of axillae, buttocks, and inguinal region. Hallmark finding is the "double comedone," with two to several comedonal surface openings with subdermal communication. Progresses to inflammatory cystic suppurative lesions.

► **Diagnostic Studies**

None. Diagnosis by history and physical examination; C&S of exudate to identify offending pathogens.

► **Diagnosis**

Rule out abscess, furuncle, carbuncle, cysts, lymphadenitis.

► **Clinical Therapeutics**

Combined therapy of antibiotics, intralesional steroids, surgery, and isotretinoin may be indicated.

► **Clinical Intervention**

Incision and drainage of painful abscesses, intralesional steroids, surgical excision of nodules or sinus tracts where indicated.

► **Health Maintenance Issues**

Psychosocial supportive therapy due to chronicity and location of disease.

## F. Lipomas

► **Scientific Concepts**
Etiology and pathogenesis unknown. Lipomas are benign fatty tumors of the subcutaneous tissue, presenting as a lobulated yellow mass surrounded by a thin capsule.

► **History & Physical**
Typically presents as a nontender, freely mobile, soft, palpable subcutaneous mass.

► **Diagnostic Studies**
None.

► **Diagnosis**
Differentiate from sarcoma by histopathology.

► **Clinical Therapeutics**
None.

► **Clinical Intervention**
Elective excision or liposuction.

► **Health Maintenance Issues**
Following diagnosis of initial occurrence, reassurance indicated for subsequent lesions unless symptomatic.

## G. Epithelial Inclusion Cysts

► **Scientific Concepts**
Typically arising from occluded follicles and pilosebaceous units, although epidermal cysts contain cheesy and fetid keratinaceous cellular debris. Epidermal inclusion cysts are lined by keratinizing squamous epithelium and have a similar clinical presentation.

► **History & Physical**
Typically appearing in young to middle-aged adults, epidermal cysts are usually less than 1 cm, firm to fluctuant cutaneous nodules that may regress without treatment but frequently recur unless surgically removed. Common sites include the head, posterior auricular folds, neck, upper trunk, and scrotum; infected cysts are typically larger, erythematous, and more painful.

► **Diagnostic Studies**
None.

► **Diagnosis**
Based on typical history and physical examination.

► **Clinical Therapeutics**
No effective oral or topical therapies available; intralesional steroids can hasten resolution of inflamed but uninfected cyst.

► **Clinical Intervention**
Infected cysts require incision and drainage of purulent material.

► **Health Maintenance Issues**
None.

## H. Melasma

▶ **Scientific Concepts**
Macular hyperpigmentation on sun-exposed facial areas associated with sunlight, pregnancy, oral contraceptives, medication, or idiopathic in nature seen 90% in women.

▶ **History & Physical**
Macular hyperpigmented symmetrical facial lesions with irregular borders in predisposed individuals.

▶ **Diagnostic Studies**
Macular hyperpigmentation accentuated with Wood's lamp examination.

▶ **Diagnosis**
Rule out postinflammatory hyperpigmentation.

▶ **Clinical Therapeutics**
Topical hydroquinone, tretinoin, glycolic acid, and low-strength topical steroids in differing combinations may reduce hyperpigmentation.

▶ **Clinical Intervention**
No clinical intervention indicated.

▶ **Health Maintenance Issues**
Strongly encourage sun avoidance and daily application of sunscreens.

## I. Urticaria

▶ **Scientific Concepts**
An acute, chronic, or chronic recurrent disorder of immunologic (IgE or complement-mediated) or physical (cold urticaria, dermographism, solar urticaria, cholinergic [exercise] urticaria, or pressure or vibratory angioedema) etiology.

▶ **History & Physical**
Rapid onset of pruritus, urticarial lesions, flushing, burning skin-colored transient papules and wheals coalescing into edematous plaques with an erythematous or white halo on sites of predilection such as pressure points, distal extremities, and trunk.

▶ **Diagnostic Studies**
No specific diagnostic test available.

▶ **Diagnosis**
Rule out SLE, Sjögren's syndrome, urticarial vasculitis.

▶ **Clinical Therapeutics**
Eliminate etiologic agents, antihistamines, oral steroids for angioedema-urticaria-eosinophilia syndrome.

▶ **Clinical Intervention**
Be prepared for emergency life support measures if anaphylaxis develops.

▶ **Health Maintenance Issues**
Avoidance of precipitating factors.

## J. Vitiligo

▶ **Scientific Concepts**

A chronic, probable autoimmune disorder with genetic and environmental precipitating factors resulting in the progressive destruction of selected melanocytes by cytotoxic T cells.

▶ **History & Physical**

In some cases attributed to trauma, illness, stress, or severe sunburn. Presents as symmetrical patterns of depigmented macules commonly involving the hands, face, skin folds, axillae, and genitalia.

▶ **Diagnostic Studies**

Wood's lamp examination accentuates clinically unapparent lesions; dermatopathology of skin biopsy is diagnostic.

▶ **Diagnosis**

Rule out pityriasis alba and other disorders of hypopigmentation such as postinflammatory hypopigmentation, mycosis fungoides, and Hansen's disease (leprosy).

▶ **Clinical Therapeutics**

Sunscreens, cosmetic makeup, topical/oral steroids, photochemotherapy (PUVA, narrow-band UVB), mini/micrografting.

▶ **Clinical Intervention**

Selective or combination therapy based on patient age, lesion distribution, previous response history, and chronicity.

▶ **Health Maintenance Issues**

Screen patients for associated endocrine disorders, particularly thyroid disease.

## BIBLIOGRAPHY

Braunwald E, Fauci AS, Kasper DL, Hauser SL, Longo DL, Jameson JL, eds. *Harrison's Principles of Internal Medicine,* 15th ed. New York: McGraw-Hill; 2001.

Dambro MR, Griffith JA. *Griffith's 5-Minute Clinical Consult, 2002.* Philadelphia: Williams & Wilkins; 2002.

Fitzpatrick TB, Johnson RA, Wolff K, Polano MK, Suurmond D. *Color Atlas and Synopsis of Clinical Dermatology,* 4th ed. New York: McGraw-Hill; 2001.

Freedberg IM, Eisen AZ, Wolff K, Austen KF, Goldsmith LA, Katz SI, Fitzpatrick TB. *Fitzpatrick's Dermatology in General Medicine,* 6th ed. New York: McGraw-Hill; 2003.

Hooper BJ, Goldman MP. *Primary Dermatologic Care.* St. Louis, MO: Mosby; 1999.

Miller AA, Simon AF. *Appleton & Lange Review for the Physician Assistant,* 4th ed. New York: McGraw-Hill; 2002.

# Ear, Nose, and Throat | 2

*Rebecca Luebke, MSBS, PA-C*

## I. HEARING IMPAIRMENT

▶ Scientific Concepts

Hearing loss as a result of auditory disorder may be classified by degree of impairment (mild, moderate, severe) or by type. Classification by type includes conductive, sensorineural, mixed, or central and depends on the site of pathology in the auditory system. **Conductive hearing loss** may be due to disorders in the external or middle ear, resulting in decreased volume for low tones and vowels. Bone conduction is usually normal and air conduction abnormal (Rinne test). Tuning fork heard more loudly in ear with conductive loss with Weber test. Conductive hearing loss may be due to middle ear stiffness or middle ear mass. In adults, conductive hearing loss is most commonly due to cerumen impaction or transient eustachian tube dysfunction associated with upper respiratory infection (URI). **Sensorineural hearing loss** may result from disorders of the inner ear, cochlea, or cranial nerve (CN) VIII. Difficulty perceiving high tones common, and equivalent loss of bone and air conduction found. **Mixed hearing loss** involves a combination of conductive and sensorineural hearing impairment, with air conduction usually worse than bone conduction. **Central hearing loss** may or may not appear as hearing loss on pure tone audiogram. Site of pathology is beyond cochlea, anywhere from cochlear nuclei to auditory cortex.

▶ History & Physical

Careful history, including the following:

1. Family history of childhood hearing impairment
2. Congenital perinatal infection (rubella, herpes, syphilis)
3. Birth weight less than 1,500 g
4. History of bacterial meningitis, particularly *Haemophilus influenzae*
5. Severe asphyxia
6. Use of ototoxic drugs (aminoglycoside antibiotics, loop diuretics, barbiturates)
7. Exposure to loud noise
8. History of head trauma
9. Complete review of systems

Physical examination includes external ear examination for evaluation of anatomic abnormalities of head and neck, otoscopy, Weber test, Rinne test.

▶ Diagnostic Studies

Testing to determine site of lesion and degree of impairment, to aid in determination of nonsurgical rehabilitation, and to determine if further testing is warranted. Pure tone audiometry (air conduction, bone conduction), speech audiometry (speech reception thresholds and speech discrimination score), impedance audiometry (tympanometry and acoustic reflexes).

▶ Diagnosis

Based on history, physical examination, and diagnostic test results.

▶ Clinical Therapeutics

Hearing aids, cochlear implants, assistive listening devices, speech reading, auditory training, speech–language training, counseling.

► **Clinical Intervention**
Possible surgical intervention with cochlear implants.

► **Health Maintenance Issues**
Avoid loud noises, wear earplugs, avoid overuse of ototoxic drugs.

## II. CERUMEN IMPACTION

► **Scientific Concepts**
The ear canal is generally self-cleaning. Impacted cerumen (wax) can often be attributed to attempts by the patient to clean canals.

► **History & Physical**
Patient may be unaware of condition or complain of hearing loss, or complain of fullness in the affected ear, ear pressure, or pain in external ear. Patient may also report drainage from the ear. Physical examination includes otoscopic evaluation as well as nose, throat, and neck (lymphadenopathy) to check for possible concomitant infection.

► **Diagnostic Studies**
Otoscopic visualization.

► **Diagnosis**
Light to dark brown cerumen filling canal, often impairing visualization of tympanic membrane (TM). May appear dry and hard.

► **Clinical Therapeutics**
Removal includes eardrops, mechanical means, suction, or irrigation. Irrigate with water at body temperature and only when TM is intact. Pretreatment with cerumen softeners may aid in removal. Follow-up for reevaluation may be indicated, particularly to check for development of infection after cerumen removal.

► **Clinical Intervention**
Usually none. Referral to a specialist for removal under microscopic guidance is indicated for TM perforation, if patient has chronic otitis media, or if unable to remove cerumen in the office.

► **Health Maintenance Issues**
Avoid use of cotton-tipped applicators and other objects inserted into ears for cleaning or scratching. Clean external canal with warm water and a washcloth over the index finger. Avoid entering ear canal.

## III. OTITIS EXTERNA (SWIMMER'S EAR)

► **Scientific Concepts**
Often follows water exposure or mechanical trauma to ear canal, allowing organism invasion. Usually caused by gram-negative organisms (*Pseudomonas, Proteus*), fungi, or *Staphylococcus aureus*. TM may be involved as its lateral surface is composed of ear canal skin. There may be, however, an acute otitis media present as well.

► History & Physical

Ear pain, pruritus, discharge, lymphadenopathy. Hearing loss if severe. Pain with tragal pressure or auricular traction. External canal erythematous and edematous, often with purulent exudate. Edema may obscure TM if severe. TM may appear erythematous but will move normally with pneumatic otoscopy unless there is concomitant otitis media.

► Diagnostic Studies

Direct visualization, palpation, otoscopy, pneumatic otoscopy, culture, Gram stain.

► Diagnosis

Made by examination and identification of causative organisms by culture and/or Gram stain.

► Clinical Therapeutics

Remove superficial debris. Topical antibiotics are most effective, particularly preparations with polymyxin or neomycin. Ciprofloxacin drops are also effective. If canal swelling accompanies infection, use combination antibiotic and steroid drops. Occasionally, oral antibiotics also used if infection extends beyond pinna, pain is severe, cervical lymphadenopathy is present, or patient is febrile. Occasionally, placement of an ear wick in the canal facilitates quicker healing by allowing the drops to remain in contact with the skin.

► Clinical Intervention

Usually none.

► Health Maintenance Issues

Ear canal must be kept dry. Use moldable earplugs if swimming. Prophylactic acetic acid or alcohol drops after swimming and showering for infection-prone patients.

## IV. MALIGNANT (NECROTIZING) OTITIS EXTERNA

► Scientific Concepts

Soft tissue infection of external ear (often persistent otitis externa). Typically caused by *Pseudomonas aeruginosa* and found in elderly, diabetic, or immunocompromised. May develop into osteomyelitis of skull base with extension to the auricle, scalp, parotid gland, middle and inner ear, and eventually the brain. May cause cranial nerve palsies or destruction, particularly in nerves VI, VII, IX, X, XI, and XII. Fatal without aggressive treatment.

► History & Physical

Hallmark is deep, boring pain in ear with granulation tissue at bony–cartilaginous junction of ear canal. Otalgia, otorrhea (foul), inflammation, hearing loss, progressive cranial nerve palsies, lymphadenopathy.

► Diagnostic Studies

Otoscopic examination, computed tomography (CT), and radionuclide scanning exhibiting osseus erosion. Magnetic resonance imaging (MRI) to evaluate intracranial involvement. Sedimentation rate and biopsies of granulation tissue may also aid in diagnosis.

► Diagnosis

Culture external auditory canal, CT for determining extent of bony destruction and soft tissue infiltration. MRI more sensitive to evaluate soft tissue involvement. Gallium scan for extent of bony involvement.

► Clinical Therapeutics

Long-term (may be several months) intravenous or oral antipseudo-monal antibiotics (ciprofloxacin hydrochloride).

► Clinical Intervention

Surgical debridement of necrotic tissue and drainage required if severe to prevent progression. Refer to otolaryngologist.

► Health Maintenance Issues

Maintain high index of suspicion in high-risk groups (e.g., diabetes mellitus, human immunodeficiency virus [HIV]).

# V. OTITIS MEDIA

## A. Acute Otitis Media

► Scientific Concepts

Middle ear infection most common in infants and children due to short length and horizontal positioning of eustachian tube. Often follows a viral URI that has caused eustachian tube edema. Fluid and mucus accumulate, resulting in a bacterial infection. Most common organisms include *Streptococcus pneumoniae, H. influenzae, Moraxella catarrhalis, Streptococcus pyogenes,* and *S. aureus. Escherichia coli* may be causative organism in infants younger than 6 weeks.

► History & Physical

Otalgia, fever, decreased hearing, discharge if TM perforates. Erythematous, bulging (when severe) or retracted TM with decreased mobility by pneumatic otoscopy. Occasional exudate or visible air–fluid levels in middle ear. May also have mastoid tenderness if infection spreads to mastoid air cells.

► Diagnostic Studies

Otoscopy and culture of any external canal exudate. Tympanocentesis for bacterial and fungal cultures indicated in seriously ill or toxic children, newborns, immunocompromised patients, or refractory infections.

► Diagnosis

Made by symptoms, signs, culture results.

► Clinical Therapeutics

Usually, amoxicillin is first-line therapy. Recommended treatment duration is typically 7–10 days, or initial observation may suffice. For resistant organisms or penicillin allergy, use erythromycin, clarithromycin, sulfa, second-generation cephalosporins, or trimethoprim-sulfamethoxazole. For resistant organisms in patients without penicillin allergy, second-line treatment may include amoxicillin/clavulanate. Quinolones may be used in adults. Analgesics and/or oral decongestants may also be needed.

► Clinical Intervention

Refer to otolaryngologist if diagnosis uncertain, treatment fails, or if complications (mastoiditis/meningitis) develop.

► Health Maintenance Issues

For recurrent infections, consider placement of tympanostomy tubes. Adenoidectomy is also potentially beneficial.

## B. Chronic Suppurative Otitis Media

► Scientific Concepts

Chronic middle ear infection due to recurrent or untreated acute otitis media. May follow trauma or other diseases. Causative organisms are different than in acute otitis media and include *P. aeruginosa, S. aureus, Klebsiella,* and other gram-negative bacilli. Chronic eustachian tube dysfunction with persistent negative middle ear pressure may lead to cholesteatoma (keratin-filled squamous epithelial-lined sac) formation. Leads to local destruction of bone with eventual invasion into cranium or inner ear.

► History & Physical

TM perforation with purulent otorrhea common. Conductive hearing loss due to TM perforation and interruption of ossicular chain. Pain and fever often absent except in acute exacerbations. Symptoms of meningitis or labyrinthitis possible if cholesteatoma invasion has occurred.

► Diagnostic Studies

Otoscopic examination, culture of purulent otorrhea. Audiogram, tympanogram, CT of temporal bone.

► Diagnosis

Based on history, physical examination, and culture results.

► Clinical Therapeutics

Removal of infected debris from external canal, topical antibiotic drops, and earplugs. Systemic antibiotics generally not indicated. Analgesics and/or oral decongestants may be needed. Definitive treatment with TM repair or reconstruction.

► Clinical Intervention

Surgical indications include necrotic bone and cholesteatoma removal.

► Health Maintenance Issues

Earplugs and early treatment of acute otitis media.

## C. Serous Otitis Media (Chronic Otitis Media with Effusion)

► Scientific Concepts

Fluid in middle ear resulting from prolonged blockage of eustachian tube and negative pressure in middle ear. Results in transudation of fluid. May follow URI, allergies, or barotrauma. More common in children.

► History & Physical

Clear or amber fluid in middle ear. TM retracted, but bony landmarks intact. Air bubbles and/or fluid meniscus may be visible behind TM, which has decreased mobility.

► **Diagnostic Studies**
Otoscopic exam, pneumatic otoscopy, tympanometry, audiogram.

► **Diagnosis**
Based on history and physical examination findings.

► **Clinical Therapeutics**
Usually self-limited. Decongestants and/or antihistamines if allergic component present. Antibiotics if bacterial involvement suspected.

► **Clinical Intervention**
If persistent (> 3–4 months) in children, consider myringotomy and/or tubes, and/or adenoidectomy to prevent speech development deficits. Rule out nasopharyngeal tumor in chronic unilateral ear effusion in adults.

► **Health Maintenance Issues**
Autoinflation exercises and decongestants prior to flying or diving.

## VI. VERTIGO

► **Scientific Concepts**
Vertigo/dizziness is difficult to assess because of varying definitions as well as numerous possible etiologies. Descriptions may include "dizziness," "spinning," "imbalance," "lightheadedness," a sensation of "ground moving," "weaving," or "rocking." Possible etiologies include peripheral or central nervous system (CNS) defects, cardiovascular disorders, psychiatric disorders, and metabolic disorders. Vertigo, hearing loss, tinnitus, and ear fullness suggest vestibular origin, either central or peripheral.

► **History & Physical**
Vertigo that is sudden in onset and severe suggests peripheral causes, while less severe and vague complaints may suggest central origin. **Peripheral lesions** are usually present with vertiginous complaints. Tinnitus, hearing loss, nausea, vomiting, or diaphoresis may accompany dizziness. Nystagmus in peripheral lesions may be horizontal or rotatory, but not vertical. Symptoms usually severe with sudden onset, lasting minutes to hours. *Benign paroxysmal positional vertigo (BPPV)* may be the etiology if the symptoms are precipitated by certain head movements, particularly when supine or getting up. It is thought to be caused by canalolithiasis in the posterior semicircular canal. BPPV is often found in the elderly. *Ménière's syndrome* involves excessive endolymphatic fluid in the inner ear (endolymphatic hydrops). Accompanying vertigo is fluctuant hearing loss, roaring tinnitus, and ear fullness. Symptoms last minutes to hours, gradually subside, only to return in months to years. Vertigo secondary to *viral labyrinthitis* occurs following a viral URI and involves infection of the cochlea and labyrinth. Hearing loss and tinnitus may also occur. Symptoms generally abate in 3 to 6 weeks. A more serious peripheral cause of vertigo is an *acoustic neuroma* (benign schwannoma of CN VIII). Symptoms may be mild and initially vague, but progress as the tumor enlarges, distinguishing it from other peripheral causes. Patients may report unilateral hearing loss and tinnitus. As the mass impinges on cerebellopontine structures, cranial nerve and brain stem deficits occur, such as facial

numbness, gait ataxia, weakness. *Ototoxic drugs* may damage the vestibular portion of CN VIII, eliciting vertigo. Streptomycin and gentamicin are known offenders. Hearing loss typically predominates. **Central lesions** generally present with brain stem symptoms in addition to vertigo. Nystagmus that is vertical or bidirectional suggests central lesion. *Multiple sclerosis* is one cause of vertigo with CNS etiology. Attacks are difficult to differentiate from peripheral causes as they may be transient, sudden, recurrent, or persistent. Slight facial numbness and voice huskiness may accompany. Another CNS cause is *vertebrobasilar insufficiency.* Initial symptoms may be solely vertigo, but later attacks usually involve brain stem abnormalities (diplopia, sensory loss, dysarthria, dysphagia, hemiparesis). *Sedatives* and *anticonvulsants* may also cause vertigo by suppressing the reticular activating system in the brain stem. **Cardiovascular origins** of vertigo are typically due to decreased cerebral perfusion. Etiologies include arrhythmias, fixed or decreased cardiac output, decreased vascular tone, or severe volume depletion. Symptoms usually worsen upon standing and improve supine. Disequilibrium or imbalance may be due to **multiple sensory deficits,** found most commonly in diabetics and/or elderly or in cerebellar disease. Exam findings include gait ataxia and other cerebellar signs. **Psychiatric illnesses** occasionally produce complaints of dizziness, particularly depression, anxiety states, and psychosis. Medications to treat these conditions may also precipitate symptoms. **Metabolic conditions** such as hypoglycemia, hypoxia, hypocarbia, and hypercarbia may cause dizziness that appears similar to that caused by decreased cerebral perfusion.

**Physical exam** should focus on eye (nystagmus), ear (including hearing acuity), cardiovascular (arrhythmias, bruits), and neurological (including cerebellar function) aspects. Remember that a few beats of nystagmus on extreme lateral gaze is normal. Testing for positional nystagmus (Dix–Hallpike maneuver) aids in diagnosis of BPPV. With the patient sitting on the table, the examiner grasps the patient's head, rotates it to the right, and then transfers him or her to the supine position with the head extended over and dropped 45 degrees below the table edge. Look for rotatory nystagmus with a 1- to 5-second delay in onset. Repeat the maneuver with the head rotated to the left. If the vertigo is due to BPPV, symptoms and nystagmus will occur when patient's head is supine and the involved ear is pointed downward.

▶ Diagnostic Studies

Audiologic testing, electronystagmography (ENG), brain stem auditory evoked response testing (if acoustic neuroma suspected), CT, MRI, stapedial reflex testing (indicates abnormal brain stem or CN VIII neurotransmission).

▶ Differential Diagnosis

See History & Physical above.

▶ Clinical Therapeutics

For BPPV, avoid precipitating positions. Repositioning maneuvers may aid in removing the particle from the posterior semicircular canal. Diuretics and low-sodium (1 g/d) diet for Ménière's syndrome. Trial of meclizine, diphenhydramine hydrochloride, dimenhydrinate, or diazepam for viral labrynthitis and other causes. Cardiovascular causes may be treated by adequate hydration, standing up slowly, and discontinuing causative drugs. Those with severe aortic stenosis should be evaluated for surgery. Chronic symptoms may require endolymphatic sac decompression, CN VIII section, labyrinthectomy, or transtympanic canal aminoglycoside injections. Treat underlying disorders accordingly.

▶ **Clinical Intervention**
Referral to neurologist if symptoms persist, are disabling, or if central vestibular disease or acoustic neuroma suspected.

▶ **Health Maintenance Issues**
None.

## VII. FOREIGN BODY IN THE EAR

▶ **Scientific Concepts**
More common in children.

▶ **History & Physical**
Hearing loss, discomfort. Foreign object visible on otoscopic examination.

▶ **Diagnostic Studies**
Otoscopy.

▶ **Diagnosis**
Based on history and physical examination.

▶ **Clinical Therapeutics**
Hook or loop for removal of firm objects. Do not irrigate if TM is perforated or if object is organic in nature (e.g., insects, beans) as water may cause them to swell. Immobilize live insects prior to removal by filling ear canal with lidocaine or mineral oil.

▶ **Clinical Intervention**
None needed unless object unable to be manually removed or infection ensues. Prophylactic antibiotics may be necessary due to trauma to ear canal and possible late infection.

▶ **Health Maintenance Issues**
Keep small objects away from young children.

## VIII. BULLOUS MYRINGITIS

▶ **Scientific Concepts**
Infection (often viral) involving the TM and deep external auditory canal. Often associated with viral URI and more common in winter. Frequently affects both ears in succession. Causative organism unknown, but *Mycoplasma pneumoniae* has been cultured.

▶ **History & Physical**
Patients complain of severe otalgia and occasionally decreased hearing. Physical exam reveals erythematous vesicles on the TM surface, which

enlarge to form bullae. Straw-colored fluid, occasionally tinged with blood, fills the bullae.

▶ Diagnostic Studies
Otoscopy.

▶ Diagnosis
Based on history and physical examination.

▶ Clinical Therapeutics
Treatment consists of topical analgesic drops containing benzocaine or lidocaine, oral analgesics if severe, and systemic antibiotics if bacterial infection suspected or cultured. Oral erythromycin if *M. pneumoniae* suspected.

▶ Clinical Intervention
If otalgia is severe, blebotomy may be performed, which involves opening the blisters with a beveled needle or myringotomy knife.

▶ Health Maintenance Issues
Usually none.

## IX. SINUSITIS

### A. Acute Sinusitis

▶ Scientific Concepts
Usually follows a viral URI. Swelling of the nasal mucosa or mechanical blockage of the osteomeatal complex prevents paranasal sinuses from draining. Results in accumulation of mucous secretions in sinuses, which become secondarily infected with bacteria. Maxillary sinuses are the most commonly infected sinuses. Edematous tissue may be due to allergic rhinitis or viral infections, while mechanical blockage may be caused by intranasal foreign bodies or tumors, deviated septum, or nasal polyps. Allergies play large role, particularly in children. Causative organisms include *S. pneumoniae, H. influenzae, S. aureus, M. catarrhalis, S. pyogenes.*

▶ History & Physical
Purulent rhinorrhea, facial pain and pressure (particularly with forward bending) over the cheeks and/or forehead, postnasal drainage, maxillary tooth pain. Examination reveals nasal inflammation, tenderness over maxillary or frontal sinuses, decreased transillumination of involved sinuses, purulent rhinorrhea. Drainage may be noted in the posterior oropharynx as well.

▶ Diagnostic Studies
Ear, nose, and throat examination (including nasal endoscopy); sinus palpation and transillumination, palpate neck for lymphadenopathy. If diagnosis questionable, sinus radiography may show mucosal thickening or air–fluid levels in sinuses. CT scans (gold standard) offer better visualization of both inflammatory changes and bone destruction. MRI if malignancy suspected.

▶ Diagnosis

Based on history, physical examination, and radiography.

▶ Clinical Therapeutics

First-line antibiotics include amoxicillin or amoxicillin with clavulanic acid. Cephalosporins also effective. For second-line therapy or penicillin allergy, consider trimethoprim-sulfamethoxazole (TMP-SMZ), macrolides, quinolones, or doxycycline. Oral or topical (nasal spray) decongestants and nasal steroid sprays to decrease inflammation and promote drainage. Little evidence to support use of therapies other than antibiotics. Reserve antihistamines and steroids for allergic components as they may dry and thicken secretions. Treatment duration longer than for typical URI treatment due to limited blood flow to sinuses. Treat for 10 to 14 days minimum.

▶ Clinical Intervention

Referral to otolaryngologist for sinus irrigation indicated when pain is severe and maxillary sinus is not draining. Avoid surgery for acute sinusitis unless infection fails to clear or complications develop. Hospital admission for IV antibiotics for persistent infection to prevent intracranial extension.

▶ Health Maintenance Issues

Normal saline nasal sprays help remove nasal crusting and secretions. Warm compresses to face, hot fluids, and inhaling steam improve ciliary function and decrease facial pain and congestion. Remove allergens.

## B. Chronic Sinusitis

▶ Scientific Concepts

Usually follows untreated or poorly treated acute sinusitis. Persistent (symptoms >3 months) low-grade infection of paranasal sinuses with chronic mucosal thickening. Consider intranasal polyps as contributory factor. Causative organisms include *S. aureus* (20% of cases), *H. influenzae, Pneumococcus,* other streptococci. Anaerobic species include *Streptococcus* and *Bacteroides* spp. Often mixed flora.

▶ History & Physical

Chronic nasal obstruction and/or drainage. Patients may present with thick, purulent discharge in morning and clearing by afternoon. Facial pain and pressure may be persistently present or only during acute exacerbations. Anosmia.

▶ Diagnostic Studies

History, physical examination (including nasal endoscopy), radiography, CT imaging of osteomeatal complex.

▶ Diagnosis

History, physical, radiographic findings. Rule out allergic rhinitis as this may mimic sinusitis. Consider cystic fibrosis in patients with nasal polyps or infection with *P. aeruginosa.*

▶ Clinical Therapeutics

First-line antibiotics include augmented amoxicillin, clindamycin, and TMP-SMZ. Prolonged course of treatment. Decongestants (topical for

2–3 days, then oral) and intranasal steroids may be used, although extent of benefit is questionable.

► Clinical Intervention

If recurrent or persistent, referral to otolaryngologist for functional endoscopic sinus surgery. Often restores physiology of sinus aeration and drainage.

► Health Maintenance Issues

Control of perennial allergic rhinitis.

## X. ALLERGIC RHINITIS

► Scientific Concepts

Seasonal allergic reactions precipitated by tree pollens in spring, grass in midsummer, and weeds in the fall. Animal dander also allergenic. Perennial conditions often triggered by dust mites and mold. Symptoms from dust mite allergy worse in morning from overnight exposure to furniture, pillows, mattresses harboring large numbers of mites. Poor control may lead to sinusitis, otitis media with effusion, or asthma exacerbation. May aggravate sleep apnea.

► History & Physical

Family history of hay fever, asthma, or atopic eczema. Inquire about pets, smokers, and type of heating system in household. Clear rhinorrhea that is more persistent than found in viral rhinitis. Seasonal variation. Pruritic eyes, nose, and palate; sneezing, tearing, postnasal drainage. Turbinate mucosa pale or violaceous and swollen with excessive crusting. Occasionally nasal polyps, which appear as yellowish boggy masses of hypertrophic mucosa. Allergic shiners (dark discoloration under eyes), allergic salute (results in crease across nasal bridge from persistently pushing up on nose to wipe secretions and open nasal passages), mouth breathing due to nasal blockage.

► Diagnostic Studies

Smear of nasal secretions reveals eosinophils. Increased immunoglobulin E (IgE) levels in serum. Eosinophils > 10% of white blood cell count.

► Diagnosis

Based on history, physical examination, nasal smear, serology. Differentiation from viral rhinitis may be sought by color of mucosa (erythematous in viral etiology; pale, violaceous in allergic).

► Clinical Therapeutics

Newer antihistamines less sedating (loratadine, astemizole, cetirizine, fexofenadine). May be combined with decongestants (oral or topical). Intranasal steroid sprays or cromolyn sodium also beneficial. More severe cases may require corticosteroids or immunotherapy.

► Clinical Intervention

For severe cases, skin testing or serum radioallergosorbent (RAST) testing to indicate causative agents. Desensitization another option for treatment. Referral to allergist if symptoms fail to resolve in 3 to 6 months, if complications develop, if quality of life is decreased, or if systemic corticosteroids are required.

### ► Health Maintenance Issues

Avoid offending allergens. Use air purifiers, dust filters, plastic coverings for pillows, mattresses. Remove dust-collecting objects such as carpet, drapes, bedspreads, wicker. Substitute synthetic materials for animal products.

## XI. EPISTAXIS

### ► Scientific Concepts

Numerous etiologies, the most common being disruption of mucosal blood vessels from trauma (nose blowing, sneezing, digital trauma, foreign bodies). May also be associated with hypertension (usually posterior bleed), ulcerations, repeated cocaine usage, nasal malignancy, bleeding diatheses such as hereditary hemorrhagic telangiectasia (Osler–Weber–Rendu syndrome), tumors (juvenile angiofibroma), and dry mucosa due to low humidity. Bleeding from the vascular plexus on the anterior septum (Kiesselbach's plexus) is most common. Posterior bleeding more serious (may lead to death) because of rapid blood loss and difficulty locating, visualizing bleeding site.

### ► History & Physical

Anterior bleed usually unilateral and arising from septum. Intermittent, brisk, arterial bleeding with blood in the posterior pharynx generally indicates posterior bleed. Localization of bleeding site necessary. Check oropharynx for blood clots. Review medications for anticoagulants, antiplatelet drugs, nasal steroid sprays, and certain herbals (*Gingko biloba* and garlic). Determine pulse and blood pressure.

### ► Diagnostic Studies

Complete blood count (CBC), prothrombin time, partial thromboplastin time, bleeding time (if recurrent or severe). Toxicology screen if intranasal substance abuse suspected. CT of sinuses only if no site found or bleeding persists.

### ► Diagnosis

History, physical examination, labs.

### ► Clinical Therapeutics

Site of bleeding will determine treatment. For all types of bleeds, patient should be sitting with head leaning forward.

***Anterior bleeds:*** Direct pressure of nasal alae, topical nasal decongestants (phenylephrine 0.125 to 1%), topical 4% cocaine as vasoconstrictor and anesthetic. Can substitute topical decongestant (oxymetazoline) and anesthetic (tetracaine) for 4% cocaine. Cauterization of bleeding site with silver nitrate, diathermy, or electrocautery. Anterior nasal packing for refractive bleeding. Dissolvable packing and nasal sponges often easier to place and more comfortable than gauze packing.

***Posterior bleeds:*** Posterior nasal packing and hospital admission.

► Clinical Intervention

Ear, nose, and throat (ENT) referral for recurrent or uncontrolled bleeding episodes.

► Health Maintenance Issues

Humidifier, lubrication with petroleum jelly or bacitracin ointment. Avoid vigorous exercise, hot or spicy foods, nasal trauma, excessive nose blowing. Trim children's fingernails.

## XII. UPPER RESPIRATORY INFECTION (VIRAL RHINITIS, COMMON COLD)

► Scientific Concepts

Acute viral infection resulting in inflammation of nasal and sinus mucosa. Caused by numerous types of adenoviruses, rhinoviruses, parainfluenza viruses, respiratory syncytial viruses, and other viruses. More common in winter months.

► History & Physical

Malaise, fatigue, low-grade fever, chills, sore throat, clear rhinorrhea, postnasal drainage, headache, sneezing, paranasal sinus pressure, plugged ears. Erythematous, edematous nasal mucosa with clear, watery discharge. Purulent discharge suggests bacterial infection.

► Diagnostic Studies

Usually none required, but a CBC with differential reveals increased lymphocytes.

► Diagnosis

Based on history, physical examination. Differential includes allergic, vasomotor rhinitis.

► Clinical Therapeutics

Oral decongestants (pseudoephedrine) if congested. Topical decongestants (nasal sprays) effective but should be discontinued after 2–3 days to prevent rebound congestion, which may be worse than original symptoms. Use antihistamines (loratadine, cetirizine, fexofenadine) for rhinorrhea. Combination decongestants, antihistamines often used. Antipyretics, analgesics, hydration, saline nasal sprays. Usually resolves in 5–10 days.

► Clinical Intervention

None usually required.

► Health Maintenance Issues

To avoid potential drowsiness with older antihistamines (diphenhydramine), choose newer agents (loratadine, fexofenadine, cetirizine).

## XIII. NASAL FOREIGN BODY

► Scientific Concepts

Foreign object lodged in nasal tissue. More common in children.

► History & Physical

Suspect if unilateral, purulent nasal drainage present. May be malodorous.

► Diagnostic Studies

Usually none needed.

► Diagnosis

Based on history, physical examination.

► Clinical Therapeutics

Mechanical removal if object visible. Avoid irrigation if object is organic as this may cause it to swell.

► Clinical Intervention

Referral to ENT if object not visible or difficult to remove.

► Health Maintenance Issues

Keep small objects away from young children.

## XIV. HERPES SIMPLEX

► Scientific Concepts

Herpes simplex virus type 1 (HSV-1) is generally responsible for upper body cutaneous disease while type 2 (HSV-2) causes genital infections. Vesicles appear anywhere on face, lips, in mouth. Vesicles quickly enlarge and eventually rupture, forming scabs. Viral shedding lasts 5–7 days until crusting over occurs. Trauma, sunlight may precipitate recurrence.

► History & Physical

Prodromal burning, itching, stinging at site where painful vesicles soon appear. Associated fever, malaise, cervical lymphadenopathy may occur. Eventual rupture of vesicles leaves brownish, honey-colored crusting. Recurrent episodes may occur throughout life as fever blisters.

► Diagnostic Studies

Tzanck smear from unroofed vesicles reveals multinucleated giant cells. Serology for HSV-1 antibodies.

► Diagnosis

Often based on history, physical examination. Differential includes aphthous stomatitis, impetigo (honey-colored crusted lesions), erythema multiforme, syphilitic chancre, and carcinoma.

► Clinical Therapeutics

Oral antiviral medications, such as acyclovir, famciclovir, or valacyclovir, may decrease severity and duration if initiated during prodromal stage. However, they are less effective once eruption occurs. Treatment duration is typically 7 to 10 days. If recurrences are frequent, daily prophylaxis with acyclovir 200 mg tid or 400 mg bid may be used. Intravenous acyclovir if immunocompromised. Topical acyclovir and pencyclovir available, but they are generally considered less beneficial than oral treatment.

► Clinical Intervention
Suspicion of ophthalmic involvement requires immediate ophthalmology referral.

► Health Maintenance Issues
Protection from sunburn, trauma.

## XV. ORAL THRUSH (CANDIDIASIS)

► Scientific Concepts
Fungal infection of oral cavity. Causative conditions include dentures, diabetes, anemia, debilitation, steroid inhalers, chemotherapy, local irradiation, corticosteroid or broad-spectrum antibiotic use. May also be found in HIV infection.

► History & Physical
Painful, creamy-white patches, which are colonies of organisms, on erythematous bases. When removed with tongue blade, leave a raw, red surface.

► Diagnostic Studies
Potassium hydroxide wet preparation of scraping reveals spores, possibly nonseptate mycelia. Biopsy shows intraepithelial pseudomycelia of *Candida albicans.*

► Diagnosis
Based on history and physical examination. Differential includes leukoplakia and lichen planus, neither of which can be removed with a tongue blade.

► Clinical Therapeutics
Nystatin mouthwash, clotrimazole troches, fluconazole, ketoconazole. Apply Nystatin powder to dentures three to four times per day for several weeks.

► Clinical Intervention
Usually none.

► Health Maintenance Issues
Rinse mouth after use of steroid inhalers.

## XVI. STREPTOCOCCAL PHARYNGITIS

► Scientific Concepts
Infection of oropharynx and tonsils by group A beta-hemolytic streptococci (GABHS).

► History & Physical
Severe odynophagia, hemoptysis, weight loss, vocal cord immobility, referred otalgia, fever, anterior cervical lymphadenopathy, malaise. Exam reveals beefy red tonsils, often with exudate, tender adenopathy, scarlatiniform rash.

► Diagnostic Studies

Throat culture positive for GABHS, CBC with leukocytosis and left shift. Rapid antigen tests are now available, but they are less sensitive than specific. A positive test may be considered equivalent to a positive culture, but a negative test requires verification with a culture.

► Diagnosis

Based on history, physical examination, culture results. Differential includes sore throat from viruses (exudate absent), *Neisseria gonorrhoeae, Mycoplasma, Chlamydia trachomatis,* mononucleosis, diphtheria (gray tonsillar pseudomembrane).

► Clinical Therapeutics

Penicillin, erythromycin (penicillin allergy, *Chlamydia, Mycoplasma*), cephalosporins, and other macrolides. Avoid ampicillin if mononucleosis suspected (causes rash). Antipyretics, analgesics, anti-inflammatories.

► Clinical Intervention

Antibiotic treatment usually prevents complications such as scarlet fever, rheumatic fever, abscess formation, poststreptococcal glomerulonephritis.

► Health Maintenance Issues

Usually none. Tonsillectomy for frequent recurrences or if chronic tonsillar hypertrophy becomes obstructive.

## XVII. ORAL CANCER/LEUKOPLAKIA

► Scientific Concepts

Any white lesion on the mucosal surface that cannot be removed by scraping can be referred to as leukoplakia. Hyperkeratosis from chronic irritation is the main cause, but approximately 2–6% are dysplastic or early invasive squamous cell carcinoma (SCC). SCC accounts for ~90% of oral cancers. Tobacco (including smokeless) and alcohol are major contributing factors. Other causes include *Epstein-Barr virus, papillomavirus,* chronic iron deficiency leading to Plummer–Vinson syndrome. Men > women.

► History & Physical

Odynophagia, dysphagia, lymphadenopathy, referred otalgia, weight loss. Complete exam of oropharynx including lips, gums, palate, lateral tongue, floor of mouth, buccal mucosa, and tonsillar fossae for white patches. These patches resemble candidiasis, but they cannot be removed by scraping.

► Diagnostic Studies

Biopsy of lesions reveals any malignant or premalignant changes.

► Diagnosis

Based on history, physical examination, biopsy results. Tumor, nodes, metastases (TNM) staging. Differential diagnoses include lichen planus, oral candidiasis, traumatic irritation, and discoid lupus.

► Clinical Therapeutics

Laser surgical excision for small lesions. Radiation as an alternative, but complications include xerostomia, mandibular necrosis. Combination resection, irradiation for large tumors. Beta-carotene, vitamin E, and retinoids may aid in regression of leukoplakia.

► Clinical Intervention

As above.

► Health Maintenance Issues

Alcohol, tobacco, smokeless tobacco abstinence.

## XVIII. EPIGLOTTITIS

► Scientific Concepts

Life-threatening inflammation of epiglottis usually caused by *H. influenzae* (type B). More commonly found in children ages 3–5 years, but can occur in adulthood. Incidence decreasing with *H. influenzae* vaccines.

► History & Physical

Odynophagia, high fever, stridor, respiratory distress. Patients often drooling, sitting up, and leaning forward. Direct visualization with tongue blade contraindicated as this may precipitate complete airway blockage because of laryngospasm and edema.

► Diagnostic Studies

Lateral neck x-ray reveals "thumb sign" or "thumbprinting" (epiglottic edema). Vital signs, blood gases to determine extent of hypoxia/airway obstruction. Blood cultures once airway secured.

► Diagnosis

Based on history, physical examination, radiographic findings.

► Clinical Therapeutics

In addition to intervention (below), third-generation cephalosporins for *H. influenzae* coverage. TMP-SMZ for penicillin allergy. Systemic steroids controversial but may decrease inflammation.

► Clinical Intervention

Laryngoscopy in operating room in presence of anesthesiologist and otolaryngologist. Cherry-red, swollen epiglottis seen. Orotracheal intubation is preferred method of treatment. On occasion, tracheostomy may be necessary.

► Health Maintenance Issues

*H. influenzae* vaccination.

## XIX. HOARSENESS

► Scientific Concepts

Hoarseness indicates laryngeal involvement. Etiologic factors include viral infections, voice overuse, smoking, inhaled irritants, allergies, benign and malignant neoplasms, recurrent laryngeal nerve damage, gastric reflux, brain stem lesion. Change in voice occurs from inflammation, irritation of vocal cords.

► **History & Physical**

Hoarseness, odynophagia, sore throat, cough, dyspnea. Complete ENT exam, indirect and direct laryngoscopy indicated if symptoms persist >2–3 weeks to rule out neoplasm.

► **Diagnostic Studies**

Indirect and direct laryngoscopy, CT, MRI, throat cultures.

► **Diagnosis**

Based on history, physical examination, diagnostic studies.

► **Clinical Therapeutics**

Acute cases usually resolve spontaneously. Voice rest. Short course of systemic steroids to decrease inflammation.

► **Clinical Intervention**

Chronic cases indicate further workup such as direct visualization and biopsy of any lesions.

► **Health Maintenance Issues**

Smoking cessation, control of gastric reflux.

## XX. LARYNGEAL CANCER

► **Scientific Concepts**

Most commonly squamous cell and majority of cases occur in those who use tobacco, smoked or smokeless. Process may be precipitated by tobacco, alcohol, radiation, drugs, diet, pollution, viral infections, and other unknown factors. Tobacco and alcohol have a synergistic effect. Five-year survival is ~50% (75% if detected early, 35% if detected late).

► **History & Physical**

Often, initial presentation is hoarseness, which advances to odynophagia and metastases to cervical nodes. Physical examination includes complete ENT exam, including cervical lymph nodes.

► **Diagnostic Studies**

Indirect mirror exam of the larynx, fiberoptic endoscope.

► **Diagnosis**

Based on history, physical examination, indirect or direct visualization, and biopsy results if tissue sample obtained.

► **Clinical Therapeutics**

Radiation therapy, conservation laryngectomy, chemotherapy, or a combination of the three.

► **Clinical Intervention**

Patients with laryngeal cancer should be followed by an oncologist for life, but more frequently in the first 2 years when the risk of recurrence is highest. Adequate rehabilitation (physical, functional, psychosocial, occupational) is essential and requires a multidisciplinary approach.

▶ Health Maintenance Issues

Preventive measures include eliminating or drastically reducing tobacco and alcohol consumption. Although currently inconclusive, other preventive efforts under investigation include antioxidants, particularly vitamin A derivatives.

## BIBLIOGRAPHY

Braunwald E, Fauci AS, Kasper DL, Hauser SL, Longo DL, Jameson, JL, eds. *Harrison's Principles of Internal Medicine,* 15th ed. New York: McGraw-Hill; 2001.

Fagnan LJ. Acute sinusitis: A cost-effective approach to diagnosis and treatment. *Am Fam Physician* 58(8):1795–1801; 1998.

Ferri FF. *Ferri's Clinical Advisor: Instant Diagnosis and Treatment.* Philadelphia: Mosby; 2002.

Gluckman JL, Farrell M. Head and neck cancer. pp. 722–724. In: Stein JH, ed. *Internal Medicine,* 5th ed. Chicago: Mosby; 1998.

Goroll AH, Mulley AG Jr. *Primary Care Medicine: Office Evaluation and Management of the Adult Patient,* 4th ed. Philadelphia: Lippincott, Williams & Wilkins; 2002.

Hoover HA. (2002, August). *Acute rhinosinusitis.* Symposium conducted at the North Carolina Academy of Physician Assistants Annual Conference, Myrtle Beach, SC.

Hoover HA. (2002, August). *Epistaxis.* Symposium conducted at the North Carolina Academy of Physician Assistants Annual Conference, Myrtle Beach, SC.

Jackler RK, Kaplan MJ. Ear, nose, & throat. pp. 227–268. In: Tierney LM, McPhee SJ, Papadakis MA, eds. *Current Medical Diagnosis & Treatment,* 41st ed. New York: McGraw-Hill; 2002.

Jahn AF, Hawke A. Infections of the external ear. pp. 2787–2794. In: Cummings CW, ed. *Otolaryngology—Head and Neck Surgery,* 2nd ed. Chicago: Mosby; 1993.

Lehrer JF, Poole DC. Diagnosis and management of vertigo. *Comprehensive Ther* 13(9):31–40; 1987.

Lucas BD, Armitage KB, Gross P, Yamauchi T. Respiratory infections: which antibiotics for empiric therapy? *Patient Care* 33(1):76–106; 1999.

Noble J, ed. *Textbook of Primary Care Medicine,* 3rd ed. St. Louis, MO: Mosby; 2001.

Trotto NE, Kaiser HB, Kaliner MA, Slavin RG. Asthma, rhinitis, sinusitis, urticaria. *Patient Care* 33(1):115–139; 1999.

# Ophthalmology 3

*J. Dennis Blessing, PhD, PA-C, and Lisa N. Reyna, MPAS, PA-C*

## I. VISUAL DEFICITS

### A. Blurred Vision

▶ Scientific Concepts

Blurred vision is a decrease in visual acuity or the inability to distinguish objects clearly. A large number of conditions can cause blurred vision. Vision disturbances can be due to an eye illness or injury, systemic illness or injury, or other organ illness or injury, and can affect one or both eyes.

▶ History & Physical

Assess normal condition of eyes including use of corrective lenses, use of contacts; injury, onset (sudden or insidious), duration, pain, tearing, redness, pruritus, discharge (type, color, amount), presence of halos, loss of vision (partial), binocular or monocular, systemic diseases (hypertension or diabetes) or other health problems, medications, prior history of ocular problems (glaucoma). Examine visual acuity; inspect orbits, cornea, sclera, conjunctiva (palpebral and bulbar), pupils and pupil reaction, extraocular movements, anterior chamber; funduscopic examination. Palpate orbital rims and globes.

▶ Diagnostic Studies

Fluorescein staining if abrasion or foreign body suspected; slit lamp examination if needed.

▶ Diagnosis

Determination of cause by history, physical examination, and diagnostic studies.

▶ Clinical Therapeutics

As indicated by diagnosis.

▶ Clinical Intervention

As indicated by diagnosis; referral when indicated.

▶ Health Maintenance Issues

Protection of eyes when potential for injury exists in work and recreational activities; sunglasses in bright sun; treatment of conditions that may have sequelae affecting vision. Control systemic conditions such as diabetes and hypertension; obtain routine screening for glaucoma.

### B. Decreased Visual Acuity

▶ Scientific Concepts

The inability to distinguish objects clearly secondary to an interruption of the light (visual) pathways to the retina.

▶ History & Physical

Assess normal condition of eyes including use of corrective lenses, use of contacts; onset (sudden or insidious), monocular or binocular, duration, pain, tearing, redness, pruritus, discharge (type, color, amount), presence of halos, loss of vision (partial), injury, systemic diseases (hypertension or diabetes) or other health problems, medications, prior history of ocular problems, ability to read print, and the distance needed to read print. Examine visual acuity; inspect orbits, cornea, sclera, conjunctiva (palpebral and bulbar), pupils and pupil reaction to include the presence of lens opacities (cataracts), extraocular movements, anterior chamber; funduscopic examination. Palpate rims and globes. Examination should concentrate on pathology that would interfere with light projection to the retina.

▶ **Diagnostic Studies**

Check visual acuity with pinhole (decreased visual acuity secondary to refractive error improves); tonometry if elevated pressures suspected; fluorescein staining if corneal defect or abrasion suspected.

▶ **Diagnosis**

Based on findings, some considerations are: need for corrective lenses, presbyopia, corneal opacity, cataracts, failure of pupils to respond, unclear aqueous humor, unclear vitreous humor.

▶ **Clinical Therapeutics**

As indicated.

▶ **Clinical Intervention**

If corrective lenses needed, then refer to an ophthalmologist or optometrist; emergent conditions (e.g., glaucoma) refer to ophthalmologist; nonemergent conditions are treated as indicated.

▶ **Health Maintenance Issues**

Routine eye exam, eye protection, patient education about expected visual changes with age, patient education about complications of systemic diseases including hypertension and diabetes.

## II. CATARACTS

▶ **Scientific Concepts**

Cataracts are opacities or discoloration of the lens of the eye due to age, disease, injury. It is a common cause of vision loss, particularly in the elderly and usually occurring after age 50, but can be congenital, or can arise from trauma or medication use.

▶ **History & Physical**

Assess normal condition of eyes including use of corrective lenses, use of contacts; injury, onset (sudden or insidious), conditions that worsen vision including bright light or poor contrast, duration, pain, tearing, redness, pruritus, discharge (type, color, amount), presence of halos, loss of vision (partial or complete), systemic diseases (hypertension or diabetes) or other health problems, medications, prior history of ocular problems. Examine visual acuity; inspect orbits, cornea, sclera, conjunctiva (palpebral and bulbar), pupils and pupil reaction, extraocular movements, anterior chamber; funduscopic examination.

▶ **Diagnostic Studies**

Usually none unless complicating conditions are suspected.

▶ **Diagnosis**

By direct examination of lens.

▶ **Clinical Therapeutics**

Usually none unless complicating conditions are present.

► Clinical Intervention

Usually none unless complicating conditions are present. Refer to ophthalmologist for evaluation and possible extraction.

► Health Maintenance Issues

Patient education about changes with age or the result of injury to eye and some complications of disease or drug use. Cataracts are one of the most successfully treated problems of vision.

## III. DIABETIC RETINOPATHY

► Scientific Concepts

Changes in the retina due to diabetes mellitus are a leading cause of blindness. The longer a person is diabetic, the more likely he or she is to develop diabetic retinopathy; higher incidence in type 1 diabetics. Three stages of diabetic retinopathy:

1. *Nonproliferative diabetic retinopathy:* Characterized by microaneurysms, hemorrhages, hard exudates, retinal edema.
2. *Preproliferative diabetic retinopathy:* Characterized by retinal nerve infarcts, venous dilation, telangiectasias.
3. *Proliferative diabetic retinopathy:* Characterized by neovascularizations, preretinal and vitreous hemorrhages, fibrous proliferation, retinal detachment.

► History & Physical

Visual history, including changes (and progression of changes) in vision, redness, pain, pattern of visual loss, injury to eye, night vision, use of corrective lenses; history of diabetes, including onset, treatment, control, and presence of other complications such as peripheral neuropathy and kidney disease. Presence of other systemic disease such as hypertension; presence of other risk factors such as obesity, medications, and compliance to therapeutic regimens and degree of control. Sudden changes in vision should prompt indepth evaluation. Examine visual acuity; complete eye exam to include detailed and careful funduscopic examination.

► Diagnostic Studies

Funduscopy and angiography (performed by ophthalmologist).

► Diagnosis

Usually by direct funduscopy.

► Clinical Therapeutics

Referral to an ophthalmologist for evaluation and intervention and recommendations for continuing care.

► Clinical Intervention

Control of diabetes and contributing diseases and factors; referral to ophthalmologist for retinopathy evaluation and treatment.

► Health Maintenance Issues

Patient education on complications of diabetes and need for reduction of risk factors and control of glucose levels. Patients must understand that, even with good glycemic control, complications may occur. Annual funduscopic examination with dilation by an ophthalmologist is a standard of care.

## IV. HYPERTENSIVE RETINOPATHY

▶ Scientific Concepts

Hypertension causes changes in the arterioles of the retina by causing thickening of the walls that result in light reflex changes (copper or silver wiring). Pressure in the arterioles may affect venous pressures at points where veins and arteries cross, thereby compressing the vein, causing dilation in the vein that predisposes it to occlusion. Hypertension also causes changes in the arteriole walls that lead to exudates and hemorrhages, which ultimately will lead to damage affecting vision.

▶ History & Physical

History should center on visual signs and symptoms, how long patient has had hypertension, how well it is controlled, other contributing disease (diabetes, thyroid), and eye health, including corrective lenses. Examination may reveal no eye changes, or mild, moderate, or severe changes that include copper wiring, silver wiring, arteriovenous nicking, venous dilation, exudates, cotton-wool spots, flame hemorrhages.

▶ Diagnostic Studies

Refer to an ophthalmologist for evaluation and treatment.

▶ Diagnosis

Findings on funduscopy.

▶ Clinical Therapeutics

Control of blood pressure, periodic checks, complications usually managed by an ophthalmologist.

▶ Clinical Intervention

Refer to an ophthalmologist.

▶ Health Maintenance Issues

Patient education to emphasize the importance of controlling hypertension and other complicating disease; annual funduscopic examination.

## V. RETINAL DETACHMENT

▶ Scientific Concepts

Detachment or separation of the retina from the choroid; retinal detachment can occur as the result of trauma or as a consequence of systemic or ocular disease; occurs more often in men than women; can be caused by ocular trauma; often due to degenerative changes in the retina; myopia increases the risk.

▶ History & Physical

History should include description of symptoms, including onset, duration, trauma, previous condition of the eye, and previous eye problems;

acute vision loss usually indicates a large detachment; history may include a "shading" of vision, flashing lights, floaters, and usually in one eye. Examine visual acuity; complete eye exam including funduscopy.

▶ **Diagnostic Studies**
Usually none except by an ophthalmologist.

▶ **Diagnosis**
By funduscopy; may reveal elevated retina, retinal folds, grayish discoloration, loss of choroidal background; findings may not be obvious.

▶ **Clinical Therapeutics**
Refer to an ophthalmologist.

▶ **Clinical Intervention**
Refer to an ophthalmologist.

▶ **Health Maintenance Issues**
None.

## VI. GLAUCOMA

▶ **Scientific Concepts**
Aqueous humor is continually produced by the ciliary body of the eye; it flows through the pupil, fills the anterior chamber, and is drained through the trabecular network to Schlemm's canal. Any increase in the pressure of any compartment of the eye is spread hydraulically throughout the eye. Glaucoma is an increase in cup/disk ratio with visual field loss (usually nasally), frequently with increased intraocular pressure. Two types of glaucoma:
1. *Open-angle glaucoma:* More common (90–95% of cases), insidious, less symptomatic.
2. *Closed-angle glaucoma:* Less common, but acute onset and an ophthalmologic emergency. Usually multiple symptoms (see History & Physical below) not found in open-angle glaucoma. Leading cause of blindness in African Americans.

▶ **History & Physical**
*Open-angle glaucoma:* Usually asymptomatic, but questions should center on vision/eye history, vision problems or symptoms, family history for glaucoma, concurrent disease (particularly diabetes and hypertension). Examination may be normal except for elevated intraocular pressure, although pressure may be below the statistical average of 21 mm Hg; may have an increase in physiologic cup to optic disk ratio with displacement of vessels to cup rim (asymmetry to opposite side); may have visual field deficits, but they are often difficult to detect.

*Closed-angle glaucoma:* Same risk factors as for open-angle glaucoma; onset is usually acute, with pain, red eye, blurred vision, halos around lights, vision loss, nausea (sometimes accompanied by abdominal pain), headache; most commonly unilateral. Pupil dilation is contraindicated. Affected eye may be red, tearing, firm to palpation; fixed mid-dilated pupil (sometimes distorted to oval shape); hazy, cloudy, or steamy cornea; increased physiologic cup to optic disk ratio; shallow anterior chamber; decreased visual acuity; marked increased intraocular pressure.

▶ Diagnostic Studies

Tonometry, visual field exam, funduscopy, goniometry.

▶ Diagnosis

Elevated pressure on tonometry; physical findings consistent with glaucoma; must recognize signs and symptoms of closed-angle glaucoma because of the emergent nature of the problem.

▶ Clinical Therapeutics

Patients with acute closed-angle glaucoma must be referred immediately to an ophthalmologist. Emergency treatment prior to referral can include topical beta-blockers, topical pilocarpine, oral carbonic anhydrase inhibitors, osmotic agents (oral glycerine or intravenous mannitol). Patients with open-angle glaucoma should be referred to an ophthalmologist and treatment based on consultant recommendations.

▶ Clinical Intervention

Referral to an ophthalmologist, emergent basis for closed-angle glaucoma.

▶ Health Maintenance Issues

Periodic checks with tonometry, visual fields, and close monitoring of cup to disk ratio for individuals with a personal and family history of glaucoma and those patients with risk factors; should be part of routine annual examination after age 40. Always screen for glaucoma (history, check depth of anterior chamber, tonometry) before use of mydriatic agents in order to prevent precipitating glaucoma attack.

## VII. INFECTIONS

### A. Conjunctivitis

▶ Scientific Concepts

Common, rarely serious, inflammation of the conjunctiva with dilation of the superficial blood vessels due to allergy, viral infection, or bacterial infection; can be highly contagious, especially among young children.

▶ History & Physical

Onset over short period of time, usually without pain, photophobia, blurred vision, or halos. Discharge in bacterial conjunctivitis is copious, purulent (yellow or green), and may cause eyelashes to mat overnight. Discharge in viral conjunctivitis is moderate and clear. Itching is prominent in allergic conjunctivitis. Presence of foreign body sensations, recent upper respiratory infections, others with disease may help determine cause of conjunctivitis; contact with any toxic substance or known allergens. Note amount and color of discharge, involvement of lids (edema), degree of conjunctival erythema or injection, pupil reaction, visual acuity, and presence of preauricular nodes. Gram stain of discharge may aid in diagnosis. Examine anterior chambers and underside of lids. Presence of preauricular nodes. Examine ears, nose, throat, neck for signs of concurrent disease. (See Table 3–1.)

### ► Diagnostic Studies

Gram stain of discharge may give indication of type of infection: segmented neutrophils indicate bacterial infection; lymphocytes indicate viral infection; eosinophils indicate allergic reaction; consider gonococcal and chlamydial infections in sexually active individuals.

### ► Diagnosis

Usually based on history and physical examination; must rule out more serious causes of red eye such as glaucoma, iritis, keratitis, corneal lesions, foreign body.

### ► Clinical Therapeutics

***Bacterial conjunctivitis:*** Antibiotic drops (no steroids). Conjunctivitis in the neonate should be treated with topical erythromycin (primarily for chlamydial infection). Gentle washing away of exudates, warm compresses to lids, avoid direct sunlight (use sunglasses), follow-up evaluation in 2–3 days.

***Viral conjunctivitis:*** Artificial tears.

***Allergic conjunctivitis:*** Topical vasoconstrictor and/or antihistamine combination and cold compresses, oral antihistamine. Topical steroids reserved for severe cases (use with care and caution).

### ► Clinical Intervention

***Viral conjunctivitis:*** Artificial tears, cold compresses to lids, avoid groups (contagious for 2 weeks), wash hands frequently.

***Allergic conjunctivitis:*** Avoid any known allergens, cold compresses to lids, consider new allergy to ophthalmic medication. At least one follow-up examination should be done.

---

### ► table 3-1

**SIGNS OF RED EYE**

| Signs | Acute Conjunctivitis | Acute Iritis | Acute Glaucoma | Corneal Lesions |
|---|---|---|---|---|
| Conjunctival injection | +/+++ | ++ | ++ | ++ |
| Discharge | +/+++ | 0 | 0 | 0/+ |
| Preauricular lymph node | 0/+ | 0 | 0 | 0 |
| Corneal opacification | 0/+ | 0 | +++ | 0/+++ |
| Corneal epithelial disruption | 0/+ | 0 | 0 | +/+++ |
| Ciliary flush | 0 | ++ | + | +++ |
| Pupil | N | Mid-dilated irregular | Small/irregular | N/small |
| Anterior chamber depth | N | N | Shallow | N |
| Intraocular pressure | N | Low | High | N |

+, present; ++, moderate; +++, severe; N, normal; 0, absent.

*Source: Goldberg JS.* The Instant Exam Review for the USMLE Step 3, *2nd ed., Stamford, CT: Appleton & Lange, 1997, p. 239.*

► **Health Maintenance Issues**

Viral and bacterial conjunctivitis are very contagious, especially among young children. Control of known allergens may help in treatment of allergic conjunctivitis. Infected individuals and close contacts should wash hands frequently.

## B. Other Infections

► **Scientific Concepts**

Bacterial infections of the eye can be serious and have serious sequelae. Corneal infections or infections of corneal ulcerations, such as from contact lens wear, can cause corneal opacification. Hypopion (pus in the anterior chamber) is an ophthalmologic emergency. Orbital cellulitis is also considered an ophthalmologic emergency, especially in infants and young children. Infection of the lacrimal ducts (dacryocystitis) is usually unilateral, related to obstruction, and caused by beta-hemolytic *Streptococcus* or *Staphylococcus aureus* in infants and persons over 40 years of age. Less serious infections, such as conjunctivitis and sty, can be treated without referral unless there are complications.

► **History & Physical**

History should include onset, duration, prior vision or visual problems, use of corrective lenses or contacts, history of injury or foreign body sensation, presence of blurred vision or decreased vision, photophobia, halos, loss of vision, pain, fever, discharge or drainage, characteristics of discharge or drainage, treatment by self or health care provider. Examine visual acuity; inspect for redness, discharge, preauricular lymphadenopathy, condition of cornea, anterior chamber, pupil, lens, conjunctiva (bulbar and palpebral), sclera, lids; extraocular movements; funduscopy.

► **Diagnostic Studies**

Fluorescein staining if indicated, tonometry if indicated (usually not done in obvious eye surface infection).

► **Diagnosis**

Based on history and examination findings. Sty (hordeolum) is a small pustule at the lid margin. Chalazion usually is a small painless mass in the lid. Corneal infections penetrate the corneal layers, and frank pus is present. Hypopion is pus in the anterior chamber; periorbital cellulitis is marked edema, erythema, warmth, and pain of the lids and periorbital soft tissues. Orbital cellulitis involves the orbit and results in restricted ocular motility with pain on attempted eye movement, and a pupillary defect is commonly present. Lacrimal gland infection generally presents with tenderness, swelling, and redness of the upper-outer lid; lacrimal duct infections present as tenderness, swelling, erythema in the nasal corner of the eye; pus can sometimes be expressed from the puncta.

► **Clinical Therapeutics**

As indicated. Orbital cellulitis, corneal infections, hypopion must be referred to an ophthalmologist for management. Lacrimal duct and gland infections are managed depending on severity of disease, usually with systemic antibiotics. Sties are treated with frequent warm compresses and topical ophthalmic antibiotic drops. Chalazion are usually treated with warm compresses. They may resolve with time. Acute infection or inflammation are treated with ophthalmic antibiotic drops or ointment. Large chalazion that put pressure on the eye or cause distortion of vision should be referred to an ophthalmologist for excision.

▶ Clinical Intervention

Referral to an ophthalmologist is indicated for serious infections.

▶ Health Maintenance Issues

Protecting eyes from exposure to potential infective agents; careful handling of contacts; hand washing before applying contacts.

## C. Herpes Simplex

▶ Scientific Concepts

The herpesvirus includes two types: herpes simplex type 1 (HSV-1) and type 2 (HSV-2). HSV-1 is the infecting agent in a vast majority of ophthalmic infections, and the cornea is the structure predominantly affected. Herpes infections of the eye and its structures are rare. The mode of transmission is by direct contact. Herpes simplex and herpes zoster infections of the soft tissues (including the lids) surrounding the eye also occur. Herpes zoster infection of the trigeminal nerve ophthalmic division may involve the cornea. Varicella should also be considered as an etiologic agent.

▶ History & Physical

Initially, a foreign body sensation, followed by increased discomfort, tearing, photophobia, conjunctival injection, decreased visual acuity. May be history of prior infection or recent viral lesions (such as fever blisters). Concurrent sexually transmitted disease (STD) should lead to consideration of HSV-2 infection and other STDs. Examine visual acuity, eyelids, conjunctiva, cornea, anterior chamber, pupils, palpebral conjunctiva of upper and lower lids, regional lymph nodes; funduscopy. Vesicles on the tip of the nose (Hutchinson's sign) may offer a clue to diagnosis and should prompt an immediate referral to an ophthalmologist.

▶ Diagnostic Studies

Fluorescein staining.

▶ Diagnosis

Identification of a branching or dendritic pattern on cornea, occasionally will appear as small punctate lesions on the cornea.

▶ Clinical Therapeutics

Immediate referral to an ophthalmologist for treatment.

▶ Clinical Intervention

Immediate referral to an ophthalmologist for treatment.

▶ Health Maintenance Issues

Avoid transmission to the eye from obvious herpes ulcerations such as fever blisters; frequent hand washing when fever blisters or other herpetic lesions are present. Exposure to sun, ultraviolet light, stress, and trauma may precipitate recurrences.

# VIII. OTHER DISORDERS OF THE EYE

## A. Keratoconjunctivitis Sicca (Dry Eye)

▶ **Scientific Concepts**

Common symptom complex, particularly in elderly. May be due to decreased tear or mucin production, surface lesions, failure to blink. May be due to ocular disease or systemic disease.

▶ **History & Physical**

A complete ocular history must be taken as well as a general history to explore for dry eyes related to other disease. Visual acuity, ocular pressures, and complete eye examination must be done. Appropriate other system examination should be done as indicated.

▶ **Diagnostic Studies**

Fluorescein staining may identify surface lesions or defects in the conjunctiva or cornea.

▶ **Diagnosis**

Based on history, physical, and lab finding.

▶ **Clinical Therapeutics**

Treatment of co-conditions. Artificial tears.

▶ **Clinical Intervention**

Referral to ophthalmologist as indicated. Close follow-up.

▶ **Health Maintenance Issues**

Patient education, protection of eyes from sun, wind, and drying or irritating conditions. Surface of eye must be kept moist.

## B. Disorders of Optic Nerve/Visual Pathways

▶ **Scientific Concepts**

Loss of vision may be in one eye or both; may be central, temporal, or nasal depending on location of lesion. Vision loss in one eye indicates a lesion of the optic nerve; bitemporal vision loss indicates a lesion of the optic chiasm; homonymous hemianopsia indicates a postchiasmal lesion.

▶ **History & Physical**

Very careful delineation of loss or reduced visual acuity, whether one or both eyes, type of defect (central, lateral, medial); pain, halos, injury, systemic disease, other neurologic signs or symptoms. Examine visual acuity; careful examination of the eyes, including visual fields and Amsler grid to map visual defect, ophthalmoscopy, complete neurological examination.

▶ **Diagnostic Studies**

Computed tomography (CT), magnetic resonance imaging (MRI) for identification of intracranial lesions.

▶ **Diagnosis**

Based on findings of history, examination, results of special studies.

▶ **Clinical Therapeutics**

Refer to an ophthalmologist, neurologist, or neurosurgeon.

► **Clinical Intervention**
Referral as above.

► **Health Maintenance Issues**
None.

## C. Strabismus

► **Scientific Concepts**
Misalignment of the eyes due to weakness of extraocular muscles; misalignment of the extraocular muscles or impaired innervation of the extraocular muscles; most commonly congenital, but can occur due to trauma, stroke, systemic disease.

► **History & Physical**
Age of onset or when first noted, family history of similar problems, injury, other neurological disorders, visual problems or complaints. Examine visual acuity; thorough eye examination with particular attention to extraocular muscles, other cranial nerve weakness, light reflex, accommodation, cover–uncover test.

► **Diagnostic Studies**
Careful eye examination with ophthalmoscopy; note corneal light reflex; cover–uncover test.

► **Diagnosis**
Based on examination findings; consider concurrent conditions in older children and adults.

► **Clinical Therapeutics**
None.

► **Clinical Intervention**
Refer to ophthalmologist for evaluation and consideration of corrective surgery or other interventions.

► **Health Maintenance Issues**
Eye examination for strabismus should be a part of every routine exam of newborns through infancy and childhood. Early detection may prevent more serious later eye problems.

## D. Disorders of the Lids

### 1. Blepharitis

► **Scientific Concepts**
An inflammatory reaction of the eyelid margins that occurs as a result of infective or noninfective reactions. Infection is commonly due to *Staphylococcus*. Noninfective is commonly a seborrheic reaction due to accelerated skin shedding and sebaceous gland dysfunction. Both can occur concurrently. Both can be chronic.

► **History & Physical**
History may indicate a chronic condition with remissions and exacerbations. The lid margins are usually red, with associated conjunctivitis and mild burning and discomfort. The eye surface may seem to be dry. There may be purulent drainage in bacterial infections. There may be a history

of exacerbations with use of eye makeup, exposure to chemicals or the elements, or excessive rubbing. A visual history should be taken. Examination should include visual acuity, which is usually unaffected by the problem. The seborrheic form of the disease is characterized by redness of the lid margins, mild edema, scaling of skin. Persistent signs despite treatment with thickening of the eye margin may indicate skin or sebaceous cyst carcinoma, which needs to be investigated carefully. The infective form of the disease will present in a manner similar to the seborrheic form with purulent material along the lids, crusting, and loss of lashes. Entropion, ectropion, and chronic conjunctivitis may also be present.

▶ Diagnostic Studies
Cultures in atypical cases, biopsy in atypical persistent cases.

▶ Diagnosis
Based on history and physical findings.

▶ Clinical Therapeutics
Eyelid margin scrubs with eyelid cleanser, warm compresses; avoid exposure to eye irritants (including makeup); discontinue contact lens until resolution; topical antibiotic eyedrops for infective form.

▶ Clinical Intervention
Referral to ophthalmologist for persistent cases.

▶ Health Maintenance Issues
Education on good eye hygiene using lid scrubs and warm compresses.

2. Ectropion/Entropion

*Ectropion:* Eversion or outward displacement of the margin of the lid.

*Entropion:* Inversion or inward displacement of the margin of the lid.

▶ Scientific Concepts
Inversion or eversion of the lids can have a number of etiologies and may occur as a consequence of aging. The primary problem to the eye is irritation of the eye surface by lashes or drying of the eye surface if lids do not completely close. The lower eyelid is most commonly affected in both conditions.

▶ History & Physical
History should center on eye complaints as well as potential causes from neurologic and systemic diseases. Examination should concentrate on eye and local conditions (inflammation, infection, injury) and systemic and neurologic etiologies (Bell's palsy).

▶ Diagnostic Studies
Usually none for entropion and ectropion alone.

▶ Diagnosis
Based on history and physical examination.

▶ Clinical Therapeutics
Treatment of injury, infection, inflammation, or other underlying cause; use of artificial tears, taping eye closed.

▶ Clinical Intervention
Surgical intervention is often needed.

▶ **Health Maintenance Issues**
Protect eyes from irritants; keep eye surface moist.

## 3. Chalazion

▶ **Scientific Concepts**
Chalazion occurs when there is blockage or low-grade inflammation of a meibomian gland of the lid, usually resulting in a painless swelling in the lid. May occasionally become acutely infected or inflamed.

▶ **History & Physical**
History is a painless, slowly growing mass in the eyelid without other symptoms. Physical examination reveals a small, nontender, firm mass in the lid.

▶ **Diagnostic Studies**
Not indicated.

▶ **Diagnosis**
Based on history and physical examination.

▶ **Clinical Therapeutics**
Antibiotics or other medications are not indicated unless there is acute infection and inflammation (rare).

▶ **Clinical Intervention**
Usually resolves without treatment. Warm compresses and eyelid margin washing may help. Large chalazion may put pressure on the globe and distort vision, which requires referral to an ophthalmologist.

▶ **Health Maintenance Issues**
Good eyelid hygiene.

## 4. Sty (Hordeolum)

▶ **Scientific Concepts**
Infection/inflammation of a lash or gland of the eyelid margin results in redness, scaling, and irritation. Sties tend to occur in crops. *Staphylococcus* is the most common causative organism, but others do occur. Contact lenses, makeup, and lid margin irritation may predispose to sty formation.

▶ **History & Physical**
History is usually that of redness and scaling of the lid. Pain is related to size of the lesion and eye irritation. Examination shows lid margin pustule(s) with localized inflammation and edema, drainage or tearing, and some eye irritation.

▶ **Diagnostic Studies**
Usually none indicated.

▶ **Diagnosis**
Based on history and physical examination findings.

▶ **Clinical Therapeutics**
Wide range of ophthalmic topical solutions: erythromycin, gentamicin, sulfacetamide.

► Clinical Intervention

Frequent hand washing, warm compresses to the eye, daily lid washing. Do not burst pustule; incision and drainage rarely needed.

► Health Maintenance Issues

Good eyelid hygiene by washing lids daily.

## IX. WOUNDS/INJURIES OF THE EYE

### A. Cranial or Ocular Injuries

► Scientific Concepts

Injury to the head or eye can affect vision and the eye. Intracranial injury may have ocular manifestations.

► History & Physical

Time, mechanism, result of injury; changes in signs and symptoms since injury; prior eye history, concomitant injury and symptoms. Initial history may be very directed due to emergent or other overriding conditions (shock, arrest, etc.). Examination may be emergent evaluation, but should include assessment of visual acuity, pupil shape and reaction, and fundi as well as direct indicators of injury (hyphema, laceration, etc.).

► Diagnostic Studies

As pertains to the eye; x-ray, CT, MRI as indicated.

► Diagnosis

Based on physical and diagnostic findings.

► Clinical Therapeutics

As indicated by diagnosis.

► Clinical Intervention

Refer to ophthalmologist. In the severely injured patient, the first goal is to save the patient's life and to limit morbidity; eye considerations may need to be secondary to that goal.

► Health Maintenance Issues

Protection of eyes during contact sports and in work settings with potential for injury.

### B. Chemical Burns to the Eye

► Scientific Concepts

Acids and bases that come into contact with the surface of the eye cause chemical burns that can destroy the eye or have lasting vision complications. Eye burns are true ophthalmologic emergencies and require immediate intervention and referral to an ophthalmologist. Base injuries are considered more dangerous because of the continued effect of the base on contacted structures despite irrigation.

► History & Physical

Usually very quick history and limited physical examination of the eye is done as treatment is initiated. Identify offending substance, time since exposure, and emergency treatment.

► **Diagnostic Studies**
Initially none.

► **Diagnosis**
By history.

► **Clinical Therapeutics**
Copious irrigation (at least one liter) with normal saline.

► **Clinical Intervention**
Emergency referral to an ophthalmologist.

► **Health Maintenance Issues**
Eye protection for all work and recreational activities that involve toxic substances.

## C. Foreign Body in the Eye

► **Scientific Concepts**
Any number of foreign bodies can lodge on the surface of the eye. The most uncomfortable are those that lodge or abrade the cornea. Some foreign bodies will lodge under the lids. Foreign body sensation may be present with surface ulcerations or injury. Foreign body sensation may persist after removal of a foreign body.

► **History & Physical**
Activity at time of foreign body, particularly if working around wood or metal, such as hammering; onset, duration, associated symptoms, effect on vision; vision history or previous eye or vision problems. Examine visual acuity if possible, cornea, anterior chamber, conjunctiva, sclera, and lids. Retract lower lid down and completely expose; upper lids must be everted and examined for foreign body; carefully examine for penetrating wound, blood in the anterior chamber; examine for fixed or distorted pupils.

► **Diagnostic Studies**
Fluorescein staining may help identify a foreign body and will demonstrate abrasions from foreign bodies; slit lamp examination will help identify foreign bodies or damage to the eye surface that are difficult to see.

► **Diagnosis**
Identify the foreign body, but always consider the multiple causes of a red eye.

► **Clinical Therapeutics**
Prompt, gentle irrigation is usually required (do not use Morgan lens). Antibiotic eyedrops are usually not indicated for acute foreign bodies, although one-time application after foreign body removal is acceptable. Anesthetic and steroid eyedrops should never be used after foreign body removal. One-time use of a cycloplegic drop may be used to relieve the discomfort following the removal of a foreign body.

► **Clinical Intervention**
Removal of surface foreign body after topical ocular anesthesia with a cotton-tipped applicator or gentle irrigation; skilled providers may use a

small-gauge needle or corneal spoon for removal. Deeply embedded and penetrating foreign bodies must be referred to an ophthalmologist. After foreign body removal, eyes may be patched for 24 hours. Patches can worsen some conditions such as foreign body, herpetic infections, and corneal ulcers, so take care to rule out these conditions or avoid the patch if any doubt. Follow-up should be in 24 to 48 hours and the eye observed for complications such as infection or formation of a rust ring.

▶ Health Maintenance Issues

Eye protection during high-risk activities, particularly hammering, sawing, and where foreign bodies may be created by the activity. Shatter-proof lenses should be a must for all corrective eyeglasses. Noncorrective safety glasses should be worn by those who do not need correction or those who wear contacts.

## D. Blunt and Penetrating Trauma

▶ Scientific Concepts

Blunt trauma is defined as trauma to the eye that does not disrupt the continuity of the eye structure. Penetrating trauma is defined as trauma that disrupts the continuity of the eye structure. Injury to the eye can result in short- or long-term problems. Blunt trauma can be as severe as penetrating trauma and must be evaluated as carefully. Initial evaluation and treatment may be key to preserving visual function, as well as cosmetic effect. Generally, evidence of internal eye trauma, disruption of the eye surface, and interference with vision are indications for referral to an ophthalmologist.

▶ History & Physical

Vision prior to injury, type of injury, mechanism of injury, first aid given, time since injury, changes since injury, concurrent injuries, and problem. Careful examination of the eye and surrounding structures, visual acuity if feasible and possible. Examine orbits, lids, conjunctiva, sclera, cornea, anterior chamber, pupils, pupillary response, extraocular movements, and do funduscopic examination. Examination should concentrate on injury and abnormal structures, disruption of eye integrity, blood in anterior or posterior chamber, retinal injury, presence of foreign bodies, and penetrating injury. Slit lamp examination.

▶ Diagnostic Studies
As indicated: skull x-rays, CT, MRI.

▶ Diagnosis
Based on findings.

▶ Clinical Therapeutics
Usually none since injuries should be referred to an ophthalmologist.

▶ Clinical Intervention

Refer to an ophthalmologist for penetrating injuries, injuries to any area of the globe and its structures, blood in the anterior or posterior chambers. Injuries to bony and soft tissues surrounding the eye should be handled in a manner that will not harm the eye.

▶ Health Maintenance Issues

Eye protection during all work and recreational activities that have even a remote possibility of causing eye injury, seat belt use while driving, etc.

## BIBLIOGRAPHY

Dambro MR, ed. *Griffith's 5-Minute Clinical Consult, 2002* Philadelphia: Lippincott, Williams & Wilkins; 2002.

Dornic D. *Ophthalmic Pocket Companion,* 6th ed. Oxford: Butterworth Heinemann; 2001.

Ferris JD. *Essential Medical Ophthalmology.* Oxford: Butterworth Heinemann; 2001.

Riordan-Eva P. Eye. In: Tierney LM, McPhee SJ, Papadakis, MA. *Current Medical Diagnosis & Treatment,* 41st ed. New York: Lange Medical Books/McGraw-Hill; 2002.

Vander JF, Gauilt JA. *Ophthalmology Secrets,* 2nd ed. Philadelphia: Hanley & Belfus; 2002.

# Pulmonary Diseases | 4

*Jill Reichman, MPH, PA-C, and Matthew McQuillan, MS, PA-C*

# I. ACUTE BRONCHITIS

*[handwritten margin note: Most common cause of bronchitis is viral. (Rhinovirus, adenovirus, influenza, parainfluenza, RSV.) m/c bacterial: Strep. pneumonia, H flu, Moraxelle Catarrholis, myroplasma pneumonie.]*

► Scientific Concepts

Acute bronchitis is characterized by inflammation of the trachea and bronchi. The most common cause is viral including rhinovirus, adenovirus, influenza, parainfluenza, and respiratory syncytial virus. The most common bacterial species to cause bronchitis include *Streptococcus pneumoniae, Haemophilus influenzae, Moraxella catarrhalis,* and *Mycoplasma pneumoniae.* Exposure to chemical and physical agents can also predispose the patient to bronchitis.

► History & Physical

The clinical presentation is similar to that of pneumonia. There may be a preceding upper respiratory tract infection (URI) with fever. Cough is characteristic of acute bronchitis, and it may be nonproductive, productive, or mucopurulent. There may be pleuritic chest pain. Associated symptoms include fever, fatigue, chest discomfort worsened by cough, and/or postnasal drip. Chest examination may be normal or demonstrate rhonchi that may clear with cough and/or occasional wheezing.

► Diagnostic Studies

Diagnostic tests are generally not indicated. However, if pneumonia is suspected, a posteroanterior (PA) and lateral chest x-ray would be appropriate.

► Diagnosis

The diagnosis is clinical. The differential diagnosis includes pneumonia and influenza.

► Clinical Therapeutics

Treatment is symptomatic; fluids, rest, and antitussive agents. Inhaled bronchodilators may be used as necessary. Antibiotics are indicated only in patients with chronic obstructive pulmonary disease (COPD), immunocompromised patients, and patients who do not respond to conservative treatment or whose condition deteriorates.

► Clinical Intervention

See Clinical Therapeutics.

► Health Maintenance Issues

Patients should be encouraged to avoid tobacco and other environmental irritants.

# II. INFLUENZA *[handwritten: Often w/ leukopenia]*

*[handwritten margin note: Influenza - virus types A, B + C of myxovirus group.]*

► Scientific Concepts

Influenza is an acute febrile respiratory illness that is usually seen in outbreaks during the winter months. Influenza is caused by influenza virus types A, B, and C of the myxovirus group. Transmission is primarily via virus-containing aerosols.

► History & Physical

Influenza is a highly contagious illness that can produce a wide range of clinical syndromes, including common cold symptoms, pharyngitis, tracheobronchitis, and pneumonia. Characteristic symptoms of influenza include cough and sore throat, but systemic symptoms such as fever, chills, myalgias, malaise, and headache predominate the presentation. Physical findings are nonspecific and may include injection of the conjunctiva, facial flushing, and pharyngeal injection. The patient appears ill.

▶ **Diagnostic Studies**

*leukopenic common*

Generally not indicated. If labs are ordered, leukopenia is common.

▶ **Diagnosis**

Diagnosis is clinical and epidemiologic. It may be difficult to distinguish influenza from other viral illnesses. During an outbreak period, a patient seen with typical symptoms is highly likely to have influenza. Specific diagnosis requires isolation of virus from pharynx or sputum but is not usually necessary. Differential diagnosis includes URI, pharyngitis, bronchitis, and pneumonia caused by other viruses or bacteria. Chest x-ray may be necessary in some cases to rule out pneumonia.

▶ **Clinical Therapeutics**

Treatment of influenza is largely symptomatic; fluids, rest, and acetaminophen. Aspirin should be avoided in children due to the association with Reye's syndrome. Amantadine and rimontadine (in adults) may be used for treatment of influenza A infection if begun within 48 hours of the onset of symptoms. There are also effective treatments for prophylaxis of influenza A infections. Zanamivir and oseltamivir are effective for the treatment of types A and B. Oseltamivir may be used for prophylaxis.

*Treatment
Amantadine -
rimontadine } adults

prophylaxis
Zanamivir / oseltamivir ✓*

▶ **Clinical Intervention**

Patients with influenza pneumonia may need to be hospitalized. Patients should stop smoking.

▶ **Health Maintenance Issues**

The prevention of influenza is an important task for primary care providers. Patients over age 65, health care or other workers in contact with the public, immunocompromised adults and children, and patients with chronic illnesses should receive yearly influenza vaccinations. Hand washing and avoidance of exposure may also help.

## III. PNEUMONIA

▶ **Scientific Concepts**

Community-acquired pneumonia in adults is a common disorder (2 to 3 million cases/year in the United States). It is most commonly caused by *S. pneumoniae*. In adults under 60 years, other causes are *Mycoplasma*, *Chlamydia*, and *Legionella*. In older patients and/or those with comorbidities, other causes are *H. influenza*, *M. catarrhalis* and other gram-negative organisms. Microbes may enter the lung by inhalation, aspiration, or hematogenous spread from an area of infection.

Hospital-acquired pneumonia is another important cause of pneumonia and is the leading cause of death due to nosocomial infections. It is defined as pneumonia that occurs more than 48 hours after admission

*Community
acquired
pneumonia
M/C = S. pneumonie
also
(<60yo) mycoplasme
Chlamydia / legionella
older h. flu
m. catarrhalis
other gram ⊖*

to the hospital. The most common causes of this type of pneumonia are *Pseudomonas aeruginosa*, *Klebsiella pneumoniae*, *Staphylococcus aureus*, and other gram-negative bacilli.

### ▶ History & Physical

Pneumonia may follow viral respiratory infections. Symptoms include fever, chills, malaise, tachycardia, tachypnea, pleuritic chest pain, cough, and sputum production. The patient may also complain of decreased appetite, weakness, and myalgia. Physical examination in bacterial pneumonia may show evidence of consolidation, dullness to percussion, increased vocal fremitus, and crackles or rales and decreased breath sounds. In early pneumonia, chest examination may be normal.

### ▶ Diagnosis

A sputum Gram stain can be attempted in patients with suspected community-acquired pneumonia. Leukocytosis with left shift is usually seen in bacterial pneumonia. Chest x-ray may show segmental, lobar, or diffuse infiltrate with air bronchograms. Blood cultures should be obtained in patients who require hospitalization and are positive in 20 to 30% of community-acquired pneumonia.

In patients with suspected hospital-acquired pneumonia, the workup should include blood cultures from two different sites and arterial blood gas or pulse oximetry. Chest x-ray is particularly important in evaluating the severity of the infection, complications, and response to treatment. In some cases, endotracheal aspiration and bronchoscopy may be necessary to obtain lower respiratory secretions for evaluation.

### ▶ Differential Diagnosis

**Viral pneumonia** is very common and is seen in children and adults. It is more prevalent during outbreaks of viral illness such as influenza. Other viruses that may cause pneumonia include respiratory syncytial virus (RSV), adenovirus, varicella, measles, and cytomegalovirus. Chest x-ray findings are variable but may show diffuse parenchymal pattern as opposed to lobar consolidation seen with bacterial pneumonia. In most cases, supportive therapy is helpful. Some viral pneumonias may be treated with antiviral agents.

*Streptococcus pneumoniae* is the most common cause of community-acquired pneumonia. Increased susceptibility is seen in persons with chronic cardiopulmonary disease. Symptoms include abrupt onset of fever, chills, productive cough, and dyspnea. Patients may appear acutely ill, and physical examination of the chest typically reveals dullness to percussion, increased vocal and tactile fremitus, and crackles or rales over the infected area. Gram stain of sputum will show gram-positive diplococci. White blood count typically shows leukocytosis with shift to the left. Chest x-ray shows a segmental lobe infiltrate. If penicillin resistance is not a concern, the treatment of choice is penicillin G. If penicillin resistance is a concern, ceftriaxone or cefotaxime, perhaps in combination with a macrolide, or fluoroquinolone may be used until susceptibility is determined.

*Staphylococcus aureus* presents similarly to pneumococcal pneumonia. A hematogenous source of infection such as an intravenous (IV) line, septic thrombophlebitis, or endocarditis may be present. It is seen in chronic care facilities and is a common cause of nosocomial pneumonia. Gram stain of sputum shows clusters of plump gram-positive cocci. Chest x-ray shows multiple nodular infiltrates, which may be associated with abscess formation. Blood cultures are usually positive. Treatment for methicillin-susceptible strains is a penicillinase-resistant antibiotic with or without rifampin or gentamicin.

**Gram-negative bacilli** usually cause pneumonia in chronically ill and/or immunocompromised individuals and is often due to aspiration of contaminated secretions. Gram-negative bacilli are a major source of hospital-acquired pneumonias. Causative organisms include *H. influenzae*, *K. pneumoniae*, *Escherichia coli*, and *P. aeruginosa*. Initial treatment in patients with severe illness usually requires a combination of an aminoglycoside or ciprofloxacin plus another drug such as ceftazidime.

*Mycoplasma pneumoniae* causes about 10–20% of all pneumonias and about 50% of pneumonias in children and young adults. Patients usually present with insidious onset of fever, myalgia, headache, malaise, and upper respiratory symptoms including sore throat and nonproductive cough. Chest x-ray findings are variable, but most patients have unilateral lower lobe segmental abnormalities that appear more severe than the clinical findings. Erythromycin and tetracycline are the standard therapy. Doxycycline and newer macrolides may also be used.

*Legionella* **pneumonia** most often presents with nonproductive cough, fever, chills, headache, malaise, and gastrointestinal symptoms such as diarrhea, nausea, vomiting, and abdominal pain. Gram stain of sputum shows polymorphonuclear leukocytes and no bacteria. Chest x-ray shows patchy or lobar infiltrate. Diagnosis can be confirmed by sputum culture or direct immunofluorescent microscopy of sputum. Erythromycin is the treatment of choice. When using oral drug therapy, newer macrolides such as clarithromycin or azithromycin or quinolones such as levofloxacin may be most effective.

**Chlamydial pneumonia** often presents with constitutional symptoms including fever, headache, and myalgias lasting up to 2 weeks. The pneumonia is usually mild. Nonproductive cough with hoarseness is common. It may be seen in closed populations such as residential institutions, among military personnel, or university students. Chest x-ray usually shows a single subsegmental infiltrate. Treatment includes tetracycline or erythromycin.

### ▶ Clinical Therapeutics

Patients with viral and mycoplasma pneumonia can usually be treated as outpatients. Healthy, young patients with bacterial pneumonia may also be treated at home provided they are watched by family or friends and have access to a health care provider or hospital. Chronically ill or immunocompromised patients, infants, or the elderly should be hospitalized for close monitoring, IV antibiotics, supplemental oxygen, hydration, aerosol treatments, and chest physical therapy.

### ▶ Health Maintenance Issues

Prophylaxis with pneumococcal and influenza vaccines is indicated for patients over 65 years of age, residents of chronic care facilities, those with chronic diseases, health care workers, and people who work with the public.

## IV. PULMONARY TUBERCULOSIS

### ► Scientific Concepts

Tuberculosis is an infectious disease caused by *Mycobacterium tuberculosis*. It is transmitted by aerosolized droplets from persons with pulmonary tuberculosis. Inhaled bacteria proliferate within alveolar macrophages and disseminate via lymphatics and the bloodstream. This stage is defined as primary tuberculosis, and most people infected are asymptomatic. The infection is usually contained but reactivation may occur months to years later. Approximately 5% will develop progressive primary tuberculosis, which causes constitutional and pulmonary symptoms. The vast majority of symptomatic patients are experiencing the reactivation of a latent infection. The majority of new cases of tuberculosis occur in foreign-born ethnic and racial minorities and new immigrants.

Tuberculosis is a major concern in acquired immune deficiency syndrome (AIDS) patients. Patients susceptible to the development of symptomatic tuberculosis include infants, children, adolescents, and the elderly. About 10% of those infected go on to develop active disease.

### ► History & Physical

Symptomatic pulmonary tuberculosis is characterized by mild malaise and fatigue, night sweats, low-grade fever, weight loss, cough, and hemoptysis. On physical exam, signs may be limited; as the disease progresses, abnormal lung findings including rales and rhonchi become more prevalent.

### ► Diagnosis

A tuberculin skin test (Mantoux) can identify individuals who have been infected with *M. tuberculosis*. The interpretation of the Mantoux test depends on the size of the area of induration and the patient's risk factors. A tuberculin reaction of 5 mm or more of induration is considered positive for persons who have had recent contact with a person with infectious tuberculosis; persons with chest x-rays with fibrotic lesions that may represent old, healed tuberculosis; persons with organ transplants and other immunocompromised patients; and persons with human immunodeficiency virus (HIV) infections. A tuberculin reaction of 10 mm or more is considered positive in persons who have a medical condition that is likely to increase the risk of tuberculosis once infected (silicosis, diabetes mellitus, chronic renal failure, etc.), recent immigrants from high-prevalence countries (Asia, Africa, and Latin America), residents of and employees in high-risk settings (correctional institutions, nursing homes, hospitals, etc.), HIV-negative IV drug abusers, and children under 4 years or any child or adolescent exposed to adults at high risk. A tuberculin reaction of 15 mm or greater is considered positive in persons with no risk factors for tuberculosis.

### ► Diagnostic Studies

The chest x-ray in primary infection shows small homogenous infiltrates. In reactivation tuberculosis, findings vary and include pulmonic infiltrates in the posterior segments of the upper lobes. The Gram stain of morning sputum or gastric aspiration is positive for acid-fast bacteria. The sputum or gastric aspiration culture is positive for *M. tuberculosis*.

▶ Clinical Therapeutics

Combinations of isoniazid, pyrazinamide, rifampin, ethambutol, and streptomycin are used to treat tuberculosis and to avoid the development of resistant strains. HIV-negative patients with previously untreated pulmonary tuberculosis can be treated with either a 6-month or 9-month regimen. The treatment of patients who are HIV positive requires the expertise of specialists. The Center for Disease Control (CDC) has published detailed guidelines that can be reviewed on the CDC website at http://www.cdc.gov/epo/mmwr/preview/mmwrhtml/00055357.htm.

Isoniazid Preventive Therapy (IPT) is indicated for the following patients who test positive: persons with HIV infection, close contacts of infected persons, recent skin test converters, persons with abnormal chest x-rays, IV drug users, persons with medical conditions that increase the risk of tuberculosis. Individuals with a positive skin test who are less than 35 years of age without clinical signs of tuberculosis should be treated with isoniazid if they are from countries with high prevalence rate, from a minority group with high risk, have low incomes, or are residents of long-term care facilities. Hepatitis is the major complication of isoniazid therapy. Regular monitoring of liver function tests is indicated for all patients on IPT or multidrug therapy. In addition, patient education regarding the early signs and symptoms of liver injury is an important part of patient management.

Multidrug-resistant tuberculosis (MDRTB) requires the attention of a clinician with expertise in this area. Treatment regimens for MDRTB are based on susceptibility testing.

▶ Clinical Intervention

The treatment of tuberculosis requires careful patient follow-up. In some cases it may be appropriate to recommend direct observation of medication ingestion in order to promote compliance. Clinicians are expected to contact their local public health office to report all cases of tuberculosis.

▶ Health Maintenance Issues

See above regarding Mantoux test and IPT.

# V. CHRONIC OBSTRUCTIVE PULMONARY DISEASE (COPD)

▶ Scientific Concepts

COPD is a chronic progressive pulmonary disease that leads to a reduction of the maximal expiratory flow rate. Chronic bronchitis and emphysema are the underlying pathologic conditions that cause COPD. Cigarette smoking is a major factor in the development of COPD. Alpha–1–antitrypsin deficiency is another cause of emphysema but is rare. Chronic bronchitis is characterized by bronchial inflammation, hyperplasia and hypertrophy of mucus glands and goblet cells, and fibrosis of lung tissue. In emphysema, the pathologic process leads to enlargement of the terminal air spaces due to alveolar destruction.

THIN
EMPHYSEMA pink puffer

Chronic bronchitis
3/12 months x 2 years

Ipratropium
decreases vagally
induced
bronchospasm

### ▶ History & Physical

The onset of COPD is often insidious. Patients present in the fifth or sixth decade of life with dyspnea on exertion, cough, and sputum production. Early in the disease process, clinical findings may be absent. As the disease progresses, physical examination may reveal the classic emphysema patient–the "pink puffer" who is thin and uses accessory muscles of respiration and has a quiet chest. Alternatively, the "blue bloater" with chronic bronchitis presents with cyanosis, peripheral edema, and a noisy chest with rales, rhonchi, and wheezes. Clinically, chronic bronchitis is defined by a productive cough for 3 of 12 months per year for 2 years.

### ▶ Diagnosis

Chest x-ray shows often shows hyperinflation of the lung fields with an increased retrosternal air space, flattening of the diaphragm, and a narrow cardiac silhouette. Parenchymal or subpleural bullae may be seen. Pulmonary function tests show a decreased forced expiratory volume in 1 second ($FEV_1$), and increased residual volume (RV), functional residual capacity (FRC), and total lung capacity (TLC). Arterial blood gases (ABGs) show hypoxia (decreased partial pressure of oxygen [$PO_2$]) and, in severe cases, hypercapnia (elevated partial pressure of carbon dioxide [$PCO_2$]). The hemoglobin may be normal or elevated.

### ▶ Clinical Therapeutics

***B2–Agonists metered-dose inhaler (MDI) (albuterol):*** Relax bronchial smooth muscle.

***Theophylline:*** Relax bronchial smooth muscle less than sympathomimetics, but have a beneficial effect on cardiac and respiratory muscles.

***Ipratropium bromide MDI:*** Decrease vagally induced bronchospasm.

***Corticosteroids:*** Reduce airway inflammation.

***Antibiotics*** *(e.g., azithromycin, trimethoprim-sulfamethoxazole [TMP-SMZ], doxycycline):* Treat infection.

Drugs are used alone or in combination dependent upon the severity of the patient's symptoms. IV theophylline and methylprednisolone may be necessary for severe exacerbations.

### ▶ Clinical Intervention

Includes the judicious use of oxygen, hydration, and pulmonary rehabilitation.

### ▶ Health Maintenance Issues

Issues to discuss with the patient are smoking cessation, clean air in the home and work environment, and administration of influenza and pneumococcal vaccines. Cough suppressants and sedatives should not be used routinely.

## VI. PNEUMOCONIOSES

Pneumoconioses are chronic fibrotic lung diseases caused by the inhalation of various inert dusts.

## A. Silicosis

► **Scientific Concepts**

Silicosis is caused by the inhalation of silica dust. The resultant fibrosis causes a decrease in lung volume, decrease in compliance, and decrease in diffusion capacity of the lungs.

► **History & Physical**

Patient's work history reveals exposure to silica (e.g., mining, quarry work, sandblasting). Simple silicosis is often asymptomatic. In complicated silicosis, patients present with dyspnea on exertion and nonproductive cough. Chest examination demonstrates tachypnea and fine crackles.

► **Diagnosis**

Chest x-ray shows eggshell calcifications of hilar and mediastinal nodes. Bilateral nodular densities progress from the periphery to the hilum. Pulmonary function tests show decrease in vital capacity, functional residual capacity, residual volume, and total lung capacity. Diagnosis can be confirmed by open lung biopsy, which will show fibrosis.

► **Clinical Therapeutics**

Treatment is supportive and may include oxygen therapy and rehabilitation.

► **Clinical Intervention**

Associated respiratory distress may be treated with bronchodilators (albuterol), chest physical therapy, and oxygen. Antibiotics (amoxicillin, TMP-SMZ, tetracycline) are indicated for superimposed infections. The incidence of tuberculosis is increased in this population. All patients should be tested for tuberculosis.

► **Health Maintenance Issues**

Avoiding inhalation of silica dust by wearing a respirator in mining, quarrying, and sandblasting.

## B. Asbestosis

► **Scientific Concepts**

Asbestosis is seen 15 to 20 years after lengthy exposure to asbestos. Pulmonary consequences are similar to those found in silicosis, with interstitial fibrosis and pleural thickening. Increased risk of malignant mesothelioma of the pleura, bronchogenic carcinoma, and tuberculosis are associated with asbestos exposure.

► **History & Physical**

Patient's work history reveals exposure to asbestos (e.g., renovation or destruction of old buildings, ship building). Patients present with dyspnea on exertion and nonproductive cough. Physical examination may reveal rales and pleural effusion. There may be clubbing of the fingers.

► **Diagnosis**

The diagnosis is most often based on a combination of a history of significant exposure to asbestos and radiographic and clinical findings that are consistent with asbestosis. Chest x-ray may show interstitial fibrosis, pleural plaques, and pleural effusions. Pulmonary function tests show decrease in vital capacity, functional residual capacity, residual volume, and total lung capacity. A computed tomographic (CT) scan may be necessary to demonstrate parenchymal fibrosis and pleural plaques. Open lung biopsy will confirm the diagnosis.

▶ Clinical Therapeutics

Treat symptomatically with oxygen. Lung transplant may be considered.

▶ Clinical Intervention

Associated respiratory distress may be treated with bronchodilators (albuterol), chest physical therapy, and oxygen. Antibiotics (amoxicillin, TMP-SMZ, tetracyclines) are indicated for infections.

▶ Health Maintenance Issues

Avoiding inhalation of asbestos dust by wearing a respirator in shipyard work, mining asbestos, boilermaking, and building restoration.

## C. Coal Workers' Pneumoconiosis

▶ Scientific Concepts

Coal workers' pneumoconiosis is caused by the inhalation of coal mine dust. It causes chronic fibrosis of the lung parenchyma leading to a decrease in lung compliance.

▶ History & Physical

Patients work history reveals exposure to coal mine dust. Exposure over years leads to a general loss of lung function, and patients present with cough, sputum production, and dyspnea.

▶ Diagnosis

Diagnosis is based on the appropriate history of exposure and characteristic chest x-ray finding. In simple disease, chest x-ray will show small nodules that predominate in the upper lung areas. In progressive massive fibrosis, the chest x-ray shows upper lobe nodules and hyperinflation of the lower lobes.

▶ Clinical Therapeutics

Treatment is supportive and includes oxygen therapy and rehabilitation.

▶ Clinical Intervention

See above.

▶ Health Maintenance Issues

The passage of the Coal Mine Health and Safety Act of 1969 mandates health standards that should reduce the risks for miners today.

## VII. PULMONARY NEOPLASMS

▶ Scientific Concepts

**Benign neoplasms** of the lung include the central bronchial adenoma and the pulmonary hamartoma commonly found in the lung periphery.

**Malignant neoplasms** of the lung are the principal cause of cancer deaths in men and women. Thirty-five percent of cancers deaths in men and 18% in women are caused by lung cancer. Carcinoma of the lung commonly presents in the 50- to 60-year-old age group. Cigarette smoking is the risk factor associated with most types of lung cancer. Ninety percent of patients with lung cancer of all types are either current or former smokers. Only bronchioalveolar carcinoma is not caused by smoking. Secondhand smoke is also a risk factor for the development of lung cancer. Asbestos is the second leading cause of lung cancer.

Clinically, malignant tumors of the lung can be divided into two categories:

**Small cell carcinomas** typically metastasize early and metastases are found on presentation. Small cell carcinoma accounts for 20–30% of malignant lung tumors. These are managed primarily through chemotherapy with or without radiotherapy. *CHEMO*

**Non–small cell carcinomas** include squamous cell carcinoma, adenocarcinoma, bronchoalveolar carcinoma, and large cell carcinoma. These neoplasms usually spread locally in the chest before metastasizing to other locations. The response of these cancers to chemotherapy is not dramatic. Squamous cell carcinoma is the most common cell type. Incidence varies from 40 to 70%. Adenocarcinoma has the greatest tendency to metastasize to the liver, brain, bone, adrenals, and lymph nodes. It accounts for 5 to 15% of malignant lung tumors and is the most common type found in lifetime smokers. Bronchioalveolar carcinoma has the best prognosis. Large cell carcinoma is an aggressive type of adenocarcinoma. Incidence varies from 1 to 10%.

### ► History & Physical

Patients may be asymptomatic when the tumor is found on routine chest x-ray. However, 75–90% of patients with lung cancer are symptomatic or may present with a new cough or a change in a chronic cough, hemoptysis, shortness of breath or dyspnea on exertion, anorexia, and weight loss. Bone pain from metastasis may be a symptom in patients with small cell carcinoma. Physical examination of the lung may be negative or one may find rales, rhonchi, and wheezes. Adenopathy may also be present. Paraneoplastic syndromes may be present in 10–20% of lung cancer patients.

### ► Diagnosis

Diagnostic studies include sputum or bronchial cell washings for cytology, chest x-rays, CT of the lung, bronchoscopy and biopsy, fine-needle biopsy, thoracentesis, and mediastinoscopy.

### ► Differential Diagnosis

Bronchitis, pneumonia, pleural effusion, tuberculosis.

### ► Clinical Therapeutics

Therapeutic options are surgery (non–small cell type), chemotherapy, and radiation therapy as indicated by location, presence or absence of metastases, and cell type.

### ► Clinical Intervention

Regular health maintenance, adequate nutrition, and pain control during therapy and after.

### ► Health Maintenance Issues

Stop smoking, avoid secondhand smoke, avoid asbestos dust.

*[Handwritten margin note: Bronchioalveolar Cancer is the only one not caused by smoking. Also has the best prognosis.]*

## VIII.  OTHER DISEASES OF THE PULMONARY SYSTEM

### A. Pleuritis

▶ Scientific Concepts

Pleuritis is characterized by inflammation of parietal pleura. The pleura may be inflamed primarily or secondarily.

▶ History & Physical

Patient presents with pleuritic pain (i.e., sharp, localized pain on deep breathing, sneezing, or coughing), cough, fever, and dyspnea. On physical examination, there may be rales, bronchial breath sounds, pleural friction rub, and decreased tactile fremitus.

▶ Diagnosis

Diagnosis is clinical; chest x-ray will be negative unless there is an underlying cause such as pneumonia.

▶ Differential Diagnosis

The differential diagnosis includes costochondritis, herpes zoster, pericarditis, and pneumonia.

▶ Clinical Therapeutics

Analgesics, anti-inflammatories, and antitussives are usually adequate treatment.

▶ Clinical Intervention

Heat and temporary splinting when coughing may provide some relief with the caution that splinting may contribute to atelectasis.

▶ Health Maintenance Issues

Smoking cessation; influenza and pneumococcal vaccines when indicated.

### B. Pleural Effusion

▶ Scientific Concepts

Defined as abnormal accumulation of fluid in the pleural space. There are five major types: transudates, exudates, empyema, hemothorax, and chylous. The classifications of transudate and exudates are to aid in the differential diagnosis.

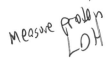

**Exudates** have at least one of the following: pleural fluid protein to serum protein ratio > 0.5; pleural fluid LDH to serum LDH ratio > 0.6; pleural fluid LDH greater than two thirds the upper limit of normal serum.

**Transudates** have none of the features listed above and are normally due to altered hydrostatic and oncotic pressures and suggest the absence of local pleural disease. Most common cause of an effusion is congestive heart failure (CHF), and more than 90% of transudates are secondary to CHF.

▶ History & Physical

May be asymptomatic if less than 200–300 mL of fluid. If effusion is larger, dyspnea, pleuritic chest pain, and dry cough are common.

▶ Diagnosis

Diagnostic thoracentesis should be performed if no cause is apparent. More than 250 mL must be present before effusion will be seen on an erect PA film. However, a lateral decubitus film can detect smaller amounts. Pleural fluid should be analyzed for total and differential white count, protein, glucose, and LDH.

▶ **Differential Diagnosis**
Includes congestive heart failure (CHF), nephrotic syndrome, pneumonia, cancer, pulmonary embolism (PE), tuberculosis, and others.

▶ **Clinical Therapeutics**
Should be directed at treating the underlying cause.

▶ **Clinical Intervention**
Thoracentesis can be therapeutic as well as diagnostic.

## C. Asthma

▶ **Scientific Concepts**
Defined as reversible (either with treatment or spontaneous) airway obstruction characterized by airway inflammation and increased airway responsiveness to a variety of stimuli.

Pathologic changes are hypertrophy of bronchial smooth muscle, mucosal edema and hyperemia, thickening of epithelial basement membrane, hypertrophy of mucous glands, acute inflammation, and plugging of airways by thick, viscid mucus. About 4–5% of the population are affected. Men and women are equally affected. Until puberty, asthma is twice as common among boys as among girls and reverses between puberty and early adulthood. Hospitalization rates are highest for children and African Americans, with death rates highest among African Americans between 15 and 24 years old.

▶ **History & Physical**
Patients exhibit a wide range of signs and symptoms, including episodic wheezing, feelings of chest tightness, shortness of breath, and cough. More severe attacks are associated with use of accessory muscles, decreased breath sounds and audible wheezing, anxiety, and apprehension. Attacks may occur spontaneously or in response to various triggers such as respiratory infections, emotional stress, weather changes, or physical activity. Amount of wheezing is not a reliable indicator for severity of episode, and absence of wheezing may be an ominous sign. Pulsus paradoxus, tachycardia, fatigue, and mental status changes may signal severe attack.

▶ **Diagnostic Studies**
Careful history, physical examination, and laboratory methods are required. Spirometry provides a means for measuring air flow. Level of airway responsiveness can be measured by inhalation challenge tests using metacholine, histamine, or exposure to a nonpharmacologic agent such as cold air.

▶ **Diagnosis**
Decreased $FEV_1$ and peak expiratory flow rate (PEFR). Physical signs vary with severity of attack.

▶ **Clinical Therapeutics**
Nonpharmacologic methods include education, relaxation techniques, controlled breathing, and a program of desensitization.

Classification of asthma (mild intermittent, mild persistent, moderate persistent, severe persistent) is useful in directing therapy and identifying patients at high risk of life-threatening attacks.

Pharmacologic treatments include bronchodilators, corticosteroids, glucocorticoids, and leukotriene modifiers.

### ► Clinical Intervention

Status asthmaticus management is similar to severe acute asthma, requiring an aggressive multidrug regimen and hospitalization. If progressive, respiratory acidosis develops and may require tracheal intubation and mechanical ventilation.

### ► Health Maintenance Issues

Discuss etiology and expectation of disease. Help patients identify potential allergens or precipitating agents in their environments. Patients should be evaluated at least every 6 months, and spirometry performed every 1–2 years once stabilized. Demonstrate proper use of MDI. Develop a patient treatment plan for severe exacerbations. Counsel patient on need for yearly influenza vaccine and pneumococcal vaccine.

## D. Pneumothorax

### ► Scientific Concepts

Pneumothorax occurs when air enters the pleural cavity, causing partial or complete collapse of the affected lung. There are generally three types: spontaneous (either primary or secondary), traumatic, and tension pneumothorax, which is a life-threatening condition caused by of excessive pressure within the pleural cavity. Tension pneumothorax primarily affects tall, thin boys between 10 and 30 years of age.

### ► History & Physical

Patients present with pleuritic chest pain that may be unilateral, dyspnea, increased respiratory rate, asymmetry of the chest, hyperresonant sound to percussion, and decreased or absent breath sounds over the area of the pneumothorax. Minimal physical findings with mild cases. Deviated trachea, severe tachycardia, hypotension with tension pneumothorax.

### ► Diagnostic Studies

Confirmed by chest x-ray, which demonstrates a visceral pleural line best revealed on an expiratory film. In tension pneumothorax, chest x-ray shows a large amount of air in the affected hemithorax and contralateral shift of mediastinal structures. Pulse oximetry or ABGs may reveal hypoxia.

### ► Clinical Therapeutics

Treatment varies with the cause and extent of the disorder. Without treatment in small (10–20%) pneumothoraces, the air usually reabsorbs. In large pneumothoraces, needle aspiration or closed drainage system is indicated. Tension pneumothorax treatment involves prompt insertion of large-bore needle or chest tube for decompression.

### ► Health Maintenance Issues

Patients who smoke should be instructed to quit smoking as recurrence rates are 50%. Also, avoidance of high altitudes, flying in unpressurized aircraft, and scuba diving.

## E. Pulmonary Embolism

▶ Scientific Concepts

Develops when a blood-borne substance lodges in a branch of the pulmonary artery and obstructs blood flow. The embolism may consist of a thrombus, air, fat, or amniotic fluid. Almost all pulmonary emboli are due to deep vein thromboses.

▶ History & Physical

Chest pain, dyspnea, and increased respiratory rate are the most frequent signs and symptoms. Can also present with apprehension, cough, hemoptysis, diaphoresis, and syncope (especially with massive pulmonary embolism). Pulmonary infarction causes pleuritic pain, moderate hypoxemia, and blood-stained sputum. Signs include tachycardia, tachypnea, crackles, and accentuation of the pulmonary component of the second heart sound.

▶ Diagnostic Studies

Blood gases reveal respiratory alkalosis, lung scan (perfusion, ventilation, or both), chest x-ray, electrocardiogram (nonspecific changes or right ventricular strain), and, in selected cases, angiography.

▶ Diagnosis

X-ray may show elevation of a hemidiaphragm and pulmonary infiltration, platelike atelectasis, oligemia in the embolized lung zone (Westermark sign), and prominence of pulmonary artery. A ventilation-perfusion lung scan may be abnormal in other diseases (COPD, asthma, CHF) as well, but an abnormal scan may support the diagnosis. Pulmonary angiography, which can detect emboli as small as 3 mm in diameter, remains the definitive test for diagnosis.

▶ Clinical Therapeutics

For acute pulmonary thromboembolism, heparin is the anticoagulant of choice. The use of thrombolytic therapy in clinical practice is controversial. Pharmacologic prophylaxis involves use of anticoagulant drugs. Low-dose subcutaneous heparin may be administered to decrease likelihood of deep vein thrombosis, thromboembolism, and fatal pulmonary embolism before and after major surgical procedures. Surgical interruption of the inferior vena cava is indicated with recurrent pulmonary embolism, which can be achieved by ligation, plication, clipping, or insertion of intraluminal filters. Prevention may be accomplished by using physical measures (external pneumatic compression of the legs, early ambulation, elevation of legs for immobilized patients, active and passive leg exercises), low-dose heparin, and antiplatelet drugs in patients at risk.

▶ Health Maintenance Issues

Identification of people at risk (prolonged bedrest, trauma, surgery, childbirth, obesity, fractures of hip and femur, advanced age, myocardial infarction, CHF, spinal cord injury); avoidance of venous stasis; early detection of venous thrombosis and hypercoagulability states.

## F. Acute Respiratory Distress Syndrome (ARDS)

▶ Scientific Concepts

Extreme form of noncardiac pulmonary edema as a result of injury to the microcirculation of the lung, following a wide variety of systemic or pulmonary insults. The mortality rate associated with ARDS is greater than 30–40%. If accompanied by sepsis, mortality rate may reach 90%. The major cause of death is multiple organ system failure often with sepsis.

▶ History & Physical

Progressive respiratory distress, increase in respiratory rate, signs of respiratory failure (labored breathing, tachypnea, intercostal retractions, and crackles). Usually occurs within 12–48 hours after the initiating event.

▶ Diagnosis

Radiologic findings show extensive bilateral diffuse consolidation of lung tissue, often sparing the costophrenic angles. Severe hypoxia persists despite increased inspired oxygen levels. Most patients demonstrate multiple organ failure (kidneys, liver, gut, central nervous system, cardiovascular system).

▶ Clinical Therapeutics

Treatment goals are to supply oxygen to vital organs and provide supportive care (mechanical ventilation, positive end-expiratory pressure, etc.) until pathologic processes have been reversed and lungs have had a chance to heal.

## G. Sarcoidosis

▶ Scientific Concepts

Multisystem granulomatous disorder of unknown etiology. Characterized by exaggerated cellular immune response manifested by noncaseating granulomatous inflammation in affected organs such as the lungs, lymph nodes, eyes, skin, liver, spleen, salivary glands, heart, and nervous system. Young adults are more frequently affected. The incidence is highest in North American blacks and northern European whites.

▶ History & Physical

Variable manifestations and an unpredictable course of progression in which any organ system can be affected. Common respiratory symptoms include cough, dyspnea, and chest discomfort. Often presents with bilateral hilar adenopathy and erythema nodosum or uveitis. Nonspecific symptoms are fever, sweating, anorexia, weight loss, fatigue, and myalgia.

▶ Diagnosis

Almost all patients have abnormal chest x-ray revealing symmetric bilateral hilar and right paratracheal adenopathy, interstitial infiltrates, or both. Diagnosis depends on compatible clinical and radiographic picture and tissue biopsy. Diagnosis usually made using transbronchial lung biopsy, bronchial lavage, the Kveim–Siltzbach skin test, and serum angiotensin-converting enzyme test.

▶ Clinical Therapeutics

Ninety percent are responsive to corticosteroids and easily controlled on modest maintenance dose when the disease has significant interference with normal life. Review of symptoms, serial radiographs, and serial measurement of ventilatory function and carbon monoxide diffusing capacity usually clearly indicate course of disease.

► **Clinical Intervention**

Approximately 50% develop permanent pulmonary abnormalities; 5 to 15% have progressive pulmonary fibrosis. Chronic fibrocystic sarcoidosis leads to a clinical picture that resembles bronchiectasis, with chronic productive cough. Hemoptysis can occur and is sometimes life threatening.

► **Health Maintenance Issues**

Pneumococcal and influenza vaccines are recommended.

# IX. SYMPTOMS REFERABLE TO THE PULMONARY SYSTEM

## A. Cough

► **Scientific Concepts**

Neurally mediated reflex that protects the lungs from accumulation of secretions and from entry of irritating and destructive substances.

► **History & Physical**

Cough receptors are located throughout the larynx, trachea, bronchi, ear canals, pleurae, stomach, nose, sinuses, pharynx, pericardium, and diaphragm. History should focus on smoking habits, environmental exposures, medications, duration and character of the cough, productive versus nonproductive, and associated symptoms of respiratory, gastrointestinal, neurologic, and heart disease.

► **Diagnostic Studies**

Diagnostic studies are obtained based on history and physical findings such as chest x-ray, spirometry, nasopharyngeal culture, barium swallow, laryngoscopy.

► **Diagnosis**

History and physical usually suggest the diagnosis.

► **Clinical Therapeutics**

Treatment should be directed at the underlying cause. Cautious use of antitussive agents is warranted. Syrups, lozenges, and topical anesthetics may be helpful. Mucolytics and expectorants are of uncertain value.

## B. Dyspnea

► **Scientific Concepts**

Generally a sign that pulmonary gas exchange is inadequate. It is a subjective sensation of discomfort associated with difficult or labored breathing.

► **History & Physical**

A comprehensive history and detailed physical examination help differentiate cardiac from pulmonary causes.

► **Diagnostic Studies**

Chest x-ray, pulmonary function tests, hemoglobin level, thyroid function studies, electrocardiogram, oximetry, and cardiopulmonary exercise testing.

▶ Diagnosis

A careful, stepwise approach to the complaint will yield a diagnosis.

▶ Clinical Therapeutics

Relieve the underlying disorder responsible for dyspnea. Supportive and therapeutic use of oxygen and pulmonary training (alter precipitating factors, pulmonary medication compliance, wear mask with cold exposure).

## C. Stridor

▶ Scientific Concepts

Collapse of the upper airways (e.g., laryngomalacia) or increased turbulence of air moving through obstructed airways produces an audible crowing sound called stridor. Impairment above the vocal cords typically produces inspiratory stridor whereas obstructions below will produce mixed or primarily expiratory stridor.

▶ History & Physical

Usually preceded by URIs that cause rhinorrhea, coryza, hoarseness, and low-grade fever.

▶ Diagnostic Studies

Chest x-ray and soft tissue neck film.

▶ Clinical Therapeutics

Usually subsides with exposure to cool moist air. Expectorants, antibiotics, bronchodilators, and antihistamines may be helpful in treating the underlying disorder.

## X. FOREIGN BODY ASPIRATION

▶ Scientific Concepts

May or may not obstruct the airway and can act as a ball valve. In 20% of cases, the object is in the upper airway; in 80%, it is in the main stem or lobar bronchus. Anatomic variations make it easier for foreign bodies to enter the right main bronchus than to enter the left. Occurs less frequently in adults than in children. The elderly and denture wearers appear to be at greatest risk.

▶ History & Physical

Classic triad is wheezing, cough, and decreased breath sounds. Other symptoms may include cough, dysphagia, stridor, pain, and dyspnea. History is usually highly suggestive, with a brief asymptomatic interval, then sudden dyspnea, coughing, and gagging.

▶ Diagnostic Studies

Laboratory evaluation is not helpful. Chest x-ray (expiratory) can be normal or show hyperinflation, atelectasis, infiltrate, or visualization of the foreign body.

▶ Diagnosis

Lateral neck x-rays for radiopaque foreign bodies in the neck. If lower airway, decubitus films in expiration may reveal more subtle degrees of hyperinflation.

► **Clinical Therapeutics**

If obstruction is complete and airway clearance maneuvers fail (e.g., Heimlich), remove object by laryngoscopy/bronchoscopy.

► **Health Maintenance Issues**

Counsel parents on anticipatory guidance measures regarding toys and feeding appropriate to the age. Most airway obstructions occur between the ages of 1 and 5 years. For total obstruction in patients less than 1 year old, back blows and chest thrusts; Heimlich maneuver for all others. Caution parents to keep small objects such as jewelry, toys, pins, peanuts, or candy out of reach.

## BIBLIOGRAPHY

Braunwald E, Fauci AS, Kasper DL, et al., eds. *Harrison's Principles of Internal Medicine,* 15th ed. New York: McGraw-Hill; 2001.

Ferri F. *Ferri's Clinical Advisor: Instant Diagnosis and Treatment.* St. Louis, MO: Mosby; 2001.

Fihn SD, DeWitt DE. *Outpatient Medicine,* 2nd ed., Chapters 19, 54, Section VII. Philadelphia: WB Saunders; 1998.

Goldman L, Bennett JC. *Cecil Textbook of Medicine,* 21st. ed. Philadelphia: WB Saunders Company; 2000.

Gorrol AH, Mulley AG. *Primary Care Medicine,* 4th ed. Philadelphia: Lippincott, Williams & Wilkins; 2000.

Rudy DR, Kurowski K. *Family Medicine.* Chapters 11, 12, 30. Baltimore: Williams & Wilkins; 1997.

Saunders CE, Ho MT. *Current Emergency Diagnosis & Treatment,* 4th ed. Chapters 5, 18, 27. Norwalk, CT: Appleton & Lange; 1992.

Stobo JD, Hellmann DB, Ladenson PW, Petty BG, Traill TA. *The Principles and Practice of Medicine,* 23rd ed. Stamford, CT: Appleton & Lange; 1996.

Tierney LM Jr, McPhee SJ, Papadakis MA, eds. *Current Medical Diagnosis & Treatment,* 42nd ed. New York: Lange Medical Books/McGraw-Hill; 2003.

# Cardiovascular Diseases 5

*Richard R. Rahr, EdD, PA-C, and Salah Ayachi, PhD, PA-C*

## I. ANGINA PECTORIS

▶ Scientific Concepts

Angina pectoris (AP) is substernal chest pain usually brought on by exertion, stress, eating, sexual activity, emotional stress, or cold weather. Episodes last from 15 to 30 minutes after the causative event, usually relieved by rest. Substernal pain is described as tightness, squeezing, burning, pressing, choking, aching, bursting, or "gaslike" pain that radiates to the neck, shoulder, or left arm. The etiology of chest pain is ischemia of the heart muscle due to narrowing of the coronary arteries, usually due to atherosclerosis. However, congenital anomalies, spasms, arterial dissection, arteritis, and aortic stenosis can cause the pain. Usually there is a family history of coronary artery disease (CAD), diabetes, hyperlipidemia, and hypertension. The risk factors for CAD contributing to chest pain are smoking, stress, inactivity, and high-fat diet. One hallmark of angina pectoris is that pain is relieved in 2 to 3 minutes by administration of nitroglycerin. Angina can occur with angiographic normal coronary arteries called Syndrome X because of poor flow reserve in the small cardiac vessels (microvasculature).

▶ History & Physical

The most salient historical finding is the onset of substernal pain with exertion and its rapid relief with rest or nitroglycerin. There is a strong family history of CAD. Patient usually has a profile of risk factors: cigarette smoking, hyperlipidemia, hypertension, obesity, and a sedentary lifestyle; a stressful occupation (e.g., airline pilots, air traffic controllers); or a recent period of strenuous activity as is seen in older people. There can be heart murmurs (Table 5–1) and palpitations (Table 5–2). AP is a historical diagnosis with advanced atherosclerosis as underlying disease. Table 5–3 lists cardiac and noncardiac causes of chest pain. The degree of cardiac involvement should be diagnosed with stress testing, angiography, thallium imagery, scintigraphic assessment, or exercise echocardiogram.

▶ Diagnostic Studies

Patients will need a baseline electrocardiogram (ECG) and echocardiogram, stress test, and perhaps exercise or stress thallium test. Exercise testing is considered the most useful noninvasive procedure for evaluating angina and to confirm the diagnosis of angina. A complete blood

▶ table 5-1

| MURMURS | | | | |
| --- | --- | --- | --- | --- |
| Type | Location | Radiation | Pitch | Sound |
| Mitral stenosis | 4th–5th ICS, LS | None | Low | Crescendo |
| Mitral insufficiency | PMI | Axilla | Med–High | Holosystolic |
| Aortic stenosis | R 2nd ICS | Carotid | Med–High | Crescendo–Decrescendo |
| Aortic insufficiency | L 3rd–4th ICS | Apex | High | Decrescendo |
| Tricuspid stenosis | 3rd–5th ICS, LS | None | Medium | Crescendo |
| Tricuspid insufficiency | 3rd–5th ICS, LS | None | Medium | Holosystolic |

ICS, intercostal space; LS, left sternal border; PMI, point of maximal impulse.

count (CBC), chest x-ray, and Holter monitor can also be useful in confirming the diagnosis. The definitive diagnosis may require coronary arteriograms to identify number and disease state of coronary vessels involved. New scintigraphic assessment of the ischemia can be a very useful test with either thallium 201 or technetium 99m sestamibi. The newest tests are: positron-emission tomography (PET) scans, ultrafast cine computed tomography (CT), cardiac magnetic resonance imaging (MRI), which may soon replace the angiogram in the near future.

### ► Diagnosis

The mainstay of a diagnosis of AP is based on historical findings with laboratory verification of underlying atherosclerosis. There are several other diseases or syndromes that mimic angina that must be considered. Costochondritis (Teitze syndrome) or anterior chest wall pain, vertebral disk disease, lung cancer, Prinzmetal's angina, Syndrome X, pneumonia, rib fracture, pneumothorax, and preeruptive shingles can also be confused for angina. Therefore, a careful history and physical are necessary to pinpoint the exact etiology (see Table 5–3).

### ► Clinical Therapeutics

There are two major approaches to treatment of AP: medical intervention and surgical/radiographic intervention. Medical treatment calls for use of short- or long-acting nitroglycerin preparations (oral tablet, spray, patch) in rapid- or long-acting form to achieve venodilation. Additional drugs, including beta blockers (propranolol, metoprolol, nadolol, atenolol), calcium channel blockers (amlodipine, diltiazem, verapamil), antiplatelet-forming drugs (aspirin), and clopidogrel are effective in reducing intensity and severity of pain.

Surgical intervention includes coronary arteriograms, angioplasty with stent placement, coronary artery bypass grafts (CABGs), and atherectomy (shave and laser procedures) to reduce the blockage and improve blood flow. Mortality rate with ejection fractions of 55% or greater is 1 to 2%; with ejection fractions of < 35%, mortality rate increases rapidly. Rate of patency 6 months after CABG is 85 to 90%, whereas with angioplasty restenosis it is 30–40% for the same period. The restenosis can be reduced to 15–20% with intracoronary artery stent placement. Stents are used in 70% of percutaneous revascularization. The major treatment intervention is to reduce smoking and dietary lipids and control blood pressure.

### ► Clinical Intervention

Unstable angina or crescendo angina occurs when chest pain becomes more frequent (requiring more nitroglycerin to relieve the pain), when it occurs at rest, or when chest pain lasts longer. Many of these patients are at risk of occlusion of the involved artery because of plaque rupture, ulceration, or hemorrhage. This could lead to an acute myocardial infarction (MI) with full occlusion, and require immediate intervention with oxygen, bedrest, monitoring, and sedation with benzodiazepines. Patient is treated with heparin or aspirin, nitroglycerin, beta blockers, calcium channel blockers, and thrombolytics. If this does not relieve the pain, coronary arteriography and revascularization are needed. In unstable angina, 10–30% of patients will have MI. The 1-year mortality rate is 10–20%. Stress testing and coronary angiography are needed in most cases to fully assess the patient.

---

**► table 5-2**

**PALPITATIONS**

- Normal
- Increased cardiac output
- Increased stroke volume
- Thyrotoxicosis
- Anemia
- Anxiety
- Exercise
- Cardiac arrhythmias—supraventricular tachycardia, ventricular tachycardia

---

**► table 5-3**

**CAUSES OF CHEST PAIN**

**Cardiac Causes**

- Angina pectoris
- Acute myocardial infarction
- Pericarditis
- Myocarditis
- Cardiomyopathy
- Valvular heart disease

**Noncardiac Causes**

- Lung mass
- Aortic aneurysm
- Disk disease
- Cholecystitis
- Esophageal disease
- Pneumothorax
- Teitze syndrome
- Peptic ulcer disease
- Anxiety states
- Musculoskeletal disease

► Health Maintenance Issues

Patients whose first episode of ischemia is silent may suddenly die. These patients have a history of hyperlipidemia, are overweight, have a strong family history of CAD, have hypertension, smoke cigarettes, and have sedentary and high-stress lifestyles. Screening programs for hypertension, hyperlipidemia, and other risk factors, as well as preexercise programs, are effective in preventing sudden death.

## II. ACUTE MYOCARDIAL INFARCTION

► Scientific Concepts

Normal function of the pumping heart requires patent arteries to provide normal blood flow. Therefore, any substantial (75% or higher) narrowing of the arteries causes disruption in this function. When coronary arteries are completely blocked by a thrombus or by severe spasm for a long period of time, an acute MI occurs. The patient who experiences severe substernal chest pain for 30 minutes, unrelieved by three nitroglycerin tablets given at 5-minute intervals, may be experiencing an MI. In 25% of MI cases, patient may experience no pain, and these infarctions are often diagnosed by routine ECG without a recallable event. Coronary artery obstruction may be due to thrombosis, vasospasms, vasculitis, dissection aneurysm, or cocaine use, increased metabolic demand (hyperthyroidism), and hypotension (shock). When the left coronary artery is involved, an anterior (left ventricle) or septal infarct occurs; involvement of the right coronary artery results in posterior-inferior, septal, or right ventricular infarct. Left circumflex artery involvement results in anterolateral or posterolateral infarct. Underlying pathogenesis is atherosclerosis with marked narrowing of the coronary arteries, which may be seen in families with a history of heart disease or other risk factors (Table 5–4).

► History & Physical

Most patients (80%) present with substernal chest pain that radiates to the jaw, left shoulder, arm, throat, precordium, or retrosternal area. Up to 20% of patients present with no pain. Typically, patients with longstanding angina pectoris will take three sublingual nitroglycerin tablets without relief. Twenty percent of patients die in the first hour after the onset of pain, before reaching the hospital. About one third of patients present with symptoms of indigestion. Many patients present with shock, congestive heart failure (CHF), syncope, or pulmonary edema. Signs of

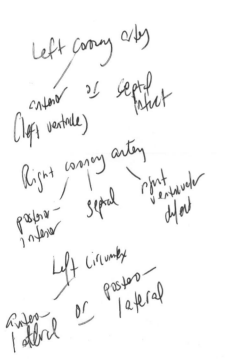

Left coronary artery
anterior or septal infarct
(left ventricle)

Right coronary artery
posterior-inferior   septal   right ventricular defect

Left circumflex
antero-lateral or postero-lateral

► table 5-4

OTHER FACTORS, MYOCARDIAL INFARCTION

- 30% of patients who undergo cardiac evaluation do not have cardiac disease.
- 25% of cases of myocardial infarction are painless.
- Nitroglycerin is mostly ineffective in ameliorating pain due to myocardial infarction.
- 20% of myocardial infarction cases die before reaching the hospital.

heart failure include jugular venous distention, orthopnea, cough, wheezing, and arrhythmias. Physical findings include edema; cyanosis; S3, S4 gallops; mitral murmur; and possibly edema and fever.

## ▶ Diagnostic Studies

The ECG is evaluated for S-T segment elevation with transmural infarction and S-T segment depression with subendocardial ischemia, T wave inversion, and Q waves. Serial cardiac enzymes (creatine kinase MB [CK-MB] and troponin T and troponin I levels) are the most reliable diagnostic markers. Baseline studies of CBC, electrolytes, chest x-ray, oxygen saturation, arterial blood gases (ABGs), and creatinine are obtained. Technetium scans, using pyrophosphate (hot spots) or thallium (cold spots), and radiolabeled antimyosin antibody fragments (takes 24–48 hours for results) are used to evaluate the size and function of the necrotic tissue.

## ▶ Diagnosis

The pattern of enzyme elevation diagnostic of infarct entails CK-MB peaking at 12–48 hours, alanine aminotransferase (ALT) at 48–72 hours, and lactate dehydrogenase (LDH) at 3–5 hours. Troponin T and troponin I peak 3–5 days following an MI and remain elevated for up to 7 days or longer. The hallmark of diagnosis is either pathologic Q wave on ECG (in cases of transmural infarcts) or elevated isoenzymes. Area of scar tissue is determined by technetium scan. Angiograms are often performed to determine the location and degree of vascular obstruction.

## ▶ Clinical Therapeutics

Treatment with tissue plasminogen activator (t-PA), streptokinase, or other thrombolytics (anistreplase, reteplase, and tenecteplase) within 1–3 hours can reduce mortality rates by reducing infarct size by 50%. A 10% reduction in mortality can be achieved with treatment up to 12 hours after infarction. Thrombolytics should not be used when there is no evidence of S-T segment changes on serial ECGs; they are contraindicated in patients with history of cerebrovascular event, marked hypertension, suspected aortic dissection, or active internal bleeding. Relative contraindications include current use of anticoagulants, recent invasive procedures, and others (prior coronary artery bypass graft, major surgery in 3 weeks, recent cardiopulmonary resuscitation [CPR], pregnancy, active peptic ulcer). All patients are admitted to cardiac care unit and given oxygen, liquid low-salt diet, and morphine for pain. Patients are given nitroglycerin to reduce preload in the acute phase; this is not useful for prophylaxis. If frequent premature ventricular contractions (PVCs) develop, lidocaine can be used to suppress arrhythmia during first 24 hours. However, lidocaine is no longer used for prophylactic suppression of ventricular arrhythmias. Angiotensin-converting enzyme (ACE) inhibitors are frequently used to reduce afterload when ejection fraction is below 35%. Up to 5% of MI patients develop ventricular fibrillation; 80% of these cases develop in the first 24 hours.

## ▶ Clinical Intervention

t-PA and streptokinase administration, angiography, angioplasty, and CABG are reserved for treatment of difficult and refractory cases. In cases of cardiogenic shock, advanced life support becomes necessary.

► Health Maintenance Issues

Risk factors for atherosclerosis or CAD must be controlled. Hyperlipidemia, stress, hypertension, lack of exercise, cigarette smoking, and obesity must all be addressed in rehabilitation phase of treatment.

## III. PRINZMETAL'S (VARIANT) ANGINA

► Scientific Concepts

Clinical syndrome in which chest pain and S-T segment elevation occur secondary to coronary artery spasm. Primarily strikes women under age 50. Affected individuals may awaken from sleep with arrhythmias or conduction disorders usually associated with right coronary artery obstruction. Diagnosis can be made from transient S-T elevation as seen on Holter monitor. Complete workup, including coronary arteriography, is needed to identify fixed lesions or by ergonovine (vasoconstrictor) test to reproduce the spasm.

► History & Physical

Patients usually present with intermittent episodes of chest pain and palpitations that occur in early morning hours. Patients tend to be younger than other cardiac patients, and frequently smoke cigarettes or use cocaine.

► Diagnostic Studies

Useful diagnostic tests include ECG, use of a Holter monitor, stress test, coronary arteriography, and echocardiography. If lesions are not observed, spasm should be suspected. Ergonovine can be given intravenously (IV) to reproduce arteriolar spasm. IV nitroglycerin is used to reverse spasm to prevent irreversible spasm and infarction.

► Diagnosis

Positive ergonovine test, in the absence of fixed lesions and transient S-T segment elevation on Holter monitoring, is diagnostic of Prinzmetal's angina.

► Clinical Therapeutics

Nitrates or calcium channel blockers are effective prophylactic agents. Patients with fixed stenosis may benefit from beta blockers.

► Clinical Intervention

Surgery may be warranted when spasms are associated with fixed stenoses.

► Health Maintenance Issues

Patients should abstain from smoking cigarettes and cocaine use.

## IV. CONGESTIVE HEART FAILURE

► Scientific Concepts

CHF is understood to be left heart failure (LHF) in which the left ventricle can no longer forcefully contract to produce an adequate stroke volume, leading to low cardiac output and tissue hypoxia. Symptoms include dyspnea, fatigue, cough, orthopnea, paroxysmal nocturnal dyspnea, and dyspnea on exertion (DOE) (Table 5–5). Physical findings include pulmonary congestion, rales, LVH, and gallops (S3, S4).

Right heart failure (RHF) occurs when failure leads to backup of blood, resulting in jugular venous distention, hepatic congestion, dependent edema, and ascites. There is rapid weight gain from fluid accumulation resulting in presacral edema and ascites (Table 5–6).

A third type of heart failure, referred to as high-output failure, is caused by the inability of the heart to meet demands associated with certain disease conditions including thyrotoxicosis, anemia, arteriovenous shunting, beriberi, or Paget's disease. This type of heart failure is easiest to correct.

Heart failure can also be described as either systolic or diastolic. Diastolic failure occurs when the atrium becomes stiff and unable to contract or becomes overstretched. May be reversed with ACE inhibitors or vasodilators. Systolic failure results in a reduced ejection fraction. Can be managed with diuretics to reduce preload, ACE inhibitors to reduce afterload, and inotropic drugs to increase myocardial contractility.

Heart failure may be caused by CAD, valvular heart disease, systemic or pulmonary hypertension, MI, cardiomyopathy, or viral myocarditis, and results in increased end-diastolic volume or preload. Increased preload leads to overstretching of cardiac muscle fibers and decreased stroke volume. Increased catecholamine release, angiotensin production, and increased vascular resistance or afterload early in heart failure further aggravate the condition.

► History & Physical

The major symptoms of LHF are dyspnea, nocturia, DOE, fatigue, orthopnea, paroxysmal nocturnal dyspnea, fatigue, and exercise intolerance. Patients with RHF complain of dependent edema, swollen abdo-

► table 5-5

CAUSES OF DYSPNEA

Pulmonary Causes

- Airway disease (asthma, chronic obstructive pulmonary disease)
- Lung parenchyma (pulmonary fibrosis)
- Pleural disease (pleural effusion or pneumothorax)
- Respiratory muscle disease (myasthenia gravis)

Nonpulmonary Causes

- Cardiac (congestive heart failure, cardiomyopathy, hypertrophic obstructive cardiomyopathy, angina pectoris)
- Anxiety (hyperventilation syndrome)
- Anemia
- Shock
- Abdominal distention
- Deconditioning
- Hypermetabolic state
- Malnutrition syndrome (hypoalbuminemia)
- Obesity (hypoventilation syndrome)

## table 5-6

### CAUSES AND LOCATION OF EDEMA

#### Causes

- Venous insufficiency
- Nephrotic syndrome
- Premenstrual syndrome
- Congestive heart failure
- Cirrhosis
- Drugs (nonsteroidal anti-inflammatory drugs, calcium channel blockers)
- Malabsorption syndrome (hypoalbuminemia)
- Pre-eclampsia, eclampsia
- Thyroid (hyperthyroidism)
- Renal (glomerulonephritis)

#### Location

- Pretibial (erect)
- Presacral (bedfast)

men, and right upper quadrant pain because of hepatic congestion. RHF patients also present with jugular venous distention, dependent edema, hepatomegaly, hepatojugular reflux, and ascites. LHF results in cyanosis, pleural effusions, wheezing, basilar rales, murmurs, and gallops (S3, S4). Cough is a common finding in LHF and in RHF precipitated by LHF.

► Diagnostic Studies

Baseline workup includes thyroid tests, ECG, chest x-ray, electrolytes, CBC, renal function studies, echocardiography, coronary arteriography, and stress testing. If cardiomyopathy is suspected, biopsy is needed to verify underlying cause(s). A new assay called BPN (B-type naturiuretic peptide) is useful adjunct to history and physical examination. The BPN is high when ventricular filling pressures are high with symptomatic heart failure.

► Diagnosis

Heart failure has many causes. Valvular heart disease may be congenital, stenotic, or regurgitant. Infectious processes and chamber dilation may be underlying causes. Myocardial diseases include CAD, MI, and myocarditis. Increased workload may be due to anemia, thyrotoxicosis, septicemia, and systemic or pulmonary hypertension. CHF can be precipitated by volume overload due to excess IV fluids.

► Clinical Therapeutics

The most common therapies include:
1. Place patient on 2.0-g sodium diet.
2. Administer diuretics, usually hydrochlorothiazide (HCTZ).
3. Administer ACE inhibitor such as captopril or enalapril.
4. Administer digoxin to patients with systolic failure or low ejection fraction.
5. Use vasodilator such as isosorbide dinitrate or hydralazine to reduce afterload.
6. Consider beta blockers for improvement of heart failure.
7. Avoid calcium channel blockers since they may worsen the condition.
8. Consider anticoagulation in LHF to prevent systemic emboli.
9. Administration of antiarrhythmics has shown to have small to no value unless targeting the specially selected patient with selected beta blockers or for ventricular arrhythmias such as frequent PVCs or ventricular tachycardia.
10. Nonpharmacological treatments—coronary revascularizations, cardiac transplant, and cardiomyoplasty (latissimus dorsi muscle wrap)—are often used with prescription.

► Clinical Intervention

The prognosis is very poor for patients with CHF, particularly if the ejection fraction is below 20%. In stable patients, the mortality rate is 10%; in unstable patients, 30–50%. About 40–50% of the deaths in heart failure are sudden, with many due to cardiac arrhythmias.

► Health Maintenance Issues

Rapid improvement of CHF can be achieved by limiting daily dietary salt intake to 2.0 g. Exercise training improves activity tolerance, but is not proven to prolong life.

# V. INFECTIVE ENDOCARDITIS

### ▶ Scientific Concepts

Patients who develop endocarditis usually have organic heart lesions resulting from open heart surgery, IV drug use, artificial valves, or congenital defects (e.g., patent ductus arteriosus). Dental or urologic procedures may precipitate these events. Patients with valvular damage due to rheumatic fever are at higher risk of developing endocarditis. They may develop fever, chills, systemic emboli, and positive blood cultures for organisms most likely to be involved—*Streptococcus viridans* (60% of cases), *Staphylococcus aureus* (20% of cases), enterococcus (5–10%), HACEK (haemophilus actinobacillus, cardiobacterium, eikenella, kingella) (5%). Small number of cases are a results of fungal infections. The most common causes of endocarditis are:

- Rheumatic fever
- Mitral valve prolapse
- Ventricular septal defect
- Tetralogy of Fallot
- Aortic coarctation
- Patent ductus arteriosus
- Hypertrophic obstructive cardiomyopathy (formerly idiopathic hypertrophic subaortic stenosis)
- Calcified valves
- Gastrointestinal procedures
- Urologic procedures
- Dental procedures
- Prosthetic valve implants
- Cardiac catheterizations
- Pacemaker implant
- Cardiac stent
- Respiratory procedures

### ▶ History & Physical

Most patients have fever and chills for about 2 weeks accompanied by cough, dyspnea, arthralgia, arthritis, diarrhea, hematuria, and abdominal and flank pain. Physical examination reveals murmurs, petechiae, splinter hemorrhages, Janeway lesions, Roth spots, pallor, Osler nodes, and splenomegaly. CBC shows leukocytosis and anemia. Patients may have hematuria, proteinuria, and renal dysfunction. Serial blood cultures ($\times 3$) taken 1 hour apart or over a 24-hour period before initiation of treatment are most important to identify organisms. Fungal cultures are negative 50% of the time. Chest x-ray shows pulmonary infiltrates or single-chamber enlargement; echocardiography is used to identify valves involved.

### ▶ Diagnostic Studies

1. Blood cultures—definitive diagnosis
2. Chest x-ray—pulmonary infiltrates
3. Echocardiography—infected valves
4. CBC—elevated white blood count, anemia
5. Urinalysis—hematuria, proteinuria

► Diagnosis
Duke University criteria for diagnosing endocarditis:
1. Major criteria:
   • Positive blood culture to identify organism involved
   • Positive echocardiography to show vegetations on valves
2. Minor criteria:
   • Predisposing condition (valve damage)
   • Fever of 38°C or higher
   • Embolic disease
   • Immunologic phenomena (e.g., glomerulonephritis, Osler node, Roth spots, rheumatoid factor)
   • Positive blood culture not meeting major criteria
   • Positive echocardiogram not meeting major criteria
Two major, one major plus three minor, or five minor yield 80% accuracy of diagnosis.

► Clinical Therapeutics
Empiric therapy (before culture results are available), give:
1. Nafcillin, 1.5 g q4h and/or
2. Penicillin, 2–3 million units q4h and/or
3. Gentamicin, 1 mg/kg q8h or
4. Vancomycin, 15 mg/kg q12h for patients allergic to penicillin
   *For cultures positive for S. viridans:*
1. Penicillin, 2–3 million units IV q4h × 4 weeks or
2. Gentamicin, 1 mg/kg q8h × 2 weeks
   *For blood cultures positive for enterococci:*
1. Penicillin as above or
2. Gentamicin as above
3. Ampicillin 2 g IV q4h—can be used if gentamicin is toxic to the patient
   *For S. aureus:*
1. Nafcillin, 2 g q4h × 4 to 6 weeks or
2. Oxacillin, 2 g q4h × 4 to 6 weeks

► Clinical Intervention
Surgical intervention for severe valve involvement and increasing heart failure.

► Health Maintenance Issues
1. Prophylactic antibiotic therapy for the following procedures:
   • Dental procedures
   • Genitourinary procedures
   • Gastrointestinal procedures
   • Cardiac catheterization
   • Pulmonary surgery
2. Prophylactic antibiotic therapy for the following conditions:
   • Prosthetic valves
   • Previous episodes of subacute bacterial endocarditis
   • Congenital heart disease
   • Hypertrophic obstructive cardiomyopathy (HOCM)
   • Mitral valve prolapse
   • Pulmonary shunt
3. Antibiotic treatment—amoxicillin 2.0 g 1 hour before the procedure.

If allergic to penicillin, use clindamycin 600 mg 1 hour before the procedure.

## VI. CARDIOMYOPATHY

▶ Scientific Concepts

Cardiomyopathy is a constellation of diseases that affect the cardiac muscle and result in CHF, arrhythmias, or sudden death. Major causes include ischemia, hypertension, valvular or congenital defects. Viral myocarditis, toxins, alcohol, nutritional deficiencies, diabetes, and connective tissue diseases may also be involved.

Cardiomyopathies may be classified into three categories: dilated, hypertrophic, and restrictive. In dilated cardiomyopathy, left ventricle is dilated and associated systolic dysfunction is present. Many dilated cardiomyopathies are idiopathic. Alcohol abuse and myocarditis have been implicated in cardiac fibrosis.

In hypertrophic cardiomyopathy (HOCM), left ventricle is small and hypercontractile, with associated left ventricular outflow obstruction. There is a genetic element to these cardiomyopathies.

The restrictive cardiomyopathies are rare and characterized by impaired diastolic filling in the face of intact contractile function. Diseases such as sarcoidosis, hemochromatosis, carcinoid syndrome, scleroderma, and amyloidosis result in restrictive cardiomyopathy. May also be a sequela of radiation therapy and myocardial fibrosis after open heart surgery.

▶ History & Physical

*Dilated cardiomyopathy:* The most common symptom is dyspnea. Paroxysmal nocturnal dyspnea (PND), orthopnea, DOE, fatigue, and edema also common findings. Physical examination findings include hypotension, rales, tachycardia, large and displaced point of maximal impulse (PMI), cool extremities, edema, jugular venous distention, ascites. Mitral murmurs and S3 gallops can be found when examining the heart.

*Hypertrophic cardiomyopathy:* Patient presents with dyspnea, chest pain, syncope with exertion; may experience palpitations and frequent cardiac arrhythmias. It is not uncommon to have young athletes experience *sudden death* after exertion. On physical examination, they are found to have enlarged PMI, S4 gallops, systolic murmurs, and bisferiens carotid pulse.

*Restrictive cardiomyopathy:* Patients present with dyspnea, fatigue, and findings consistent with right-sided failure. Physical examination reveals edema, jugular venous distention, ascites, and enlarged heart.

▶ Diagnostic Studies

Echocardiography may help to identify valvular damage, ventricular aneurysms, and dilated ventricles. A thallium-201 scan may identify cardiac ischemia. In addition to echocardiography, Doppler ultrasound and cardiac catheterization are used to diagnose hypertrophic cardiomyopathy. ECG and chest x-ray are used to detect LVH, MI, and other cardiac diseases.

ECG and chest x-ray are used to document heart enlargement. Echocardiography may also be used to assess cardiac enlargement defects. Appropriate laboratory studies must be performed in order to identify underlying diseases causing cardiomyopathy (cardiac biopsy).

▶ Diagnosis

***Dilated cardiomyopathy:*** Combine data from ECG, chest x-ray, echocardiogram, catheterization, and thallium scan.

***Hypertrophic cardiomyopathy:*** Chest x-ray, ECG, Doppler ultrasound, and cardiac catheterization are needed to measure intracardiac pressures such as left ventricular end-diastolic pressure.

***Restrictive cardiomyopathy:*** In addition to chest x-ray, ECG, echocardiography, and catheterization, a heart muscle biopsy may be used to diagnose this type of cardiomyopathy.

▶ Clinical Therapeutics
1. Dilated cardiomyopathy:
   • Discontinue alcohol use.
   • Correct any endocrine causes (e.g., thyroid, diabetes, adrenal medullary, and/or anterior pituitary disorders).
   • Treat autoimmune diseases, if applicable.
   • Treat edema with diuretics or other drugs for CHF.
2. Hypertrophic cardiomyopathy:
   • Beta blocker as initial drug for outflow obstruction
   • Calcium channel blockers
   • Surgical intervention for excision of septum
   • Dual-chamber pacing
   • Implant defibrillator to prevent sudden death
3. Restrictive cardiomyopathy (little useful therapy is available):
   • Diuretic for CHF; overuse can worsen symptoms
   • Steroids for sarcoidosis
   • Transplantation, if possible

▶ Clinical Intervention
The major intervention involves diuretics and placement of defibrillator to prevent sudden death. Cardiac muscle biopsy may be needed to identify exact diagnosis and prognosis.

▶ Health Maintenance Issues
1. Minimize the use of alcohol and reduce exposure to toxins.
2. Limit salt intake to ameliorate CHF.
3. ACE inhibitors may be used to improve survival and quality of life.

## VII. PERICARDITIS

▶ Scientific Concepts
Acute pericarditis is a common disorder that may be due to any of several causes, including viruses (coxsackievirus, echovirus, influenza, Epstein–Barr virus, human immunodeficiency virus [HIV]), uremia, radiation, drug toxicity, hemopericardium, autoimmune syndrome, tuberculosis, varicella, hepatitis, mumps, neoplasms, Lyme disease, and following MI (Dressler's syndrome). The sequelae of pericarditis include

pericardial effusion and restriction of diastolic filling. Bloody or serous pericardial effusion and restricted diastolic filling can evolve into a medical emergency because of constrictive pericardial tamponade.

▶ History & Physical

Patients with pericarditis present with pleuritic chest pain that is relieved by sitting. Pain may be substernal and radiate to shoulders, back, neck, or epigastrium. They complain of dyspnea, fever, chills, and fatigue. Physical examination reveals a pericardial friction rub, usually heard best along the left sternal border. ECG changes include generalized S-T segment elevation and late T wave inversion that will evolute over 2 to 6 weeks before coming back to normal. Echocardiography reveals pericardial effusion. Chest x-ray shows cardiomegaly. Patient with constrictive pericarditis can present with CHF, jugular venous distention (with inspiration called Kussmaul's sign), ascites, edema, hepatic congestion, dyspnea, weakness, fatigue, arrhythmias, and pulsus paradoxus (drop of 10 mm Hg blood pressure with inspiration).

▶ Diagnostic Studies
1. ECG—ST-T changes
2. Chest x-ray—enlarged (water bottle) heart
3. ECG—pericardial effusion
4. MRI—pericardial effusion
5. CBC—leukocytosis

▶ Diagnosis
1. Echocardiography is an excellent tool for diagnosis of pleural effusion and tamponade.
2. Pulsus paradoxus confirmed by blood pressure is important for diagnosis of tamponade.
3. CT and MRI reveal pericardial thickening.
4. Chest x-ray shows pericardial calcification in 50% of cases of constrictive pericarditis.

▶ Clinical Therapeutics
1. Viral pericarditis:
   • Aspirin, 650 mg q4 to 6 h or other nonsteroidal inflammatory prescription, or
   • Indocin, 100–150 mg qd in divided doses or
   • Short course of steroids in unresponsive cases
2. Pericardial effusion:
   • Pericardiocentesis
   • Pericardiectomy in cases of chronic disease (e.g., uremia, neoplasia)
3. Constrictive pericarditis:
   • Gentle diuresis
   • Pericardiotomy or pericardial window surgery

▶ Clinical Intervention

Cardiac tamponade and constrictive pericarditis may require immediate surgical intervention to evacuate accumulated fluids and/or pericardium.

▶ Health Maintenance Issues

Time is needed for rest and recovery.

# VIII. AORTIC COARCTATION

## ► Scientific Concepts

Aortic coarctation is a localized narrowing of the aortic arch just distal to the origin of the left subclavian artery, which results in decreased blood flow to the kidneys, increased release of renin, and secondary hypertension. Defect is usually congenital and requires surgical repair in childhood years. Narrowing is often located at the level of the ligamentum arteriosum, and may have aortic valve (stenosis, regurgitation) involvement. Resulting increased collateral circulation through intercostal arteries produces "notching" of the ribs seen on chest x-ray. It is not unusual for coarctation patients to have a congenital cerebral aneurysm that can rupture.

## ► History & Physical

Classic symptoms are dyspnea, edema, PND, and DOE as seen with heart failure. Major physical findings are significant increases in blood pressure in vessels proximal to defect, blood pressure discrepancy between arms and legs, weak or absent femoral pulses, and harsh systolic murmur auscultable in the back.

## ► Diagnostic Studies

Chest x-ray shows left ventricular hypertrophy (LVH), enlarged aortic knob, and lower pulmonary artery and notching (scalloping) of the ribs. ECG shows LVH. Arteriography is used to locate and assess degree of obstruction. Echocardiography is used to identify aortic structures and degree of atrioventricular (AV) involvement.

## ► Diagnosis

Aortography and catheterization with pressure gradient readings are primary methods of diagnosis. MRIs and Doppler ultrasound can be used to estimate severity of obstruction.

## ► Clinical Therapeutics

Surgical correction is indicated for all patients younger than 20 years of age. For patients under 40 years of age, surgical intervention is recommended if there are signs and symptoms of refractory hypertension or if severe LVH is present. After age 50, balloon angioplasty may be used because surgical mortality is greatly increased. Only 75% of patients show amelioration of hypertension after surgery. Complications of balloon angioplasty may include aortic tears requiring immediate intervention. Corrective surgery has an operative mortality of 1–4% for patients under 20 years old. However, untreated coarctation can lead to cerebral hemorrhage, aortic dissection, and frequent bouts of infectious endarteritis.

## ► Health Maintenance Issues

Salt intake must be carefully monitored. Subacute bacterial endocarditis prophylaxis may be necessary to prevent further valve damage.

# IX. CARDIAC ARRHYTHMIAS AND CONDUCTION DISORDERS

▶ Scientific Concepts

Specialized myocardial fibers make up the conduction system. The sinoatrial (SA) and AV nodes are both capable of generating and conducting electrical impulses; normally, the SA node sets the pace (pulse) at 60 to 100 impulses per minute. When it generates impulses at less than 60, *sinus bradycardia* develops, and when the rate exceeds 100, the condition is called *sinus tachycardia*. Variation in rate associated with respiratory cycles is termed *sinus arrhythmia*.

If the SA node fails to initiate the impulse, the AV node (junction) becomes dominant and initiates a slower rhythm. Under certain circumstances, an ectopic atrial impulse develops. If transmission of the impulse through the AV node is impeded, an AV block results. AV blocks vary in severity and clinical significance from transient and benign blocks to severe, second-degree AV blocks (type II), and complete heart block, which can be fatal if left undetected and untreated.

When the conduction system is damaged at the level of the right and/or left branch of the bundle of His, bundle branch blocks (BBBs) develop. These may be partial (incomplete) or complete. These types of conduction derangements may coexist with other conduction anomalies as well as arrhythmias.

Under certain conditions, when the SA node fails to generate impulses, a focus of activity develops in one of the atria and "paces" the heart at a slightly slower rate than does the SA node. Activity may develop in the same site (focus) in the atria but may also develop in different foci, yielding a wandering atrial pacemaker. In either case, an *atrial escape rhythm* protects against prolonged SA node arrest.

When a single impulse arises prematurely in an atrial focus, a premature atrial complex (PAC) develops, which interrupts and resets normal sinus rhythm pattern. PACs may be conducted into AV node and ventricles eliciting early QRS complexes or may be blocked when they reach these structures during their refractory period. As with atrial escape beats, PACs may originate from a single focus or from multiple atrial pacemaker sites (multifocal atrial tachycardia).

When three or more PACs occur consecutively, there is atrial tachycardia, which may last a few seconds or may be sustained for hours or days. One of two processes may be responsible for this tachyarrhythmia: (1) enhanced automaticity by physiologic disturbances or (2) impulse reentry, both of which suppress SA node pacemaking activity.

Abnormalities of the cardiac rhythm can result in sudden death, syncope, near syncope, dizziness, and palpitations due to the reduced cardiac output with the underlying cardiac muscle perfusion. Arrhythmias are usually detected by patients' symptoms brought on by cardiac muscle ischemia, MIs, electrolyte imbalances, hormone imbalances, hypoxia, drug effects, or vasovagal responses. Therefore, there is a need to have long-term, 24-hour monitoring to correctly identify the arrhythmia. Many of the supraventricular arrhythmias are benign, but the high grade heart blocks and ventricular arrhythmias have very serious complications and prevent the normal cardiac perfusion needed to sustain life.

► History & Physical

*Sinus bradycardia* is a normal finding in physically well-conditioned persons, but may also be the result of pathologic processes. Similarly, *sinus tachycardia* is a normal response both to physiologic and pathologic conditions. Its etiology must be determined. Individuals with first-degree AV blocks (P-R interval > .20 seconds and constant) are often asymptomatic until the block is aggravated by drugs, such as digitalis, or by vagotonic influences, at which time patient may complain of dizziness or lightheadedness.

Patients with Wenckebach (Mobitz type I) AV block may develop lightheadedness, weakness, and fatigue, and may require pharmacologic and/or electronic therapy. Mobitz type I may be seen in patients with acute MI or myxedema, either singly or in conjunction with other conduction disturbances, but may also be seen in individuals with increased vagal tone who are otherwise normal.

Patients treated with drugs such as digitalis, procainamide, quinidine, lidocaine, propranolol, or tricyclic antidepressants such as amitriptyline (Elavil), all of which depress conduction, may be at risk of developing Mobitz type II AV block due to interference with conduction. Mobitz type II can develop into complete (third-degree) AV block. Patients may present with lightheadedness and syncopal episodes.

Patients with supraventricular tachycardia (i.e., rhythms driven by pacemakers above common bundles) may complain of palpitations (see Table 5–2) and lightheadedness, and may experience syncope.

► Diagnostic Studies

The ECG provides important clues in identifying the various impulse generation and/or conduction disorders. The His bundle electrogram is a record of electrophysiologic events in the conduction pathways and offers additional insights into these processes. His electrography is an invasive procedure. The Holter monitor is very useful to get a 24-hour reading of the ECG rhythm to make an exact diagnosis and the frequency of the abnormal rhythm.

► Diagnosis

See Table 5–7.

► Clinical Therapeutics

Therapeutics should treat underlying condition(s). Pathologic conditions that produce sinus bradycardia include decreased metabolic activity (myxedema, hypothermia) and increased intracranial pressure (cerebral edema, subdural hematoma). Conditions that produce sinus tachycardia include hyperthyroidism, fever, anemia, heat exposure, shock, CHF, acute MI, pulmonary emboli, hypoxia, hypercapnea, smoking, pain, anxiety, adrenergic agonists, and vagolytic agents.

A first-degree AV block that accompanies MI, myocarditis, drug intoxication, or other cardiac problems of recent onset should be evaluated thoroughly. Second-degree AV blocks develop with more severe depression of AV nodal conduction because of disease or by vagotonic influences (i.e., carotid pressure, vomiting) causing failure of some impulses to traverse the AV node or reach and activate the ventricles. The result is missed beats and an atrial rate higher than that of ventricles. Wenckebach (Mobitz type I) is usually transient and reversible, but may progress to

► table 5-7

### ELECTROCARDIOGRAPHIC EVALUATION

#### Atrioventricular Blocks (AVBs)

| AVBs | PR Interval | Dropped Beat(s) | P:QRS Ratio |
|---|---|---|---|
| 1° | > 20 sec | No | 1:1 |
| 2° Type 1 | Normal to prolonged | Yes | Variable (ex: 3:2, 4:3, 5:4) |
| Type II | Normal, constant | Yes | |
| 3° | Variable | Yes | Variable |

#### Complete Bundle Branch Blocks (C-BBBs)

| Type | PR Interval | QRS Interval | QRS Shape | Check in Lead(s) |
|---|---|---|---|---|
| C-RBBB | normal | > 0.12 s | "M" shape | $V_1$ |
| C-LBBB | normal | > 0.12 s | "Rabbit ears" | $V_5$ and $V_6$ |

#### Premature Complexes

| Type | P Wave | QRS | Compensatory Pause | Cause(s) |
|---|---|---|---|---|
| PAC | Abnormal | Normal | No | Smoking, caffeine, alcohol, stress |
| PJC | None, inverted | Normal | No | Diseases, enhanced automaticity |
| PVC | None | Abnormal | Yes | Drugs, toxins, electrolyte disturbance |

#### Arrhythmias

| Type | Rate Beats/Min | Rhythm | P Wave | QRS |
|---|---|---|---|---|
| PAT | 150–250 | Regular | Upright | Normal |
| SVT | 150–250 | Regular | None | Normal |
| PJT | 150–250 | Regular | Inverted Retrograde | Normal |
| Aflutter | 250–350 | Usually Regular | Sawtooth Baseline | Normal |
| Afib | > 350 | Irregular | Undulating Baseline | Normal |
| PVT | 150–250 | "Regular" | — | Abnormal pattern |
| Vflutter | Irregular | Irregular | — | None identifiable |

PAC, premature atrial complex; PJC, premature junctional complex; PVC, premature ventricular complex; PAT, paroxysmal atrial tachycardia; SVT, supraventricular tachycardia; PJT, paroxysmal junctional tachycardia; Aflutter, atrial flutter; Afib, atrial fibrillation; PVT, paroxysmal ventricular tachycardia; Vflutter, ventricular flutter (between tachycardia and fibrillation).

more severe block. Type II AV block differs from type I in that, in addition to AV node block, there is an intermittent block in one bundle branch and a complete block in the other. This form of AV block can progress to third-degree AV block or asystole requiring CPR and/or transcutaneous pacing. In third-degree AV block, there is complete dissociation between atria and ventricles; atrial rate (usually normal) exceeds ventricular rate, which may be in the 40–60 beats per minute range, if there is a junctional escape beat, or 30–40 beats per minute if ventricular pacemaker is below AV junction. This condition requires immediate electronic pacing.

Tachyarrhythmias require suppression of the "irritable" focus with antiarrhythmic drugs; in emergent cases, electrocardioversion may be required. However, in cases of arrhythmias due to reentry phenomena, surgical ablation of the anomalous bypass tract may ameliorate the condition. Carotid massage and the Tilt test can be used to distinguish AV nodal reentrant tachyarrhythmias.

► Health Maintenance Issues

A number of conduction problems may be attributed to hyper-responsiveness to physiologic stimuli; others are due to pharmacologic agents and/or ischemic, inflammatory, and degenerative processes. While some of these are not amenable to modification, judicious use of pharmacologic agents goes a long way toward preventing some of these problems.

## X. PERIPHERAL VASCULAR DISEASE

► Scientific Concepts

Peripheral vascular disease (PVD) is narrowing of arteries supplying blood to upper and lower extremities. Lower-extremity disease is more common with decreased blood flow due to narrowing of aorta, iliac, and femoral arteries. The disease manifests itself by cramping, affecting calf muscles upon walking two blocks or less. PVD affects males more than females, is due to atherosclerosis, and is aggravated by smoking (Buerger's disease). In 10–20% of patients with suspected PVD, a definitive diagnosis cannot make the underlying cause.

► History & Physical

The onset of PVD is gradual. Over time, patients have thinning of skin and loss of hair on lower extremities. There is elevation pallor and dependent rubor of lower legs. Later findings included ulceration and gangrene of one or both lower legs. In severe cases, patients experience pain at rest during the night. Patients with severe arterial occlusive disease will have the six Ps: pain, pallor, pulselessness, paraesthesia, paralysis, and poikilothermia.

If calf pain develops after walking two blocks, disease is considered mild; it is considered moderate and severe when pain develops after one and one-half blocks, respectively. Severe disease calls for immediate surgical intervention. Calf pain is relieved by rest. In later stages of the disease, dorsalis pedis pulses may not be palpable and need to be verified by Doppler.

► Diagnostic Studies

MRI and Doppler ultrasonographic studies, with and without exercise, may be used to measure blood flow. Arteriograms are used to locate areas of blockage if bypass or angioplasty procedures are contemplated.

► Diagnosis

Diagnosis of blockage or narrowing can be achieved by using MRI, Doppler ultrasonograph, or arteriograms.

► Clinical Therapeutics

Medical treatment involves use of aspirin, 325 mg qd, or pentoxifylline, 400 mg tid, or cilostazol 100 mg bid (newest prescription) to ameliorate blood flow (platelet aggregation and/or vasodilation). Patients may undergo bypass surgery; 75 to 80% of grafts remain patent after 5 years. Laser, thermal, mechanical, or balloon angioplasty with stent placement can be used to improve blood flow. Lumbar sympathectomy has been used in a few cases to increase flow.

▶ Clinical Intervention

Patients who experience pain at rest or at night are at high risk for gangrene. These individuals are candidates for immediate surgical intervention. The surgical operative mortality is 2–5%. In the management of the acute arterial embolism patient, there is a 5–25% amputation rate.

▶ Health Maintenance Issues

Abstinence from tobacco products tends to allow development of collateral blood flow. Similarly, exercise and lowering of dietary fat reduce risk of arteriosclerosis and generate a better prognosis.

## XI. AORTIC ANEURYSM

▶ Scientific Concepts

Pathologic dilation of a blood vessel is an aneurysm. Most common area is abdominal or thoracic aorta. The principal cause is arteriosclerosis. However, syphilitic aortitis, media necrosis, and bacterial infections can cause the defect. True aneurysm involves all three layers—intima, media, and adventitia—whereas a pseudoaneurysm usually involves intima and media, but spares the adventitia.

Aortic aneurysm classification is based on location (abdominal vs. thoracic) and pattern of dissection (ascending vs. descending). Untreated, an aneurysm of 6 cm or greater carries mortality risk of 50% in 2 years. Surgery is recommended for aneurysms > 6 cm in diameter. The risk factors for aneurysm are: diabetes mellitus, tobacco use, elevated cholesterol, hypertension, positive family history, and homocystinuria.

▶ History & Physical

The pain of thoracic aneurysm has a tearing quality and radiates to the back. Patient may experience syncope, weakness, tracheal deviation, hoarseness, claudication, and CHF. The mediastinum may appear wide in the presence of a thoracic aneurysm. Patients with abdominal aneurysms have a pulsatile mass and almost always have an abdominal bruit.

▶ Diagnostic Studies

The usual labs include ECG, chest x-ray, transthoracic and transesophageal echocardiography, and ultrasonography; the latter is the most cost effective. CT and MRI are also useful. In some instances, an aortogram is obtained before surgery.

▶ Diagnosis

Diagnosis is established when aorta diameter is ≥ 4 cm. Surgery is performed if diameter is smaller and patient is symptomatic. Aortic dissection with tearing pain is a life-threatening condition.

▶ Clinical Therapeutics

In high-risk patients, treatment may include use of beta blockers when aortic diameter is 4–6 cm. Physicians believe that the beta blockers will slow the rate of progression of the dissection. The operative mortality rate for an abdominal aortic aneurysm is from 2–8%.

▶ Health Maintenance Issues

Since underlying cause of all aneurysms is arteriosclerosis, patients need to be counseled to control blood pressure, lower dietary fat, abstain from smoking, and increase physical activity.

## XII. THROMBOPHLEBITIS

▶ Scientific Concepts

Thrombophlebitis refers to partial or complete occlusion of veins in upper or lower extremity by inflammatory processes. Predisposing factors include trauma, CHF, surgery, bedrest, pregnancy, hypercoagulopathic states, use of oral contraceptives, and neoplasms, especially of lower extremity veins. Thrombophlebitis may result in sudden death because of embolization of clots into lungs.

▶ History & Physical

Patients with thrombophlebitis complain of tender, hot, and visible calf veins. In more extensive cases, pain may involve entire leg, including the thigh. Those who present with dyspnea, hemoptysis, syncope, tachycardia, and pleuritic chest pain may have pulmonary emboli. Patients with CHF, on oral contraceptive agents, or with history of varicose veins have higher incidence of thrombophlebitis.

There are 800,000 new cases of thrombophlebitis each year; 80% involve deep calf veins and 25% popliteal and femoral veins. Fixed splitting of $S_1$ and supraventricular arrhythmias are common with pulmonary emboli.

▶ Diagnostic Studies

Dual Doppler ultrasound and contrast venography are used to evaluate blood flow. Prothrombin time (PT), partial thromboplastin time (PTT), and international normalized ratio (INR) are used to measure clotting time to detect hypercoagulopathic states. Ventilation-perfusion scans are used to detect pulmonary thromboemboli. Special tests can be performed to detect deficiencies or excesses of antithrombin II, fibrinolytic proteins C and S, lupus anticoagulant, and homocystinuria. PTT is used to measure effectiveness of heparin in treating venous stasis.

▶ Diagnosis

Differential diagnosis of thrombophlebitis includes cellulitis, muscle strain or trauma, ruptured Baker's cyst, and obstruction of lymphatics.

▶ Clinical Therapeutics

Treatment of deep and superficial thrombophlebitis is often a judgment call. Following are guidelines for deep and superficial thrombophlebitis. All patients who are anticoagulated need to be observed carefully for bleeding.

***Superficial thrombophlebitis:*** If disease process is localized and not near saphenous femoral vein junction, local heat and bedrest with elevation are usually effective in limiting the thrombosis. A nonsteroidal anti-inflammatory drug can be used to relieve the symptoms. If the process is extensive or begins to involve the saphenous vein junction, or if the junction is involved initially, ligation of saphenous vein at saphenofemoral junction is indicated. Removal of the involved vein could result in more rapid recovery. Anticoagulation therapy is usually not warranted unless thrombophlebitis is rapidly progressing.

***Deep vein thrombophlebitis:*** All patients with extensive thrombophlebitis are placed on bedrest and leg elevation (10–15 degrees) to level of heart and slightly flexed. Rapid IV infusion (bolus) of heparin at 5,000–10,000 units followed by continuous infusion of 1,000–1,500 units qh until PTT is two times normal over 7–10 days may be used. A second option is to give IV heparin by heplock at 5,000 units over 8–12 hours for 7–10 days until PTT is two times normal. Warfarin is given before the termination of heparin treatment and continued for up to 3 months. To prevent venous stasis, patient may be treated with aspirin, 80–325 mg qd.

► Clinical Intervention

In cases of severe pulmonary embolization resulting in significant hemodynamic changes, surgery may be necessary. In cases of recurrent emboli, vena cava filter or plication may be indicated to prevent embolization. Most patients are back to normal activity by 3–6 weeks.

► Health Maintenance Issues

Patients with varicose veins should be encouraged to participate in reasonable exercise activities and to wear thromboembolic disease hose to prevent venous pooling and reduce risk of embolization.

## XIII. RHEUMATIC FEVER

► Scientific Concepts

Rheumatic fever is a very rare disease in the United States due to screening and treatment of beta-hemolytic streptococcal pharyngitis. The disease usually strikes children aged 5–15 years. Pharyngitis usually precedes rheumatic fever by 1–3 weeks. Valvular heart disease is common when condition is not treated. Mitral valve is affected in 75–80% of cases, aortic valve is affected 30% of the time, and tricuspid and pulmonary valves are affected 5% of the time.

► History & Physical

Patients with rheumatic fever present with major physical findings, including carditis, rigidity of valve cusps, fusion of commissures, shortening and fusion of chordae tendinea, valvular stenosis, valvular cusp lesions, pericarditis, pericardial friction rub, prolonged P-R interval on ECG, cardiomegaly, CHF, hepatomegaly, sinus tachycardia, erythema marginatum, subcutaneous nodules, Sydenham's chorea, and migratory polyarthritis. Minor physical findings include fever and polyarthralgia. Laboratory findings include P-R prolongation on ECG, elevated erythrocyte sedimentation rate (ESR), and positive and rising streptococcal titers. Two major findings or one major and one minor finding are required for the diagnosis of rheumatic fever. Patients with long-standing CHF can present with rales, ascites, edema, jugular venous distention, orthopnea, PND, and DOE at two blocks. Final diagnosis is made using Jones criteria (Table 5–8).

► table 5-8

### JONES CRITERIA FOR DIAGNOSIS OF RHEUMATIC FEVER

| Major Findings | Minor Findings |
| --- | --- |
| Carditis | Arthralgia |
| Polyarthralgia | Fever |
| Chorea | Elevated sedimentation rates |
| Erythema marginatum | C reactive protein |
| Subcutaneous nodules | Prolonged P-R interval on electrocardiogram (lead II) |

### ► Diagnostic Studies

In the acute phase of the disease, the following are observed: rise in antistreptolysin-O (ASO) titer and ESR, cardiomegaly and heart failure signs, prolonged P-R interval, arrhythmias, and pericarditis changes on ECG. Diagnosis is established when two major or one major and one minor Jones criteria are met. Both ASO titer and ESR must be elevated in the acute phase as well. The differential includes rheumatoid arthritis, osteomyelitis, endocarditis, systemic lupus erythematosus, sickle cell anemia, chronic meningococcemia, and Lyme disease.

### ► Clinical Therapeutics

Patients are treated with bedrest; aspirin, 600–900 mg q4h; and benzathine penicillin, 1.2 million units one time, intramuscularly, or procaine penicillin 600,000 units qd for 10 days. Patients with penicillin allergy may be treated with erythromycin, 250 mg PO tid for 10–14 days. Patients with associated severe pericarditis and CHF are also treated with 40–60 mg corticosteroids for 2 weeks (value unproven), then tapered. The immediate mortality rate in acute treatment is 1–2%. Thirty percent of the children infected with rheumatic fever will die within 10 years. Sixty-six percent of the patients who have had rheumatic fever will have detectable valvular abnormalities within 10 years of contact.

### ► Clinical Intervention

Patients are followed and treated for CHF. As with subacute bacterial endocarditis, antibiotic prophylaxis is given for genitourinary, dental, surgical, and obstetric procedures.

### ► Health Maintenance Issues

Acute sore throats with cervical lymphadenopathy require rapid strep screen and treatment. Patients are advised to complete the entire course of antibiotics.

## BIBLIOGRAPHY

Andreoli TE, Bennett JCM, Carpenter CJC, Plum F. *Cecil Essentials of Medicine,* 5th ed. Philadelphia: WB Saunders; 2001.

Barry MM, Amidon TM. Heart. In: Tierney LM Jr., McPhee SJ, Papadakis MA, eds. *Current Medical Diagnosis & Treatment,* 41th ed. New York: Lange Medical Books/McGraw-Hill; 2002.

Bickley LS, Hoekelman RA. *Bates' Guide to Physical Examination and History Taking,* 8th ed. Philadelphia: Lippincott; 2003.

DePilippi CR, Runge MS. Evaluating the chest pain patient: Scope of the problem. *Cardiol Clin* 17:307–326; 1999.

Johnson PA, Goldman L, Sacks DB, et al. Cardiac troponin T as a marker for myocardial ischemia in patients seen at the emergency department for acute chest pain. *Am Heart J* 137(6):1137–1144; 1999.

Massie BM. Systemic hypertension. In: Tierney LM Jr., McPhee SJ, Papadakis MA, eds. *Current Medical Diagnosis & Treatment,* 41th ed. New York: Lange Medical Books/ McGraw-Hill; 2002.

Skillings J. Therapeutic options in angina pectoris. *Clinical Advisor for Physician Assistants* June:29–37; 1999.

# Gastroenterology and Nutrition 6

*Nancy Ivansek, MA, PA-C*

## I. ESOPHAGUS

### A. Esophagitis

▶ Scientific Concepts

There are many causes including gastric acid reflux, infection (*Helicobacter pylori*, viral) or medication irritation. Usually the results of prolonged or too frequent relaxation of or decreased lower esophageal sphincter (LES) tone. Contributing factors include obesity, caffeine, high-fat diet, and pregnancy. Ulceration, erosion, and stricture formation are complications. Barrett's esophagus is considered a premalignant lesion and is present in up to 10% of patients with chronic reflux.

▶ History & Physical

Heartburn is typical symptom, most often occurring 30–60 minutes after eating. Other less specific signs and symptoms include substernal chest pain, regurgitation, water brash, cough, hoarseness, dysphagia, odynophagia, and asthma.

*[handwritten margin note: "? pain in swallowing solids & liquids"]*

▶ Diagnostic Studies

Upper endoscopy (esophagogastroduodenoscopy [EGD]) with biopsy if Barrett's suspected, 24-hour pH monitoring, manometry, barium swallow, and upper gastrointestinal (UGI) radiography. (Most sensitive testing is 24-hour pH monitoring.)

▶ Diagnosis

Often made on visual inspection; biopsy important if Barrett's suspected; abnormal number of reflux events on 24-hour monitoring or decrease LES tone on manometry.

▶ Clinical Therapeutics

Antacids offer rapid relief but the duration of action is less than 2 hours. Histamine (H$_2$) blockers (e.g., cimetidine, ranitidine) reduce acid, but proton pump inhibitors (e.g., omeprazole, lansoprazole) offer superior efficacy. Promotility agents (e.g., metoclopramide, cisipride) work by increasing LES pressure and enhance esophageal acid clearance and gastric emptying. Metoclopramide has many neuropsychiatric side effects and cisipride is no longer available in the United States.

▶ Clinical Intervention

Antireflux surgery for refractive cases, periodic endoscopic exam for screening in patients with Barrett's.

▶ Health Maintenance Issues

Most important admonition is to avoid lying down within 3 hours of eating. Weight loss if obese; reduce fat, citrus, caffeine, chocolate and alcohol; eliminate peppermint; stop smoking; elevate head of bed.

### B. Motor Disorders

▶ Scientific Concepts

May result from stroke, multiple neurologic disorders, aperistalsis, achalasia (failure of LES to relax), diffuse esophageal spasm, or scleroderma.

► **History & Physical**

Dysphagia (solid and/or liquid), sticking sensation, odynophagia, chest pain, heartburn, hoarseness.

► **Diagnostic Studies**

Barium esophagraphy, upper endoscopy, and esophageal manometry of LES.

► **Diagnosis**

Disordered peristalsis, increased LES pressures on manometry.

► **Clinical Therapeutics**

Prokinetic agents, anticholinergics, nitrates, calcium channel blockers, or beta agonists are effective in approximately 50%.

► **Clinical Intervention**

Balloon dilation, injection of botulinum toxin, surgical myotomy, and treatment of underlying conditions as indicated.

► **Health Maintenance Issues**

Eating more slowly and taking smaller boluses of food and warm liquids at the start of a meal may facilitate swallowing.

## C. Neoplasm

► **Scientific Concepts**

Usually develops in persons between 50 and 70 years of age. Overall ratio men to women 3:1. Two histologic types: adenocarcinoma and squamous cell carcinoma. In the United States, squamous cell more common in African Americans; adenocarcinoma in Caucasians. Squamous cell has high incidence in China and southeast Asia. Risk factors include heavy smoking, alcohol abuse, geography, vitamin deficiency, history of lye ingestion, achalasia, Barrett's esophagus. Diagnosis usually late, after metastasis/extension.

► **History & Physical**

Ninety percent have solid food dysphagia. Odynophagia; weight loss; coughing on swallowing; anorexia; chest or back pain. Bleeding rare.

► **Diagnostic Studies**

Upper endoscopy with biopsy very reliable, UGI barium study, ultrasound, computed tomography (CT) to evaluate for extension into adjacent structures.

► **Diagnosis**

Biopsy pathology establishes diagnosis.

► **Clinical Therapeutics**

Treatment depends upon the tumor stage. Combined radiation and chemotherapy is superior to radiation alone.

► **Clinical Intervention**

Surgical resection of the esophagus provides durable relief of dysphagia. For reasonably well-nourished patients without other serious comorbid conditions.

► **Health Maintenance Issues**

Five-year survival rate is less than 15%.

## D. Injury/Hemorrhage

▶ **Scientific Concepts**

External or iatrogenic trauma may rupture (Boerhaave syndrome); foreign body may obstruct trachea; caustic ingestions will produce scarring, motility disturbances, and predispose to cancer. Severe vomiting may cause Mallory–Weiss tear in mucosa with brisk bleeding.

▶ **History & Physical**

History of trauma or instrumentation, alcoholism, portal hypertension. History of large meal followed by forceful vomiting.

▶ **Diagnostic Studies**

Urgent upper endoscopy.

▶ **Diagnosis**

Evaluate extent of injury, identify bleeding points, locate foreign body.

▶ **Clinical Therapeutics**

Initial treatment is supportive; intravenous fluids, analgesic, and transfusion if indicated to prevent circulatory collapse.

▶ **Clinical Intervention**

Extraction of foreign body, endoscopic sclerotherapy of varices. Most Mallory–Weiss tears stop bleeding spontaneously. Vomiting should not be induced following caustic ingestion.

▶ **Health Maintenance Issues**

Long-term follow-up after caustic ingestion; alkali causes worse damage.

## II. STOMACH

### A. Gastritis/Duodenitis

▶ **Scientific Concepts**

Acute or chronic inflammation, localized or generalized, caused by drugs (nonsteroidal anti-inflammatory drugs [NSAIDs], aspirin, alcohol), caustic substances, stress related to severe illness, burns, postsurgical, or infection (most commonly *H. pylori*).

▶ **History & Physical**

Anorexia, epigastric pain, nausea, vomiting, hematemesis; erosive gastritis is usually asymptomatic.

▶ **Diagnostic Studies**

Upper endoscopy with biopsy is most sensitive.

▶ **Diagnosis**

Gastritis is not a clinical diagnosis. Diagnosis is made based on endoscopic and histological evaluation.

▶ **Clinical Therapeutics**

$H_2$ blockers given twice daily or daily; proton pump inhibitors (PPIs).

► Clinical Intervention

Remove or discontinue offending agents. If NSAID cannot be stopped, misoprostol may lessen reoccurrence in nonchildbearing age patients. Fluids and/or blood transfusion may be indicated in acute conditions.

► Health Maintenance Issues

Periodic endoscopic screening in chronic conditions; stop smoking.

## B. Peptic Ulcer Disease

► Scientific Concepts

Occurs as a break in the gastric or duodenal mucosa when normal mucosal defensive factors are impaired or overwhelmed by acid and pepsin. Hemorrhage, perforation, penetration, peritonitis can occur. Three major causes are recognized: NSAIDs, chronic *H. pylori,* and acid hypersecretion. Stricture, pyloric stenosis, and obstruction are late consequences. Gastric ulcers have malignancy potential, duodenal do not. Hemorrhage can be rapid and fatal when ulcer erodes arterial vessel.

► History & Physical

Periodic epigastric pain radiating to back or left upper quadrant, often at night; nausea, vomiting, hematemesis, melena. Pain may be exacerbated or relieved with food. Abrupt increase in pain signals perforation. NSAID ulcers are often painless.

► Diagnostic Studies

Upper endoscopy with antral biopsy for *H. pylori* is diagnostic procedure of choice. Noninvasive, relatively inexpensive evaluation for presence of *H. pylori* is now available in the form of serologic and breath (C-urea breath test) testing.

► Diagnosis

History can be highly suggestive, but definitive diagnosis is made during endoscopy.

► Clinical Therapeutics

If hospitalized, intravenous (IV) $H_2$ blockers with or without antacid. For outpatient setting, PPIs are more effective and have better compliance. Recommendations for *H. pylori* eradication include clarithromycin, metronidazole, amoxicillin, tetracycline, PPIs, and bismuth.

► Clinical Intervention

Nothing by mouth, possible nasogastric (NG) suction, fluids, transfusion, endoscopic sclerotherapy for active bleed, surgery for rebleed. Significant nonhemorrhagic ulcer may need hospitalization for bowel rest and IV $H_2$ blockers. Consider pH monitoring. Outpatients may be managed with twice-daily PPIs, antacids for breakthrough pain, and avoidance of evocative foods (e.g., caffeine, alcohol, citrus).

► Health Maintenance Issues

Aggressive prophylactic IV $H_2$ blockage in severely ill/intensive care unit patients; remove offending agents; stop smoking. Contribution of psychosocial stress is controversial. Rescope in 6 to 8 weeks to document healing of gastric ulcers. Bland/milk diets no longer felt to be helpful. Some evocative foods may need to be eliminated during healing.

## C. Nonulcer Dyspepsia

► Scientific Concepts

Up to two thirds of patients have no obvious cause for their dyspepsia symptoms. Symptoms may arise from increase visceral afferent sensitivity, delayed gastric emptying, and impaired accommodation to food complicated by psychosocial stressors. Patients have lifelong functional complaints interfering with work and social life. Typically, there are periods of resolution and exacerbation.

► History & Physical

Symptoms may be indistinguishable from peptic ulcer disease or gastroesophageal reflux disease. Patients with peptic ulcers tend to be over 45 years. Patient will have intermittent upper abdominal pain, gnawing, burning, and aching, with bloating, belching, and nausea. Often have extragastrointestinal complaints and show signs of anxiety or depression.

► Diagnostic Studies

Optimal cost-effective diagnostic approach is controversial. Upper endoscopy, indicated for all patients over 45.

► Diagnosis

Diagnosis is one of exclusion. Endoscopy will rule out structural versus functional cause.

► Clinical Therapeutics

All medications used in ulcer disease have been used with varying success. Prokinetic agents show some promise.

► Clinical Intervention

Avoid overevaluation and treatment once diagnosis is made.

► Health Maintenance Issues

A stable physician–patient interaction is key; reassurance and allaying fears (e.g., cancer) is therapeutic. Food diaries may reveal dietary or psychosocial exacerbators.

## D. Neoplasm

► Scientific Concepts

Gastric adenocarcinoma is second most common cancer worldwide. Incidence in the United States is declining. Men are affected twice as often as women. Tobacco use and consumption of overly processed foods and nitrites contribute to risk. Premalignant conditions include gastric polyp, pernicious anemia, atrophic gastritis, previous gastrectomy.

► History & Physical

Usually asymptomatic until quite advanced. Presenting symptoms include dyspepsia epigastric pain, early satiety, weight loss, anorexia, and vomiting. Bleeding rare.

► Diagnostic Studies

Endoscopy with cytology brushing and biopsy. UGI may not detect small or superficial lesions.

► Diagnosis

On pathology, all gastric ulcers need biopsy and follow-up.

▶ Clinical Therapeutics

For adenocarcinoma, chemotherapy has not been shown to prolong life but may provide palliation.

▶ Clinical Intervention

Surgery with follow-up radiation is therapy of choice.

▶ Health Maintenance Issues

Prognosis depends on stage. Five-year survival with adenocarcinoma is approximately 12%. Disease is diagnosed late after spread or extension. Prognosis with lymphoma is better.

## III. SMALL BOWEL

### A. Small Bowel Obstruction

▶ Scientific Concepts

The most common causes of obstruction are adhesions (more frequent in patients with prior abdominal surgery). Other causes are: external or internal hernias, stricture, endometriosis, volvulus, intussusception, and rarely neoplasm. Adynamic or paralytic ileus occurs following open abdominal surgery, peritonitis, pancreatitis, cholecystitis, or pneumonia. Exacerbated by narcotics.

▶ History & Physical

Symptoms depend on location. Proximal obstruction presents with minimal distention, diffuse abdominal pain, nausea, and protracted vomiting. Pain is more crampy and distention greater the more distal the lesion. Mechanical obstructions produce hyperactive bowel sounds; they will become absent late in the course and are an ominous sign. Bowel sounds characteristically absent in ileus. Dehydration and obstipation may occur. Careful examination for abdominal wall hernias.

▶ Diagnostic Studies

Plain abdominal films; acute abdominal series, kidney, ureter, bladder (KUB). Barium radiography can confirm location. The cause should be identified, but often these resolve spontaneously with decompression.

▶ Diagnosis

Plain films reveal ladderlike pattern of dilated small bowel with multiple air–fluid levels, dilated proximal loops, and lack of air in rectum. Barium studies to document transit time to cecum.

▶ Clinical Therapeutics

Fluid replacement and stabilization of patient, electrolyte correction with mechanical obstruction. Discontinue narcotics and anticholinergics with ileus.

▶ Clinical Intervention

Bowel rest, NG decompression, barium studies may be therapeutic as well as diagnostic. Surgical intervention is determined by the underlying disorder; correction of mechanical obstruction prior to intestinal ischemia leading to necrosis, perforation, and peritonitis.

► Health Maintenance Issues

Prompt presentation to health care provider with onset of symptoms.

## B. Irritable Bowel Syndrome

► Scientific Concepts

Classified as a functional idiopathic disorder with no organic component to the symptoms complex. Up to 20% of adult population have symptoms compatible with the diagnosis. Entity characterized by more than 3 months of lower abdominal pain and bowel complaints occurring continuously or intermittently. Probably representing clinical manifestations of a heterogeneous group of disorders.

► History & Physical

Intermittent crampy abdominal pain and distention relieved/altered by defecation, stools looser and more frequent, mucus with the stool, feeling of incomplete evacuation. Symptoms do not interfere with sleep. Physical examination essentially normal, though some with mild tenderness to palpation.

► Diagnostic Studies

With careful history, few studies required. Complete blood count (CBC), serologic tests, serum albumin, erythrocyte sedimentation rate (ESR), and stool occult blood tests should be normal. If diarrhea present, check thyroid function and stool for ova and parasites. Younger patients need flexible sigmoidoscopy; those over 40 require full colonoscopy.

► Diagnosis

Physical examination and endoscopic examination normal.

► Clinical Therapeutics

Two thirds of patients respond to education and reassurance. No one agent superior to placebo. Depending on symptoms, antispasmodics, antidiarrheal, anticonstipation, or psychotropic agents may be useful.

► Clinical Intervention

None required or appropriate.

► Health Maintenance Issues

A dietary/symptom log may help identify triggers. Dietary fiber must be increased gradually, often with recommended supplements such as psyllium. Reassurance, avoidance of overtesting and medicating. Address any psychiatric or psychological disorder.

## C. Infectious Gastroenteritis

► Scientific Concepts

Most enteric infections result from oral–fecal transmission. The toxins are either preformed, in which the illness occurs within hours after ingestion, or toxins form after adherence or penetration into bowel wall. Symptoms then occur after several days. Norwalk virus is the most common cause of infectious gastroenteritis/diarrhea in the United States.

► History & Physical

Travel, food, recent antibiotic treatment, concurrent household illness, and sexual history important. Acute, crampy abdominal pain with watery diarrhea, rarely with blood.

► Diagnostic Studies

Stool culture, *Clostridium difficile* titer, colonoscopy with biopsy when indicated.

► Diagnosis

Often made by history, stool culture for enteric pathogens and/or biopsy.

► Clinical Therapeutics

Avoid empiric antibiotics in immune-competent adult, especially with *Salmonella.* Travelers' diarrhea, cholera, pseudomembranous colitis, *Campylobacter,* and all sexually transmitted infections require appropriate antibiotic therapy. Fluid replacement, oral or IV, necessary in most cases. Ciprofloxacin or another fluoroquinolone is recommended treatment for *Campylobacter, Shigella* and *Yersinia* as well as traveler's diarrhea. Metronidazole is used to treat *C. difficile.*

*[handwritten margin note: Metronidazole for C. dificile]*

► Clinical Intervention

None required.

► Health Maintenance Issues

Education regarding food-borne organisms and necessity of proper hand washing, food handling, and cooking. Adequate community sanitation. Prophylaxis is recommended when traveling to some endemic areas (e.g., cholera). However, it is generally not recommended for common travelers' diarrhea.

## D. Inflammatory Bowel Disease (IBD)

► Scientific Concepts

IBD refers to both regional enteritis (Crohn's disease [CD]) and ulcerative colitis (UC). There are many similarities but treatment and prognosis differ; thus, it is important to make correct diagnosis. Etiology uncertain but both probably immune/autoimmune disorder with familial and environmental factors. Important to rule out infectious causes as source of chief complaint.

Crohn's is transmural granulomatous disease affecting any part of gastrointestinal (GI) tract from mouth to anus. Nearly all patients have involvement of terminal ileum. Extraintestinal manifestations (skin, eye, joint) are common and may be presenting complaint. "Skip areas" of normal GI tissue are characteristic. Complications include fistulae, perianal disease, stricture, malnutrition, growth retardation, and carcinoma.

UC is inflammatory disease of mucosa and submucosa only. Usually develops in a continuous pattern, with rectum nearly always involved. Islands of pseudopolyps seen on endoscopy and destruction of haustral markings on x-ray (leaving colon appearing flat) are characteristic. Complications include toxic megacolon, hemorrhage, perforation, and rarely stricture. Cancer more prevalent than with Crohn's disease.

► History & Physical

CD presents with colicky right lower quadrant (RLQ) pain and diarrhea with fever and weight loss. Physical examination finds tender RLQ and possible mass, often perianal disease. Bleeding rare. UC patients often present with bloody diarrhea, crampy lower abdominal pain, and fecal urgency; fever and weight loss variable. Individuals characteristically have periods of symptomatic flare-ups and remissions.

*[Handwritten margin note: "Cobblestoning" and String sign w/ Crohn's disease. Loss of haustral marking w/ U.C.]*

▶ Diagnostic Studies

Stool culture, ova and parasite exam, other labs (CBC, electrolytes, ESR, C reactive protein [CRP]) nonspecific but reflect severity of disease, inflammation. Barium studies and colonoscopy are indicated and have characteristic findings as above, but must be avoided when patient is acutely ill.

▶ Diagnosis

Stool with mucus, blood, and/or white blood cells; edematous, friable colonic mucosa. On x-ray, cobblestoning and string sign with CD. Loss of haustral markings with UC.

▶ Clinical Therapeutics

Sulfasalazine, 5-aminosalicylate acid enemas, steroid enemas, systemic steroids, methotrexate, antibiotics, antidiarrheals. Folic acid in UC decreases risk of cancer development.

▶ Clinical Intervention

Total colectomy in UC for refractive cases and cases of toxic megacolon. In CD, surgery should be avoided unless patient has obstruction, perforation, severe bleed, or intractable disease unresponsive to other therapies.

▶ Health Maintenance Issues

Psychosocial aspects are many, support groups widely available, family counseling may be needed. All patients with active IBD require colonoscopy every 1 to 2 years to screen for cancer.

## E. Ischemic Bowel Disease

▶ Scientific Concepts

Mesenteric ischemia typically occurs both acutely and chronically in patients over 45 with history of arteriosclerosis, coronary artery disease, myocardial infarction, congestive heart failure, peripheral vascular disease, or after stroke or abdominal aortic aneurysm repair. Ischemic colitis occurs in patients with similar profile but develops secondary to decreased perfusion of smaller vessels of intestinal wall. Focal ischemia often results from episodes of hypotension. Intestinal angina occurs with repeated bouts of ischemia. Infarction followed by perforation may result.

▶ History & Physical

Classically "pain out of proportion" to physical findings. Severe crampy abdominal pain, often worse postprandially. Presentation may be similar to IBS. Initially, abdominal examination may be normal or include decreased bowel sounds, mild distention, and tenderness progressing to a rigid, acute surgical abdomen.

▶ Diagnostic Studies

CBC, amylase, lipase, lactic acid, and Doppler ultrasound. Arteriography is the gold standard.

▶ Diagnosis

High index of suspicion for diagnosis because specific signs and symptoms do not often appear. Increased white blood count (WBC), amylase, and lactic acid. Evidence of significant narrowing/occlusion of vessels on imaging. Diagnosis often made at laparotomy.

▶ Clinical Therapeutics
Bowel rest, fluids, antibiotics.

▶ Clinical Intervention
Most require urgent surgical intervention.

▶ Health Maintenance Issues
Vigilance is required in patients with vascular disease presenting with abdominal pain.

## F. Neoplasm

▶ Scientific Concepts
Benign and malignant tumors are rare. Adenomatous is most common tumor. Carcinoid is most common, neuroendocrine tumor; most are malignant. Adenocarcinomas account for 30 to 40 of small bowel cancers and are very aggressive. Lymphoma has better prognosis.

▶ History & Physical
Often asymptomatic. Symptoms include obstruction, GI bleed (occult or frank), dysphagia. Characteristic symptomatic carcinoid presents with facial flushing and diarrhea.

▶ Diagnostic Studies
UGI with small bowel follow-through, abdominal CT, EGD for proximal lesions. Using an enteroscope, biopsies can be obtained.

▶ Diagnosis
Histological exam of surgical specimen.

▶ Clinical Therapeutics
Depend on staging. Advanced disease often treated with chemotherapy and radiation. Lymphoma responds more favorably to chemotherapy.

▶ Clinical Intervention
Surgical resection and staging.

▶ Health Maintenance Issues
None.

# IV. COLON/RECTUM

## A. Constipation

▶ Scientific Concepts
Symptom of delayed transit time and reduced water content in stool. Associated with excessive difficulty or straining at defecation. Often due to lack of exercise, inadequate fiber in diet, pregnancy, tumor, volvulus, intussusception, rectocele, obstruction, hypothyroidism, medications, or psychiatric disorder. May result from laxative abuse with lifelong dependence.

▶ History & Physical
Bowel movements occur infrequently (less than every other day), overly hard, and difficult and painful to pass.

▶ Diagnostic Studies

Colonoscopy, barium enema to rule out structural abnormality. Thyroid function if hypothyroidism suspected.

▶ Diagnosis

Constipation is a symptom, not a disease; therefore, underlying causes need investigation.

▶ Clinical Therapeutics

Increase fluid and fiber, fiber supplements if necessary, occasional stool softener or laxative. Treat underlying disorder.

▶ Clinical Intervention

If severe, soap suds (or alternative) enema, or manual disimpaction providing that obstruction requiring surgical intervention has been ruled out.

▶ Health Maintenance Issues

Attention to adequate diet and fluids, increase physical activity, discontinue offending medications. Reassure that bowel function is variable.

## B. Appendicitis

▶ Scientific Concepts

Inflammatory condition secondary to obstruction, followed by bacterial proliferation, edema, and vascular compromise. If untreated, necrosis, perforation, and peritonitis may occur. Age of increased occurrence is bimodal at 10 to 30 and over 60, with equal male/female prevalence.

▶ History & Physical

Pain may be sudden in onset. Initially, periumbilical pain migrating to RLQ (McBurney's point) over several hours and possibly days; nausea, vomiting, anorexia, and fever. Physical examination reveals tender RLQ, diminished or absent bowel sounds, guarding and rebound as peritonitis develops. Pain with flexion of iliopsoas or rotation of obturator muscles and exacerbation of pain with rectal exam also supports the diagnosis of appendicitis.

▶ Diagnostic Studies

Careful history, with attention in female patients to date of last menstrual period and possibility of pregnancy. Lab studies to include CBC, urinalysis, urinary chorionic gonadotropin. CT becoming gold standard; abdominal ultrasound to rule out gynecological source for RLQ pain (most critically, ectopic pregnancy).

▶ Diagnosis

Most often, clinical diagnosis is made on history and physical and confirmed in operating room. Diagnosis more difficult in pregnant females, patients on steroids, and elderly, who may not have pain, fever, or elevated WBC. Mortality is increased in the elderly.

▶ Clinical Therapeutics

Preoperative antibiotics, fluids.

▶ Clinical Intervention

Strictly surgical disease, no role for nonsurgical treatment. May be performed as traditional open procedure or laparoscopically.

► Health Maintenance Issues
None.

## C. Diverticular Disease

► Scientific Concepts
Common disorder of Western civilization with low-fiber diet. Not true diverticular, when formed only by mucosa and submucosa where blood vessels penetrate colon wall. Most prevalent in narrower sigmoid colon. Complications include progression to diverticulitis with microperforation, bleeding, abscess, peritonitis, and fistula formation to bladder/vagina.

► History & Physical
Often asymptomatic. Crampy lower abdominal pain, usually left lower quadrant (LLQ), with alternating constipation/diarrhea. With diverticulitis, fever and pain become more constant, lower gastrointestinal (LGI) bleed becomes more likely.

► Diagnostic Studies
Barium enema, colonoscopy, sigmoidoscopy. Avoid these studies in acute phase or if perforation is suspected. CT is preferred study.

► Diagnosis
Diverticula easily seen on barium x-ray or endoscopy. Will see blood and/or pus as signs of inflammation with diverticulitis.

► Clinical Therapeutics
High-fiber diet, bowel rest. Add antibiotic if diverticulitis diagnosed. Quinolones, broad-spectrum penicillins with metronidazole most commonly used.

► Clinical Intervention
Surgical resection for abscess, stricture, fistula, or persistent blood loss.

► Health Maintenance Issues
Maintain proper bowel function with adequate fiber, fluid, and exercise.

## D. Colon Carcinoma

► Scientific Concepts
Currently second leading visceral neoplasm in males and females in the United States. Contributing factors include low-fiber, high-fat/red meat diets; exposure to environmental toxins; and prolonged exposure to bile acids. Risk factors include advanced age; personal or family history (first-degree relative) of colon, genital, or breast cancer; familial polyposis; > 10-year history of IBD. Most tumors are thought to arise in an adenomatous polyp.

► History & Physical
Adequate history taking important to establish risk factors and initiate screening since signs and symptoms are often vague and occur late. LGI bleeding (either occult or frank), weight loss, change in bowel habits or stool caliper, change of appetite, malaise. Occasionally, palpable mass felt on physical examination. Right-sided lesions, though less common, present even later. A digital rectal exam discovers almost 15% of colorectal cancers.

▶ **Diagnostic Studies**

Fecal occult blood tests (FOBT) can detect blood in stool but have a low specificity for colorectal cancer. Flexible sigmoidoscopy, barium enema, followed by complete colonoscopy. If symptoms are suspicious or patient is high risk, proceed with formal colonoscopy. Initial labs include CBC, liver function test, and, if lesion confirmed, carcinoembryonic antigen, and CA19-9.

▶ **Diagnosis**

Apple-core lesion on x-ray, mass on endoscopy biopsied and confirmed by pathology. Extent of disease and prognosis determined by Duke's classification.

▶ **Clinical Therapeutics**

Chemotherapy dependent on Duke's stage of disease.

▶ **Clinical Intervention**

All require surgical intervention either with resection or, in some cases of lower rectal tumors, ablation with yttrium aluminum garnet laser. Radiation often adjunctive.

▶ **Health Maintenance Issues**

Decrease fat and red meat in diet, increase fiber and antioxidants (beta carotene; vitamins A, C, E; and estrogen all reduce risk). Avoid constipation. Participate in recommended screening procedures dependent on age and risk factors. Guidelines suggest yearly occult blood testing after 40 and periodic sigmoidoscopy or colonoscopy after age 50 in the low-risk individual. When risk factors such as family history, ulcerative colitis, or familial polyposis exist, screening must begin earlier and be more aggressive. Occult blood testing can be misleading, with many false negatives and positives, yet still an inexpensive and somewhat useful initial approach. Sensitivity improves with serial testing (three to six specimens recommended).

## E. Hemorrhoids

▶ **Scientific Concepts**

Arise secondary to increased pressure exerted on anus from straining, obesity, lifting, with pregnancy when hormone changes exacerbate, or with alcoholism secondary to cirrhosis. Internal hemorrhoids occur above dentate line and originate from superior hemorrhoidal vessels; they may bleed but are not painful unless prolapsed or thrombosed. External hemorrhoids arise from inferior hemorrhoidal venous plexus and are typically more symptomatic.

▶ **History & Physical**

Bright red rectal bleeding with bowel movement, pain, sense of fullness, pruritus, mucus in stool. Will appear purple with or without erosion when thrombosed.

▶ **Diagnostic Studies**

Visual exam, anoscopy.

▶ **Diagnosis**

Friable, edematous, tender, rectal mass with or without erosion, maceration.

▶ Clinical Therapeutics

Steroid and/or anesthetic creams, suppositories (to decrease swelling and inflammation and/or to promote evacuation), warm sitz bath.

▶ Clinical Intervention

Thrombosed hemorrhoids require urgent evacuation and excision. Partial or complete hemorrhoidectomy if refractive or recurrent as indicated.

▶ Health Maintenance Issues

Proper bowel function requires adequate fluid, fiber, and exercise. Avoid straining. Some patients may require stool softeners.

## F. Anal Fissure

▶ Scientific Concepts

Tearing of anoderm secondary to straining with hard stool. Sphincter now exposed and goes into spasm, which fails to relax with next defecation, so injury becomes more extensive and may lead to anal ulcer. Occurs at the anterior and posterior midline position; if found elsewhere, consider Crohn's, tuberculosis, malignancy, abscess, or sexually transmitted infection.

▶ History & Physical

Abrupt-onset, intense rectal pain with bowel movement, blood on tissue; constipation often follows due to fear of recurrent pain.

▶ Diagnostic Studies

Visual examination, anoscopy often difficult if unanesthetized.

▶ Diagnosis

Observation of linear tear.

▶ Clinical Therapeutics

Bulk agents, stool softeners, hydrocortisone suppositories/cream, sitz bath.

▶ Clinical Intervention

Occasionally require sphincterotomy.

▶ Health Maintenance Issues

Maintain good bowel function with fluid, fiber, and exercise.

## G. Anorectal Abscesses and Fistulae (Fistula-in-Ano)

▶ Scientific Concepts

Perianal abscesses result from obstruction, stasis, and finally infection of cryptoglandular tissue. Hard stool, diarrhea, foreign bodies, and anal intercourse may all be traumatic and begin this process. Fistulous tracts are inflammatory, originate in the abscess, and communicate to skin. Proper history is important to rule out underlying contributory conditions (e.g., diabetes, IBD, engagement in anal sexual activity).

▶ History & Physical

Acute pain and swelling worsening with ambulation and defecation. Pus drains from fistulous ostia. Fever and chills may accompany. Urgent problem in the diabetic and immunocompromised patient.

► Diagnostic Studies

Visual examination, palpation of tender, red mass; anoscopy transrectal ultrasound (generally requires anesthesia).

► Diagnosis

By inspection on physical examination.

► Clinical Therapeutics

Broad-spectrum antibiotics, IV are often required.

► Clinical Intervention

Surgical drainage of abscess done urgently, preferably in operating room. Fistula-in-ano requires excision of fistulous tract; not emergent condition.

► Health Maintenance Issues

Avoid rectal trauma; seek prompt attention in patient with diabetes or malignancy or immunocompromised patient.

## H. Pilonidal Disease

► Scientific Concepts

May occur congenitally due to malformations in sacrococcygeal area. Sinus formation and small skin pits develop. Hair (after puberty) invades and acts as foreign body creating draining sinus.

► History & Physical

Pain, swelling, and purulent drainage from ostia in gluteal cleft. Most always found with embedded hairs. Does not communicate with anorectum, which differentiates it from fistula-in-ano.

► Diagnostic Studies

None.

► Diagnosis

Inspection on physical examination.

► Clinical Therapeutics

Antibiotic to cover skin flora.

► Clinical Intervention

Sitz bath, surgical incision, drainage with either primary closure or marsupialization. May recur when primarily surgically closed.

► Health Maintenance Issues

Patient may need to keep area shaved to prevent recurrence once treated.

## V. GALLBLADDER

► Scientific Concepts

Cholecystitis occurs both acutely and chronically as result of inflammation of gallbladder lining secondary to obstructive stones/sludge or infection. When stones are present, most are composed of cholesterol, having precipitated out of an inadequate bile salt pool. Factors predisposing to stones include multiple pregnancies, rapid weight loss, oral contraceptives, ileal disease (Crohn's), and genetics. The remaining stones are pigmented of bilirubin from excessive hemolysis. Except in the diabetic, asymptomatic stones do not require therapy.

▶ **History & Physical**

Patients complain of epigastric to right upper quadrant (RUQ) sharp, wavelike pain, which may radiate around and into back, often with nausea and vomiting. Episodes last approximately 3 hours. On palpation of the RUQ, patient may stop inspiration abruptly and involuntarily guard (Murphy's sign). Attacks frequently begin postprandially. May present with fever, chills, and ileus.

▶ **Diagnostic Studies**

Gallbladder ultrasound preferred. If negative but clinically suspicious, nuclear scan (hepato-iminodiacetic acid [HIDA]) may be added. Some centers do oral cholecystograms. Both studies add cholecystokinin to stimulate contraction and image gallbladder function. WBC and liver function profile (LFP: alanine transaminase [ALT], aspartate transaminase [AST], alkaline phosphatase, bilirubin).

▶ **Diagnosis**

Labs may all be modestly elevated. Presence of stones, sludge (thickened bile is semiobstructing), thickened gallbladder wall, dilated cystic/common duct, grossly enlarged bag, and/or reduced contraction support diagnosis.

▶ **Clinical Therapeutics**

Oral bile acid therapy (ursodeoxycholine) appropriate only in patients completely unfit for surgery due to limited efficacy. IV antibiotics and fluid resuscitation preoperatively in acute setting. Antispasmodics may be helpful in the less acute patient awaiting surgery.

▶ **Clinical Intervention**

Cholecystectomy—vast majority done laparoscopically.

▶ **Health Maintenance Issues**

In the mildly symptomatic, low-fat diet and antispasmodics will provide temporary relief. In general, gallbladder disease cannot be prevented.

## VI. PANCREAS

### A. Pancreatitis

#### 1. Acute Pancreatitis

▶ **Scientific Concepts**

In the industrialized world, 70–80% is due to alcohol abuse or gallstones. Other etiologies include trauma, drugs, hyperlipidemia, post endoscopic retrograde cholangiopancreatography (ERCP)/surgery, hypercalcemia, infection, and tumor. Severity ranges from mild, isolated, self-limited to severe, life-threatening condition with massive hemorrhage and autodigestion of abdominal contents.

► **History & Physical**

Fulminating, continuous, abdominal pain, may radiate to back and flanks. Nausea, vomiting, fever often present. Tachycardia, tachypnea, and hypotension when severe.

► **Diagnostic Studies**

Serum amylase, lipase, liver function test (LFTs), CBC, plain abdominal films, abdominal ultrasound, CT, ERCP.

► **Diagnosis**

Amylase and lipase elevated in majority, but levels do not correlate with severity. Elevated 6-hour urinary amylase is the gold standard. Alkaline phosphatase and bilirubin elevated with biliary obstruction. Plain film shows isolated air–fluid level near pancreas (sentinel loop); ultrasound will identify ductal dilatation and stones. CT may define pancreatic changes.

► **Clinical Therapeutics**

Aggressive fluid replacement, IV antibiotics, pain control avoiding morphine (elevates ampullary pressure), and hyperalimentation in some cases.

► **Clinical Intervention**

Bowel rest with or without NG tube drainage, ERCP for stone extraction. Vigilant monitoring of status and development of complications, including pancreatic pseudocyst and progression to hemorrhagic pancreatitis.

► **Health Maintenance Issues**

Sobriety is mandatory for alcohol-induced disease. Discontinue offending medications and treat hyperlipidemia.

## 2. Chronic Pancreatitis

► **Scientific Concepts**

Ninety percent due to chronic alcohol ingestion, anatomical anomalies (pancreas divisum), familial, ductal obstruction from previous scarring, fibrosis, or stent placement. Ten to 30% of cases are idiopathic.

► **History & Physical**

Periodic or continuous periumbilical pain radiating straight through to back, malnutrition, weight loss, steatorrhea, and diabetes mellitus.

► **Diagnostic Studies**

ERCP, ultrasound, CT plain abdominal films. Labs may or may not be useful.

► **Diagnosis**

Calcification may be seen on plain films or ultrasound. CT delineates inflammatory changes; ERCP reveals ductal dilatation/stricture.

► **Clinical Therapeutics**

Analgesia, usually requiring opioids, replacement of pancreatic enzymes, insulin if hyperglycemic.

► **Clinical Intervention**

Pain control difficult. Partial pancreatectomy in severe cases. Surgery may also be required for complications, most commonly pseudocyst drainage.

► Health Maintenance Issues

Sobriety is mandatory to halt progression.

## B. Pancreatic Neoplasm

► Scientific Concepts

Nearly all tumors are adenocarcinomas, being dense, firm, fibrotic, thus easily able to invade adjacent structures. These characteristics are usually responsible for presenting symptoms. Advanced age, male sex, smoking, chronic pancreatitis, and exposure to dichlorodiphenyltrichloroethan (DDT) are risk factors.

► History & Physical

Few characteristic signs of primary disease. May complain of vague, dull, upper abdominal pain, weight loss, anorexia, diarrhea, and jaundice. Painless jaundice is presumed to be pancreatic cancer until proven otherwise.

► Diagnostic Studies

CT, magnetic resonance imaging (MRI), ERCP, CT-guided percutaneous biopsy, exploratory laparotomy may be necessary. CA19-9 and 242 tumor markers are reasonably specific.

► Diagnosis

Confirmed only by histologic examination of biopsy specimen.

► Clinical Therapeutics

Chemotherapy and radiation for palliation only. No curative therapeutics.

► Clinical Intervention

Less than 15% amenable to surgical resection (Whipple procedure); even those have poor 5-year survival. Aggressive pain control with permanent IV catheter, nerve block.

► Health Maintenance Issues

Measures are supportive and palliative. Tumors are aggressive, fast growing, and fatal.

## VII. LIVER

### A. Hepatitis

► Scientific Concepts

Inflammatory condition of liver parenchyma leading to necrosis. Causes include viral types A–G, alcohol, drugs, toxins, autoimmune and hereditary disorder, cytomegalovirus, Epstein–Barr virus, and not-yet-identified non-A non-B virus. Types A and E are endemic in underdeveloped countries and are spread via oral–fecal route. They cause only acute hepatitis and do not become chronic or exist in carrier state. Types B and C are spread parenterally. Types G appears as a coinfection with C. IV drug users, promiscuous individuals, homosexual males, and health care workers exposed to blood/blood products are at risk. Hepatitis B and C may result in acute, chronic, or asymptomatic carrier states and may progress to cirrhosis and hepatocellular carcinoma. Type D only coexists with B as a "superinfection," increasing morbidity and mortality. Alcohol alone is generally not a causative factor when consumed at levels less than 80 g/d in males and 40 g/d nonpregnant females. However, other co-existing conditions (e.g., viral hepatitis, drug use, malnutrition) may accelerate alcoholic fatty liver and proceed to fulminant hepatitis. Drugs may present as direct hepatotoxins or may indirectly interfere with normal liver metabolism. Drugs may also cause idiosyncratic reactions. Hemochromatosis (common), Wilson's disease (rare), and alpha-1-antitrypsin deficiency all may result in hepatitis.

### ► History & Physical

History to include age, gender, race, travel, immunizations, occupation, sexual preferences/behaviors, IV drug use, medications, and family history. Presenting symptoms nonspecific, often flulike, malaise, fatigue, fever, arthralgia, arthritis, rash, jaundice, dark urine, pale stools, upper abdominal fullness/pain. Physical findings may not be present or, depending on severity, include hepatosplenomegaly, lymphadenopathy, ascites, and the stigmata of chronic alcoholism.

### ► Diagnosis Studies

LFP including alkaline phosphatase, bilirubin, ALT, AST, and gamma-glutamyl transpeptidase (GGT). CBC, viral serology, alcohol/drug (illicit and legitimate) screen. Liver biopsy often indicated.

### ► Diagnosis

ALT and AST, both absolute levels and their ratios, can help identify likely cause. Alcoholics often present with depleted serum protein levels, anemia, macrocytic and target red blood cells, elevated GGT. Elevated bilirubin and alkaline phosphate indicate either biliary or intrahepatic obstruction. Appropriate viral serology can identify the specific virus and status of infection. Rapid return to normal LFP following withdraw of offending drug confirms chemical hepatitis. Biopsy specimen can demonstrate progression to cirrhosis.

### ► Clinical Therapeutics

Supportive care, adequate fluid and nutrition, avoidance of liver toxins mainstay of therapy for all types of hepatitis. No additional measures needed for viral types A and E. Interferon is effective in reducing severity, complications, and long-term sequelae in types B and C. Must be instituted early. If infection becomes fulminant, patient will require protein restriction and lactulose to prevent hepatic encephalopathy, high-dose corticosteroids, and an exchange transfusion. Autoimmune hepatitis may respond to steroids. Hemochromatosis and Wilson's disease require long-term chelation therapy and phlebotomy. Nonimmunized individuals with accidental or inadvertent exposure to blood/body fluids should receive hepatitis B immune globulin immediately. Infants exposed perinatally, household contacts, and sexual partners should also be offered post-exposure prophylaxis when not previously immunized.

### ► Clinical Interventions

Liver transplantation is mandatory if patient fails to respond to aggressive therapy and continues to deteriorate.

▶ Health Maintenance Issues

Appropriate immunizations for patients traveling to endemic areas for types A and B. Type A vaccine indicated for military personnel, lab workers, homosexual males, IV drug users, day care workers, and primate handlers. Type B vaccine to all infants, health care workers, patients on dialysis, those with high-risk behaviors, regular recipients of blood product, and inmates. Avoidance of occupational and environmental toxins (e.g., organic solvents). Moderate alcohol consumption is permitted in the nonalcoholic individual; however, strict abstinence is mandatory in the alcoholic. Proper nutrition with vitamin supplementation also helpful.

## B. Cirrhosis

▶ Scientific Concepts

Defined as presence of fibrosis with creation of excessive extracellular matrix. This interferes with normal blood flow through liver, impairing nutrient/metabolite exchange and reducing synthesis of hepatic products. Initially, liver enlarges, firm nodules form, liver then gradually becomes shrunken. Most frequent causes are alcohol consumption and viral hepatitis. Others include drugs, toxins, autoimmune complexes, biliary obstruction, congestive heart failure, and some metabolic or genetic abnormalities. Ultimate complications of portal hypertension, GI hemorrhage, and liver failure are fatal.

▶ History & Physical

History suspicious for any type of hepatitis or family history. Onset may be dramatic if late stage. Early presentation is more subtle with complaints of malaise, fatigue, easy bruising. On examination, ascites, jaundice, striae, hepatomegaly with mild tenderness. Liver may be enlarged and firm or shrunken and nonpalpable. Splenomegaly, muscle wasting, mental confusion/encephalopathy are late manifestations. When advanced to portal hypertension, signs include hemorrhoids, caput medusa, esophageal varices, and splenomegaly. No clinical findings are diagnostic.

▶ Diagnostic Studies

LFP, 5′ nucleotidase, albumin, protime, bleeding time, viral hepatitis panel, serum ammonia, abdominal ultrasound, CT, ERCP; ultimately liver biopsy will confirm diagnosis. EGD may demonstrate esophageal varices. Because of the increased risk of coagulopathy, the biopsy is best done with laparoscopic direct visualization.

▶ Diagnosis

Mild elevation of hepatocellular enzymes, decreased albumin and coagulation proteins. (Prothrombin time is reliable monitor of liver function.) Definitive diagnosis made by pathologic examination of biopsy specimen.

▶ Clinical Therapeutics

All therapy aimed at treating sequelae of cirrhosis. Sodium and fluid restrictions combined with low-dose diuretics can reduce ascites. Encephalopathy can be treated with protein restriction and lactulose and in some cases zinc supplementation (reduce ammonia). Beta blockade (a reduction of heart rate of about 25%) to reduce portal pressures.

► Clinical Intervention

Sclerotherapy/banding of esophageal varices, placement of Laveen or Denver shunt to drain ascites (controversial, last-ditch effort at palliation), placement of transjugular intrahepatic portosystemic shunt (TIPS) (connects hepatic and portal veins). All are palliative and are not predictably effective. Liver transplantation may be appropriate for the alcohol-abstinent patient.

► Health Maintenance Issues

Treatment for alcoholism if appropriate; avoid alcohol in all cirrhotic patients; eliminate offending drugs/toxins; address high-risk behaviors; limit acetaminophen. With early intervention, fibrosis may be halted, thus avoiding the ultimately fatal complications.

## C. Hepatocellular Carcinoma (Hepatoma)

► Scientific Concepts

Uncommon primary tumor in United States, accounts for 50% of malignancies in parts of South Africa and Asia. Etiology is unknown, but preexisting cirrhosis secondary to chronic type B or C viral hepatitis, alcoholism, hemochromatosis, and alpha-1-antitrypsin deficiency are all significant risk factors. Others include long-term treatment with exogenous androgens, schistosomiasis, and clonorchiasis. Unlike primary hepatoma, metastatic liver disease is common. In non–third world countries, 50% of patients dying with malignancies will have liver metastases. Benign hepatic cysts and hemangiomas are common and require no treatment unless painful due to size or bleeding.

► History & Physical

History of cirrhosis or other risk factors. Patient presents with fatigue, malaise, rapid weight loss, abdominal pain. Ascites may be bloody; enlarged liver may be tender and firm. Bruit heard over liver is highly suggestive. Jaundice is uncommon finding.

► Diagnostic Studies

LFP, alpha-fetoprotein, gallium scan, CT, angiography, and cautiously performed liver biopsy. Tumors are highly vascular, and patient often has coexisting coagulopathy.

► Diagnosis

Abrupt increase in alkaline phosphatase in previously stable cirrhotic patient, increase alpha-fetoprotein, filling defect on gallium scanning, tumor blush on angiogram.

► Clinical Therapeutics

No effective treatment currently available. Prognosis poor, with life expectancy generally less than 6 months.

► Clinical Intervention

Surgery rarely indicated and only when confirmed to one lobe.

► Health Maintenance Issues

Avoidance of risk factors for cirrhosis. Proper immunizations, early identification and treatment of hemochromatosis and alpha-1-antitrypsin deficiency. Careful follow-up in patients with chronic hepatitis B and C.

## D. Abscess

▶ Scientific Concepts

Pyogenic abscesses most commonly are secondary to biliary disease (e.g., acute cholecystitis, ascending cholangitis). The bacteria, frequently gram negatives and anaerobes, may also gain entry from contiguous organs or penetrating trauma. *Entamoeba histolytica* is the only parasitic pathogen and is spread via fecal–oral route. Persons at high risk are institutionalized individuals and homosexual males. Asymptomatic carriers found in the United States. *Candida* is a source of liver abscess in the immunocompromised patient.

▶ History & Physical

History of risk factors, surgical history. Presenting complaints of malaise, RUQ pain, fever/chills, mild hepatomegaly. Jaundice found in 25%.

▶ Diagnostic Studies

LFP, CBC blood culture, chest x-ray, abdominal ultrasound, CT with IV contrast, serology (immunoglobulin M enzyme-linked immunosorbent assay [IgM ELISA]) if parasitic infection is consideration.

▶ Diagnosis

Elevated white blood count, mildly elevated LFP, increased gamma-glutamyl transpeptidase (GGTP), blood culture positive in 50%. Round/oval defects on ultrasound, air–fluid levels within liver. Amebic abscess more typically single than multiple.

▶ Clinical Therapeutics

Broad-spectrum IV antibiotics to cover gram negatives and anaerobes in pyogenic abscess. For amebic abscess, metronidazole followed by iodoquinol (intestinal amebicide) is recommended.

▶ Clinical Intervention

CT-guided percutaneous drainage of pyogenic abscess is indicated. Open surgical drainage may be required when primary treatment fails. Therapeutic aspiration indicated when amebic abscess large and in danger of rupture with resulting pulmonary and anaphylactic complications.

▶ Health Maintenance Issues

Good sanitation, avoid high-risk behaviors, prompt treatment of acute biliary disease.

## VIII. HERNIA, EXTERNAL

▶ Scientific Concepts

A hernia is a defect in the normal musculofascial continuity of the abdominal wall allowing its contents to protrude. The most common types are direct and indirect inguinal, umbilical, and incisional. Femoral, obturator, and Spigelian occur rarely. The groin hernias occur more frequently in males and are described depending on their anatomic location in reference to the inferior epigastric and femoral vessels. Both groin and umbilical hernias may be congenital or acquired. When acquired, they are due to greater intra-abdominal pressures than the strength of the abdominal wall, allowing the defect to enlarge. Small or large bowel, omentum, or bladder then protrudes through the defect. Severity can range from an easily reducible and painless hernia (these are usually large defects) to incarcerated (unable to reduce) to strangulated. With strangulation, obstruction occurs, the blood supply is lost, and necrosis ensues. Urgent surgical correction is required. Incisional hernias can occur through fascia wherever previous incision has been made. They may result from inadequate surgical technique in the closure or, more often, a wound infection.

### ▶ History & Physical

The patient describes sudden or gradual onset of a bulge in the groin, scrotum, or umbilicus. However, often a bulge is not apparent and the patient complains of dull, throbbing pain radiating to thigh, scrotum, and lower back. The pain is worse with activity and improves with rest. A sudden increase in pain, change to a colicky nature, nausea, or vomiting with decreased bowel sounds indicates an obstruction regardless of location.

On examination, the umbilical hernia will protrude when the patient coughs or lifts head while supine. The defect is palpable. Groin hernias often visible but may be detected only by placing the index finger into the inguinal canal, having patient cough or bear down, then feeling bulge of soft tissue pressing against the examining finger. Best performed with patient upright.

### ▶ Diagnostic Studies

None usually required, though some obscure types (e.g., obturator, internal, paraesophageal) may need CT or barium studies.

### ▶ Diagnosis

A physical examination will detect the hernia, although the clinician will not necessarily be able to distinguish among the types of groin hernias until surgery.

### ▶ Clinical Therapeutics

There is no role except for temporary pain management until repair can be made.

### ▶ Clinical Intervention

There are several surgical approaches to groin hernias, most commonly using mesh reinforcements in some manner. Laparoscopic repair in large multicenter prospective studies has proved superior in terms of recovery, risk of recurrence, and number of wound infections. Incisional and umbilical hernia repairs may or may not require mesh. In the patient unsuitable for surgery, a truss may provide some support and pain relief.

### ▶ Health Maintenance Issues

Infant groin hernias should be identified and corrected as early as possible. Use of good body mechanics in heavy work can reduce incidence of groin hernia. Umbilical hernias in adults are often secondary to or aggravated by obesity. Weight loss and improved abdominal wall strength will benefit these patients. Surgical repair is recommended for most to avoid complications. The small, painful hernia is the one at greatest risk and is easier to repair early on.

# IX. NUTRITIONAL REQUIREMENTS AND ASSESSMENT

▶ Scientific Concepts

Forty nutrients are required by the human body. Nutrients are essential if they cannot be synthesized by the body and if a deficiency causes an abnormality that is reversed when the deficit is corrected.

▶ Essential Nutritional Elements

The following are required for normal nutritional functioning:
- Water
- Energy source (i.e., carbohydrates)
- Water-soluble vitamins
- Fat-soluble vitamins
- Essential amino acids
- Minerals
- Essential fatty acids

▶ Daily Requirements

The amount of a particular element needed by the body is defined as the recommended daily allowance (RDA). RDA levels have been established by the Food and Nutrition board of the National Academy of Science to express the amount of a nutritional item needed to maintain a healthy state. Many factors may influence the specific nutritional requirements of an individual, including the composition of a diet, various disease states, and physiologic factors (i.e., pregnancy).

▶ Levels of Specific Nutrients

Vitamins are a group of organic compounds needed to conduct metabolic functions. Vitamins are divided into water-soluble—thiamin, riboflavin, niacin, $B_6$, $B_{12}$, folate, panothenic acid, biotin, and ascorbic acid—and fat-soluble—A, D, E, and K. Fat-soluble vitamins can accumulate and cause toxic syndromes. Deficiencies of both water- and fat-soluble vitamins cause specific syndromes that will be discussed later in this chapter. Safe and adequate levels for all vitamins can be found in any standard textbook of nutrition or medicine. See Table 6–1 for a summary of selected vitamin functions and sources.

Minerals are inorganic compounds needed for proper metabolic function. The minerals are divided into major—calcium, magnesium, phosphorus, sodium, potassium, and chloride—and minor groups—iron, zinc, copper, manganese, molybdenum, fluoride, iodine, cobalt, chromium, and selenium—by the amount needed each day. The body needs energy to support growth, function, and repair. Energy is provided by dietary protein, fat, and carbohydrates.

Protein is needed to provide for structural integrity and function. The nine essential amino acids are needed to synthesize other needed proteins. Supplemental nitrogen should be available to provide for proper protein synthesis. Amount of protein needed in diet depends in part on

## ► table 6-1

### SUMMARY OF VITAMIN ACTIONS AND SOURCES

| Vitamin | Type | Important Action | Sources |
|---|---|---|---|
| A | Fat soluble | Retinal function, wound healing; under investigation for prevention of cancer/heart disease | Pigmented vegetables |
| D | Fat soluble | Acceleration of phosphorus and calcium absorption in gastro-intestinal tract | Sunlight, fresh fruits, milk |
| E | Fat soluble | Thought to protect cell membranes and structures as antioxidant, ? role in prevention of cancer, heart disease and cataracts | Vegetables, seed oil |
| K | Fat soluble | Promotes hemostasis by assisting in function of coagulation factors; synthesized by bacteria in intestine | Leafy green vegetables |
| Thiamine (B$_1$) | Water soluble | Cofactor in carbohydrate oxidation | Meat, milk, eggs |
| Riboflavin (B$_2$) | Water soluble | Cofactor in oxidation reduction reactions | Meat, dairy products, fish |
| Niacin | Water soluble | Involved in oxidation reduction reactions, can be used to lower blood lipids | Cereals, vegetables, dairy products |
| Pyridoxine (B$_6$) | Water soluble | Metabolism of amino acids | Meat, starchy vegetables |
| C (ascorbic acid) | Water soluble | Synthesis of collagen, antioxidant, wound healing, absorption of iron | Fresh fruits and vegetables |

quality of protein consumed. Animal sources provide the highest quality protein, followed by legumes and other plant sources.

Fat is the densest calorie source of energy for the body. The primary role of dietary fat is to provide essential fatty acids (specifically linoleic acid needed for prostaglandin synthesis).

Carbohydrates should supply 55 to 60% of the energy requirements in the average U.S. diet. Sources of carbohydrate include simple sugars, complex carbohydrates (starches), and fiber. Insoluble dietary fiber can assist in lowering levels of cholesterol and improving colonic function.

### ► History & Physical

History, physical examination, and laboratory testing are necessary to assess nutritional status. History questions should be directed at what meals are eaten each day and general composition of meals. Specific attention should be directed toward groups that are at traditionally high risk for nutritional deficiency: pregnant and nursing women, the poor, the elderly, and adolescents. Patient-generated dietary logs may be kept for days to weeks so as to better access nutritional patterns, problems, and deficits.

The targeted physical examination is directed at observation of muscle wasting, fat stores, and signs of nutrient deficits. Observation of body habitus to detect such conditions as obesity can be measured using reference charts with "ideal height–weight" guidelines that have been produced by actuarial organizations. Anthropomorphic measurements are felt to be more reliable. A commonly performed anthropomorphic measurement is skin fold thickness analysis of triceps and arm muscle circumference. Several sophisticated options are available to conduct anthropomorphic measurement including bioimpedance and underwater weighing. A measurement also used to gauge obesity is the body mass index (BMI). It is calculated by dividing the weight in kilograms by height in meters squared. A BMI between 25 and 30 classifies an individual as overweight; if the BMI is over 30, the individual is considered obese.

▶ Diagnostic Studies

Serum albumin has been used to serve as a marker for protein calorie malnutrition. Malnutrition will cause abnormally low levels of albumin, as will other disease states (e.g., liver disease). Lab workup for nutritional assessment often includes measures of immune function. Total lymphocyte count and reactions to common skin antigens (e.g., purified protein derivative), although nonspecific, can be useful prognostically. Serial weights should be measured. Dieticians can perform calorie counts to more objectively monitor elements of nutritional intake. Other investigations for specific deficiencies (e.g., vitamin $B_{12}$) will be discussed in other sections.

▶ Diagnosis

While laboratory investigations may provide some helpful clues to diagnosis, most are nonspecific and one must keep in mind that other nonnutritional processes may be responsible for alterations in laboratory values.

▶ Clinical Therapeutics
None.

▶ Clinical Intervention
None.

▶ Health Maintenance Issues

Health care providers should encourage patients to eat a balanced diet following recommendations set in the "Food Guide Pyramid" as established by the U.S. Department of Agriculture. Diets whose concepts are not founded on clinically proven nutritional data should be avoided. Patients should be cautioned that excessive consumption of some vitamins and minerals might be harmful.

## A. Protein Calorie Malnutrition

▶ Scientific Concepts

Protein malnutrition occurs as a result of relative or absolute deficiency of protein as an energy source. Two distinct syndromes are classically described in relation to malnutrition—kwashiorkor syndrome (deficiency of protein but adequate total energy) and marasmus (both protein and total energy deficiencies). In the United States, most causes of malnutrition are secondary, related to another disease process. Secondary malnutrition may occur due to:
• Increased utilization of calories (e.g., burns)
• Decreased intake (e.g., oral trauma)
• Malabsorption (e.g., diarrhea)

Malnutrition affects every major organ system. Chief clinical effects may include decreased production of proteins by liver and decreased cardiac contractility resulting in electrocardiographic shifts. Increased wound healing time and depressed immunologic functioning (depressed T-lymphocyte activity) may result. Muscle wasting and pulmonary problems due to decreased vital capacity and tidal volume may occur.

▶ History & Physical

Clinician should seek history of unintentional weight loss, poor dietary intake, or history of clinical circumstances that may produce malnutrition from secondary cause. Most obvious finding on physical examination would be weight loss in adult patient. Children will manifest failure to thrive. Skin will usually be dry and hair thin. Edema may be present from low protein levels. In more extreme cases, face and extremities will exhibit loss of fat stores.

▶ Diagnostic Studies

Look for decrease in serum albumin level and lymphocyte count.

▶ Diagnosis

Watch for development of risk factors in susceptible patients. Do not overlook diagnosis in patients who are hypermetabolic.

▶ Clinical Therapeutics

Correct underlying deficiencies in electrolytes and infections first. Then begin process of replacing energy and proteins. Calories and protein intake must be advanced slowly while observing patient carefully. Most adults can tolerate 30 kcal/kg and 0.8–1 g of protein. Later, advance patient to 40 kcal. Vitamins and minerals can be added initially. The addition of fat calories is variable but usually occurs later in recovery.

▶ Clinical Intervention

Patients may need parenteral feeding if enteral is not available. Enteral feedings always preferable if that route is available.

▶ Health Maintenance Issues

Vigilance as to which patients are at risk. Providing adequate nutritional support to hospitalized patients may prevent development of protein calorie malnutrition.

## B. Vitamin Deficiencies

▶ Scientific Concepts

Vitamins serve as cofactors to allow metabolic reactions to occur. Clinically, most vitamin deficiencies occur as part of protein calorie malnutrition or in concert with other vitamin deficiencies rather than as single entity.

### 1. Vitamin A Deficiency

▶ History & Physical

One of the most common vitamin deficiency syndromes in developing nations. Seek history of concurrent malabsorption, alcoholism, or oil laxative abuse. Night blindness is earliest symptom. Xerosis, hyperkeratinization, and loss of taste may result. Small white spots may appear on conjunctiva (Bitot's spots). More serious ocular findings such as blindness are late findings.

▶ Diagnostic Studies

Serum levels for vitamin A.

▶ **Diagnosis**

Problems with dark adaptation, night blindness may be only finding in early disease.

▶ **Clinical Therapeutics**

Treat with vitamin A, 30,000 IU/d for 1 week. Higher doses needed for more advanced disease.

▶ **Clinical Intervention**

None needed.

▶ **Health Maintenance Issues**

Recognize patients at risk and encourage proper diet.

## 2. Vitamin D Deficiency

▶ **History & Physical**

Vitamin D deficiency is uncommon in the United States. Vitamin D deficiency has classic characteristics and is known as *rickets*. Features include skeletal deformities such as genu valgus and varum. Other abnormalities include enlarged spleen, liver, and skull, along with thoracic deformities. Those at risk for vitamin D deficiency are urban elderly, particularly those living in cold, northern climates. Lack of sunlight, staying indoors, and diet poor in vitamin D–enriched products and calcium (fortified milk) add to the risk. Certain anticonvulsants render vitamin D inactive. Other anticonvulsants may interfere with calcium absorption.

▶ **Diagnostic Studies**

Serum calcium and phosphate levels, possibly radiography in severe cases.

▶ **Diagnosis**

Vitamin D deficiency should be considered in patients with hypocalcemia. One must also determine reason for vitamin D deficiency, such as malabsorption or resistance to action of vitamin D.

▶ **Clinical Therapeutics**

Administration of vitamin D and calcium.

▶ **Clinical intervention**

None needed.

▶ **Health Maintenance Issues**

Importance of vitamin D calcium supplementation to patients at risk.

## 3. Vitamin E Deficiency

▶ **History & Physical**

Vitamin E functions as antioxidant. Seek history of malabsorption, cystic fibrosis, biliary atresia, or chronic cholestatic liver disease. Physical examination includes areflexia of decreased proprioception, vibratory sense changes, gait disturbances.

▶ **Diagnostic Studies**

Serum vitamin E levels should be measured.

▶ **Diagnosis**

Typical clinical symptoms with low levels of serum vitamin E.

► **Clinical Therapeutics**
The standard therapeutic dose of vitamin E for replacement therapy has not been established. The antioxidant benefit comes with doses of 100 to 400 units/d. Vitamin E can increase vitamin K requirements resulting in bleeding tendencies.

► **Clinical Intervention**
None required.

► **Health Maintenance Issues**
Observe patients at risk for development of clinical deficiency.

## 4. Vitamin K Deficiency

► **History & Physical**
Vitamin K stores in the body are small, thus deficiencies may develop quickly. Broad-spectrum antibiotics may hamper the production of vitamin K by intestinal bacteria. Patients with history of poor dietary intake also at risk. No specific findings on physical examination.

► **Diagnostic Studies**
Abnormally prolonged prothrombin time (PT) and partial thromboplastin time (PTT).

► **Diagnosis**
Patient with risk factors and typical pattern of coagulation abnormalities. Therapeutic trial of vitamin K when diagnosis is in question.

► **Clinical Therapeutics**
Subcutaneous vitamin K at 15 mg.

► **Clinical Intervention**
None required.

► **Health Maintenance Issues**
Recognize patients at risk; ensure proper diet.

## 5. Thiamine (Vitamin B₁) Deficiency

► **History & Physical**
In United States, most thiamine deficiency cases result from excessive alcohol abuse. Signs and symptoms of deficiency include anorexia, muscle cramps, paresthesias, and irritability. Patients are prone to develop cardiovascular and nervous system abnormalities. Classic signs of heart failure may be present. On neurologic examination, search for peripheral sensory neuropathy that is more pronounced in the upper extremities. Patients with advanced disease may develop one of the two classic syndromes associated with thiamine deficiency. Wernicke's encephalopathy consists of nystagmus, truncal ataxia, and confusion. Korsakoff's syndrome includes amnesia, confabulation, and impaired learning.

► **Diagnostic Studies**
Most common utilized test is measurement of erythrocyte thiamine transketolase. The clinical response to a trial of thiamine is usually diagnostic.

► **Diagnosis**
Consider thiamine deficiency in alcoholic patient with typical symptoms.

▶ **Clinical Therapeutics**

Administer thiamine parentally, approximately 50–100 mg/d for several days; followed by oral doses of 5–10 mg/d. Concomitant administration of other water-soluble vitamins is also advised.

▶ **Clinical Intervention**

None needed.

▶ **Health Maintenance Issues**

Attempt interventions in alcoholic patients aimed at abstinence from alcohol and proper diet to prevent development of thiamine deficiency.

## 6. Riboflavin (Vitamin B₂) Deficiency

▶ **History & Physical**

Most patients have a concurrent condition that causes riboflavin deficiency. Diets inadequate in protein and calories, alcoholism, and medication interaction are common causes. Clinical signs include cheilosis, angular stomatitis, glossitis, and dermatitis.

▶ **Diagnostic Studies**

Riboflavin deficiency is usually treated empirically.

▶ **Clinical Therapeutics**

Usually treated with diet inclusive of meat, fish, and dairy. If necessary, administer oral preparation at 5–15 mg/d until symptoms resolve.

▶ **Clinical Intervention**

None needed.

▶ **Health Maintenance Issues**

Maintain proper diet for patient to prevent deficiency; treat coexisting nutritional problems.

## 7. Niacin Deficiency

▶ **History & Physical**

Niacin deficiency is most commonly caused by alcoholism and nutrient–drug interactions. Can occur in inborn metabolism errors. Niacin deficiency presenting with dermatitis, diarrhea, and dementia is referred to as *pellagra*. Dermatitis is symmetric and characterized by appearance of desquamated and hyperpigmented lesions. Any diarrhea that is present may also accompany stomatitis or glossitis. Dementia is nonspecific, manifested by loss of memory, hallucinations, and finally psychosis.

▶ **Diagnostic Studies**

No specific lab tests will confirm.

▶ **Diagnosis**

Typical clinical syndrome and response to therapeutic trail.

▶ **Clinical Therapeutics**

Oral niacin 10–150 mg/d in conjunction with adequate tryptophan. High doses are associated with cutaneous flushing. Pretreatment with aspirin helps reduce the flushing.

▶ **Clinical Intervention**

None needed.

► **Health Maintenance Issues**

Maintenance of balanced diet. Pellagra was once believed to be linked to diet in which corn supplied most of the calories. Although there is a relationship, interplay of intake of corn and development of pellagra is now recognized to be more complex.

## 8. Pyridoxine (Vitamin B$_6$) Deficiency

► **History & Physical**

A history of ingestion of isoniazid, penicillamine, or oral contraceptives is important as interactions with medications is one of the most common causes of pyridoxine deficiency. Alcoholism may also be a contributing factor. Physical examination may reveal weakness, cheilosis, stomatitis, and dermatitis. More significant deficiency may result in sensory neuropathy, anemia, and seizures.

► **Diagnostic Studies**

Measure pyridoxine phosphate levels in the blood.

► **Clinical Therapeutics**

Treat with pyridoxine orally in doses of 10 to 20 mg/d. Vitamin B$_6$ is routinely prescribed when patients are receiving medications that interfere with metabolism of this vitamin.

► **Clinical Intervention**

None needed.

► **Health Maintenance Issues**

See Clinical Therapeutics above.

## 9. Ascorbic Acid (Vitamin C) Deficiency

► **History & Physical**

Patients at risk for vitamin C deficiencies are those who smoke cigarettes, are poor, or have chronic illnesses. Scurvy will develop in patients who have moderate or severe deficiency of vitamin C. Classic findings in scurvy are perifollicular hemorrhage, petechiae, and purpura. As disease progresses, hemorrhages occur into gums, joints, and even intracerebrally. Mild vitamin C deficiency may manifest only as lethargy and fatigue. Wound healing also impaired.

► **Diagnostic Studies**

Diagnosis is made on clinical grounds or by using plasma ascorbic acid levels.

► **Diagnosis**

Made from typical clinical appearance.

► **Clinical Therapeutics**

Begin treatment with 300 to 1,000 mg/d of ascorbic acid.

► **Clinical Intervention**

None needed.

► **Health Maintenance Issues**

Counseling about proper nutrition.

## C. Obesity

► **Scientific Concepts**

Defined as a weight in excess of 20% of ideal body weight (although some definitions vary). Ideal weight can be read off a table that relates to gender, frame size, height, and weight. BMI is a useful tool to relate to height and weight in a clinically useful way. A BMI of 20–25 $kg/m^2$ is considered healthy. Once BMI increases to a value of 30 $kg/m^2$, obesity is present. It is now recognized that may factors may play a role in development of obesity. Genetic factors, environmental factors, and dietary intake all play a role to some extent in development of obesity. Obesity increases risk of developing many diseases, including gallbladder disease, joint problems, diabetes mellitus, cardiovascular disease, and several forms of cancer.

### ▶ History & Physical

Dietary histories relayed by patients tend to underreport calorie ingestion. Food intake logs kept by patients over a period of days may help to portray more accurately. Take drug history, seeking medications associated with weight gain, such as steroids. Be alert for congenital syndromes associated with obesity that may be present and recognizable from physical examination (e.g., Prader–Willi), although in practice these syndromes are rare. Measure the BMI to confirm clinical assessment of body fat. Ascertain waist circumference. If circumference is >100 cm in men and 90 cm in women, there is associated risk of low high-density lipoprotein (HDL) levels and high triglycerides.

### ▶ Diagnostic Studies

Measurement of blood lipids, serum glucose, etc., for comorbid conditions.

### ▶ Diagnosis

Diagnosis is made from clinical presentation and determination of BMI.

### ▶ Clinical Therapeutics

Use of medications to treat obesity should be reserved primarily for patients who have a BMI > 30 $kg/m^2$. There are many appetite suppressants currently available. Two major categories of medications are serotonergic agents and noradrenergic agents. Use of amphetamine for weight loss is no longer advisable.

### ▶ Clinical Intervention

Nonpharmacologic therapies to assist obese patient may help to induce or maintain weight loss. Exercise is an important adjunct to assist patient in maintaining normal weight. Behavior modification therapy may provide assistance in initial weight loss and eating behavior. Diet therapy may also be used to reduce overall fat and calorie intake. More frequent, small feedings with high-carbohydrate and fiber-containing foods will help maintain satiety. Patient must also be aware that location of eating may promote consumption of high-fat foods or excessive intake. This includes buffet style or cafeteria settings.

Surgery is a consideration for those with BMI of 40 $kg/m^2$ or 35 $kg/m^2$ (or greater) with significant comorbidity factors. Recommended procedure is the Roux-en-Y anastomosis.

### ▶ Health Maintenance Issues

Weight regain is a significant issue to the obese patient who has been successful in losing weight. A regime of exercise and supportive environment will be helpful to maintain a more desirable weight for a patient.

## BIBLIOGRAPHY

Barton S. *Clinical Evidence.* London: BMJ Publishing; 2001.

Gorroll AH, Mulley AG Jr. *Primary Care Medicine: Office Evaluation and Management of the Adult Patient.* Philadelphia: Lippincott; 2000.

Holmes N. *Physician Assistant's Clinical Companion.* Springhouse, PA: Springhouse; 2001

Richter J. *Healing Horizons in Acid Reflux Disease.* Cleveland: Quintiles Medical Communication; 2001

Tierney LM Jr., McPhee SJ, Papadakis MA, eds. *Current Medical Diagnosis & Treatment,* 42nd ed. New York: Lange Medical Books/McGraw-Hill; 2003.

# Renal Diseases  7

*Brenda L. Jasper, MPAS, PA-C*

## I. RENAL FUNCTION

► Scientific Concepts

The nephron is the functional unit of the kidney, with approximately 1.0 million nephrons per kidney. Each nephron consists of a glomerulus and tubule. Responsible for fluid and electrolyte maintenance, excretion of waste products of metabolism, and secretion of hormones.

## A. Measurement of Renal Function

► Scientific Concepts

*Blood urea nitrogen (BUN):* Produced from metabolism of amino acids in the liver. BUN is not as useful in predicting glomerular filtration rate (GFR) because it is influenced by other factors. It is increased in states of increased tissue breakdown (gastrointestinal [GI] bleeding, corticosteroids), high dietary protein intake, and prerenal azotemia. It is decreased in malnutrition and liver disease.

*Creatinine:* Produced from metabolism of creatine in skeletal muscle and dietary meat consumption. Daily production is fairly constant. Plasma creatinine varies inversely with the GFR; as the GFR decreases, the creatinine increases. In general, a doubling of serum creatinine represents loss of one half of the GFR (i.e., rise in plasma creatinine from 1.0 mg/dL to 2.0 mg/dL represents 50% loss of renal function, and subsequent doubling of plasma creatinine represents an additional 50% loss of the remaining renal function). Therefore, the initial rise in plasma creatinine is clinically important as this represents a significant fall in the GFR.

*GFR:* Direct measure of renal function based on filtration of plasma across the glomerulus. Most accurate determination would be measurement of insulin clearance or radiolabeled compounds. These substances are freely filtered and not secreted by the tubules, giving a more precise measurement of GFR, but are not used in clinical practice. Estimations of the GFR and whether the GFR is changing or stable are most relevant in clinical practice.

*Creatinine clearance (CrCl):* Clinical measurement of creatinine filtered across glomerulus and secreted by tubule. A direct measure of GFR is not clinically feasible; therefore, CrCl is used to estimate the GFR. CrCl is calculated by obtaining a 24-hour urine collection for creatinine and measuring of serum creatinine using the following formula:

$$CrCl = \frac{\text{urine creatinine} \times \text{volume (mL/min)}}{\text{plasma creatinine}}$$

Normal creatinine clearance in men is 120 ± 25 mL/min; women, 95 ± 20mL/min. Estimation of CrCl by plasma creatinine in a patient with stable plasma creatinine is:

$$CrCl = \frac{(140 - \text{age}) \times \text{weight in kilograms}}{\text{plasma creatinine} \times 72}$$

In women, multiply result by 0.85 due to decreased muscle portion of body weight.

## B. Urinalysis

### 1. Hematuria

▶ **Scientific Concepts**

Detection of hemoglobin in urine, gross or microscopic. May originate from any site in the urinary tract.

▶ **History & Physical**

Evaluate for gross hematuria, recent illness such as upper respiratory infection (postinfectious glomerulonephritis, immunoglobulin A [IgA] nephropathy), urinary symptoms suggestive of infection or stones, other systemic illnesses (systemic lupus erythematosus, vasculitis, bleeding disorder, sickle cell trait or disease), family history of kidney disease (hereditary nephritis, polycystic kidney disease), and prostatic disease. Rule out hematuria secondary to menstrual bleeding in women.

▶ **Diagnostic Studies**

*Urinalysis:* Two or more red blood cells per high-power field in centrifuge urine specimen. Red sediment with clear supernatant indicates hematuria. Heme-positive red supernatant indicates hemoglobinuria (intravascular hemolysis) or myoglobinuria (muscle damage). Heme-negative red supernatant indicates porphyria, ingestion of beets, or phenazopyridine use. Cells are dysmorphic in glomerular bleeding and of uniform size and shape in nonglomerular bleeding.

*Other diagnostic studies:* Intravenous pyelogram (IVP), renal sonogram, cystoscopy, urine cytology; computed tomographic (CT) scan may detect small tumors; renal angiography to detect arteriovenous malformations. If no cause identified, follow and reevaluate.

▶ **Diagnosis**

Identify site of bleeding as either glomerular or extraglomerular. A three-tube test may help determine source of bleeding. Hematuria may be transient or persistent, with transient hematuria most common; source not found in most cases. Tumors of genitourinary (GU) tract, infections, and benign prostatic hypertrophy (BPH) should be ruled out as causes.

▶ **Clinical Therapeutics**

Treat infection or underlying disease if identified.

▶ **Clinical Intervention**

Renal biopsy can identify form of glomerulonephritis associated with hematuria (IgA nephropathy, hereditary nephritis, or membranoproliferative glomerulonephritis) but reserved for those cases associated with deterioration in renal function, proteinuria, or unexplained hypertension.

▶ **Health Maintenance Issues**

Microscopic hematuria is a common finding and can be transient; careful history and appropriate testing should be done on all older patients due to increased risk of malignancy. Persistent hematuria requires an evaluation.

2. Proteinuria

▶ Scientific Concepts

Increased permeability of glomerular capillary wall to albumin or low-molecular-weight proteins; normal protein excretion < 150 mg protein per day.

▶ History & Physical

Identify any history of systemic illness associated with proteinuria (diabetes mellitus, systemic lupus erythematosus, etc.), past history of poststreptococcal glomerulonephritis, or family history of renal disease.

▶ Diagnostic Studies

*Random urine specimen:* Urine dipstick sensitive for albumin; sulfosalicylic acid detects all proteins including nonalbumin proteins such as immunoglobulin light chains. Three separate specimens to confirm. If under age 25, rule out orthostatic proteinuria. Screen for microalbuminuria with urine albumin to creatinine ratio (> 30 mg/g or 0.03 mg/mg indicates microalbuminuria) or dye-impregnated strips (20–200 µg/min or 30–300 mg/d indicates microalbuminuria).

*24-hour urine for protein excretion:* < 1 g/d usually indicates benign form of isolated proteinuria, > 1 g/d is indicative of glomerular disease, and > 3.0 g/d indicates nephrotic range proteinuria.

*Renal sonogram or IVP:* Rule out structural lesions. Renal biopsy reserved for those with evidence of abnormal renal function, >2 g/d proteinuria, or associated hematuria.

▶ Diagnosis

*Benign orthostatic (postural):* Increased protein excretion when upright, normal protein excretion when supine. Most often seen in adolescents. Proteinuria usually < 1 g/d and often disappears over years and is not generally associated with renal damage.

*Transient (intermittent):* Most commonly seen. Benign form that often resolves on repeat exams. Can be seen with exercise, fever, and acute illness.

*Persistent:* Ongoing protein excretion of 1–2 g/d. More likely associated with underlying renal disease. Prognosis better in those under age 25.

▶ Clinical Therapeutics

Treatment of underlying glomerular disease, if present, is key. Angiotensin-converting enzyme (ACE) inhibitors work by lowering efferent arteriolar resistance and have effect on glomerular capillary permeability. Nonsteroidal anti-inflammatory drugs (NSAIDs) occasionally used for heavy proteinuria but with limited success. Used only when renal function is not impaired because they lower GFR and can lead to acute renal failure or hyperkalemia.

▶ Clinical Intervention

Dietary protein restriction (in select patients, 0.6–0.8 g/kg/d plus protein added to match urinary protein losses), reduction in blood pressure.

### 3. Cells

- *Red cells:* Can be present from any site in urinary tract. Red cell morphology can help identify site. Cells are dysmorphic in glomerular bleeding, uniform shape in nonglomerular bleeding.
- *White cells:* Pyuria indicative of infection; eosinophils may be clue to interstitial nephritis.

### 4. Casts

- *Hyaline:* Mucoprotein composition; not associated with renal disease. Can be seen in volume depletion and with diuretic use.
- *Red cell:* Indicative of glomerular disease, usually glomerulonephritis or vasculitis.
- *White cell:* Seen in pyelonephritis and other tubulointerstitial disorders.
- *Broad/waxy:* Form in tubules that have been dilated; seen in chronic or advanced renal failure.

### 5. Osmolality

- Urine osmolality can vary under influence of antidiuretic hormone (ADH) released from the posterior pituitary gland. Useful in clinical settings of hypernatremia, hyponatremia, polyuria, and when differentiating prerenal disease from acute tubular necrosis.

### 6. Volume

- *Anuria:* Urine volume less than 100 mL/d.
- *Oliguria:* Urine volume less than 400 mL/d.
- *Polyuria:* Urine volume exceeding 3 L/d.

## II. INFECTIOUS DISEASES AND INFLAMMATORY CONDITIONS OF THE KIDNEY/URINARY TRACT

### A. Urinary Tract Infections (UTIs)

▶ Scientific Concepts

***Uncomplicated UTI:*** Not associated with anatomic or structural deformity in urinary tract, recent surgery involving urinary tract, catheters, or other GU procedures. Community-acquired infections mostly seen in females, rare in males. Eighty to 85% are secondary to *Escherichia coli.* Long-term sequelae are rare.

***Complicated UTI:*** Associated with anatomic abnormalities, obstructive uropathy, or abnormal bladder function. Risk factors include catheters, renal calculi, GU procedures, and pregnancy. Frequently asymptomatic; organisms are more diverse and are often more resistant to antibiotics. Recurrence rates are high if underlying problem not addressed. Duration of therapy is 7–14 days.

### 1. Lower Urinary Tract Infections (Bladder, Prostate, Urethra)

▶ History & Physical

Symptoms include frequency, urgency, dysuria, voiding small amounts, suprapubic pain, cloudy urine, occasional hematuria.

▶ Diagnostic Studies

- Microscopic exam of urine for pyuria, hematuria, and Gram stain.
- Urine culture colony count of 100,000 colony-forming units of bacteria per milliliter of urine has been standard of diagnosis. However, in uncomplicated UTI, 30–50% of symptomatic women have lower quantitative counts isolated. In this population, any quantitative count of an organism with pyuria and clinical symptoms is sufficient for diagnosis. Urine should be midstream specimen in sterile container after proper cleaning of external genitalia. *E. coli* most common organism in uncomplicated UTIs. *Proteus* organisms seen in patients with staghorn calculi. *Pseudomonas* and *Candida* more likely nosocomial infections or in patients with indwelling catheters.
- Prostate secretions for white blood cells (WBCs), bacteria, and culture.
- Urethral or cervical discharge for Gram stain and culture (bacterial or viral) to identify organism; gram-negative intracellular diplococci in gonococcal urethritis; Tzank test for herpes simplex virus; ligase chain reaction (LCR) test for *Chlamydia*.
- Radiodiagnostics are not indicated for uncomplicated cystitis or urethritis in women. Cystoscopy, voiding cystourethrogram (VCUG), and IVP reserved for complicated or chronic cases and should be considered in infants or males with first infection.

▶ Diagnosis

***Cystitis:*** Symptoms generally sudden in onset. Patient may present with any symptoms of lower UTI. Risk factors include gender (mostly female), age (18–40), sexual intercourse, delayed postcoital voiding, and pregnancy. *E. coli* is most common organism.

***Urethritis:*** Often presents with dysuria, pyuria, or urethral discharge. Urine culture shows low bacterial count or no bacteria. Often associated with sexually transmitted diseases (STDs) such as *Chlamydia trachomatis*, *Neisseria gonorrhoeae*, or herpes simplex virus.

- *Chlamydial urethritis:* Asymptomatic or symptoms of urethritis, cervicitis, or pelvic inflammatory disease. Discharge usually clear or mucoid and watery. Undetected or untreated chlamydial infections are one of the leading causes of female infertility in the United States. In males, chlamydial infections may cause epididymitis or prostatitis.
- *Gonococcal urethritis:* Usually associated with urinary symptoms, purulent urethral discharge, and gram-negative intracellular diplococci. In women, may be asymptomatic or associated with vaginitis, cervicitis, Bartholin's glands inflammation, or chronic salpingitis. In men, urethral pain and creamy, purulent discharge may be present; may involve prostate or epididymis. Culture for organism or obtain LCR assay of urine or discharge for diagnosis.
- *Herpes simplex virus (type 2):* Typically associated with tender grouped vesicles on an erythematous base. Virus lies latent in presacral ganglion, then reactivates. Viral shedding can by asymptomatic following initial infection or occur during a recurrence.

***Prostatitis***

- *Acute bacterial:* Signs and symptoms include sudden onset of fever and chills. Urinary symptoms may include dysuria, frequency, urgency. Suprapubic, perineal, and low back pain may be present. Obstructive symptoms with prostatic enlargement. Prostate is tender, warm, and swollen on digital rectal exam. Most common organism is enteric gram-negative bacilli (*E. coli* and *Pseudomonas*); enterococci and staphylococci less common. Systemic bacteremia can result if an acutely inflamed prostate is massaged.

- *Chronic bacterial:* Signs and symptoms include relapsing UTIs and urinary symptoms of dysuria, frequency, and urgency. Dull perineal, suprapubic, or low back pain may be present. Prostate feels normal to indurated on exam.
- *Nonbacterial:* Most common form of chronic prostatitis. Cause is unknown. Signs and symptoms are similar to chronic bacterial prostatitis. Cultures of urine and prostate secretions are sterile. Diagnosis is one of exclusion.
- *Prostatodynia:* Form of chronic noninflammatory prostatitis. Symptoms similar to chronic prostatitis. No WBCs or organisms in cultures.

### ► Clinical Therapeutics

#### Acute cystitis and coliform urethritis

- *Short course of antibiotics:* Three-day therapy more effective than single dose and is the usual treatment for uncomplicated cystitis. Trimethoprim-sulfamethoxazole (TMP-SMZ), trimethoprim, nitrofurantoin, or fluoroquinolones may be used. Amoxicillin less effective than other agents for short-course therapy.
- *Exceptions:* Pregnant women, those with multiple recent infections, symptoms more than 7 days, recurrent symptoms after initial 3-day antibiotic course, those with complicating factors (diabetes), and the elderly should receive a 7-day antibiotic regimen.

**Recurrent cystitis:** Single postcoital antibiotic dose or bedtime dose of antibiotic daily to three times weekly can reduce number of cystitis episodes. Encourage postcoital voiding.

#### Urethritis associated with STDs

- *Chlamydial:* Sexual partners must be treated. Azithromycin, 1 g PO single dose, or doxycycline, 100 mg bid for 7 days; erythromycin or tetracycline, 500 mg qid can also be used.
- *Gonococcal:* Sexual partners must be treated. Ceftriaxone, 125 mg intramuscularly (IM) or single dose of cefixime or fluoroquinolone orally can be used. Avoid penicillin and tetracycline due to increased resistance of organisms. Due to frequent concomitant chlamydial infection, single-dose azithromycin 1 g or doxycycline 100 mg bid for 7 days should be given.
- *Herpes simplex virus:* Oral acyclovir, 200 mg five times daily × 7–10 days or until resolved, to reduce the frequency and severity of recurrent episodes. Topical acyclovir six times daily can be added and may help reduce both viral shedding and the interval to healing. Maintenance therapy with acyclovir 400 mg twice daily for recurrent genital infections. Famciclovir and valacyclovir can also be used for recurrent genital herpes episodes.

#### Prostatitis

- *Acute bacterial:* Often associated with cystitis. Antibiotic therapy dependent on organism cultured in urine or prostatic secretions. Initial treatment usually parenteral antibiotics (ampicillin plus aminoglycoside).

Once afebrile for 24–48 hours, oral TMP-SMZ or fluoroquinolone can be used. Treatment course is 30 days.

- *Chronic bacterial:* Usually caused by gram-negative enteric bacteria. Difficult to treat; can use TMP-SMZ or fluoroquinolone for 6–12 weeks.
- *Nonbacterial:* Treat with erythromycin or tetracycline for 6 weeks if *Chlamydia* suspected; otherwise fluoroquinolone for several weeks. Sitz baths, alpha-adrenergic blocking agents, and anti-inflammatory agents may provide symptomatic relief.

▶ Clinical Intervention

Sexually active young adults are at increased risk of STDs. Patient education is key to prevention. Treat to prevent complications of pelvic inflammatory disease and sterility.

## 2. Upper Urinary Tract Infections (Kidney)

▶ History & Physical

Presents as an acute illness; obtain history for evidence of recurrent infection, childhood infections, or stones. Signs and symptoms include flank, low back, or abdominal pain; fever and chills; tachycardia; headache; nausea and vomiting; malaise; costovertebral angle tenderness; dysuria, frequency, urgency may or may not be present. In children, symptoms may be absent or nonspecific. In chronic pyelonephritis, symptoms may be absent, nonspecific, or related to infection.

▶ Diagnostic Studies

Laboratory findings include leukocytosis in acute pyelonephritis. BUN/creatinine are normal or elevated. Microscopic exam of urine may reveal pyuria, WBC casts, hematuria, and proteinuria. If acutely infected, Gram stain for bacteriuria. Urine culture for identification of causative organism, usually gram-negative bacteria. Blood culture is positive in 10–20% of patients with acute pyelonephritis. Radiodiagnostics are used to identify underlying pathology such as reflux, renal calculi, or other factors interfering with urine flow. Abdominal film to evaluate for radiopaque calculi and soft tissue evaluation. IVP reveals blunting of calyces and cortical scarring in chronic pyelonephritis. Voiding cystourethrogram in young children to evaluate for vesicoureteral reflux; retrograde cystogram may be helpful. Renal ultrasound and CT may identify obstruction or perinephric abscesses.

▶ Diagnosis

*Acute pyelonephritis:* Inflammation of the renal parenchyma. Spread of bacteria from bladder to kidneys; may result in sepsis. Responds to oral antibiotics in majority of cases; failure to respond should prompt further investigation. Generally not associated with long-term morbidity.

*Chronic pyelonephritis:* Renal scarring due to recurrent or persistent infection. Associated with anatomic abnormalities of the urinary tract including vesicoureteral reflux, obstruction, and renal calculi. Most commonly seen in children with vesicoureteral reflux resulting in renal scarring and damage (reflux nephropathy).

▶ Clinical Therapeutics

*Acute pyelonephritis:* Outpatient therapy for compliant, clinically stable (nontoxic) patient is 10- to 14-day course of antibiotic based on urine sensitivities. TMP-SMZ or a fluoroquinolone may be initial choice. Inpatient therapy for more acutely ill patient requires IV antibiotics (third-generation cephalosporin, fluoroquinolone, ampicillin plus gentamycin) pending urine and blood cultures. Once afebrile and stable, change to appropriate oral antibiotic and complete 10- to 14-day course. If fever or bacteriuria persist beyond 48–72 hours, evaluate for underlying urinary tract abnormality.

***Chronic pyelonephritis:*** Difficult situation; may develop resistant organisms. Renal damage is irreversible and may progress to end-stage renal failure. Goal is to prevent recurrent infection and glomerulosclerosis. If possible, eliminate any risk factors such as lesions obstructing urine flow, catheters, or calculi. Treat symptomatic episodes initially with 10–14 days of appropriate antibiotic. Relapsing bacteriuria may respond to a 6-week course of antibiotics. Suppressive therapy with continuous prophylactic low-dose antibiotics in certain patients, especially children, may decrease renal scarring and reflux; choices include TMP-SMZ, nitrofurantoin, or methenamine mandelate. Surgical correction indicated for severe vesicoureteral reflux, structural abnormalities, or when other complicating factors are present.

▶ **Clinical Intervention**

Prompt detection and treatment of UTIs in children and surgical repair of any underlying anatomic abnormalities to prevent further damage. Management of other complicating factors such as infected stones. Vesicoureteral reflux has familial tendency; may want to screen siblings.

▶ **Health Maintenance Issues**

***Asymptomatic bacteriuria:*** All pregnant women should be treated with at least 7-day course of antibiotics due to increased risk of fetal prematurity and maternal pyelonephritis. May indicate vesicoureteral reflux in preschool and young girls; treatment and urological evaluation is indicated. In men and nonpregnant women (especially elderly) without evidence of obstructive uropathy or vesicoureteral reflux, no treatment indicated. Not usually seen in males until after age of 60 years.

***Catheter-associated bacteriuria:*** Associated with asymptomatic and symptomatic UTIs; asymptomatic bacteriuria in patient with a catheter is not usually treated. In the hospital setting, urosepsis related to catheter bacteriuria is the most common source of gram-negative bacteremia. Recurrent episodes of infections are common if catheter not removed. Increased risk of *Candida albicans* infection. Asymptomatic candiduria should be treated with catheter change with or without antifungals. Disseminated candiduria requires systemic antifungal therapy. No indication for antibiotic prophylaxis in patient with chronic catheter.

## B. Epididymitis

▶ **Scientific Concepts**

Inflammation of the epididymis as a result of bacterial ascent from the lower urinary tract. Can be sexually transmitted or non–sexually transmitted. Sexually transmitted type usually seen in younger men and is associated with either gonococcal or chlamydial urethritis. Non–sexually transmitted type seen in older men and associated with gram-negative bacterial UTIs or prostatitis.

► **History & Physical**

Symptoms of urethritis or cystitis may be present, as well as fever, scrotal pain, and swelling. Epididymis may be tender, warm, or swollen. Scrotal pain may radiate along spermatic cord. Lower abdominal tenderness or flank pain on the involved side and prostate tenderness may be present.

► **Diagnostic Studies**

Leukocytosis and left shift on complete blood count (CBC), Gram stain of urethral discharge, urinalysis for pyuria or bacteriuria, urine culture, scrotal ultrasound, radionuclide scanning.

► **Differential Diagnosis**

Testicular tumors, torsion of spermatic cord, testicular trauma, orchitis. Phren's sign (pain from epididymitis improved with elevation of scrotum above pubic symphysis) may aid in differential but not specific.

► **Clinical Therapeutics**

Antibiotic therapy based on offending organism. Sexually transmitted types are treated with antibiotic to cover *N. gonorrhoeae* (when present) then 10-day course of tetracycline or erythromycin to cover *C. trachomatis*. Sexual partners must be treated. Non–sexually transmitted types are treated for 14 days with broad spectrum antibiotic.

► **Clinical Intervention**

Bedrest with scrotal elevation, oral analgesics. Once treated, non–sexually transmitted epididymitis requires urinary tract evaluation to rule out other pathology.

► **Health Maintenance Issues**

Delayed or inadequate therapy can lead to complications, including orchitis, abscesses, or impaired fertility.

## III. URINARY TRACT OBSTRUCTION AND TUMORS

### A. Urinary Tract Obstruction

► **Scientific Concepts**

Can occur at any site in urinary tract and may be congenital or acquired disorder with either structural or functional obstruction. Classified by degree, duration (acute, subacute, chronic), and site of obstruction.

► **History & Physical**

Obtain patient history. Symptoms vary with degree of obstruction. In setting of obstruction, anuria implies complete bilateral obstruction or obstruction of a single functioning kidney. Pain is more likely associated with acute obstruction; can vary in intensity/location. Chronic obstruction may present with no or vague symptoms. Urinary symptoms may include polyuria, nocturia, frequency, hesitancy, and decreased urinary stream. Palpable mass or distended bladder may be present as well as prostatic enlargement on rectal exam.

► **Diagnostic Studies**

Laboratory tests may reveal acute or chronic renal failure; abnormal blood chemistry. Urinalysis may be normal or have few red cells, white cells, or minimal proteinuria. Bacteria suggestive of underlying infection. Urine cytology to evaluate for malignancy. Urine volume may be normal, increased, or decreased. Anuria suggests complete bilateral obstruction. Plain film of abdomen to identify radiopaque stones. Postvoid bladder scan or bladder catheterization to evaluate for urinary retention or neuropathic bladder. Ultrasound may reveal hydronephrosis or tumors. CT can further identify cause of obstruction. IVP to evaluate upper urinary tract obstruction. Useful in patients with cysts and staghorn calculi. In patients with renal insufficiency, limited due to risk of radiocontrast nephrotoxicity. Retrograde pyelography to evaluate and visualize ureter and collecting system. Used when other testing is inconclusive and in patients with contrast allergy. Cystoscopy or urodynamic studies to evaluate bladder and rule out lower urinary tract obstruction.

▶ Diagnosis

***Congenital anomalies of urinary tract:*** Ureteropelvic junction obstruction most common and seen more in boys than girls. Can be detected by ultrasonography in utero. Treatment is surgery or close monitoring in select patients.

***Obstructing calculi:*** Must have bilateral obstruction or obstruction of single functioning kidney to cause renal failure.

***Urethral stricture:*** Seen with trauma (urethral instrumentation) or infections (gonococcal, infections secondary to indwelling catheters). Treatment includes dilation, urethrotomy with endoscope, or surgical repair.

***Renal tumors***

- *Renal cell carcinoma:* Most common neoplasm of kidney. More common in men, usually in fifth to seventh decades of life. Often found incidentally by sonogram or CT scan. Classic presenting triad of gross hematuria, flank pain, and palpable mass present in only 10 to 15% of patients. Most present with gross or microscopic hematuria. Acquired cystic disease of the kidney, which can develop in patients with end-stage renal disease, is a risk factor. CT scan is best method to evaluate suspected renal lesion and is more sensitive than ultrasound or IVP. Treatment is radical nephrectomy. Radiation therapy may be used for metastatic disease. Chemotherapy of limited value as tumor is very resistant; immunotherapy is promising. Survival rate is poor for those with positive lymph nodes and metastases.
- *Sarcoma:* Less than 3% of all malignant renal tumors. Treatment is radical nephrectomy.
- *Wilms' tumor (nephroblastoma):* Most common urologic tumor in children. Usually presents around age of 3 years; both familial and nonfamilial forms. Associated with congenital anomalies, including genitourinary malformations and aniridia. Asymptomatic abdominal mass is usual presentation; abdominal pain, hematuria, nausea and vomiting, anorexia, hypertension, and anemia may be present. Diagnosis made by ultrasound, CT scan, or magnetic resonance imaging (MRI). Treatment includes surgery, radiation, and chemotherapy, depending on staging of tumor pathology. Metastatic disease to regional lymph nodes, lung, and liver may occur. Prognosis based on tumor type and staging.

- *Metastatic tumors:* Primary tumors including lung, breast, and lymphoma can metastasize to kidney. Prognosis usually poor.

***Renal pelvis and ureteral tumors:*** Uncommon tumors with male predominance. Transitional cell carcinoma most common. Increased risk in smokers, analgesic abuse, and those with occupational exposure to certain chemicals. Painless gross hematuria is often the presenting symptom; flank pain from ureteral obstruction. Diagnosis by IVP or retrograde studies. Treatment is surgical excision; chemotherapy and radiation of limited value.

### Bladder carcinoma

- *Transitional cell carcinoma:* Greater than 90% of all bladder cancers with male:female ratio of 3:1. Median age of diagnosis is 65 years. Most present with painless gross hematuria. Diagnosis made by cystoscopy and biopsy. Associated with the following environmental factors: occupational exposure (aniline dyes, rubber, leather, dry cleaning), analgesic abuse, radiation therapy, and cyclophosphamide therapy. Smoking increases risk by 50%. Treatment is based on staging of tumor. Transurethral resection of tumor, intravesical immunotherapy or chemotherapy (intravesical bacillus Calmette–Guérin [BCG]), radiation, chemotherapy (cisplatin or combination chemotherapy), or partial or radical cystectomy are options.
- *Squamous cell carcinoma:* Associated more with bladder irritation from chronic catheters and chronic infections. More frequent in Egypt due to chronic infection with *Schistosoma haematobium.* Treatment is based on tumor stage.

## B. Neuropathic Bladder

### ▶ Scientific Concepts

Normal bladder capacity 400–500 mL. Nerve supply from both autonomic and somatic nervous systems.

### ▶ History & Physical

Obtain history and physical with neurologic examination and palpation of bladder. Signs and symptoms may vary with cause: in spastic neuropathic bladder–involuntary urination, vague lower abdominal discomfort, autonomic dysreflexia, frequency, nocturia, urgency, double voiding; in flaccid neuropathic bladder–urine retention and overflow incontinence.

### ▶ Diagnostic Studies

BUN/creatinine; urinalysis; urodynamic studies—uroflowmetry, cystometric evaluation, urethral pressure measurement, electromyography; cystoscopy, retrograde cystogram; x-ray studies—VCUG, IVP, sonogram, CT scan.

### ▶ Diagnosis

***Spastic neuropathic bladder:*** Partial or severe neural damage above the conus medullaris (T12). Associated with reduced bladder capacity, involuntary bladder contractions, high voiding pressures, detrusor hypertrophy, sphincter spasticity (ureteral reflux). Causes include spinal cord injuries; autonomic dysreflexia may be present.

*Mildly spastic neuromuscular dysfunction:* Weakened cerebral regulation causing symptoms of urinary frequency, nocturia, urgency, and incontinence. Causes include brain tumors, Parkinson's disease, multiple sclerosis, dementia, cerebrovascular accidents, and partial spine injuries.

*Flaccid neuropathic bladder:* Damage to peripheral innervation of bladder or sacral cord segments S2-4. Associated with large bladder capacity and residual urine, lack of voluntary bladder contractions, low voiding pressures, mild hypertrophy of bladder wall, and decreased tone of external sphincter. Causes include trauma, tumors, congenital anomalies, posterior spinal cord lesions, radiation or surgical damage, and neuropathies (diabetes, pernicious anemia).

► Clinical Therapeutics
*Spastic:* Low-dose anticholinergic medications and parasympatholytic drugs (oxybutynin chloride, dicyclomine hydrochloride, methantheline bromide, tolterodine).

*Flaccid:* Parasympathomimetic drugs (bethanechol chloride).

► Clinical Intervention
*Spastic:* Bladder training, Foley catheter, condom catheter, sphincterotomy in males, sacral rhizotomy, neurostimulation of sacral nerve roots (bladder pacemaker), urinary diversion.

*Flaccid:* Bladder training, intermittent catheterization, surgery for BPH if bladder outlet obstruction present.

## C. Enuresis

► Scientific Concepts
Involuntary passage of urine at night or while sleeping usually due to delayed maturation of central nervous system. Usually defined as bedwetting after age 3 years; 10% of children over 3 years may have enuresis.

► History & Physical
Urine stream is normal. Not associated with UTIs. Frequency and urgency may be present. Physical and urological exam normal.

► Diagnostic Studies
Daytime incontinence needs further investigation. Urological evaluation usually not indicated unless other organic disease (obstruction, urethral stenosis, ureteral reflux, neuropathic bladder) or infection is suspected.

► Differential Diagnosis
Obstruction, ureteral reflux, infection, neurogenic disease, urethral stenosis.

► Clinical Therapeutics
Imipramine drug of choice. Others include parasympatholytic drugs, sympathomimetic drugs, desmopressin nasal spray (antidiuretic hormone preparation), and psychotherapy.

► Clinical Intervention
Limit evening fluids, empty bladder at bedtime, awaken to void at night; mechanical devices such as alarm pads on bed may be helpful.

► Health Maintenance Issues

Bladder training should not start until after age 18 months. Anxiety of parents may be transferred to child. Psychological fear may cause enuresis. Most cases resolve by age 10 years.

## D. Testicular and Prostate Disease

### 1. Testicular Carcinoma

► Scientific Concepts

Two to three cases per 100,000 males in the United States per year. Ninety to 95% are germ cell tumors (seminoma, nonseminoma), others are nongerminal tumors (Leydig cell, Sertoli cell, gonadoblastoma). Most common germ cell tumor in bilateral primary testicular carcinoma is seminoma. In the United States, more frequent in white males and those of higher socioeconomic classes. More common on right side than left due to higher incidence of cryptorchidism on right. Risk is higher in those with history of cryptorchidism (especially intra-abdominal testis); tumor is usually a seminoma. Surgery to relocate the testis into scrotum does not decrease risk of malignancy but aids in future examinations for tumors. Other risk factors include maternal exogenous estrogen during pregnancy, trauma, and testicular atrophy due to infection.

► History & Physical

Signs and symptoms include painless enlargement of testis, testicular mass (usually firm and nontender), and testicular heaviness. Occasionally, pain from testicular hemorrhage, abdominal masses, lymphadenopathy, or gynecomastia present. Ten percent of tumors are asymptomatic on presentation; found after trauma, by partner, or on routine exam. Metastatic symptoms of back pain, dyspnea, cough, nausea, vomiting, anorexia, bone pain, and leg swelling due to venous obstruction may be present.

► Diagnostic Studies

Increased alpha fetoprotein (AFP) in nonseminomatous germ cell tumors (not in seminomas), increased human chorionic gonadotropin (hCG), increased total lactic dehydrogenase (LDH) and LDH isoenzyme-1, anemia, increased liver function tests, scrotal ultrasound, metastatic evaluation (chest x-ray, CT abdomen/pelvis, possibly CT of chest), 24-hour urine for CrCl if chemotherapy needed.

► Differential Diagnosis

Epididymitis, epididymoorchitis, hydrocele (transillumination of scrotum helpful), spermatocele, varicocele, epidermoid cyst.

► Clinical Therapeutics

Dependent on tumor type and staging. Radiation therapy or chemotherapy; seminomas are very radiosensitive.

► Clinical Intervention

Inguinal exploration with radical orchiectomy. Retroperitoneal lymph node dissection or modified version for nonseminomatous germ cell tumor.

► Health Maintenance Issues

If no lymph node dissection, then surveillance with monthly follow-up for first 2 years, bimonthly in third year, then at regular intervals with repeat tumor markers at each visit and chest x-ray and CT scan every 3–4 months. Those with retroperitoneal lymph node dissection or radiation also require regular follow-up at 3-month intervals for 2 years, every 6 months for 5 years, then yearly with physical exam, repeat AFP, hCG, LDH, and chest x-ray. Survival rate dependent on tumor type and stage; rates improving with advances in combination chemotherapy.

## 2. Prostate Carcinoma

▶ Scientific Concepts

Most common cancer in American males. Nearly 200,000 new cases diagnosed in 2000, and there are many more occult prostate cancers that are not clinically recognized. Incidence increases with age; uncommon under the age of 40 years, however, incidence increases to one in eight in men 60–79 years of age. Most tumors are adenocarcinomas. Environmental, dietary, genetic, and hormonal factors may all play a role in etiology.

▶ History & Physical

Most patients are asymptomatic and are found to have abnormal prostate by digital rectal exam. Urinary obstructive symptoms can occur but are more likely due to BPH. Symptoms of metastatic disease (cord compression, pathologic fractures) may be present.

▶ Diagnostic Studies

Digital rectal exam and prostate-specific antigen (PSA) with age-specific reference ranges. PSA useful for detecting, staging, and monitoring response to therapy, as well as evaluating for recurrence of tumor. Serum acid phosphatase is more predictive of metastases. BUN/creatinine is elevated if obstruction present. Alkaline phosphatase and serum calcium are elevated with bone metastases. Obtain prostate biopsy by transrectal ultrasound guidance. Transrectal ultrasound to image prostate can be used in staging of prostate cancer. MRI used to evaluate prostate and lymph nodes. Radionuclide bone scan used to rule out bone metastases.

▶ Differential Diagnosis

Benign prostatic hyperplasia, prostatitis, prostatic fibrosis, prostatic calculi or cysts.

▶ Clinical Therapeutics

Treatment determined by tumor grade and stage as well as the patient's life expectancy and morbidity of treatment. Locally extensive cancers are at increased risk for local and distant relapse with radiation or surgery alone; other therapies under investigation include surgery or radiation with androgen deprivation (luteinizing hormone-releasing hormone [LHRH] agonists, estrogens, antiandrogens, orchiectomy), cryosurgery, advanced radiation, and hormonal therapy alone. Metastatic prostate cancer can be treated with testicular androgen deprivation (LHRH agonists, estrogens, orchiectomy) and adrenal androgen blockage with an antiandrogen (flutamide, bicalutamide). Treatment of hormone refractory disease is difficult; palliative measures for pain control. Antiandrogen therapy must be stopped. Chemotherapeutic agents of limited value; ongoing studies with use of estramustine, ketoconazole, and mitoxantrone.

► **Clinical Intervention**

Based on TNM staging system (primary tumor, regional lymph nodes, distant metastases), age, and health of patient. Watchful waiting may be alternative in those with other medical illnesses or in older men (generally if life expectancy <10 years) and those with small-volume or well-differentiated cancers. Localized disease and minimal extracapsular disease may respond to radiation therapy or prostatectomy.

► **Health Maintenance Issues**

Increased risk in African Americans, those with positive family history of prostate cancer, and possibly in those with prior vasectomy. High dietary fat intake may increase risk.

## 3. Benign Prostatic Hyperplasia

► **Scientific Concepts**

Most common benign tumor in men. Primary etiology unclear; hormonal and age-related factors possible. Increased frequency in men over 50 years of age.

► **History & Physical**

Urinary symptoms may include frequency, nocturia, hesitancy, dribbling, urgency, decreased force and caliber of urinary stream, incomplete bladder emptying, and urinary retention. Symptoms generally progressive over years. A symptom index system has been designed to help select therapy. Obtain a careful history to rule out other urinary tract problems. Physical examination should include digital rectal exam, palpation of bladder, and genital exam to exclude structural deformity.

► **Diagnostic Studies**

Digital rectal exam, urinalysis may help establish other diagnosis; serum BUN/creatinine, ultrasound, uroflowmetry and postvoid residual urine, serum PSA, and cystoscopy. Cystoscopy not recommended for routine evaluation; useful when hematuria is present to exclude other structural abnormalities or prior to surgical therapy.

► **Clinical Therapeutics**

*Alpha-1-adrenergic blockers:* Alpha-1 adrenoreceptors are present in prostate and base of bladder and are increased in prostatic hyperplasia; blocking these receptors, especially subtype alpha-1a, can reduce bladder outlet resistance. Alpha-1-adrenergic blockers are approved for treatment of BPH, increase urinary flow, and improve prostate symptom scores. Monitor for hypotension, lightheadedness, and dizziness. Terazosin, doxazosin, and prazosin are all alpha-1 selective, whereas tamsulosin is selective to alpha-1a receptors. Selective blockade of alpha-1a receptors produces fewer systemic side effects.

*5-alpha-reductase inhibitors:* Finasteride acts to decrease dihydrotestosterone, reduce obstructive symptoms, increase urinary flow rate, and lower PSA level. Shown to reduce prostate volume; however 6 months of therapy needed for maximum benefit.

*Combination therapy:* Ongoing studies using alpha-blockers and 5-alpha-reductase inhibitors are underway.

*Phytotherapy:* Use of plants or plant extracts including saw palmetto berry and others. Efficiency and safety not tested in controlled studies.

▶ Clinical Intervention

*No therapy:* Close monitoring may be reasonable when symptoms not severe.

*Transurethral resection of prostate (TURP):* Mainstay of therapy but invasive; for moderate to severe symptoms. Complications include retrograde ejaculation, postoperative failure to void, TUR syndrome (intraoperative fluid absorption), hemorrhage, UTI, bladder neck contracture, urethral stricture, incontinence, impotence, and obstruction necessitating second TURP.

*Transurethral incision of prostate:* Used in cases of moderate to severe bladder outlet obstructive symptoms when prostate is normal or small.

*Open prostatectomy:* Reserved for cases in which prostate gland is large (weight is more than 100 g) or when other surgical procedures are required at the same time. Surgical approach may be suprapubic or retropubic.

*Minimally invasive procedures:* Laser prostatectomy (transurethral laser-induced prostatectomy), transurethral needle ablation of prostate, transurethral electrovaporization of prostate, microwave hyperthermia, transurethral balloon dilation of prostate, high-intensity focused ultrasound, urethral stents.

▶ Clinical Intervention for Urinary Tract
  Obstruction and Tumors

Relieve obstruction with catheter, suprapubic cystostomy, ureteral catheter, or nephrostomy tube. Postobstructive diuresis may occur. Close monitoring, pharmacological management, surgery, chemotherapy, radiation.

## IV. NEPHROLITHIASIS

▶ Scientific Concepts

Renal calculi are more common in men, occur more often in hot and dry climates, are often recurrent, and usually present in third to sixth decade of life. Metabolic, hereditary, and infectious etiologies play a role in stone formation. Ninety percent pass spontaneously, especially if <4 mm in size.

▶ History & Physical

Obtain history including onset of symptoms, timing of first stone and subsequent stones, previous evaluations (radiodiagnostics, stone analysis, hospitalizations), and family history of renal calculi. Evaluate for other known diseases associated with stone formation including primary hyperparathyroidism, renal tubular acidosis, medullary sponge kidney, and sarcoidosis.

Signs and symptoms of dysuria, frequency, and urgency may or may not be present. Hematuria may be gross or microscopic. Nausea and vomiting are occasionally associated. Renal colic results from pressure and dilatation of urinary system. It is abrupt in onset, increases in intensity over a period of time, reaches a plateau, then remains constant and severe. May begin in flank and radiate downward to groin, testicle, or vulva. Stones lodged at ureterovesicle junction may present with irritant voiding symptoms rather than renal colic. Asymptomatic stones are often found on x-ray. Stones are radiopaque except for uric acid stones.

### ▶ Diagnosis

**Calcium stones:**  Ninety percent of stones are a mixture of calcium oxalate or calcium oxalate/calcium phosphate. Risk factors include:

- *Low urine volume:* Urine saturation by crystalloids increases as urine volume decreases. Preventive goal in stone formers is to excrete at least 2 L of urine per day.
- *Hypercalciuria:* Usually idiopathic but primary hyperparathyroidism, renal tubular acidosis, sarcoidosis, and vitamin D excess are some other causes. Idiopathic hypercalciuria is most common cause of hypercalciuria. Familial tendency, usually seen in men. Serum calcium normal, parathyroid hormone (PTH) level normal or low. High intestinal calcium absorption leads to increased urinary calcium excretion. Primary hyperparathyroidism is seen more in middle-aged or older women. Associated with elevated serum calcium and PTH levels. Hypercalciuria is the result of increased production of 1,25-dihydroxyvitamin D by kidney in response to PTH. Parathyroid adenoma is cause in 95% of cases; others due to parathyroid hyperplasia.
- *Hyperuricosuria:* May result from excessive dietary purine intake. Increased uric acid crystals in urine act as a surface for calcium oxalate deposition.
- *Hyperoxaluria:* Increased urinary excretion of oxalate can cause calcium oxalate stone formation. Seen with increased production of oxalate (primary hyperoxaluria, excess vitamin C intake) or increased absorption of oxalate either dietary or intestinal (Crohn's disease, malabsorption, ileal surgery).
- *Hypocitraturia:* Citrate combines with calcium in the renal tubular lumen to form a soluble complex. Low levels of citrate in the urine predispose to calcium stone formation. Hypocitraturia may result from chronic metabolic acidosis (chronic diarrhea, renal tubular acidosis), hypokalemia, or acetazolamide therapy.

**Uric acid stones:**  Nonopaque by radiologic study. Associated mainly with acid urine pH (as seen in gout, idiopathic uric acid stones, chronic diarrhea associated with ileostomy or laxative abuse) and an increased urinary uric acid concentration (dietary purine intake, rapid cell turnover, or massive nucleolysis following chemotherapy).

**Cystine stones:**  Reduced renal tubular reabsorption of cystine. Seen only with hereditary disorder of cystinuria.

**Struvite stones:**  Form as a result of urease-positive bacterial urine infection (often *Proteus* or *Providencia*). Contain both struvite (magnesium ammonium phosphate) and calcium phosphate and are often seen as large staghorn calculi in renal collecting system. Urine pH high, usually > 8.0. Can lead to chronic renal failure (if bilateral), persistent infection, or abscess. Infection difficult to resolve due to bacteria in stones.

► Diagnostic Studies

*Urinalysis:* Hematuria is commonly seen; may be microscopic or gross. Bacteriuria and crystalluria may be present. Cystine and struvite crystals are specific; other crystals can be seen in normal urine but may be significant if found in a patient with suspected stones.

*Metabolic investigation:* Laboratory tests may include serum calcium, serum phosphorus, PTH level, uric acid, creatinine, BUN, electrolytes, serum protein, and urinalysis. Twenty-four-hour urine collection for measurement of urinary excretion of calcium, phosphate, uric acid, oxalate, citrate, cystine, creatinine, pH, sodium, and urine volume. Must collect all urine in 24-hour period. One or two collections are recommended (weekday and weekend). Should be done in the patient's normal outpatient setting (not while hospitalized), with patient eating and drinking usual amount of food and beverages (not on any unusual diets), and with the patient participating in usual activities. Stone analysis.

*Abdominal film:* Identify radiopaque but not radiolucent (uric acid) stones.

*Renal sonogram:* Identify stones in renal pelvis and kidney. Non-obstructing stones in the ureter may not be seen.

*IVP:* Locate site of obstruction and identify structural or anatomical abnormalities.

*Spiral CT:* Becoming test of choice due to higher sensitivity, faster scan times, and no need for IV contrast.

► Clinical Therapeutics
**Treatment of calcium stones**
- *Hypercalciuria state:* Idiopathic—increase fluid intake. Restrict dietary sodium (high sodium intake in diet will increase renal calcium excretion and decrease the effect of thiazide diuretics). Dietary protein restriction (especially animal protein) may decrease calciuria. Dietary calcium restriction is not advised; should maintain moderate calcium intake of at least two to three servings daily as a low-calcium diet can lead to bone loss and also increase oxalate excretion. Thiazide diuretics used to decrease urine calcium excretion. Primary hyperparathyroidism—parathyroid surgery for adenoma or hyperplasia.
- *Hyperuricosuria state:* Reduce purine intake in diet. Pharmacological management with allopurinol.
- *Hyperoxaluria state:* Reduce excess oxalate in diet (colas, citrus juices, chocolate, tea) and reduce vitamin C supplements. In cases of intestinal disease, treatment includes calcium supplements to bind intestinal oxalate, low-fat diet, and cholestyramine.

*Treatment of uric acid stones:* Increase urine volume to 3 L/d. Alkalization of urine with bicarbonate; uric acid is more soluble in alkaline urine. Goal is urine pH 6.0 to 7.0. Reduce purine intake in diet. Allopurinol if hyperuricosuria is >1,000 mg/24 h. Acetazolamide can raise urine pH by causing bicarbonaturia.

*Treatment of cystine stones:* Goal is to increase urine volume to help dissolve excess cystine in urine. Need urine volume of ≥ 4 L daily and increased urine volumes at night. Goal is urinary cystine concentration of

<250 mg/L. Penicillamine can help prevent cystine precipitation. Alkalization of urine is beneficial.

***Treatment of struvite stones:*** Treat any associated metabolic stone disease. Suppress infection using long-term antibiotics with high tissue penetration. Achieving sterile urine is not generally successful. Percutaneous nephrolithotomy and extracorporeal shock wave lithotripsy are preferred treatment of choice. Surgery is a last resort measure for struvite stones causing obstruction, severe pain, serious infections, or substantial bleeding; stones can recur after surgical removal.

► Clinical Intervention

Increase fluid intake to at least 2 L/d. During acute episodes, strain all urine and provide analgesics. Urological management options include cystoscopy with retrieval by stone basket, extracorporeal shock wave lithotripsy, and percutaneous nephrolithotomy.

► Health Maintenance Issues

Without intervention, 40% of patients will have recurrent stones in 5 years. Identify associated risk factors, including diet (increased dietary intake of animal protein, purines, oxalate, sodium), climate (increased frequency in hot and dry areas), family history, medication use (triamterene, acetazolamide), and conditions associated with stone formation (medullary sponge kidney, horseshoe kidney, polycystic kidney disease, etc.). Patient education on preventive measures can decrease stone recurrence rate.

## V. RENAL FAILURE

### A. Acute Renal Failure

► Scientific Concepts

Acute decline in renal function over a period of hours to days; may or may not be reversible. Results in an accumulation of waste products including urea nitrogen and creatinine in the blood. In general, increase in creatinine of 0.5 to 1.0 mg/dL, decrease in the calculated creatinine clearance of 50%, or a decline in the renal function requiring dialysis. A doubling of serum creatinine represents 50% loss of GFR. Prerenal azotemia and acute tubular necrosis (ATN) account for most of cases of acute renal failure.

► History & Physical

Identify onset of renal dysfunction—in hospital versus outpatient, acute illness versus chronic systemic process. Previous labs or history of elevated creatinine helpful in establishing timing of renal disease. Evaluate for history of trauma, drugs, drug overdose, or recent illness. Physical examination findings can vary. Decreased skin turgor, postural hypotension and tachycardia, and dry mucous membranes may indicate volume depletion. Edema, rales, elevated jugular venous pressure, ascites, and gallop rhythm may indicate cardiac failure, cirrhosis, or nephrotic syndrome. Fever and rash may indicate acute interstitial nephritis. Livedo reticularis, cyanotic toes, or digital ulcers may indicate atheroembolic disease. Distended bladder or enlarged prostate may indicate obstruction.

▶ Diagnostic Studies

Elevated BUN/creatinine, urine volume (anuric, oliguric, normal), urinalysis (casts, protein, hematuria, cells), urine sodium and osmolality, serum tests for specific illness (antineutrophil cytoplasmic antibody [ANCA], antinuclear antibody [ANA], etc.). Radiodiagnostics include: abdominal plain film, renal ultrasound, IVP, renal angiogram, CT scan, renal scan, cystoscopy, retrograde pyelogram. Renal biopsy in those cases of acute renal failure of unknown etiology and to identify specific disease processes to help guide therapy.

▶ Differential Diagnosis

Prerenal versus ATN: Prerenal disease is a result of decreased renal perfusion. ATN is a result of intrinsic insult to the renal tubules from either ischemia or nephrotoxins. Urine and laboratory diagnostic indices:

***Prerenal:*** BUN/creatinine ratio > 20:1, normal urinalysis, urine sodium < 20 mEq/L, urine osmolality > 500 mOsm/kg, fractional excretion of sodium < 1%.

***ATN:*** BUN/creatinine ratio < 20:1, urinalysis reveals muddy brown granular casts and renal tubular epithelial cells and casts, urine sodium > 40 mEq/L, urine osmolality < 350 mOsm/kg, fractional excretion of sodium >1%.

▶ Diagnostic Categories

***Prerenal:*** Result of decreased renal perfusion.

- *Volume depletion:* Presents with signs of hypovolemia on examination. Causes may include GI losses (vomiting, diarrhea, bleeding), renal losses (diuretics, osmotic diuresis), and third-space losses (burns, tissue trauma from crush injury, pancreatitis). Treatment is fluid replacement.
- *Heart failure:* Associated with severe cardiac dysfunction (systolic or diastolic). Goal is to improve cardiac function (reduce ischemia or improve cardiac output with digitalis, vasodilators, ACE inhibitors, dopamine, dobutamine).
- *Cirrhosis:* Associated with a decrease in effective tissue perfusion. Increased renal vasoconstriction leads to acute renal failure in hepatorenal syndrome.
- *Hypotension:* Associated with shock or treatment of severe hypertension.
- *Bilateral renal artery stenosis:* Decreased renal perfusion due to renal artery disease. Use of ACE inhibitors in a patient with bilateral renal artery stenosis or renal artery stenosis in a patient with one functioning kidney can cause renal failure. ACE inhibitors lower systemic and intrarenal blood pressure. Because GFR is maintained by angiotensin II–mediated efferent arteriolar constriction, blocking angiotensin II formation with ACE inhibitors decreases GFR and may cause renal failure. Diuretics can enhance this effect.
- *NSAIDs:* NSAIDs reduce renal vasodilator prostaglandin synthesis. In prerenal states such as volume depletion, heart failure, nephrotic syndrome, or cirrhosis, NSAIDs can cause acute renal failure. In states of volume depletion, vasoconstrictors are activated and renal prostaglandins are needed to help compensate for the decreased perfusion to the kidneys. Blocking prostaglandin synthesis with NSAIDs can result in renal failure; reversible with removal of offending agent. NSAIDs can

also cause an acute interstitial nephritis, nephrotic syndrome, and may be a risk factor in analgesic nephropathy.

- *Nephrotic syndrome:* Urinary protein losses cause hypoalbuminemia and plasma volume depletion. Characterized by proteinuria (3.0 g/d or greater), hypoalbuminemia, edema, hyperlipidemia, and a hypercoagulable state.

***Intrinsic renal disease:*** Disorders within the kidney involving the blood vessels, glomeruli, tubules, or interstitium causing impaired renal function.

### Tubular disease

- *ATN:* Associated with a sudden decline in renal function lasting 7–21 days, followed by gradual improvement back to baseline. Tubular injury related to renal insult, usually ischemia or a nephrotoxin. Postischemic ATN is seen with severe prerenal disease such as hypotension and shock. Nephrotoxic ATN is seen with drugs, radiocontrast, and heme pigments.
- *Aminoglycoside nephrotoxicity:* Most common cause of antibiotic-associated renal injury in hospitalized patients. Drug accumulates in the renal cortex. Seen in 7–36% of patients on aminoglycosides, and is related to dose and duration of therapy. Findings include an increase in the BUN and creatinine occurring 5–7 days into course of therapy. Toxicity risk minimized by maintaining drug levels in therapeutic range and monitoring serum creatinine. In addition to dose and duration, other risk factors include: volume depletion, sepsis, elderly patients, underlying renal disease, exposure to other nephrotoxins (radiocontrast, drugs). ARF is usually reversible when drug discontinued but may take weeks. Tobramycin is the least nephrotoxic.
- *Radiocontrast nephrotoxicity:* Associated with an increase in the creatinine within 24 hours after the radiocontrast study. Creatinine peaks at 3–7 days, then quickly returns to baseline in most cases. Risk factors include: preexisting renal insufficiency (creatinine > 1.5 mg/dL), diabetic nephropathy, volume depletion, severe congestive heart failure, and elderly patients. Risk of renal failure is low when creatinine < 1.5 mg/dL but increases with more advanced renal insufficiency and also with amount of contrast used, number of studies performed, and concomitant medications (ACEI, NSAIDs). Prevention in high-risk patients includes IV hydration before, during, and after the study as well as avoiding other nephrotoxic agents and limiting amount of contrast. Role of nonionic agents is limited. Has not been shown to benefit patients with normal renal function but may offer small benefit in those with creatinine > 1.5–2.0 mg/dL. In those patients with chronic renal failure, the use of acetylcysteine (600 mg twice daily the day before and day of procedure) in addition to IV hydration and nonionic agents appears to protect the kidneys from contrast-induced nephrotoxicity.
- *Cisplatin:* Direct tubular toxin. Toxicity can be limited with IV hydration, specifically isotonic sodium chloride. Renal magnesium wasting commonly seen.
- *Heme pigments associated with ATN:* Seen with rhabdomyolysis (myoglobinuria) or intravascular hemolysis (hemoglobinuria). Rhabdomyolysis is caused by trauma (tissue ischemia), infections, toxins

(ethanol, toluene, ethylene glycol), intense exercise, seizures, and drugs (cocaine, heroin, hepatic hydroxymethyl glutaryl coenzyme A (HMG CoA) reductase inhibitors, fibric acid derivatives). Lab findings include myoglobinuria; urine dipstick positive for blood but no or few red blood cells (RBCs) seen on microscopy; urine red to brown with pigmented granular casts; plasma normal in color; markedly elevated plasma creatine kinase; elevated serum creatinine out of proportion to BUN; elevated uric acid, potassium, and phosphorus levels; and decreased serum calcium. Treatment includes IV isotonic fluids, forced alkaline diuresis with sodium bicarbonate (alkalinizes urine and increases solubility of heme proteins), mannitol, and furosemide. Treat hyperkalemia and hyperphosphatemia. Hemoglobinuria associated with intravascular hemolysis can be seen in transfusion reactions with mismatched blood, drugs, and infections. Lab findings include hemoglobinuria; urine red to brown with pigmented casts; plasma pink in color; low haptoglobin; and elevated levels of LDH, bilirubin, potassium, phosphorus, and plasma hemoglobin.

- *Multiple myeloma:* Characterized by overproduction of monoclonal immunoglobulin light chains by malignant plasma cells. Cause is unknown; median age at diagnosis is approximately 65 years. Renal failure is due to tubular obstruction from casts and tubular cell toxicity. Presentation may include acute or chronic renal failure, proteinuria, anemia, weakness, bone pain (especially back), pathologic fractures, lytic lesions on x-ray, and hypercalcemia. Diagnosis confirmed by abnormal paraprotein found in serum or urine protein electrophoresis, immunoelectrophoresis of blood or urine for monoclonal light chains (Bence Jones proteins), bone marrow biopsy, or renal biopsy. Treatment includes hydration, alkalinization of urine, correction of hypercalcemia, decrease production of immunoglobulins (chemotherapy and steroids), plasmapheresis, or dialysis.

### Interstitial disease

- *Interstitial nephritis:* Characterized by interstitial inflammation, edema, and renal tubular cell damage; glomeruli and blood vessels not usually involved. May be acute or chronic. Can be due to hypersensitivity to a drug (penicillin, methicillin, NSAIDs, sulfonamides, rifampin, cimetidine, diuretics), related to infections (acute pyleonephritis, systemic infections), associated with immunologic disorders (systemic lupus erythematosus, cryoglobulinemia), or idiopathic. Presentation may include rash, arthralgias, or fever. Lab findings include eosinophiluria by Hansel stain, mild proteinuria, hematuria, pyuria, WBC casts, and peripheral eosinophilia. Renal dysfunction can be mild to severe and may require dialysis. Diagnosis based on clinical and laboratory findings. Renal biopsy to confirm diagnosis when in question. Treatment is supportive; stop suspected drugs. Steroid therapy controversial; may offer some benefit in drug-induced ATN. Recovery over weeks to months, although renal function may not return to baseline.

### Glomerular disease

- *Glomerulonephritis (GN):* Term for inflammation of the glomerulus. Nephritic syndrome is associated with hypertension, edema, active urine sediment with hematuria, RBC casts, and proteinuria. RBC casts indicative of GN. Nephrotic syndrome associated with > 3.0 g/d proteinuria, hypoalbuminemia, hyperlipidemia, and edema. Lab tests include urinalysis (hematuria, proteinuria, cells, casts), BUN/creatinine, 24-hour protein and CrCl, urine and protein electrophoresis, complement levels, antistreptolysin-O (ASO) titer and other disease-specific tests (antiglomerular basement membrane antibody [anti-GBM antibody], ANCA, ANA, cryoglobulin, hepatitis screen), renal sonogram, and renal biopsy.

- *Poststreptococcal glomerulonephritis:* Caused by a nephritogenic strain of group A beta-hemolytic streptococci and may occur after pharyngeal or skin infection. Most commonly seen in children and otherwise healthy young adults; course more benign in children. Has latent period of 7–21 days from infection to onset of nephritis. Presenting signs and symptoms may include abrupt onset of hematuria (cola-colored urine), edema (usually periorbital), hypertension, oliguria, nonnephrotic range proteinuria, and RBC and other cellular casts. Lab tests include throat or skin culture positive for group A streptococci, decreased serum complements, and elevated titers for ASO, anti-DNAaseB, and antihyaluronidase. Treatment mainly supportive; appropriate antibiotics. Antihypertensives, sodium restriction, and diuretics may be indicated. In children, disease usually self limiting.

- *Rapidly progressive glomerulonephritis (RPGN):* Associated with loss of renal function over days to weeks. Diagnosis confirmed by renal biopsy, which shows crescents in glomeruli; immunofluorescence and electron microscopy to determine specific type of disease (Wegener's granulomatosis, Goodpasture's disease, immune complex glomerulonephritis, idiopathic). Treatment includes antihypertensives, steroids, and cytotoxic agents or plasmapheresis depending on diagnosis; dialysis if needed.

- *Goodpasture's disease:* Form of rapidly progressive GN associated with pulmonary hemorrhage and anti-GBM antibodies. Incidence higher in males and often presents in second and third decades. In 20–60% of cases, preceded by an upper respiratory infection. Lab tests include positive circulating anti-GBM antibodies, iron deficient anemia, normal complements, and pulmonary infiltrates on chest radiograph. Renal biopsy identifies deposition of immunoglobulin G (IgG) along glomerular basement membrane (GBM). Treatment includes steroids, cyclophosphamide, and plasma exchange (remove circulating anti-GBM antibodies). Dialysis when needed.

**Vascular disease**

- *Vasculitis:* Systemic condition associated with inflammatory changes in vessel walls thought to be related to immune response mechanisms. Causes include temporal arteritis, polyarteritis nodosa, Kawasaki disease, Wegener's granulomatosis, and Henoch–Schönlein purpura. Presenting symptoms vary and are related to vessels and organs involved; may include fever, arthralgias, myalgias, headache, abdominal pain, and weight loss. Diagnosis based on physical exam and symptoms, specific serologic laboratory tests (ANCA, circulating immune complexes, complement levels), and microscopic evaluation of vessels from renal or other tissue biopsies. Treatment is dependent on disease and severity; corticosteroids and cytotoxic agents are choices.

- *Malignant hypertension:* Presents with severe headache, blurred vision, dizziness, and confusion. Diagnostic findings are blood pressure > 200/130 mm Hg; retinopathy (hemorrhages and exudates); papilledema; increased creatinine, hematuria, proteinuria, and RBC casts. Presence of papilledema is required to make diagnosis. Initial treatment goal is to reduce diastolic blood pressure gradually to range of 100–110 mm Hg to minimize target organ ischemia; initial drug choices may include IV sodium nitroprusside and nitroglycerine due to their short onset of action and duration allowing more precise titration of blood pressure. IV labetalol, nicardipine, and enalapril also used.

- *Atheroembolic disease:* Atheromatous plaque causing obstruction of medium or small renal arteries. Presentation may include livedo reticularis, cyanotic toes, painful ulcerations of digits, fever, abdominal pain, anorexia, and GI bleeding due to bowel infarction. Usually associated with disruption of plaque during angiography or surgical procedure. Renal dysfunction can be mild to acute renal failure; onset of renal failure is typically slow and progressive over 30–60 days; may or may not recover some renal function. Diagnosis based on history and suspicion as well as physical exam. Eosinophilia and mild proteinuria may be present. Differential diagnosis includes contrast-induced renal failure, vasculitis, ATN, interstitial nephritis, and renal artery stenosis. Treatment is supportive; pain control, management of digital ischemic areas, amputation, avoid anticoagulant therapy, avoid further angiography procedures, and dialysis if needed. Those at increased risk for thromboembolic disease are elderly patients with extensive atherosclerotic and hypertensive disease, smokers, male gender, and those over the age of 70 years.

***Postrenal:*** Obstruction of the urinary tract leading to reduced GFR. Causes include: urethral obstruction, bladder outlet obstruction due to prostate (hyperplasia, tumors), bladder dysfunction, tumors (bladder, pelvic malignancy, retroperitoneal fibrosis), and bilateral ureteral obstruction (calculi). Symptoms depend on location and cause of the obstruction. Urine volumes may vary. Ureteral obstruction must be bilateral or occur in setting of one functioning kidney to cause renal failure. Physical exam may detect prostatic enlargement, distended bladder, or mass. Laboratory findings include elevated BUN/creatinine. Renal sonogram to rule out hydronephrosis or hydroureter. Bladder catheterization for postvoid residual urine may establish a diagnosis. Treatment guided by the underlying cause. Bladder catheter, ureteral stents, and nephrostomy tubes may be indicated to relieve acute obstruction.

## B. Chronic Renal Failure

### ▶ Scientific Concepts
Progressive decline in renal function, generally over months to years. Loss of nephrons may lead to end-stage renal disease (ESRD). Diabetes mellitus and hypertension most common causes of ESRD.

### ▶ History & Physical
History of medication or other drug use, obstructive symptoms, past renal disease, hypertension, diabetes mellitus, proteinuria, hematuria,

family history of renal disease or other illnesses. Most patients are asymptomatic until renal disease is advanced (CrCl < 10–15 mL/min). Symptoms may include fatigue, weakness, feeling cold, anorexia, nausea, vomiting, metallic taste, hiccup, sleep disturbance, irritability, restless legs, twitching, pruritus, decreased concentration, dyspnea, edema, or chest pain (pericarditis). Uremia is used to describe this spectrum of clinical symptoms and is indicative of severe renal insufficiency. Physical examination findings: may appear chronically ill, sallow complexion, skin excoriations, ecchymoses, retinopathy, uremic odor to breath, hypertension, rales, cardiomyopathy, pericardial rub, edema, drowsy, lethargic, confused, asterixis, myoclonus, rash, arthritis, palpable kidneys, prostate exam.

### ▶ Diagnostic Studies

*Laboratory data:* BUN/creatinine, anemia (normocytic, normochromic), metabolic acidosis, hypocalcemia, hyperphosphatemia, serum albumin, proteinuria, hematuria, urine casts, 24-hour urine for protein and creatinine clearance, other markers of specific disease (ANA, serum protein electrophoresis, ANCA, etc.). Obtain prior labs to document chronic nature of disease and aid in estimating progression of renal failure.

*Radiodiagnostics:* Renal ultrasound (small echogenic kidneys, polycystic kidneys, chronic obstruction), abdominal x-ray, IVP, renal scan, CT/MRI, renal angiogram, renal osteodystrophy on x-ray.

*Renal biopsy:* Tissue diagnosis in unexplained acute and chronic renal failure associated with systemic disease to help determine extent of renal involvement and guide treatment. Relative contraindications include a solitary kidney, bleeding disorder, multiple cysts, or severe uncontrolled hypertension.

### ▶ Diagnostic Categories

*Prerenal:* Conditions leading to prolonged decreased tissue perfusion (severe heart failure, cirrhosis).

*Intrinsic renal*

#### Tubular disease

- *Polycystic kidney disease (PCKD):* Autosomal dominant inherited disorder that occurs 1 in every 400–1,000 live births. Accounts for 5–10% of all cases of end-stage renal failure. Characterized by enlargement of the kidneys with multiple cysts and slow deterioration in renal function over years, with 25–45% of patients progressing to end-stage renal failure by middle age or later. Cysts also found in liver, pancreas, and spleen but not associated with liver failure. Renal calculi, infections, and cyst hemorrhage may occur. Cerebral aneurysms may be associated with this disease in 5–10% of patients. Ruptured cerebral aneurysms may occur in certain families.

  Diagnosis based on positive family history, physical exam, genetic testing, abdominal or flank pain, hematuria or UTIS, finding of hypertension (80% of patients), renal insufficiency (mild or advanced), and minimal proteinuria. Renal calculi and cyst hemorrhage may develop. Renal sonogram (test of choice) or CT scan to confirm cysts. Screening for PCKD with renal ultrasound may be done in those with positive family history; more likely to diagnose in those over age 30. Age-dependent criteria now established. Magnetic resonance angiography of the brain indicated if family history of cerebral aneurysm is present.

Treatment is supportive; blood pressure control (ACE inhibitors), cyst drainage for severe pain. Dietary protein restriction of limited benefit; recommend 1.0–1.1 g/kg/d. Dialysis or renal transplant for those with ESRD. Risk factors for disease progression include a younger age at diagnosis, hypertension, race (increased progression of disease in African Americans), and kidney size. Complicating factors may include bleeding from cysts, UTIs, infected cysts, pain, renal calculi, and cerebral hemorrhage.

- *Medullary sponge kidney:* A benign disorder characterized by development of cysts in terminal collecting ducts. Most patients are asymptomatic at presentation. Associated with increased incidence of renal calculi and UTIs. Diagnosis made by IVP that reveals brushlike appearance to calyces. Renal function is normal. No specific treatment except for UTIs and stone complications.

### Interstitial disease

- *Analgesic abuse:* Less than 1% of cases of ESRD in the United States. Increased risk with analgesics containing *both* aspirin and phenacetin (no longer available), acetaminophen, NSAIDs, combination analgesics, and possibly aspirin. Risk related to dose and duration of drug use. Clinical presentation is typically middle-aged women with chronic pain and daily analgesic use over a long period of time. May have hematuria or flank pain secondary to papillary necrosis, elevated BUN/creatinine, hypertension, or mild proteinuria. An increased risk of transitional cell carcinoma (especially bladder) is associated with phenacetin.

  Diagnosis based on suspicion or history of analgesic use; interstitial nephritis and renal papillary necrosis are pathologic findings. IVP may detect papillary necrosis and sonogram or CT scan may show an irregular renal contour. Treatment is to discontinue analgesics (especially combinations of aspirin and acetaminophen) and control hypertension.

  *Other causes of interstitial disease:* Chronic pyelonephritis, multiple myeloma.

### Glomerular disease

- *Diabetic nephropathy:* The major cause of ESRD, accounting for approximately 44% of dialysis patients. Marked glomerular sclerosis leads to renal failure. Glomerular disease is usually not detected until diabetes is present for 10 years. Lab findings of elevated BUN/creatinine; obtain 24-hour urine for protein and creatinine clearance. Microalbuminuria can be detected by radioimmunoassay prior to positive dipstick protein and is predictive of gross proteinuria and eventual renal insufficiency. Microalbuminuria is usually seen between 7 years after onset of type 1 diabetes and dipstick proteinuria is seen after 10–20 years of type 1 diabetes, followed by progressive decline in renal function over years with ESRD occurring within 5–15 years of onset of proteinuria. Type 2 diabetics may initially present with proteinuria due to prolonged length of time from onset of disease to diagnosis. Type 1 diabetics with diabetes more than 5 years should have microalbuminuria screening yearly. Type 2 diabetics should have initial screening for proteinuria by dipstick at diagnosis. If no proteinuria present, should be immediately screened for microalbuminuria and yearly thereafter. Microalbuminuria can be measured by spot albumin-to-creatinine ratio or 24-hour urine collection.

Diagnosis: In those patients with type 1 diabetes, if diabetes is present at least 10 years and is accompanied by proteinuria and retinopathy, a renal biopsy generally is not indicated unless other disease is suspected by history or exam. For type 2 diabetes, if no retinopathy is present, may need to evaluate for and rule out other forms of renal disease.

Treatment involves strict glycemic control, especially early on in disease as well as blood pressure control. ACE inhibitors beneficial in reducing intraglomerular pressure and microalbuminuria; non-dihydropyridine calcium channel blockers are also useful but with less effect on decreasing urine protein excretion. Blood pressure goal in patients with proteinuria is 130/80 mm Hg. Dietary protein restriction may be helpful. Dialysis (hemodialysis or peritoneal) and renal transplant for those with ESRD.

- *Membranous nephropathy:* Most common cause of nephrotic syndrome in adults presenting with proteinuria and no other obvious systemic illness. Cause is often idiopathic. Males > females, usually over 30 years of age. Can be associated with malignancy in those patients presenting over age 60. Associated with an increased risk of arterial and venous thrombosis, especially renal vein thrombosis. Disease is an immune-mediated process with immune complexes found in glomerular capillary walls. Course is variable and depends on serum creatinine, biopsy findings, age, sex, and amount of proteinuria; only 20 to 30% develop progressive renal failure, remainder have remission, stable, or very slow progression of renal disease. May be associated with other systemic illness or medication 20–30% of the time.

  Diagnosis: Proteinuria (often nephrotic), microscopic hematuria, hypertension, edema, anasarca, anorexia, hyperlipidemia, hypoalbuminemia, lipiduria, normal or elevated BUN/creatinine.

  Treatment: In those with normal renal function and nonnephrotic proteinuria, controlling blood pressure and reducing proteinuria with ACE inhibitors helpful. Dietary protein restriction may be beneficial. Treat hyperlipidemia. Anticoagulants for those who have had a thrombotic event. Immunosuppressive therapy with corticosteroids and cytotoxic agents for those with progressive renal disease or severe nephrotic syndrome.

- *Focal glomerulosclerosis:* Characterized by segmental sclerosing lesions in glomeruli. Primary idiopathic and secondary forms (reflux nephropathy, human immunodeficiency virus [HIV]-associated nephropathy, morbid obesity) have been identified. Seen in children and adults. Most progress to ESRD, usually 5–20 years from presentation.

  Diagnosis: Proteinuria, microscopic hematuria, and hypertension may be seen. Diagnosis confirmed by renal biopsy.

  Treatment is controversial. ACE inhibitors may be used to decrease proteinuria. Corticosteroids or other immunosuppressive drugs in patients with nephrotic syndrome, elevated creatinine, or significant findings on biopsy.

- *Lupus nephritis:* Disease associated with deposition of immune complex in tissues. Renal involvement varies from mild to ESRD. Physical examination findings include a malar rash, photosensitivity, oral ulcers, arthritis, serositis, and hypertension.

  Diagnosis: BUN/creatinine, proteinuria, hematuria, cellular casts in urine, lupus erythematosus cell prep, anti-DNA antibody, double-stranded DNA, anti-Sm antibody, positive ANA, antiphospholipid antibody. Obtain renal biopsy to define renal pathology (class I–VI) and guide treatment.

  Treatment consists of corticosteroids for active lupus nephritis to promote remission of renal disease. Steroids and cytotoxic drugs (cyclophosphamide) are used for more aggressive renal disease.

- *IgA nephropathy (Berger's disease):* Most common form of primary glomerulonephritis worldwide. Characterized by IgA deposition in mesangium of glomeruli. It is most common in children and young adults; male:female ratio 2:1 to 3:1. May present with hematuria 1–2 days following recent URI symptoms; hematuria may recur months to years later associated with pharyngitis, febrile state, or vigorous exercise. Other presentations include asymptomatic microscopic hematuria and proteinuria (< 1 g/d) or Henoch–Schönlein purpura.

  Diagnosis: Increased serum IgA levels (not specific), increased circulating IgA-containing immune complexes, elevated BUN/creatinine, proteinuria. Renal biopsy is the standard for diagnosis.

  Treatment for acute disease may include steroids, cytotoxic agents, anticoagulants, and plasmapheresis. Chronic disease treatment involves control of hypertension (ACE inhibitors), sodium and protein restriction, and steroids. Immunosuppressives are of unclear benefit. Dialysis and renal transplantation for those with ESRD. IgA nephropathy is a chronic disease with progressive worsening of renal function in 40% of patients, with half of those developing ESRD within 20 years from presentation. One third of patients have persistent microscopic hematuria and minimal proteinuria but no renal failure.

- *Amyloidosis:* Two forms of amyloidosis. Primary form is due to overproduction of monoclonal immunoglobulin light chains. Secondary form involves deposition of nonimmunoglobulin serum amyloid A protein. Amyloid deposits are found mainly in glomeruli and stain positively with Congo red. Other organ involvement (cardiac, GI, pulmonary) may be seen.

  Diagnosis: Proteinuria, renal insufficiency, monoclonal light chains in blood or urine, renal biopsy, rectal, gingival, or fat pad biopsy.

  Treatment of primary amyloid includes melphalan, prednisone, and autologous stem cell transplant. Treat underlying disease process in secondary amyloid; colchicine may be helpful. Dialysis or renal transplantation for those with ESRD.

- *Minimal change nephropathy (Nil disease):* Presents as nephrotic syndrome. May occur in children or adults. In children, peak age of onset 24–36 months and males > females. Usually not associated with hypertension, hematuria, or renal dysfunction.

  Diagnostic findings include: nephrotic range proteinuria, hypoalbuminemia, edema, hypercholesterolemia, and oval fat bodies in urine. Renal biopsy confirms diagnosis. In children, initiate treatment with a trial of steroids before renal biopsy.

Treatment is corticosteroids. For steroid-resistant or frequent relapsing cases, may use chronic low-dose steroids, cyclophosphamide, chlorambucil, or cyclosporine. In those patients who are unresponsive to therapy, management of edema with salt restriction and diuretics. ACE inhibitors or NSAIDs can be used to decrease proteinuria. Prognosis is good with complete remission or partial remission; relapses occur in 75 to 85% of patients. Relapses in most children disappear 10 years after onset of disease. Chronic renal failure rare in patients responsive to steroids. Complications are related to use of steroid drugs and cytotoxic agents.

### Vascular disease

- *Hypertensive nephrosclerosis:* Second leading cause of ESRD. Vascular and glomerular damage usually occurs over years. Risk of chronic renal failure secondary to hypertension is much more likely in blacks, especially African Americans males. Most patients are asymptomatic on presentation.

  Diagnosis: Elevated BUN/creatinine, urinalysis benign or with minimal protein.

  Treatment focused on management of hypertension. Must rule out other possible causes of renal disease. Dialysis or renal transplantation for those with ESRD.

- *Renovascular hypertension (renal artery stenosis):* Hypertension as a result of renal artery stenosis. This form of hypertension accounts for 1% of all cases of hypertension and is the result of increased renin release. Causes of renovascular hypertension are fibromuscular hyperplasia (young patients) or, more commonly, atherosclerotic disease (70–80%). Risk factors include: patients with sudden-onset hypertension below age 20 or over age 50, accelerated hypertension, presence of abdominal bruits, other atherosclerotic disease, acute decline in renal function after use of ACE inhibitor, difficult-to-control hypertension, or asymmetry of kidney size on ultrasound.

  Diagnosis: Renal artery Doppler, magnetic resonance angiography (MRA), captopril renal scan, renal angiography (gold standard of diagnosis), renal vein renin levels. Asymmetric kidneys on renal sonogram may be clue to diagnosis.

  Treatment includes hypertension control (ACE inhibitor may cause acute renal failure in those with bilateral renal artery disease), renal artery angioplasty, renal artery stent, or surgical revascularization.

***Postrenal:*** Obstructive uropathy represents approximately 3 to 5% of causes of ESRD. Congenital anomalies and neuropathic bladder are other causes of postrenal failure. Prolonged time before diagnosis is made contributes to chronic renal failure.

### ▶ Clinical Therapeutics

Slow progression with efforts to control hypertension, control blood glucose, and reduce urinary protein excretion with ACE inhibitor. Drug dosing in chronic renal failure:

- Dose medications on estimation of creatinine clearance by Cockcroft and Gault equation:

$$CrCl = \frac{(140 - age) \times weight\ (in\ kg)}{72 \times serum\ creatinine}$$

**Multiply result by 0.85 in females**

- Caution with use of NSAIDs and ACE inhibitors (can decrease GFR) in those with known renal disease.

▶ Clinical Intervention

Slow progression with dietary protein restriction. Avoid radiocontrast material and other nephrotoxins. Monitor labs for metabolic acidosis, hyperphosphatemia, hyperuricemia, hyperkalemia, hypocalcemia, and anemia. Dialysis and renal transplantation for those with ESRD.

***ESRD:*** Preparation includes early nephrology referral to begin teaching, counseling, dialysis preparation information, and management of abnormal blood chemistries, uremic symptoms, and comorbid conditions (hypertension, lipids, anemia). Spare nondominant arm from venipunctures in anticipation of future dialysis access. Recommendations for arm access are when CrCl < 25 mL/min, serum creatinine > 4 mg/dL, or within 1 year of anticipated dialysis. Permanent dialysis access should be placed at least 3 to 6 weeks prior to start of dialysis for synthetic grafts and several months in advance for primary arteriovenous fistulas. For acute hemodialysis access, temporary cuffed or noncuffed catheters are placed. These should preferably be inserted in the internal jugular vein as use of subclavian vein can lead to stenosis and prevent future placement of permanent access in affected arm (femoral vein may also be used). For chronic dialysis access, choices include a primary arteriovenous fistula (preferred), synthetic arteriovenous graft, or peritoneal dialysis catheter.

### *Dialysis*

Indications for dialysis include fluid overload, congestive heart failure, pericarditis, progressive uremic symptoms (especially neurologic or GI), encephalopathy, uremic coagulopathy, and cases of severe hyperkalemia or metabolic acidosis resistant to management. In general, CrCl < 10 mL/min in a patient with other symptoms; earlier in diabetics.

- *Hemodialysis:* Most common form of renal replacement therapy. Requires creation of permanent access (primary arteriovenous fistula or synthetic arteriovenous graft); noncuffed temporary or tunneled cuffed dialysis catheters are not recommended for long-term dialysis. Hemodialysis involves diffusion of solutes across a semipermeable dialyzer membrane and fluid removal by the hydrostatic pressure gradient. Usual treatment 3–4 hours, three times weekly on fixed schedule at an outpatient dialysis unit.

  Key management goals include blood pressure control with fluid removal and antihypertensives, erythropoietin for anemia, nutritional support to maintain serum albumin (low serum albumin associated with increased mortality), dietary restriction (potassium, phosphorus, fluids), measurement of dialysis adequacy by urea reduction ratio or urea kinetic modeling, and monitoring of psychological status (decreased employment rates, increased disability and depression).

  Complications include vascular access difficulties (clotting, stenosis, malfunction, infected catheters), hypotension on dialysis, muscle cramps, allergic reactions, renal osteodystrophy from secondary hyper-parathyroidism, and disequilibrium syndrome (neurologic symptoms or seizures related to rapid removal of urea). In United States, gross annual mortality is 20–22% for all dialysis patients. Risk is higher for diabetics and elderly; nutrition and compliance are key factors.

- *Peritoneal dialysis:* Requires insertion of a peritoneal catheter into the abdomen. Involves diffusion of solute across peritoneal membrane and fluid removal due to hyperosmotic dialysate fluid. Technique involves instillation of an electrolyte and dextrose solution (dialysate) into peritoneum over a period of time then removal of the fluid on a continuous cycle. Done by patient at home, either intermittently (chronic ambulatory peritoneal dialysis [CAPD]) or with a continuous cycler machine (continuous cycle peritoneal dialysis [CCPD]) nightly.

- Key management goals include regulation of blood pressure with volume removal or antihypertensives, anemia control with erythropoietin, increased protein requirements due to protein loss in dialysate, psychosocial factors (more independent with care, responsible for own dialysis), and measurement of dialysis adequacy (peritoneal membrane kinetics). Complications include peritonitis, exit site or catheter tunnel infection, peritoneal membrane failure, and renal osteodystrophy.

### Renal transplantation

- *Pretransplant evaluation:* May be done before patient is on dialysis. Involves general health assessment, including active illnesses and infectious diseases as well as systemic examinations including dental, ophthalmologic, urologic, cardiac, pulmonary, GI, immunologic, and psychosocial evaluations. Blood work including blood ABO group type, human lymphocyte antigen (HLA) histocompatibility tissue typing, HIV and hepatitis screening, panel-reactive antibodies, and recipient–donor cross-match are obtained. Once a patient is deemed a candidate for renal transplant, he or she is placed on the United Network for Organ Sharing (UNOS) waiting list; average length of wait for cadaveric kidney is 27 months but may vary depending on the patient's ABO blood group.

   Contraindications include serious infections, active malignancies (those treated and free of disease for 2 years may be a candidate), ongoing substance abuse, other end-organ disease (i.e., severe cardiac disease), and noncompliant patient. Age alone is not a contraindication unless significantly advanced or other illnesses present.

- *Donor:* Donor kidney source may be cadaveric, living related donor, or living unrelated donor.

- *Post transplant:* Immunosuppressives are the key to successful renal transplantation and are evolving constantly. There are three phases of immunosuppressive therapy—induction (initial), maintenance, and rejection treatment. Drug regimens vary; generally given in combination as cyclosporine or tacrolimus (FK506), azathioprine or mycophenolate mofetil, and corticosteroids. Rejection is decreased by attempts to match major histocompatibility antigens. Can be hyperacute (within 24 hours), acute (within first 3 months), or chronic. Acute rejection often reversible with corticosteroids or anti–T cell antibody therapy. Chronic rejection is usually irreversible, progressive, and the most common cause of late graft loss. Occasionally, recurrent disease in graft may cause loss of transplant kidney.

Management post transplant involves careful measure of renal function and immunosuppressive drug levels (avoid toxicity and side effects), monitor for rejection (oliguria, fever, tenderness over graft, declining renal function, hypertension), and monitor for consequences of immunosuppression. Survival rates are improving. One-year patient survival is 98% for living related and 95% for cadaveric donor transplants. One-year graft survival is 95% for living related and 90% for cadaveric donor transplants. Renal transplantation improves quality of life, increases life expectancy in diabetics and the young, and is the most cost-effective method of care for those with ESRD.

# VI. ELECTROLYTE IMBALANCES

## A. Hyponatremia

*hyponatremia = $< 135$ mg/L*

► Scientific Concepts

Serum sodium concentration $< 135$ mEq/L. Frequently seen in hospitalized patients.

► History & Physical

Signs and symptoms vary depending on the severity and rate of decline of serum sodium as well as age of patient. Sudden development of severe hyponatremia may cause serious central nervous system symptoms. Nausea, anorexia, malaise, headache, altered sensorium, lethargy, seizures, brain edema and herniation, and Cheyne–Stokes respirations may be present.

► Diagnostic Studies

Serum sodium, electrolytes, plasma osmolality (low in true hyponatremia, normal or high in pseudohyponatremia), urine osmolality (true hyponatremia suppresses ADH release resulting in urine osmolality $< 100$ mOsm/kg), urine sodium ($< 10$ mEq/L in volume depletion, $> 20$ mEq/L in syndrome of inappropriate antidiuretic hormone [SIADH]).

► Diagnosis

***Hyponatremia with hypovolemia:*** Extrarenal losses (urine sodium $< 10$ mEq/L) may be due to GI losses (vomiting, diarrhea) or third-space losses (pancreatitis, peritonitis, burns, severe muscle injury). Renal volume loss (urine sodium $> 20$ mEq/L) may be due to excessive diuretics—especially thiazides (clue is hypokalemic metabolic alkalosis associated with potassium-losing diuretics); salt-losing nephropathy—usually associated with advanced renal disease; mineralocorticoid deficiency (Addison's disease)—hyponatremia and hyperkalemia present; or osmotic diuresis (glucose, urea, mannitol)—both water and electrolyte loss.

***Hyponatremia with volume overload:*** Seen in edematous states including cardiac failure, cirrhosis, nephrotic syndrome, and renal failure. Urine sodium $< 10$ mEq/L (if not on diuretic therapy). In renal failure, urine sodium may be $> 20$ mEq/L due to renal tubular dysfunction and inability to conserve sodium.

***Hyponatremia with euvolemia:*** SIADH is associated with low plasma osmolality, high urine osmolality, and high urine sodium ($> 20$ mEq/L).

May be seen with carcinoma (especially oat cell carcinoma of lung), pulmonary infection or acute disease, central nervous system disorders (stroke, infections, tumors, acute psychosis), or drugs (chlorpropramide, carbamazepine, several tricyclic antidepressants and serotonin reuptake inhibitors, and others).

Postoperative hyponatremia results from administration of excess hypotonic fluids in setting of increased ADH levels due to surgery or postoperative pain.

Primary polydipsia is a condition in which there is increased water intake beyond ability of the kidney to excrete (usually > 10 L/d). Associated with normal plasma osmolality and urine osmolality < 100 mOsm/kg. May be seen in patients with psychiatric disease.

Hypothyroidism, usually severe. Glucocorticoid deficiency (secondary adrenal insufficiency).

***Hyponatremia with increased extracellular fluid osmolality:*** Water moving from intracellular to extracellular space without a change in total body water. Hyperglycemia is associated with an increased plasma osmolality. For each 100 mg/dL rise in blood glucose, serum sodium decreases by 1.6 mEq/L. Mannitol administration is associated with an increased plasma osmolality. Water is pulled into extracellular space diluting the serum sodium.

***Pseudohyponatremia:*** Plasma osmolality normal in pseudohyponatremia. Hyperlipidemia and hyperproteinemia cause pseudohyponatremia. High levels of lipids and proteins occupy larger portion of plasma volume, therefore less water and sodium per liter of plasma (measurement of sodium using ion-specific electrodes reduces this effect). Plasma sodium concentration in relation to plasma water is normal.

Glycine irrigation during urologic surgery is another cause of pseudohyponatremia. A dilutional fall in serum sodium occurs due to absorption of fluid.

▶ Clinical Therapeutics

Demeclocycline antagonizes effect of vasopressin on kidney. Used to treat SIADH when it is not responsive to fluid restriction. Hypertonic saline is indicated for severe hyponatremia (usually sodium < 120 mEq/L) with central nervous system symptoms; given with furosemide.

▶ Clinical Intervention

In volume-depleted states, correct extracellular volume depletion with isotonic saline. In euvolemic states, treat underlying condition, remove offending drug, and/or fluid restrict. Restrict fluid intake to less than urine output plus insensible losses. In volume-expanded states, treat underlying condition, water and salt restriction.

▶ Health Maintenance Issues

Rate of correction for hyponatremia is dependent on duration and severity of hyponatremia and patient symptoms. Rapid correction of hyponatremia can cause central pontine myelinolysis. In acute hyponatremia (duration < 48 hours and sodium < 120 mEq/L), correct more quickly due to increased risk of neurologic complications. For symptomatic hyponatremia, rate of correction is 1.0 to 2.0 mEq/L/h. Hyponatremia of indeterminate duration should be corrected at 1.0 to

2.0 mEq/L/h not to exceed 12 to 15 mEq/L over the first 24 hours. Those with moderate symptoms can be corrected at a rate of <0.5 mEq/L/h while those with more severe symptoms should be corrected at the higher rate above. Aim for serum sodium 130 to 135 mEq/L over the first 48 hours of treatment to avoid overcorrection. Chronic hyponatremia (duration > 48 hours and no symptoms) can be corrected more slowly.

## B. Hypernatremia

### ▶ Scientific Concepts

Serum sodium concentration > 150 mEq/L. Represents a disorder of water balance. Protective mechanism against hypernatremia is thirst and vasopressin secretion. Most commonly the result of impaired thirst or inability to get fluids in the setting of water loss (especially infants, elderly).

### ▶ History & Physical

Signs and symptoms are primarily neurologic. Lethargy, weakness, coma, twitching, seizures, and irritability may be present. The severity of symptoms is more dependent on the rate of developing hypernatremia (acute vs. chronic) and duration rather than the serum sodium level.

### ▶ Diagnostic Studies

Serum sodium, electrolytes, urine sodium, increased plasma osmolality, urine osmolality (inappropriately low in central and nephrogenic diabetes insipidus; high or maximally concentrated in sodium overload, insensible water loss, and hypodipsia).

### ▶ Diagnosis

*Hypernatremia with hypovolemia:* Extrarenal losses from GI tract (diarrhea) or excessive sweating can cause hypernatremia. With GI losses, the urine is hypertonic and urine sodium < 10 mEq/L is due to renal sodium and water conservation.

Renal losses from osmotic diuresis (glucose, urea, mannitol) or loop diuretics. Urine sodium > 20 mEq/L with renal losses.

*Hypernatremia with euvolemia:* Extrarenal losses from insensible water losses (fever, respiratory, burns).

Renal losses from central diabetes insipidus or nephrogenic diabetes insipidus can cause hypernatremia. In central diabetes insipidus, there is inadequate vasopressin release and hypotonic urine with increased plasma osmolality. In nephrogenic diabetes insipidus, there is impaired kidney response to vasopressin. This can be secondary to renal or other diseases and drugs (lithium, demeclocycline).

Hypothalamic disorders including reset osmostat (higher plasma sodium level seen as normal) or hypodipsia.

*Hypernatremia with volume overload:* Hypertonic salts (hypertonic saline, large amounts of sodium bicarbonate) and ingestion of sodium (high-sodium enteral feedings).

### ▶ Clinical Therapeutics

Goal is to correct cause. Volume-expanded states without advanced renal disease respond to diuretics. Diuretics cause renal loss of sodium and water; must replace urine water loss with free water. Central diabetes insipidus (DI) responds to vasopressin.

▶ Clinical Intervention

Fluid replacement based on calculation of water deficit. In volume-depleted states, isotonic saline should be administered to the hypotensive patient until extracellular fluid volume is restored, then hypotonic saline may be given to correct plasma osmolality.

▶ Health Maintenance Issues

Avoid overly rapid correction of chronic hyponatremia to prevent brain edema. Acute symptomatic hypernatremia may be corrected quickly over several hours. Chronic symptomatic hypernatremia should be corrected with goal to lower serum sodium concentration by 1.0 to 2.0 mEq/L/h until symptoms resolve then continue to correct water deficit over 24–48 hours.

## C. Hypokalemia

▶ Scientific Concepts

Serum potassium concentration < 3.5 mEq/L. Potassium is the major intracellular cation.

▶ History & Physical

Signs and symptoms depend on level of serum potassium and include the following systems: cardiac (arrhythmias, electrocardiogram changes—flat T waves and prominent U waves, increased sensitivity to digitalis), neuromuscular (muscle weakness, cramps, paresthesias, rhabdomyolysis, ileus), and renal (polyuria, polydipsia).

▶ Diagnostic Studies

Serum potassium, urine potassium, serum electrolytes, serum magnesium, glucose, urine sodium and chloride, evaluate for acid–base disorders, plasma renin and aldosterone levels, and blood pressure.

▶ Diagnosis

*Extracellular to intracellular redistribution of potassium:* Insulin administration/excess, metabolic alkalosis, catecholamine excess, respiratory alkalosis, beta-adrenergic agonists, and hypokalemic periodic paralysis (hereditary disorder).

*Potassium losses:* Extrarenal losses including GI (diarrhea, laxative abuse), extreme sweating, and extensive burns.

Renal losses including diuretics, vomiting (release of aldosterone in response to volume depletion causing renal potassium loss), excess mineralocorticoid (Cushing's syndrome, licorice), renal tubular acidosis, hypomagnesemia, and primary hyperaldosteronism.

*Decreased potassium intake:* Uncommon cause of hypokalemia because of potassium content in various foods and ability of kidney to conserve potassium efficiently.

▶ Clinical Therapeutics

Correct underlying cause. If hypomagnesemia present, this must be corrected for potassium balance to be restored. Various types of potassium salts are available for replacement therapy. In cases of hypokalemia with metabolic alkalosis or unclear cause, use only potassium chloride. For hypokalemia with metabolic acidosis, use a bicarbonate salt. Potassium-sparing diuretics can be used in those with primary hyper-aldosteronism. Caution when used in those with renal insufficiency.

▶ Clinical Intervention

Route of potassium replacement may be oral or IV. Oral is preferred route of replacement. Usual rate of IV replacement is no greater than 10 mEq/h; in urgent cases, no greater than 15 to 20 mEq/h in a central vein. Potassium concentration of IV fluids should be no greater than 40 mEq/L due to risk of phlebitis unless infused into a large vein. Avoid glucose solutions and alkali as these can further decrease serum potassium by causing intracellular shift of potassium.

▶ Health Maintenance Issues

Monitor serum potassium levels in those on diuretics, especially those on cardiac glycosides or with cardiovascular disease; mild hypokalemia may predispose to arrhythmias.

## D. Hyperkalemia

▶ Scientific Concepts

Serum potassium concentration > 5.0 mEq/L. Potassium is the major intracellular cation. Hyperkalemia is often iatrogenic.

▶ History & Physical

Signs and symptoms depend on level of serum potassium. May present with nonspecific complaints or GI symptoms. Often asymptomatic until level 6.5 mEq/L or greater. May include cardiac (electrocardiogram changes—peaked T waves, prolonged PR interval, widening of QRS, arrhythmias) and neuromuscular (paresthesias, weakness, tingling) systems.

▶ Diagnostic Studies

Serum potassium, serum electrolytes, BUN/creatinine, evaluate for acid–base disorders, urine pH, plasma aldosterone and cortisol levels, rule out pseudohyperkalemia; history and physical examination.

▶ Diagnosis

*Increased intake:* Transient hyperkalemia unless renal potassium excretion is impaired.

*Transcellular redistribution:* Insulin deficiency, acidosis (especially hyperchloremic metabolic acidosis), cell breakdown (rhabdomyolysis, tumor cell lysis), digoxin toxicity, nonselective beta-adrenergic blocker, and hyperkalemic periodic paralysis (rare hereditary disorder).

*Impaired renal excretion:* Renal failure with oliguria, mineralocorticoid deficiency (Addison's disease, hyporeninemic hypoaldosteronism, drugs including NSAIDs, ACE inhibitors, angiotensin II antagonists, heparin), and renal tubular dysfunction (hyperkalemic type I distal renal tubular acidosis, drugs including potassium sparing diuretics and trimethoprim).

*Pseudohyperkalemia:* Traumatic blood draw with hemolysis, excessive fist clenching or tourniquet pressure with blood draw, thrombocytosis, and marked leukocytosis.

▶ Clinical Therapeutics

Reserved for severe hyperkalemia or if electrocardiographic changes present. Evaluate and correct causes such as pseudohyperkalemia and transcellular redistribution of potassium. Antagonize cell membrane effects with IV calcium gluconate. Shift potassium intracellularly with sodium bicarbonate, glucose/insulin, and beta-2-adrenergic agonists. Remove excess potassium with cation exchange resin (Kayexalate, oral or enema) or loop diuretics.

▶ Clinical Intervention

Remove excess potassium by dialysis, either hemodialysis or peritoneal dialysis (slower method of potassium removal); dietary potassium restriction.

▶ Health Maintenance Issues

Identify those patients at risk for hyperkalemia (renal insufficiency, mineralocorticoid deficiency). Use caution with certain drugs (NSAIDs, ACE inhibitors, trimethoprim, potassium-sparing diuretics) in this population.

## VII.  ACID–BASE DISORDERS

### A.  Respiratory Acidosis

▶ Scientific Concepts

Hypercapnia as result of decreased alveolar ventilation.

▶ History & Physical

Signs and symptoms associated with acute-onset respiratory acidosis include somnolence, confusion, myoclonus, asterixis, coma, papilledema, bradypnea, and hypopnea.

▶ Diagnostic Studies

Decreased arterial pH, increased partial pressure of carbon dioxide ($PCO_2$), increased serum bicarbonate.

▶ Differential Diagnosis

Respiratory center depression (sleep apnea, brain stem infarct, sedative overdose), neuromuscular disorders (multiple sclerosis, amyotrophic lateral sclerosis, Guillain–Barré syndrome, poliomyelitis), restrictive disorders (pneumo/hemothorax, kyphoscoliosis, acute respiratory distress syndrome), and acute or chronic pulmonary disease (interstitial fibrosis, chronic obstructive pulmonary disease [COPD], bronchospasm).

▶ Clinical Therapeutics/Interventions

Treat underlying cause and improve ventilation. Consider naloxone if sedative overdose suspected.

### B.  Respiratory Alkalosis

▶ Scientific Concepts

Hypocapnia as a result of increased rate of pulmonary carbon dioxide excretion. Hyperventilation is most common cause. Normal in pregnancy and high altitudes.

▶ History & Physical

Signs and symptoms include lightheadedness, anxiety, paresthesias, tachypnea, and hyperpnea.

▶ Diagnostic Studies

Increased arterial pH, decreased $PCO_2$, decreased serum bicarbonate.

▶ Differential Diagnosis

Hyperventilation and other causes of hypoxia (high altitude, severe anemia), central nervous system events (infarction, trauma, tumor, infection), sepsis with endotoxin, drugs (salicylates, progesterone), pulmonary disease (pneumonia, pulmonary edema, or embolism), and excessive mechanical ventilation.

▶ Clinical Therapeutics/Interventions

Treat underlying cause and maintain oxygenation.

## C. Metabolic Acidosis

▶ Scientific Concepts

Anion gap helpful in determining cause. Anion gap = (Na) − ($HCO_3$ + Cl); normal anion gap is $12 \pm 4$ mEq/L.

▶ History & Physical

Signs and symptoms are related to underlying disorder and may include diarrhea, oliguria, anuria, Kussmaul respirations, hypotension, arrhythmias, and lethargy.

▶ Diagnostic Studies

Decreased arterial pH, decreased $PCO_2$, decreased serum bicarbonate; anion gap, electrolytes, urine or serum ketones, and serum lactate.

▶ Differential Diagnosis

Metabolic acidosis with increased anion gap seen in ketoacidosis, lactic acidosis, drug intoxications (ethylene glycol, methanol, salicylates), and advanced renal failure. Metabolic acidosis with normal anion gap seen with GI bicarbonate loss (diarrhea and drainage of small bowel or pancreatic secretions), renal bicarbonate loss (acetazolamide, renal tubular acidosis), and inorganic acid ingestion (ammonium chloride, sulfur).

▶ Clinical Therapeutics/Interventions

Treat underlying disorder; sodium bicarbonate administration for moderate to severe metabolic acidosis. For ketoacidosis, treat with fluids, correct electrolytes and glucose; insulin for diabetic ketoacidosis; thiamine for alcoholic ketoacidosis. For lactic acidosis, goal is to restore tissue perfusion and oxygenation; sodium bicarbonate for severe acidosis. Treatment for drug intoxication is based on specific drug ingested. Ethylene glycol and methanol poisoning are treated with ethanol infusion and hemodialysis. Salicylate overdose is treated by alkalinization of urine and may require hemodialysis.

## D. Metabolic Alkalosis

▶ Scientific Concepts

Elevated plasma bicarbonate. Generated by loss of hydrogen ion or chloride and maintained by decreased renal bicarbonate loss.

### ► History & Physical

Signs and symptoms include weakness, neuromuscular irritability, and symptoms of volume depletion.

### ► Diagnostic Studies

Increased arterial pH, increased $PCO_2$, increased serum bicarbonate; decreased potassium and chloride; anion gap may be increased; urine chloride.

### ► Differential Diagnosis

In volume-depleted states (low urine chloride), consider gastric acid loss (vomiting, nasogastric suction) or renal loss from diuretics (urine chloride low after diuretic stopped). In volume-repleted states (high urine chloride), consider mineralocorticoid excess (hyperaldosteronism, Bartter's syndrome, Cushing's syndrome, licorice excess) or severe hypokalemia.

### ► Clinical Therapeutics/Interventions

If present, correct extracellular volume deficit with chloride-containing solutions or treat other underlying disorders. Acetazolamide can be used in volume-expanded patients. Rarely, dilute hydrochloric acid infusion required.

## BIBLIOGRAPHY

Braunwald E, et al., eds. *Harrison's Principles of Internal Medicine,* 15th ed. New York: McGraw-Hill; 2002.

Greenberg A, ed. *Primer on Kidney Diseases,* 3nd ed. San Diego: Academic Press; 2001.

Rose BD, ed. *Up to Date,* Version 10.1; 2002.

Schena FP, et al., eds. *Nephrology.* London: McGraw-Hill; 2001.

Schrier RW, ed. *Manual of Nephrology,* 5th ed. Philadelphia: Lippincott, Williams & Wilkins; 2000.

Tanagho EA, McAninch JW, eds. *Smith's General Urology,* 15th ed. New York: McGraw-Hill; 2000.

Tierney LM Jr, McPhee SJ, Papadakis MA, eds. *Current Medical Diagnosis & Treatment,* 42nd ed. New York: Lange Medical Books/McGraw-Hill; 2003.

# Male Genitourinary Disorders $\Big| 8$

*Raymond L. Eifel, MS, PA-C*

## I. BENIGN CONDITIONS

### A. Hydrocele/Varicocele

▶ Scientific Concepts

A hydrocele is a collection of fluid between the tunica vaginalis and the testicle. It is the most common benign mass, occurring in 1% of adult males. It is caused by any process that stimulates production of serous fluid (i.e., tumor, inflammation, trauma).

A varicocele is a tortuous enlarged spermatic vein above the testicle, occurring almost always on the left, as the left spermatic vein is 8–10 cm longer than the right vein and is susceptible to valvular incompetence. Occurs in ~15% of adolescent and adult males. A varicocele is associated with testicular atrophy in adults and alterations in semen quality secondary to an increased temperature in the associated testis, often resulting in infertility for the male.

▶ History & Physical

With either condition, the patient is generally asymptomatic. On physical exam of the hydrocele, a smooth, cystic-feeling mass will be appreciated around the testicle, but not the spermatic cord. A hydrocele will transilluminate. The patient with a varicocele will present with a soft mass or swelling above the testicle that may worsen when the patient is asked to stand and decrease when the patient lies down. Observation of a "bag of worms" in the scrotum is common.

▶ Diagnostic Studies

A scrotal ultrasound is indicated for a hydrocele if the testicle does not transilluminate, if testicular palpation is not possible, or with a varicocele that is sudden in onset and does not reduce in size in the supine position. If a tumor is suspected, in addition to ultrasound, get testis tumor markers (alpha-fetoprotein [AFP]; beta-human chorionic gonadotropin [β-hCG]).

▶ Differential Diagnosis

When scrotal discomfort or a solid mass lesion is suspected, the practitioner should consider testicular torsion (a surgical emergency), epididymitis, and testicular tumor.

▶ Clinical Intervention

Small asymptomatic hydroceles often require no intervention other than patient reassurance. Larger symptomatic hydroceles require surgical excision. Needle aspiration of the hydrocele is generally unsuccessful as the fluid usually reaccumulates and the hydrocele recurs. Needle aspiration is a treatment option for a patient who is a poor surgical candidate. Refer to a urologist for follow-up.

### B. Paraphimosis/Phimosis

▶ Scientific Concepts

Paraphimosis occurs when the foreskin of the penis has been retracted and remains trapped behind the glans penis with secondary swelling and pain. Failure to reduce the foreskin after insertion of a urethral catheter is a common cause. If left untreated, it can progress to penile necrosis. Phimosis is a narrowing or constriction of the penile foreskin in an uncircumcised adult male, commonly caused by poor hygiene and chronic infection.

► **History & Physical**

With paraphimosis, the patient will present with pain around the glans penis; he may report recent insertion of a urethral catheter. Upon exam, the foreskin will be drawn back behind the glans, often with considerable swelling. With phimosis, since the patient cannot retract the foreskin, he may complain of a urine stream that sprays or discharge secondary to infection.

► **Diagnostic Studies**

With phimosis, if infection is present, perform culture and sensitivity (C&S) of the discharge.

► **Diagnosis**

Made with history and physical exam.

► **Clinical Therapeutics**

Phimosis is best treated with mild soap, water, and drying after retracting the foreskin fully. Local application of antibiotic ointment (i.e., bacitracin) or steroid-based creams may be beneficial.

► **Clinical Intervention**

Paraphimosis should be reduced immediately. A topical anesthetic or penile block may be indicated. If a manual reduction cannot be performed, an emergency dorsal slit or circumcision may be necessary. These latter two items also apply to the treatment of phimosis, although the treatment of an active infection should be completed prior to performing a dorsal slit in this group. Urology consult is indicated.

► **Health Maintenance Issues**

Hygiene is key to treatment and prevention of infections secondary to phimosis. Complications of phimosis include continued infections (balanitis), paraphimosis, and penile carcinoma.

## II. INFECTIOUS CONDITIONS

### A. Epididymitis/Orchitis

► **Scientific Concepts**

Unilateral inflammation of the epididymis resulting in scrotal pain. Inflammation is usually unilateral but may spread to both testicles and the scrotal wall. Hydrocele formation occurs in some situations. Caused by urinary pathogens, sexually transmitted diseases (STDs), and sterile inflammation. Orchitis is generally secondary to an extension of an associated epididymitis, producing an epididymoorchitis.

► **History & Physical**

Highest incidence is in young, sexually active men. Older age groups are next with urinary tract infections (UTIs). Rarely occurs in prepubertal boys. Scrotal elevation and support improve pain. Physical findings include urethral discharge, UTI symptoms, pain and inflammation extending from the posterior epididymis to the scrotal wall. Fever and chills can occur with severe infection and abscess formation.

▶ Diagnostic Studies

Urinalysis, Gram stain of urethral discharge, urethral culture. Cultures should be done for gonorrhea and chlamydia. Ultrasound of scrotum; radionuclide scan.

▶ Diagnosis

Differential diagnosis includes testicular torsion, orchitis, mumps orchitis, tumor, hydrocele, varicocele, spermatocele, trauma, postvasectomy congestion.

▶ Clinical Therapeutics

Epididymitis and orchitis are treated identically and should be treated for gonococcal/nongonococcal organisms (doxycycline, ceftriaxone, ciprofloxin, norfloxin). With bacteriuria, treat for urinary pathogens (trimethoprim-sulfamethoxazole [TMP-SMZ], tetracycline, ciprofloxacin, norfloxacin).

▶ Clinical Intervention

Appropriate analgesia (nonsteroidal anti-inflammatories [NSAIDs] for mild to moderate pain, opiates for severe pain). Additionally, scrotal elevation and cold packs may help with pain. Pain improves within 1–3 days, but swelling may take several weeks to resolve. Sterility sometimes a complication.

▶ Health Maintenance Issues

Screening in patients with high-risk behaviors (i.e., multiple partners, no barrier methods practiced, change in sexual partner in last 6 to 12 months). Counsel, educate, and encourage the use of condoms. Discuss issues of promiscuity, abstinence, and risk behavior management.

## B. Urethritis

▶ Scientific Concepts

Urethral inflammation, discharge, and painful urination are hallmarks of the urethral syndrome. Predominantly an STD in sexually active postpubertal males. Can also be seen in other UTIs such as cystitis, prostatitis, and epididymitis. Causative organisms, in order of incidence, include *Neisseria gonorrhoeae, Chlamydia trachomatis, Ureaplasma, Trichomonas,* cytomegalovirus, herpes simplex virus, human papillomavirus, other bacteria.

▶ History & Physical

Higher incidence seen in males < 35 years old, multiple sexual partners, and prior history of STDs. Avoidance of condoms considered high risk. Contact with a known carrier is best actively treated, even if asymptomatic. Symptoms include dysuria, urethral discharge, and suprapubic tenderness. Associated symptoms of proctitis, pharyngitis, and conjunctivitis are sometimes seen. Inguinal lymphadenopathy can be present.

▶ Diagnostic Studies

Culture or rapid reagins of urethral discharge, Gram stain, urinalysis, urine culture, and wet prep. Viral cultures are indicated if physical examination indicates.

▶ Diagnosis

Differential diagnosis includes STDs, UTIs, trauma, foreign bodies (i.e., venereal warts, polyps), Reiter's syndrome.

► Clinical Therapeutics

Current recommended drug treatment is ceftriaxone, 250 mg intramuscularly (IM), plus doxycycline, 100 mg bid × 7 days. Alternate regimens include macrolides and fluoroquinolones. Metronidazole is used in cases of trichomoniasis. Increasing incidence of drug resistance should be noted. Treat sexual partners, and consider posttreatment repeat of positive cultures.

► Clinical Intervention

None, except surgical treatment of underlying causes (i.e., polyps, condyloma). Medical management of associated conditions (i.e., Reiter's syndrome).

► Health Maintenance Issues

Counseling regarding sexual abstinence, condom use, and risks related to multiple sexual partners is essential. Stress importance of compliance to treatment regimens, avoidance of intercourse until treatment completed, and communication to partners.

## III. TESTICULAR TORSION

► Scientific Concepts

Acute ischemia of testis caused by twisting of cord and vascular supply. Torsions can occur involving the entire testicular structure as well as within the tunica vaginalis.

► History & Physical

History of trauma (20%), prior history of testicular pain. Exercise, cold temperature, and sexual stimulation may play a role. Peak occurrence at age 14, but occurs in all age groups. Two thirds of cases occur in second decade. Scrotal enlargement, pain, redness, and edema are common. Accompanying nausea, vomiting, and fever may occur.

► Diagnostic Studies

Urinalysis, CT or ultrasound, Doppler ultrasound, and radionuclide testicular scintigraphy with technetium.

► Diagnosis

Differential diagnosis includes epididymitis, orchitis, hernia, hematoma, hydrocele, varicocele, tumor, infiltrate, and abscess.

► Clinical Therapeutics

Pain management and rapid diagnosis are essential. Testicular salvage is related to length of time torsion persists. Manual reduction of torsion may be successful; this can be facilitated by 1% lidocaine injection.

► Clinical Intervention

Rapid surgical exploration of scrotal contents is essential for testicular salvage. Removal of necrosed testis may be indicated. Fixation of testis recommended.

► Health Maintenance Issues

High level of suspicion in young age groups. No screening measures are available to determine risk. Open communication with young male patients about testicular exam should take place. This is to facilitate better communications with parents and providers. Reporting of testicular problems is often delayed to a point of poor outcome.

## IV. ERECTILE DYSFUNCTION (ED)

► **Scientific Concepts**

Erectile dysfunction (impotence) is defined as the inability to maintain an erect penis sufficient for coitus. Erectile dysfunction (ED) is described as two types. Psychogenic ED, which occurs primarily for psychological reasons (performance anxiety, depression), is the primary cause for ED in men under 35 years old. Organic ED is more likely in men over age 50 and is secondary to a preexisting organic disease. Primary organic causes for ED include vascular, endocrine, neurologic, and end organ failure (i.e., priapism or Peyronie's disease). Other common causes of ED include drug-induced impotence (antihypertensives, psychotropics), alcoholism, cigarette smoking, and postsurgical changes after pelvic surgery.

► **History & Physical**

Question patients regarding medical and surgical history, atherosclerotic risk factors, history of pelvic or spinal trauma. Interview for recent life crises, medication changes, and sexual history. Physical exam should include external genitalia, prostate, and peripheral pulses.

► **Diagnostic Studies**

Fasting blood glucose (diabetes), serum testosterone. Additional studies may include penile duplex ultrasound, nocturnal penile rigidity monitoring, psychological and neurological evaluations.

► **Differential Diagnosis**

Differential will include many potential causes including medical (diabetes mellitus, neurologic disease, hypertension, hyperlipidemia), behavioral (alcohol abuse, cigarette smoking, depression), surgical (postradical prostatectomy), traumatic (back or spinal injury, pelvic or penile fracture), or medication induced.

► **Clinical Therapeutics**

Treat the underlying cause if identified. Therapies to assist in erections include vacuum erection devices, intraurethral injection (alprostadil), oral medication (sildenafil), or testosterone replacement therapy, although this latter treatment is contraindicated for men with known or suspected prostate cancer.

► **Clinical Intervention**

A urological consult is indicated for surgical interventions that may include arterial revascularization of the arteries in the penis, a plication or excision of the tunica albuginea for an individual with Peyronie's disease, or an implantation of a penile prosthesis.

► **Health Maintenance Issues**

Stop smoking and alcohol abuse, weight loss (if the patient is obese), practice "safe sex," continued counseling potentially with spouse/ significant other if there is a clear psychological etiology.

## V. PRIAPISM

▶ Scientific Concepts

Penile erection, often painful, not related to sexual stimulation. Incidence/prevalence in the United States is unknown.

▶ History & Physical

Penile erection that is painful and prolonged (> 6 hours) without sexual desire. Patients will often delay seeking treatment because of embarrassment. On physical exam, the corpora cavernosa may be partially to fully rigid, with a flaccid glans. Eventual loss of sexual function may occur in up to 50% of the cases.

▶ Diagnostic Studies

There are no primary diagnostics for priapism. However, appropriate diagnostics for disease processes involved are indicated. A sickle cell evaluation for hemoglobin S should be performed in all African American patients with priapism. Complete blood count (CBC) should be completed to rule out leukemia.

▶ Differential Diagnosis

Causes for priapism are numerous. Blood dyscrasias (leukemia, sickle cell), vascular thrombosis, pelvic masses (hematoma, neoplasm), spinal cord tumors, urinary calculi and infections, and drugs (trazodone, chlorpromazine, some antihypertensives).

▶ Clinical Therapeutics

Generally pharmaceutical management involves pain management and observation.

▶ Clinical Intervention

In sickle cell, hydration and exchange transfusion are appropriate. If a neurogenic cause is determined, caudal or spinal anesthesia is appropriate. Urologic referral for surgery. Placement of shunts or invasive release of congestion in cavernosum/spongiosum. Treat other underlying causes.

▶ Health Maintenance Issues

Proper screening and management of blood disorders. Familial history is vital in the screening of these blood disorders. Atherosclerotic disease should be noted in the differential diagnosis (i.e., lipid disorders, smoking, hypertension, diabetes).

## VI. PROSTATE DISORDERS

## A. Benign Prostatic Hypertrophy (BPH)

▶ Scientific Concepts

Benign prostatic hypertrophy (BPH) has unknown etiology but appears to be hormonally influenced. It is characterized by a progressive enlargement of the prostate gland (transitional zone) resulting in an obstructive uropathy whose signs and symptoms include decreased force of stream and frequent urination. Rarely affects males younger than age 40; the mean age in which men develop symptoms is between 60 and 65 years.

### ▶ History & Physical

Increased frequency, urgency, nocturia, weak stream, hesitancy, and dribbling are characteristics. An enlarged prostate is palpable on rectal examination. A distended bladder, secondary to urinary retention, may be identified when the lower abdomen is examined. The International Prostate Symptom Score (I-PSS) is recommended to grade BPH and monitor treatment. Total score ranges from 0 to 35; the greater the BPH symptoms, the higher the score.

### ▶ Diagnostic Studies

Urinalysis may reveal hematuria and infection characteristic of UTIs. Elevated blood urea nitrogen (BUN) and creatinine may reflect urinary retention.

### ▶ Diagnosis

Diagnosis based on the history and clinical examination of the patient, while excluding other causes of obstructive uropathy. These include prostate cancer, acute prostatitis, urethral stricture, or neurogenic bladder. Prostate-specific antigen (PSA) may be elevated in BPH (>4 ng/mL but <10 ng/mL). Intravenous urography, uroflowmetry, and cystourethroscopy can narrow the diagnosis. Consider postvoid residual volumes.

### ▶ Clinical Therapeutics

Phytotherapy (saw palmetto) is a nonpharmacologic option that may provide some patients with benefit. The mechanism for this action is unknown. The first line of therapy with a pharmacologic agent includes the use of alpha-1 blockers like terazosin, doxazosin, and tamsulosin, which relax prostate smooth muscle. Tamsulosin is the only alpha-1 blocker that is selective in its action, therefore hypotensive responses seen with terazosin and doxazosin are not seen with tamsulosin. 5-alpha-reductase inhibitors (finasteride), which block testosterone conversion, are utilized in treatment of BPH to decrease the volume of the gland.

### ▶ Clinical Intervention

Surgical treatment for complications or recurrent symptoms. Transurethral resection of the prostate (TURP) is the most common operation requiring little more than an overnight stay in the hospital. The most common side effect of a TURP is retrograde ejaculation. Other therapies include laser, ultrasound, microwave. Stents are best used for patients who are poor surgical candidates.

### ▶ Health Maintenance Issues

BPH is a natural process of aging in men; their health care provider should inform them about anticipated signs and symptoms. Medications should be checked. BPH symptoms can result from probanthine or phenylephrine use.

## B. Prostate Cancer

### ▶ Scientific Concepts

The second most common cause of cancer death in males. Increased incidence with age. Majority of prostate cancer localized to peripheral zone (~70%). Etiology is unknown; however, genetic, endocrine, diet, and environmental factors are suspected. Most are adenocarcinomas.

▶ History & Physical

Risk factors include family history, African American males, and age > 50 years old. Most men with prostate cancer are asymptomatic. Weight loss or bone pain suggests late stage with metastases. Rectal examination reveals a firm, indurated, rock hard, nontender, localized area.

▶ Diagnostic Studies

PSA, although not solely specific to prostate cancer, is useful in narrowing the diagnosis and monitoring treatment. Transrectal ultrasound (TRUS) with needle biopsy confirms the diagnosis. Magnetic resonance imaging (MRI) and radionuclide bone scan verify metastases.

▶ Diagnosis

Once a definitive diagnosis is made, the Gleason pathology grading and tumor, node, metastases (TNM) staging system are applied for prognosis and determining treatment.

▶ Clinical Therapeutics

Treatment is based on the above classification system identifying localized disease or metastases. Radiation therapy by external beam (XRT) or radioactive seed implants (brachytherapy) placed into the prostate through the perineum are treatment options. Hormone treatment offers androgen deprivation to sensitive tumors.

▶ Clinical Intervention

Bilateral orchiectomy provides radical antiandrogen effects. The main surgical therapy is radical prostatectomy, which has the side effects of serious incontinence (2–3%) and impotence (<25%).

▶ Health Maintenance Issues

The role of prostate screening poses a serious dilemma. PSA was not designed to be a screening tool. Prostate screening remains controversial because PSA is not specific to prostate cancer. Annual digital rectal examination is recommended in males at 50 years of age.

## C. Prostatitis

▶ Scientific Concepts

Classified as acute or chronic bacterial. Usually caused by gram-negative rods (*Escherichia coli*) or gram-positive organisms (*Enterococcus*). Bacteria ascend up the male urethra. Nonbacterial prostatitis is relatively common and is an inflammatory disease of unknown cause. Viruses and atypical microorganisms (mycoplasma) should be considered if bacterial organisms are eliminated.

▶ History & Physical

History of UTI. Perineal, suprapubic, and lower back pain. Dysuria, frequency, urgency, and obstructive symptoms. Fever may be present. Digital rectal examination reveals a boggy, tender, indurated prostate that is warm to palpation. Aggressive massage of prostate is cautioned with acute prostatitis because of the risk of sepsis.

► **Diagnostic Studies**

Digital rectal examination. Urine is collected in series of initial void, midstream, and postprostatic massage collections. Prostatic secretions are also sent for culture and sensitivity as is the urine. Analysis reveals hematuria, many bacteriuria (> 100,000 colony-forming units [CFU]/mL), or pyuria (> 10 white blood cells per high-power field [WBC/HPF]). Cultures and sensitivity to identify offending organism. CBC shows elevated WBC.

► **Diagnosis**

History, physical, and urinalysis should establish the diagnosis. Consider urethritis, cystitis, pyelonephritis, and epididymitis in the differential diagnosis.

► **Clinical Therapeutics**

Treat with broad-spectrum systemic antibiotics until sensitivities are known. TMP-SMZ is often the antibiotic of choice. Several weeks of antibiotic therapy are essential. Follow-up urinalysis and culture are needed after antibiotic treatment to test for cure. Consider NSAIDs and sitz baths daily for symptomatic relief.

► **Clinical Intervention**

Chronic prostatitis may require 6 weeks to 3 months of antibiotic therapy to suppress recurrent UTIs.

► **Health Maintenance Issues**

Age > 50 years old, frequent catheterization, and most males with urethritis age 15–30 years old are at risk of prostatitis.

## VII. URINARY TRACT INFECTIONS

► **Scientific Concepts**

Any UTI in an adult male mandates a thorough workup. In males aged 3 months to 50 years, incidence of UTI is low; therefore, the possibility of anatomical abnormalities must be entertained in this age group. UTIs are rare in young men. Female to male ratio, 30:1. Males who are homosexual, noncircumcised, or have a partner with vaginal colonization have a greater incidence. Not until the age of 60 years does the incidence of UTI in men begin to approach that of women. This increase is considered a result of diseases associated with the prostate or instrumentation. In any male that presents with a UTI, an upper tract origin must also be considered (i.e., infected calculus).

► **History & Physical**

Age > 50 years. Dysuria, frequency, urgency, hematuria, and nocturia. Flank pain and costovertebral angle tenderness if upper UTI. If a young man is frequently diagnosed with a UTI, it is possible that an STD has been overlooked. Recurrent UTIs may have been treated with an antimicrobial to which the organism was resistant. Review for underlying causes including diabetes and patients who may be immunocompromised.

► **Diagnostic Studies**

Dipstick with positive nitrate and leukocyte esterase tests. Urinalysis and culture. Use midstream catch for culture and sensitivity. Standard is > 100,000 CFU/mL. Microscopic spun urinalysis under HPF prior to culture, look for bacteria or WBCs. Send for C&S. Check previous culture and sensitivities in cases of resistance. In younger men, urethral smear for chlamydia and *N. gonorrhea* should be completed.

► **Diagnosis**

UTI is a simple diagnosis. The workup for a UTI is often complex, focused on obstructive uropathy. Cystourethroscopy, intravenous urography, and uroflowmetry are indicated in male UTI. Treat the cause.

► **Clinical Therapeutics**

Gram-negative rods (*E. coli*) most common pathogen. TMP-SMZ for simple UTI. Broad-based antibiotic selection initially, then focused on sensitivities to urine culture growth. The length of treatment is longer in men than women to avoid the development of a prostate infection. Follow-up culture indicated if complicated UTI. Alpha-1 blockers indicated if patient has high urinary postvoid residual (> 100 mL).

► **Clinical Intervention**

Nosocomial infections are related to indwelling catheter. Straight catheterization recommended. Recurrent infections are often due to urological abnormalities or chronic bacterial prostatitis. Referral to a urologist is indicated.

► **Health Maintenance Issues**

Good hydration. Increase fluids especially with certain drugs (e.g., sulfas). Void regularly. Avoid coffee, alcohol, spicy foods, and cigarette smoking (cigarette smoking is a major risk factor for the development of bladder cancer). Use of cranberry juice is inconclusive; possible mechanism that keeps bacteria from adhering to the bladder wall may be useful in men with a high postvoid residual.

## VIII. TRAUMA

### A. Ureteral Trauma

► **Scientific Concepts**

Uncommon urologic injury. Associated with blunt multisystem or penetrating trauma (i.e., gunshot wound, stab wound). Iatrogenic injury seen with instrumentation during surgery as a result of ligating or crushing a ureter with a clamp or ligature.

► **History & Physical**

High index of suspicion required based on mechanism of injury. Flank and lower abdominal pain, oliguria, anuria, fever, with or without hematuria. Postsurgical findings are nonspecific. Additional findings to those listed above include palpable abdominal mass, elevation in BUN, sepsis, persistent drainage from operative sites.

▶ Diagnostic Studies

Diagnosis identified with intravenous pyelogram (IVP).

▶ Diagnosis

Consider with any associated injury to the genitourinary area. Missed diagnosis can result in urine leak, ileus, fever, sepsis, or ureterocutaneous fistula.

▶ Clinical Therapeutics

Minor injury may divert urine by ureteral stenting. Foley catheter to decompress bladder and monitor urine output. Broad-spectrum antibiotics to prevent infection.

▶ Clinical Intervention

Major injury demands early diagnosis and repair. Ureteroureterostomy is most common operative repair. Prompt urological consult indicated.

▶ Health Maintenance Issues

Anticipatory guidance. The best treatment is prevention of trauma. Avoid alcohol, drugs, and conflict. Mostly due to penetrating trauma and iatrogenic injury. Inform patients of risk as part of patient consent for surgery.

## B. Urethral Trauma

▶ Scientific Concepts

Blunt injury occurs with greater frequency than penetrating. High index of suspicion with deceleration mechanism of injury. Associated pelvic fractures. Disruption may be complete or partial.

▶ History & Physical

Blunt perineal trauma, usually in the form of a straddle injury from a bicycle with resulting pelvic fracture, is often mechanism of injury. Blood at the tip of the urethral meatus is the classic presentation. Hematuria, anuria, perineal edema, or tender and distended lower abdomen and "high-riding" prostate on digital rectal examination.

▶ Diagnostic Studies

Retrograde urethrogram is mandated for the evaluation of a urethral injury.

▶ Differential Diagnosis

Differential diagnosis includes both lower and upper urinary tract injuries.

▶ Clinical Therapeutics

Do not insert Foley or straight catheter until retrograde urethrogram is performed to confirm that the urethra is normal. Insertion of a Foley catheter may worsen an incomplete injury. If extravasation of contrast is noted, a suprapubic catheter is then placed to decompress the bladder. Prompt urological consult is indicated.

▶ Clinical Intervention

Primary repair with stenting for small lacerations or delayed primary repair with suprapubic cystostomy for complex injury. Complications include stricture, impotence, and incontinence.

▶ **Health Maintenance Issues**

Most commonly seen with blunt injury associated with automobile accidents.

## C. Bladder Trauma

▶ **Scientific Concepts**

Bladder trauma may present as an intraperitoneal or extraperitoneal perforation or both. Intraperitoneal injuries occur during severe, blunt, lower abdominal trauma, generally when the bladder is full. The increased bladder is acute and the bladder perforates at it weakest point, the dome. An extraperitoneal injury may be associated with a pelvic fracture, where the displaced pelvis perforates the bladder.

▶ **History & Physical**

History of lower abdominal trauma. Anuria, oliguria, and gross or microscopic hematuria. Localized suprapubic or diffuse abdominal pain. Tenderness to percussion or palpation. Intraperitoneal rupture will result in acute abdomen secondary to peritonitis.

▶ **Diagnostic Studies**

Hemorrhagic shock may result from associated injuries. Follow serial hemoglobin/hematocrit. Retrograde urethrogram to rule out suspected urethral injury if indicated by blood at tip of meatus. If negative, Foley catheter insertion to decompress bladder. Urinalysis dipstick to identify microhematuria if gross hematuria is not noted. Pelvic x-ray may show associated pelvic fracture. Cystography to note extravasion. Cystogram is radiologic study of choice. IVP to rule out kidney or ureteral injury often will miss bladder injury.

▶ **Diagnosis**

Bladder trauma is a diagnosis of exclusion, eliminating other genitourinary tract injuries. A missed diagnosis can increase mortality and morbidity.

▶ **Clinical Therapeutics**

Conservative management is indicated for bladder contusions with Foley catheter decompression and irrigation of clots. Intravenous fluid resuscitation as needed. Broad-spectrum antibiotics. *Caution:* bladder decompression > 1,000 cc should never be allowed without adequate intravenous fluid replacement. Historically, gradual bladder decompression has been emphasized.

▶ **Clinical Intervention**

Extraperitoneal ruptures may be managed conservatively with catheter decompression or require surgery for repair and drainage. In either type of management, the indwelling Foley will be left in place between 7 and 14 days with broad-spectrum antibiotic coverage. A cystogram should be performed prior to catheter removal to check for extravasation of contrast material. If the study is positive for extravasation, the catheter must remain for an additional 2 weeks. Intraperitoneal ruptures mandate surgical exploration, repair with absorbable sutures, and drainage through a suprapubic tube for bladder decompression during healing.

▶ **Health Maintenance Issues**

See previous trauma topics about prevention and anticipatory guidance.

## BIBLIOGRAPHY

Berkow R, Beers MH. *The Merck Manual of Diagnosis & Therapy,* 17th ed. Rahway, NJ: Merck & Company; 1999.

Currey R. Epididymitis: Recognition & management. *PA Today* 6(12):10–13; 1998.

Hanno PM, Wein AJ. *Clinical Manual of Urology,* 2nd ed. New York: McGraw-Hill; 1994.

Howes DS. (2002, January 14). Urinary Tract Infection, Male. eMedicine Journal, 3. Retrieved August 10, 2002 from http://www.emedicine/emerg/topic625.htm.

Macfarlane M. *Urology,* 3rd ed. Philadelphia: Lippincott, Williams & Wilkins; 2001.

Resnick MI, Novick AC. *Urology Secrets,* Philadelphia: Hanley & Belfus; 1995.

Tanagho EA, McAninch JW. *Smith's General Urology,* 15th ed. New York: McGraw-Hill; 2000.

Walsh PC, Retik AB, Vaughan, ED Jr., Wein AJ. *Campbell's Urology,* 7th ed. Philadelphia: WB Saunders; 1998.

Weiss R, Fair WR. *Management of Prostate Diseases,* 2nd ed. New York: Professional Communications; 1997.

Wieder, JA. *Pocket Guide to Urology.* Caldwell, ID: Griffith Publishing; 1999.

# Obstetrics and Gynecology  9

*Constance Goldgar, MS, PA-C, Paula Phelps, MHE, PA-C, and Dawn Morton-Rias, PD, RPA-C*

## I. VAGINA/VULVA

### A. Vaginal Infections and Sexually Transmitted Diseases

Vaginal infections are among the most common gynecological disorders of women. Complaints range from mild itching of the vagina or vulva with or without discharge to severe swelling of the labia and vulva, profuse discharge, itching, and pain. Many vaginal infections are sexually transmitted and may be chronic and/or recurrent. Asymptomatic infection is common.

#### 1. *Trichomonas vaginalis*

▶ Scientific Concepts

Caused by protozoa, may be carried symptomatically or asymptomatically by men and women; transmitted sexually.

▶ History & Physical

Profuse, frothy, gray-greenish, malodorous leukorrhea worse after menstruation, with or without secondary vulvar pruritus. Dysuria and urinary frequency are common. Vulvar and/or labial swelling or inflammation, cervical petechiae (strawberry spots).

▶ Diagnostic Studies

Trichomonads visualized on saline wet mount, potassium hydroxide (KOH) prep under darkfield, phase contrast, ordinary microscope or identified on Pap smear. Vaginal pH is usually > 5.0.

▶ Diagnosis

Rule out other etiologic agents.

▶ Clinical Therapeutics

Metronidazole, 2 g PO one dose or 500 mg bid 7 days for both partners.

▶ Health Maintenance Issues

Patient education, use of condoms, avoid high-risk sexual behaviors. Patient and partner should be advised to avoid alcohol or vinegar during treatment as they may interact with metronidazole, causing severe nausea, vomiting, sweating, weakness, and other complications.

#### 2. Condyloma Acuminata (Genital Warts)

▶ Scientific Concepts

Many types, transmitted via direct contact with human papillomavirus (HPV) through mucous membranes or skin abrasions. Incubation period may be 1–6 months. Infection with HPV (especially subtypes 16 and 18) is associated with cervical cancer.

▶ History & Physical

May be symptomatic or subclinical, may include pruritus, burning, pain, bleeding, and dyspareunia. Single or multiple exophytic warts from a few millimeters to large fleshy lesions covering the entire genitalia or flat grey lesions.

▶ **Diagnostic Studies**

May be identified on appearance, Pap smear, colposcopy, or biopsy of a condyloma. Application of 3–5% acetic acid causes warts to turn white; may aid in diagnosis.

▶ **Diagnosis**

Rule out other genital ulcer disease including chancroid, condyloma lata of secondary syphilis, *Molluscum contagiosum,* and genital herpes.

▶ **Clinical Therapeutics**

Trichloroacetic acid (TCA), podophyllum resin (podophyllin), applied by health professional. Podifilox or imiquimod may be applied by patient. Podophyllum resin is not approved for use during pregnancy; TCA is approved for use in pregnancy. Larger warts may require laser treatment, cryotherapy with liquid nitrogen, electrocautery, or surgical excision.

▶ **Clinical Intervention**

HPV is highly contagious and is implicated in a high percentage of cervical dysplasias and cervical cancer; warts may grow rapidly during pregnancy, may predispose infant to genital warts or laryngeal papillomatosis.

▶ **Health Maintenance Issues**

Patient education, use of condoms, avoid high-risk sexual behaviors. Consider screening for human immunodeficiency virus (HIV) infection. If topical therapy is instituted, patient must follow directions carefully to avoid inflammation.

3. **Herpes Simplex Virus**

▶ **Scientific Concepts**

Two primary types, type 2 (80–90%), type 1 (10–20%), mucosal contact with herpes simplex virus (HSV)-infected secretions/lesions, asymptomatic shedding, or perinatal transmission. This virus is frequently found in association with other sexually transmitted diseases (STDs).

▶ **History & Physical**

May be symptomatic or subclinical. Prodromal symptoms include tingling, irritation, pruritus, or vaginal discharge. Primary episode associated with pain, dysuria, and dyspareunia with lesions; inguinal lymphadenopathy; fever and multiple tender, vesicular lesions at site of infection. Recurrent outbreaks tend to be slightly less severe.

▶ **Diagnostic Studies**

Identification of multinucleated giant cells in Wright–Giemsa stain, viral culture, serological assay, enzyme-linked immunosorbent assay (ELISA)/Western blot.

▶ **Diagnosis**

Rule out other genital ulcer disease, chancroid, HPV, and syphilis.

▶ **Clinical Therapeutics**

Currently no cure; acyclovir, famciclovir, and valacyclovir PO for up to 5 days offers symptomatic relief, may diminish severity of recurrences. Current treatment of primary episode: acyclovir, 200 mg PO five times daily (or 800 mg three times daily) for 7–10 days; famciclovir, 250 mg PO tid 7–10 days; or valacyclovir, 1 g PO bid 7–10 days. The therapy for a recurrent outbreak is a 5-day regimen of: acyclovir, 200 mg PO bid, tid, or qid or 400 mg PO bid; famciclovir 125 mg bid; valacyclovir 500 mg bid. To suppress outbreaks in patients with severe recurrences, the recommended suppressive doses taken continuously are: acyclovir 400 mg bid; famciclovir 125–250 mg bid; or valacyclovir 500 mg qd.

▶ Clinical Intervention

Clinical picture may be exacerbated by other serious illness, immuno-compromise, or stress. Epidemiologic link to cervical cancer; high mortality rate in neonatal disease.

▶ Health Maintenance Issues

Patient education, use of condoms, avoid high-risk sexual behaviors. Consider screening for HIV infection.

4. *Chlamydia*

▶ Scientific Concepts

Currently the most common STD in the United States, causing non-gonococcal cervicitis in women and urethritis in men. Causative agent *Chlamydia trachomatis*. Sequelae of infection include infertility, pelvic inflammatory disease (PID), and ectopic pregnancy. Perinatal transmission associated with neonatal chlamydial conjunctivitis and pneumonia. Risk factors for screening include age (sexually active females < 25 years), increased number of sexual partners, and prior history of STDs.

▶ History & Physical

The majority of lower genital tract chlamydial infections are asymptomatic, detected by routine screening. Patients may present with no signs or symptoms, mild to severe vaginal discharge, dysuria, pelvic pain, urethritis, and infection of Bartholin glands to cervicitis with muco-purulent cervix.

▶ Diagnostic Studies

Urinalysis positive for > 500 polymorphonuclear neutrophils (PMNs)/ 1,000 and Gram stain positive for polymorphonuclear lymphocytes (PMLs) without gonococci are nonspecific tests for *C. trachomatis*. Cell culture that detects organisms from the endocervical swab demonstrates specificity close to 100% and has been the "gold standard" but delays diagnosis 3–7 days. Direct immunofluorescence techniques (MicroTrak): amplified chlamydia test (AMP-CT, Gen Probe), which detects chlamydia in the urine; enzyme immunoassay (Chlamydiazyme); and chlamydia polymerase chain reaction (PCR) and ligase chain reaction (LCR), which amplify deoxyribonucleic acid (DNA), are newer, more sensitive, and specific approaches for detection of chlamydia.

▶ Diagnosis

Rule out infection of other etiologic origin. Untreated infection associated with multiple complications.

▶ Clinical Therapeutics

Azithromycin (Zithromax), 1 mg PO; doxycycline, 100 mg PO bid for 7 days; or ofloxacin, 300 mg PO bid for 7 days. If pregnant: erythromycin, 500 mg PO qid for 7 days. If PID develops, treat with ceftriaxone, 250 mg intramuscularly (IM) one dose, and doxycycline, 100 mg PO bid for 7 days, or ofloxacin, 400 mg PO bid, and metronidazole, 500 mg PO bid.

► **Health Maintenance Issues**

Patient education, use of loose-fitting clothing, use of condoms, avoid high-risk sexual behaviors, concurrent treatment of all partners, and delay sexual relations until treatment is complete.

## 5. Lymphogranuloma Venereum

► **Scientific Concepts**

Caused by one of the aggressive L1–L3 serotypes of *C. trachomatis*. More common in tropical and subtropical nations. More common in women than men; incubation period 7–21 days.

► **History & Physical**

In early phase, vesicopustular eruption progressing to inguinal and vulvar ulceration, pronounced inguinal lymphadenopathy, positive "groove sign" (line between lymph nodes), fever, joint pain, and body aches. Strictures and narrowing of the vagina or rectum common complication of ulcerations.

► **Diagnostic Studies**

Isolation of *C. trachomatis* via culture or microimmunofluorescent and complement fixation tests, if available.

► **Diagnosis**

Rule out other ulcerative infectious disease. Diagnosis correlates well with degree of suspicion.

► **Clinical Therapeutics**

Treatment includes doxycycline, 100 mg PO bid for 21 days (preferred); tetracycline, 500 mg PO qid for 21 days; or erythromycin, 500 mg PO bid for 21 days.

► **Clinical Intervention**

Concurrent abscesses may require incision and drainage. If untreated, long-term complications include perianal scaring, vaginal, anal, rectal, and sigmoid strictures, requiring surgical intervention including colostomy. Consider screening for HIV infection.

► **Health Maintenance Issues**

Risk increases with unprotected sexual activity. Prevention achieved with use of condoms and avoidance of high-risk behaviors.

## 6. Bacterial Vaginosis

Previously referred to as *Gardnerella vaginalis,* the most common cause of bacterial vaginitis and vaginal discharge in sexually active patients.

► **Scientific Concepts**

Polymicrobial condition involving interactions between several components of the vaginal flora, especially anaerobes, elevation of vaginal pH, and production of amines.

► **History & Physical**

Grey/white, malodorous, creamy, noninflammatory vaginal discharge, little to no vulvar irritation or pruritus, most pronounced symptom is odor; discharge and signs of inflammation may or may not be evident.

▶ **Diagnostic Studies**

Wet mount and Gram stain reveal "clue cells" (unstained exfoliated epithelial cells with a large number of gram-negative bacteria); an amine odor ("fishy") is present when 10% potassium hydroxide solution is added to a drop of the vaginal discharge. This is considered a positive "whiff test"; cultures are not generally useful.

▶ **Diagnosis**

Presence of three to four of the following: clue cells on microscopic examination; white, noninflammatory, adherent discharge; vaginal fluid pH > 4.5; positive "whiff test."

▶ **Clinical Therapeutics**

Metronidazole, 500 mg PO bid for 7 days or single dose of 2 g PO; metronidazole vaginal gel, 0.075% per vagina qd or bid for 5 days; or clindamycin, 300 mg bid for 7 days. In pregnancy, treatment of choice is metronidazole, 250 mg PO tid for 7 days (second and third trimester). Clindamycin is not recommended during pregnancy.

▶ **Clinical Intervention**

Obstetric and gynecologic complications associated with untreated bacterial vaginosis in pregnancy include premature rupture of membranes (PROM), chorioamnionitis and PID in the nonpregnant female.

▶ **Health Maintenance Issues**

Patient education: although bacterial vaginosis is a non–sexually transmitted disease, the clinician may use this opportunity to discuss use of condoms and avoidance of high-risk sexual behaviors.

## 7. Gonorrhea

▶ **Scientific Concepts**

STD caused by direct contact with *Neisseria gonorrhoeae*. May be asymptomatic in infected female patients. Incubation period is 2–8 days following infection.

▶ **History & Physical**

No symptoms to mild to severe purulent vaginal discharge, pelvic pain, urethritis, dysuria, urinary frequency, infection of Bartholin glands, fever, signs of nonspecific vaginitis to cervicitis with mucopurulent cervix, pain on pelvic examination, and adnexal tenderness. Other symptoms may include anorectal inflammation, pharyngitis, tonsillitis, conjunctivitis, and disseminated infections such as septic arthritis, endocarditis, meningitis, polyarthralgias, tenosynovitis, and dermatitis.

▶ **Diagnostic Studies**

Routine cervical, urethra, pharynx, and rectum sampling for culture using Thayer–Martin medium. Becoming more common is a LCR assay, which can detect both *N. gonorrhea* and *C. trachomatis*. Gram-stained smear will identify gram-negative intracellular diplococci with PMLs.

▶ **Clinical Therapeutics**

With the emergence of resistant strains, treatment of choice is a single dose of ceftriaxone, 125 mg IM, plus doxycycline, 100 mg PO bid for 7 days; doxycycline or tetracycline, 500 mg qid for 7 days, should be given routinely because of high risk of coexisting chlamydial infections.

► **Clinical Intervention**

Evaluate for extragenital infection.

► **Health Maintenance Issues**

All partners should be treated; patient education and follow-up including safe sex practices should be provided. Sexual activity should not be resumed until a follow-up culture is negative. Consider screening for concomitant infections such as syphilis, chlamydia, or HIV infection.

## 8. Chancroid

► **Scientific Concepts**

STD more common in the tropics and Southeast Asia. Caused by *Haemophilus ducreyi,* chancroid is a cofactor for HIV transmission and has been found in coexistent syphilis and herpes infections. Incubation period is short, with lesions appearing 3–5 days following exposure.

► **History & Physical**

Symptoms include the presence of painful, vesicopustular lesions, progressing to nonindurated, saucer-shaped weal that produce a profuse, foul-smelling discharge, found on the external genitalia, perineum, thigh, or cervix. Lymphadenopathy, buboes in the lymph nodes, and abscess formation are common.

► **Diagnostic Studies**

The diagnosis is clinical, with cultures and smears less reliable; *H. ducreyi* is difficult to isolate.

► **Diagnosis**

Rule out other ulcerative disorders including lymphogranuloma venereum, herpes, and syphilis.

► **Clinical Therapeutics**

Azithromycin, 1 g PO in one dose, or ceftriaxone, 250 mg IM in one dose.

► **Health Maintenance Issues**

Sitz baths and meticulous hygiene are beneficial, use of condoms and avoidance of high-risk behaviors encouraged. Consider screening for HIV infection.

## 9. Syphilis

► **Scientific Concepts**

STD caused by direct sexual contact with the spirochete, *Treponema pallidum.* Infection in utero, via needle sticks and blood transfusion uncommon. A diagnosis of another STD is considered a risk factor for syphilis, and previous treatment does not confer immunity against future infections.

► **History & Physical**

*Primary* lesion (chancre, painless indurated ulcer) at site of inoculation approximately 10 to 90 days after contact. Heals spontaneously. *Secondary* stage heralded by a maculopapular rash approximately 6 weeks post healing of primary lesion. Associated with malaise, fever, generalized lymphadenopathy, condyloma lata (moist papules), and alopecia. *Latent* phase occurs approximately 2–6 weeks post resolution of the rash, considered infectious for first 1–2 years in latency. One third of all un-treated patients develop *tertiary* syphilis, which is associated with serious cardiovascular and central nervous system (CNS) sequelae.

▶ **Diagnostic Studies**

Serologic tests. *Nontreponemal tests*—rapid plasma reagin [RPR], Vene-real Disease Research Laboratory [VDRL], automated reagin test [ART]. *Treponemal tests* used in follow-up to positive nontreponemal tests (micro-hemagglutination test for *T. pallidum* [MHATP], fluorescent treponemal antibody-absorption test for syphilis [FTA-ABS]). Darkfield microscopy may be used in evaluating chancres, condyloma lata, and mucous patches; useful in diagnosing primary and secondary syphilis. PCR is specific for detection of *T. pallidum* in amniotic fluid, neonatal serum, and spinal fluid.

▶ **Diagnosis**

Positive RPR/VDRL and follow-up FTA. Rule out other ulcerative disorder.

▶ **Clinical Therapeutics**

Primary, secondary, and early latent (< 1 year) are treated with peni-cillin G benzathine (Bicillin), 2.4 million units IM in single dose. Alter-native for penicillin-allergic, nonpregnant patient is doxycycline, 100 mg PO bid for 2 weeks. Tertiary or late syphilis is treated with penicillin G benzathine (Bicillin), 2.4 million units IM 1/wk × 3 consecutive weeks, or tetracycline hydrochloride, 500 mg PO qid 14 days, or doxycycline, 100 mg PO bid 2 weeks.

▶ **Clinical Intervention**

Pregnancy does not alter the course of the infection. Risk of fetal infec-tion correlates with degree of exposure to spirochetemia and gestational age. The earlier the fetus is exposed, the greater the risk of premature delivery or stillbirth. Infected neonates may not develop symptoms until weeks or months later and may include lymphadenitis, hepatospleno-megaly, osteochondritis, and irregular epiphyseal juncture on x-ray. Treat-ment in pregnancy as above, except if penicillin-allergic, then desensitize patient with gradually increasing doses of oral penicillin and proceed with treatment as above.

▶ **Health Maintenance Issues**

Partners should be treated; patient education and follow-up. Con-sider screening for HIV infection.

## 10. Atrophic Vaginitis

▶ **Scientific Concepts**

Most common cause of vaginal discharge in the postmenopausal woman. Estrogen deficiency precipitates thinning of vaginal mucosa.

▶ **History & Physical**

Symptoms include dysuria, pruritus, burning, soreness, bleeding, and dyspareunia. Thin, erythematous mucous membranes; loss of rugae; and watery discharge are common. Vaginal pH 7.0.

▶ **Diagnostic Studies**

Serum follicle-stimulating hormone (FSH), luteinizing hormone (LH), wet mount, and Pap smear.

► Diagnosis

Rule out other cause of vaginal discharge, STD, urinary tract infection (UTI), foreign body, allergen.

► Clinical Therapeutics

Exogenous estrogen (topical or systemic) and lubricants.

► Health Maintenance Issues

Avoid irritants, encourage lubrication with sexual activity. Increased sexual activity may improve condition.

## 11. Candidiasis

► Scientific Concepts

Mycotic vaginitis is the second most common cause of symptomatic vaginal discharge. Infections typically caused by yeasts (*Candida albicans,* most commonly), which may be precipitated by cyclic hormones including oral contraceptives, diabetes mellitus, chemical irritation, immunocompromise, pregnancy, or recent antibiotic therapy.

► History & Physical

Thick, white vaginal discharge; mild to severe vulvar pruritus and burning; red, swollen vulva and vaginal mucosa; white exudate on cervix or vaginal mucosa.

► Diagnostic Studies

Wet mount or KOH prep slide with visualization of budding yeast or hyphae, or culture on Nickerson's medium.

► Diagnosis

Classic clinical presentation is common.

► Clinical Therapeutics

Topical application of antifungal cream or vaginal suppositories such as miconazole, terconazole, clotrimazole, butoconazole, or nystatin at bedtime for 3 days or at bedtime for 7 days; systemic treatment with fluconazole or ketoconazole.

► Clinical Intervention

Treat underlying condition. Further evaluation is necessary for recurrent or recalcitrant infections with potential for prolonged treatment.

► Health Maintenance Issues

Provide health education and referral for evaluation of recurrences.

## B. Prolapse of Vaginal Walls

► Scientific Concepts

Defects in pelvic support structures may result in prolapse of urethra (urethrocele), bladder (cystocele), rectum (enterocele), or uterus (uterine prolapse). Loss of muscle tone may be attributed to advancing age, pregnancy, multiple or difficult childbirth, or increased intra-abdominal pressure. May progress after menopause.

► History & Physical

Symptoms related to degree of prolapse and structures involved. When descent is limited to the upper two thirds of the vagina, it is said to be first degree; second degree is present when the structure approaches the vaginal introitus, and third degree involves descent outside of the vaginal opening. Symptoms include fullness, pressure, urinary symptoms including incontinence, frequency, urgency, incomplete voiding; relaxed vaginal outlet.

▶ Diagnostic Studies

Diagnosis is by physical and pelvic exam. Q-tip test (assessment of degree of upward motion of a cotton tipped applicator placed in the urethra when the patient strains), urodynamic testing, and evaluation of urinary function are diagnostic studies employed to assess pelvic relation including cystocele.

▶ Diagnosis

Rule out urethral obstruction. Herniation of other structures may be simultaneously diagnosed.

▶ Clinical Therapeutics

Medical measures include vaginal pessaries, Kegel isometric exercise, and estrogen replacement therapy. Treatment with anticholinergic drugs (propantheline bromide), beta-sympathomimetic agonists (metaproterenol sulfate), musculotropic drugs (flavoxate hydrochloride), diazepam, and bromocriptine mesylate have been effective in providing improvement, depending on the problem. Surgical interventions may be employed depending on anatomical defect. Vaginal hysterectomy or Moschowitz procedures may be offered if the defect causes secondary urinary retention, obstruction, or other significant complication.

▶ Clinical Intervention

Kegel exercises may be recommended. If pessary is placed, regular removal and replacement are recommended.

▶ Health Maintenance Issues

Patient education plays an important role in treatment and management. Nonmedical treatment interventions include biofeedback and bladder training.

## C. Vulvar and Vaginal Neoplasms

### 1. Vulvar Carcinoma

▶ Scientific Concepts

A disease classically occurring in women over 50 years of age, but now seen in younger women as well. Associated with HPV infection.

▶ History & Physical

Patients may be asymptomatic or present with a long history of pruritus, pain, bloody discharge, vulvar mass, or rash, which may range from leukoplakia, as in Paget's disease, to hyperpigmentation, as in Bowen's disease. Vulvar pruritus is the most common presenting complaint.

▶ Diagnostic Studies

The visibility of the region lends itself to early detection and treatment. Toluidine blue staining of the vulva and incisional biopsy of any lesion or suspicious areas as well as computed tomographic (CT) scan to rule out metastatic disease are most helpful.

► **Diagnosis**

Suspicious lesions should be biopsied; prognosis is worse with pelvic lymph node involvement. Early vulvar intraepithelial neoplasia (VIN) may be classified as VIN I (mild dysplasia), II (moderate dysplasia), or III (severe dysplasia or carcinoma in situ).

► **Clinical Intervention**

Assess tumor size, node involvement, and metastasis (TNM staging). Good surgical outcome with radical vulvectomy; less extensive surgery for early disease. Radiation therapy prior to surgery for more advanced disease. Chemotherapy not useful.

► **Health Maintenance Issues**

Careful and regular pelvic exams and early detection and treatment provide best opportunity for recovery.

## 2. Vaginal Carcinoma

► **Scientific Concepts**

Relatively rare disease. Etiology unknown, yet chronic irritation from pessary use, prior existence of preinvasive carcinoma in situ (CIS), and HPV have been implicated. Squamous cell carcinoma accounts for the majority of invasive vaginal cancer. Clear cell adenocarcinoma, usually related to diethylstilbestrol (DES) exposure before 18 weeks' gestation in utero, and vaginal melanoma account for a small percentage of vaginal carcinomas.

► **History & Physical**

Early stages (preinvasive carcinoma of the vagina) generally asymptomatic. Abnormal painless vaginal bleeding or ulcerated lesions as noted on routine exam, illustrating need for continued regular Pap smears in the postmenopausal female and those who have undergone hysterectomy. Vaginal bleeding or discharge are the most common symptoms of invasive vaginal cancer.

► **Diagnostic Studies**

Abnormal Pap smear, incisional biopsy of gross lesion, colposcopy to identify smaller lesions.

► **Diagnosis**

Biopsy to rule out other causes of red ulcerated or white hyperplastic lesions of the vagina.

► **Clinical Intervention**

Staging based on extent and structural involvement. Primary treatment radiotherapy, then surgical or vaporization with carbon dioxide laser or 5-fluorouracil cream.

► **Health Maintenance Issues**

Must rule out other gynecologic cancer as vaginal cancer may represent metastasis of cervical cancer. The larger the mass, the worse the prognosis. Lymph node involvement and tumor location are important prognostic factors.

## II. FALLOPIAN TUBES

► Scientific Concepts

PID is a general term for acute, subacute, recurrent, or chronic infection of the oviducts and ovaries often with involvement of adjacent tissues. PID has become increasingly recognized and may frequently be due to a coexisting infection with either *N. gonorrhoeae* or *C. trachomatis* or both. Pathways of dissemination include lymphatic (i.e., postpartum and postabortal), endosalpingo, and peritoneal spread of microorganisms as in intrauterine device (IUD)-related infections, and in rare cases hematogenous routes such as tuberculosis.

► History & Physical

Insidious or acute onset of lower abdominal cramps and pelvic pain, mild to severe purulent vaginal discharge, urethritis, dysuria, urinary frequency, fever > 38°C (100.4°F), leukocytosis, erythema of the vaginal mucosa, purulent cervicitis, with rebound tenderness, inguinal lymphadenopathy, adnexal tenderness and pain on motion of cervix (chandelier sign), palpable tubo-ovarian abscess (~15% of cases), pelvic abscess (may include infection), and unilateral tenderness of Bartholin glands.

► Diagnostic Studies

Beta-human chorionic gonadotropin (hCG) and cultures obtained from the cervix, urethra, anus, and pharynx when appropriate. Cervical cultures, including for *N. gonorrhoeae,* grown on a Thayer–Martin agar plate and kept in a carbon dioxide–rich environment are diagnostic for *N. gonorrhoeae.* Gram-stained smear may identify gram-negative intracellular diplococci with leukocytes or endocervical culture or antigen test for *Chlamydia* may be positive. Culdocentesis is generally productive of a cloudy fluid, which should also be cultured with sensitivity. Blood work may reveal increased white blood cells (WBCs) with a left shift and an increased sedimentation rate. Laparoscopy and pelvic sonogram may reveal a tubo-ovarian mass.

► Diagnosis

Rule out ectopic pregnancy, acute abdomen, ovarian torsion, and ovarian mass. Concomitant signs of infection suggest PID.

► Clinical Therapeutics

Hospitalization may be necessary, if a surgical emergency (i.e., appendicitis and ectopic pregnancy), pelvic abscess is present, patient is pregnant, patient is an adolescent, severe illness precludes outpatient management, or if the patient fails to respond to outpatient therapy with 72 hours of initial treatment. Inpatient regimens include cefoxitin, 2 g intravenously (IV) q6h, plus doxycycline, 100 mg PO bid or IV q12h. Post hospital discharge, treatment is doxycycline, 100 mg PO bid for a total of 10–14 days. Outpatient regimens include ofloxacin, 400 mg PO bid for 14 days, and metronidazole, 500 mg PO bid for 14 days, or ceftriaxone, 250 mg IM in one dose, plus doxycycline, 100 mg PO bid 14 days, or cefoxitin, 2 g IM, with probenecid, 1 g PO. Surgical intervention such as colpotomy (drainage of cul-de-sac) or salpingo-oophorectomy may be necessary.

▶ Clinical Intervention

Patients with suspected pelvic abscess who fail to respond to antibiotic therapy may require surgical intervention, CT-guided percutaneous drainage, colpotomy drainage, or exploratory laparotomy.

▶ Health Maintenance Issues

Acute or chronic PID may result in infertility, chronic pelvic pain, and increased incidence of ectopic pregnancy.

## III. CERVIX

### A. Abnormal Pap Smear

▶ Scientific Concepts

Widespread use of the Pap smear and early cytologic detection of abnormal preinvasive cervical lesions have resulted in early intervention and management of dysplastic cervical lesions. Rule out fungal, bacterial, viral, or other infection and benign inflammatory changes. Sexually transmitted viruses may induce malignant transformation of lesions. It is currently thought that a very high percentage of cervical dysplasias and cancers are associated with HPV infection.

▶ History & Physical

Risk factors include cervical mucosa previously altered by HPV, repeated STDs, cervicitis, cigarette smoking, multiple sexual partners, early age at first intercourse, and DES exposure. May be asymptomatic, cervix appearing normal; cervical discharge and/or postcoital bleeding possible. HPV infection is a major risk factor.

▶ Diagnostic Studies

Pap smear findings as reported in common descriptive conventions (Table 9–1). Cultures, colposcopy, colposcopically directed punch biopsy, and endocervical curettage are essential for further evaluation and treatment.

## ▶ table 9-1

### COMMON DESCRIPTIVE CONVENTIONS

| Class System | CIN System | Bethesda II System |
|---|---|---|
| Class I | Negative | Negative |
| Class II | Atypia or inflammatory changes | Atypical squamous cells of undetermined origin (ASCUS) cellular changes with or without atypia |
| Class III, mild to moderate dysplasia | Mild to moderate cervical intraepithelial neoplasia (CIN I or II) | Low-grade squamous intraepithelial lesion (LGSIL) and high-grade (HGSIL) |
| Class IV, severe dysplasia | Severe cervical intraepithelial neoplasia (CIN III) | HGSIL |
| Class V | Suggestive of cancer or carcinoma in situ (CIS) | Squamous cell cancer |

▶ Diagnosis

Abnormal findings on Pap smear warrant further evaluation.

▶ Clinical Therapeutics

Depends on etiology and extent; treat underlying infection; electro-cautery, cryotherapy, laser vaporization, loop electrosurgical excision, cone biopsy, chemotherapy agents.

▶ Clinical Intervention

Close follow-up of abnormal Pap smears is necessary. Cytopathologists consider a Pap smear to be a medical consultation and will often make recommendations as to follow-up. Also several algorithms exist to aid the clinician in management of abnormal Pap smears. Once the diagnosis of cervical intraepithelial neoplasia has been made and the lesions have been treated, then follow-up Pap smears are needed to detect recurrence. Current recommendation is that Pap smears are repeated every 3 months for a minimum of 1 year after treatment. ThinPrep technique reduces clinician variability in slide handling and decreases smears with atypical squamous cells of undetermined significance (ASCUS).

▶ Health Maintenance Issues

Cervical screening with annual Pap smear is recommended at the onset of sexual activity or age 18. Patient education and counseling on importance of regular Pap testing and prompt and appropriate treatment of any cervical lesion. Once a low-risk patient has documented three normal consecutive annual Pap smears, some clinicians advise patients may go every 1–3 years between Pap smears.

## B. Cervicitis/Endocervicitis

▶ Scientific Concepts

Nonspecific term to describe infectious process; may be localized to the cervix; may be caused by same etiologic agents as vaginal infections, HPV, STDs, and PID. Risk factors include early coitus and multiple partners.

▶ History & Physical

May be asymptomatic to complaints of yellow vaginal discharge, post-coital bleeding, and dyspareunia. Infective agent may be identified on abnormal Pap smear.

▶ Diagnostic Studies

Pap smear, cervical culture, enzyme assays, colposcopy, and serology to rule out syphilis.

▶ Diagnosis

Identify causative or infective agent.

▶ Clinical Therapeutics

Depends on etiology and extent; treat underlying infection. Treatment may include electrocautery, cryotherapy, laser vaporization, loop electro-surgical excision, cone biopsy, or topical chemotherapeutic agents.

▶ Clinical Intervention

Close follow-up, with repeat Pap smear following treatment, in 3–4 months for the next year, then every 4 to 6 months during the second year; annual colposcopy for 2 years.

► **Health Maintenance Issues**

Patient education and counseling on importance of regular Pap testing and prompt and appropriate treatment of any cervical lesion. Screen pregnant women for infectious cervicitis because of risk to fetus.

## C. Cervical Polyps

► **Scientific Concepts**

Benign, pedunculated multiple or single growths, which vary in size. More common in multiparous women. Most originate from the endocervix, composed of vascular connective tissue stroma and covered by epithelium.

► **History & Physical**

Usually symptomatic, may include leukorrhea, postcoital bleeding, menorrhagia, postmenopausal bleeding, or bloody discharge. Soft, red, pedunculated growths may be visible extending from cervical os or endocervix.

► **Diagnostic Studies**

Pap smear and biopsy; rule out endometrial polyp. Some may be visible via hysterography or identified via dilatation and curettage (D&C).

► **Diagnosis**

Microscopic examination and biopsy of polyp confirms diagnosis. Rule out cervical neoplasia, chronic cervicitis, or prolapsed submucosal myoma.

► **Clinical Therapeutics**

Treat accompanying vaginal infection, if any.

► **Clinical Intervention**

Most polyps are removed surgically with concurrent antibiotic therapy if infection occurs. Close follow-up and repeat Pap smear regularly.

► **Health Maintenance Issues**

Prevention of vaginal and cervical infections that can precede cervical polyps. Patient education and counseling on importance of regular Pap testing.

## D. Cervical Cancer

► **Scientific Concepts**

Common but treatable cancer in women, which begins as cervical dysplasia and progresses over time into malignancy in the exo/endo-cervix; hematogenous spread or local spread via the lymphatics. Regional pelvic lymph nodes are generally affected and metastasis is to the lungs, brain, bone, and liver.

► **History & Physical**

Risk factors include early coitus, multiple sexual partners, cervical mucosa previously altered by HPV, repeated STDs or cervicitis, cigarette smoking, and DES exposure. May be asymptomatic; intermenstrual or postcoital bleeding most common early symptoms. Later-stage symptoms include change in urinary or bowel habits or function, bone pain, weakness, weight loss, and anemia. Cervix may appear normal to ulcerative with friable lesion(s).

▶ Diagnostic Studies

Abnormal Pap smear findings (see Abnormal Pap Smear), cultures, colposcopy, colposcopic biopsy, cone biopsy, magnetic resonance imaging (MRI), abdominal CT scan, lymphangiography, intravenous pyelogram (IVP), and sigmoidoscopy with biopsy aid in diagnosis and staging.

▶ Diagnosis

Rule out other ulcerative cervical disorders including cervicitis, condyloma acuminata, syphilis, and chancroid.

▶ Clinical Therapeutics

Proper technique in performing the Pap smear is essential for early diagnosis and treatment. Treatment may include surgical intervention such as partial, extended, or radical hysterectomy; radiation (most effective and widely used); or chemotherapy (least effective). Pelvic exenteration (radical hysterectomy with surgical removal of rectum, bladder, and/or vulva) may be necessary.

▶ Clinical Intervention

Excellent prognosis with early identification and treatment.

▶ Health Maintenance Issues

Preventive measures include avoidance of high-risk behaviors and known risk factors. Patient education and counseling on importance of regular Pap testing and prompt and appropriate treatment of any cervical lesion.

## IV. UTERUS

### A. Leiomyoma of the Uterus

▶ Scientific Concepts

Commonly known as *uterine fibroids,* leiomyomas are benign local proliferations of smooth muscle cells that are hormonally responsive to estrogen. Common to women over age 30, and more common in African American and Asian women; uterine fibroids constitute the most common indication for surgery for women in the United States. Uterine fibroids may be subserosal (outside of the uterine wall), intramural (within the myometrium), or submucosal (within the endometrium). It is uncertain whether uterine fibroids have malignant potential, with studies suggesting degeneration to a leiomyosarcoma occurring rarely, perhaps 1 in 1,000 cases.

▶ History & Physical

Most women with fibroids (50 to 65%) will be asymptomatic. Of those with clinical symptoms, abnormal uterine bleeding is the most common symptom; depending on size and location, symptoms can include abdominal pressure, dyspareunia, dysmenorrhea, menorrhagia, rectal pressure, complications in pregnancy (e.g., infertility, habitual abortion, premature labor), and anemia. Uterine fibroids may be multiple, and the uterus is generally irregularly enlarged.

▶ **Diagnostic Studies**

Uterine size may be assessed with bimanual pelvic exam; pelvic ultrasound is the most common means of diagnosis. MRI, hysterosalpingography (HSG), saline infusion ultrasonography, and hysteroscopy are additional tools for imaging the size and location of uterine fibroids. Leiomyoma may also be identified during cesarean section.

▶ **Diagnosis**

Pregnancy, endometrial hyperplasia or carcinoma, ovarian neoplasia, tubo-ovarian mass, and diverticula are included in the differential of a woman with an enlarged uterus.

▶ **Clinical Therapeutics**

In the past, the primary treatment was surgical (hysterectomy). More recently, myomectomy has been performed for fertility considerations. Depending on severity of pain, anemia, urinary symptoms, or concomitant complications of leiomyoma, conservative therapy (observation) is recommended. However, a myoma should not go untreated if it obscures the evaluation of the adnexae. Leiomyomas are estrogen-dependent; hence, reduction of uterine size, fibroids, and complication associated with leiomyoma diminish in the postmenopausal period. Gonadotropin-releasing hormone (GnRH) agonists, 50–500 μg daily or 3- to 6-mg implant q3mo may retard growth. Common clinical effect of GnRH is short-lived; regrowth following discontinuation of therapy.

▶ **Clinical Intervention**

Observation is the mainstay. Treatment is individualized depending on symptoms, complications, and interest in future conception.

▶ **Health Maintenance Issues**

Leiomyomas are time limited. Patient education and empowerment are important for patient management.

## B. Endometrial Polyps

▶ **Scientific Concepts**

Mass of estrogen-sensitive proliferative tissue (like leiomyoma) that projects outward from cervical os. Rule out endometrial carcinoma versus submucosal myoma. Fundal in origin. Can undergo neoplastic changes.

▶ **History & Physical**

Patient generally complains of recurring menorrhagia, premenstrual and postmenstrual bleeding. On pelvic exam, uterus is normal size. Sudden bleeding in the postmenopausal female with crampy pain could be infarction of a polyp. If still bleeding after D&C, think polyp.

▶ **Diagnostic Studies**

Ultrasound not useful; MRI is helpful, but hysteroscopy is the most useful test.

▶ **Diagnosis**

Rule out endometrial and cervical carcinoma with biopsy.

► Clinical Therapeutics

Surgical excision is the treatment of choice, either by hysteroscopic resection or D&C. One must look specifically for endometrial polyps (often overlooked).

► Clinical Intervention

Polyps may recur and should be excised.

► Health Maintenance Issues

Patient education and routine follow-up indicated.

## C. Endometrial Hyperplasia and Cancer

► Scientific Concepts

Endometrial hyperplasia is the abnormal proliferation of glandular and stromal elements of the endometrium resulting in histologic alterations in the cell architecture and/or cytologic atypia. Endometrial hyperplasia and endometrial adenocarcinoma are common. Endometrial hyperplasia may be considered a precancerous state. With simple hyperplasia (also known as mild hyperplasia), fewer than 1% of these lesions will progress to carcinoma. With complex hyperplasia (also known as moderate hyperplasia without atypia), if untreated, approximately 3% will progress to cancer. Atypical simple hyperplasia (moderate hyperplasia with atypia) untreated may progress to carcinoma in 8% of cases, and atypical complex hyperplasia (severe) progresses to carcinoma if untreated in 29% of cases. Endometrial carcinoma is the most common gynecologic malignancy. Histologic grade and depth of myometrium invasion are the most important prognostic factors. Adenosquamous, clear cell squamous, and papillary serous carcinoma have worse prognoses than the more common adenocarcinoma. Incidence increases with age, 45 to 65 most common age group.

► History & Physical

Abnormal or excessive uterine bleeding is the most common clinical presentation. Risk factors are the same for both endometrial hyperplasia and endometrial carcinoma and are related to prolonged and/or unopposed estrogen exposure (e.g., obesity, nulliparity, early menarche, late menopause, and exogenous estrogen without progesterone). Other risk factors include hypertension, diabetes mellitus, and tamoxifen use. Physical examination occasionally reveals an enlarged uterus secondary to endometrial hyperplasia.

► Diagnostic Studies

Pap smear is rarely positive. D&C and endometrial biopsy are most useful. CA-125 may be elevated. With atypical complex hyperplasia on biopsy, approximately 25% of patients will have coexistent endometrial carcinoma. Other diagnostic studies including chest x-ray, CT scan, bone scan, mammography, and barium enema to rule out metastasis. Test for occult blood because of association with colorectal cancer.

► Diagnosis

Rule out atypical hyperplasia, endometriosis, or other gynecologic cancer.

► Clinical Therapeutics

Treatment for endometrial hyperplasia depends on histology and patient's age. Medical therapy for endometrial hyperplasia is progestin:

medroxyprogesterone or oral progesterone for 3 months followed by rebiopsy. Chemotherapeutic agents such as cisplatin and adriamycin may be used to treat endometrial carcinoma. Surgical staging, hysterectomy, and regional radiation are the mainstay. Best outcome associated with early detection and minimal invasion.

▶ **Clinical Intervention**
Atypical complex hyperplasia is often treated by hysterectomy due to high risk of cancer and typical age of patient. Surgical treatment of endometrial carcinoma is related to degree of invasion and node involvement. Obese, hypertensive, or anovulatory females may reduce risk with weight loss or by taking oral contraceptives.

▶ **Health Maintenance Issues**
Estrogen replacement therapy should also include progestational agents. Recurrence of cancer most common within the first 2 years following treatment. Pap smear every 3 months for 2 years and endometrial biopsy recommended.

## D. Dysfunctional Uterine Bleeding

▶ **Scientific Concepts**
Dysfunctional uterine bleeding (DUB) includes menorrhagia, metrorrhagia, menometrorrhagia, amenorrhea, and/or anovulatory cycles not due to other causes such as pregnancy, systemic disease, or cancer. DUB represents abnormal hormonal regulation rather than the cyclical fluctuating gonadotropins and hormones. Occurs commonly with anovulation in adolescence and near menopause.

*Amenorrhea:* Primary—absence of menarche by the age of 18, generally due to congenital abnormalities or genetic disorders (e.g., absent uterus or vagina, imperforate hymen, testicular feminization). Secondary—absence of menses for three to six successive cycles in a woman who has previously experienced menarche, most commonly due to pregnancy. An occasional cause is continued hypothalamic suppression after discontinuing oral contraceptives, hormonal imbalance, or excessive weight loss.

*Menorrhagia:* Heavy, prolonged menstrual flow that may be due to submucosal myomas, endometrial hyperplasia, malignant tumors.

*Metrorrhagia (intermenstrual bleeding):* Bleeding that occurs at any time between menstrual periods. Endometrial polyps, hyperplasia, endometrial and cervical carcinomas are pathologic causes. In recent years, exogenous estrogen administration has become a common cause of this type of bleeding.

*Menometrorrhagia:* heavy bleeding that occurs between periods and may also be associated with heavy periods. Pathologic causes as in metrorrhagia.

*Oligomenorrhea:* Menstrual periods that occur more than 35 days apart. Estrogen-secreting tumors will produce oligomenorrhea prior to other patterns of abnormal bleeding.

▶ **History & Physical**
Uterine bleeding unrelated to menses, absence of menses, or irregular bleeding in the absence of other systemic symptoms or disorders.

Basal body temperature record determining ovulation may be useful. Examination may be unremarkable; note evidence of hirsutism or virilization. Abdominal mass and irregular uterus suggests myoma; symmetrically enlarged uterus is more typical of adenomyosis or endometrial cancer.

### ▶ Diagnostic Studies

Obtain Pap smear. Endometrial biopsy is gold standard for determination of ovulation. Complete blood count (CBC) with platelet, prothrombin time (PT), partial thromboplastin time (PTT), pregnancy, and thyroxine/thyroid-stimulating hormone (TSH). Consider FSH/LH and androgens as indicated. D&C in those who have higher risk for endometrial hyperplasia. D&C can be diagnostic and therapeutic.

### ▶ Diagnosis

Rule out other medical conditions.

### ▶ Clinical Therapeutics

Treat underlying cause. Investigate hormonal status, correct anovulatory cycles with hormones or oral contraceptives; surgical measures to correct endometriosis, myoma, and other surgical disorders. After exclusion of organic disease and pregnancy, treat with any combined progestin–estrogen oral contraceptives. In acute unstable situations, treat with estrogen, 25 mg IV q4h. When bleeding stops, and thereafter, induce shedding with 10 mg medroxyprogesterone qd for 10–13 days. Long-term management is achieved with low-dose oral contraceptives. Ovulatory DUB may be treated with nonsteroidal anti-inflammatory drugs (NSAIDs) alone or in conjunction with progestin–estrogen therapy.

### ▶ Clinical Intervention

D&C, hysteroscopy, and endometrial ablation may be therapeutic as well as evaluative of organic lesions. Hysterectomy may be recommended in severe cases and if preservation of fertility is not desired, and when other treatments have failed. Estrogens should not be administered to perimenopausal women or those at risk for endometrial cancer.

### ▶ Health Maintenance Issues

Most anovulatory cycles in young women can be successfully managed. Uterine bleeding in the perimenopausal female requires full evaluation due to risk of cancer in this age group.

## V. OVARY

### A. Ovarian Cysts

#### ▶ Scientific Concepts

The growth and regression of intraovarian structures appear to predispose the ovary to multiple abnormalities of structure and function. They may be solid, cystic, or mixed. Etiology unknown.

*Functional tumors* (producing sex hormones) include follicular cysts, lutein cysts, theca-lutein cysts, and polycystic ovary. Follicular cysts are caused by the failure of the ovarian follicle to rupture in the course of follicular development and ovulation. The cyst is formed by one or more layers of granulosa cells. Lutein cysts form when the corpus luteum becomes cystic or hemorrhagic or fails to degenerate after 14 days. Development of theca-lutein cyst is accompanied by increase in beta-hCG. Examples include hydatidiform mole, choriocarcinoma, or ovulation induction with gonadotropins. Polycystic ovary (Stein–Leventhal syndrome) is characterized by multiple inactive follicle cysts of the ovary, androgen excess, and chronic anovulation. Inflammatory ovarian tumors include salpingo-oophoritis and tubo-ovarian abscess and result from inflammation of tube or ovary or tubo-ovarian cysts. Neoplastic epithelial tumors include stromal or germ cell tumors. Epithelial tumors, serous tumors, mucinous tumors, and endometroid tumors possess the highest potential for malignancy. Stomal tumors are derived from sex cords, fibromas, and Sertoli– Leydig cell tumors (germ cell tumors), and dermoid cysts are derived from embryonic germ cells. Calcifications are common. Benign cystic or germ cell tumors are the most common ovarian neoplasms. Epithelial neoplasia is the most common malignant ovarian tumor. Stromal neoplasia is uncommon. During the reproductive years, 70% of all noninflammatory tumors are functional, 20% are neoplastic, and 10% are endometriomas. After menopause, one half of all ovarian tumors are malignant.

► History & Physical

Ovarian tumors and cysts are often clinically silent except for nonspecific pressure, low pelvic pain, dyspareunia. Functional cysts may cause menstrual abnormalities. Ruptured cysts are painful, sometimes so painful that it is easy to confuse with appendicitis or other causes of an acute abdomen. Adnexal mass and uterine enlargement may be noted (4- to 8-cm tumor on bimanual exam). Regression following menses. Benign tumors are characteristically unilateral, cystic, and mobile. Malignancies are usually solid, fixed, and nodular; may cause ascites.

► Diagnostic Studies

Pelvic exam, CBC, beta-hCG, and transabdominal or transvaginal ultrasound most important. Abdominal CT, barium enema, colonoscopy, or IVP may be indicated.

► Diagnosis

Rule out ovarian malignancies, uterine myoma, diverticulitis, ectopic pregnancy, other causes of abdominal pain.

► Clinical Therapeutics

Observation or monophasic oral contraceptives for 4–6 weeks.

► Clinical Intervention

If cyst is < 6 cm, observation; regression likely. If > 6 cm or cyst persists more than 6–8 weeks, cystectomy or wedge resection recommended.

► Health Maintenance Issues

Risk of ovarian cancer increases with age; annual pelvic exam is recommended.

## B. Ovarian Malignancy

► Scientific Concepts

A variety of malignancies arise from ovarian epithelium, stromal, or germ cells. Ovarian cancer accounts for over 50% of gynecologic cancer deaths. Risk increases with age, positive first-degree family history, low parity, infertility, and high-fat diet.

▶ History & Physical

Often asymptomatic, pelvic pressure, vague gastrointestinal (GI) symptoms, fullness, or abdominal distention may be the only signs or symptoms.

▶ Diagnostic Studies

Pelvic ultrasound, serum CA-125, CT scan, carcinoembryonic antigen (CEA), liver function studies, and barium enema as warranted.

▶ Diagnosis

GI or other malignancy or tubo-ovarian abscess.

▶ Clinical Therapeutics

Surgical staging, excision, and debulking are critical.

▶ Clinical Intervention

Concurrent use of chemotherapy (cisplatin, carboplatin, paclitaxel, or cyclophosphamide) may be indicated. Alternative drugs include etoposide, 5-fluorouracil, adriamycin, or other alkylating agents.

▶ Health Maintenance Issues

Follow-up with routine monitoring of CA-125 is recommended. Attention to potential protective factors is encouraged, and annual pelvic exams are recommended.

## VI. MENSTRUAL DISORDERS

### A. Dysmenorrhea

▶ Scientific Concepts

Dysmenorrhea (pain associated with menses), categorized as primary (idiopathic) or secondary. Dysmenorrhea represents a source of disability for many.

*Primary:* No identifiable cause of pain, normal pelvic organs. Etiologic theory: excess prostaglandin produced in the endometrium. Smooth muscle stimulant causes increased uterine contractions resulting in increased intrauterine pressure. Usual onset late teens to early 20s, declines with age.

*Secondary:* Clinically identifiable cause (e.g., endometriosis, leiomyomas, or other structural abnormalities). With endometriosis, leiomyomas becomes worse with age during the childbearing years. Neither affected by childbearing.

▶ History & Physical

*Primary:* History is more characteristic, recurrent month after month, first 1–3 days of menstruation, pain in lower abdomen and suprapubic area, radiation to back and thighs. Other symptoms include nausea, vomiting, diarrhea, fatigue, low backache, and headache. Physical and pelvic examinations are usually normal, with perhaps generalized tenderness throughout pelvis.

***Secondary:*** Symptoms less severe and more general in nature. Complaints of menorrhagia with pain suggest myomas or polyps. History and physical findings suggest underlying disorder (abdominal fullness, rectal pain, etc.).

### ▶ Diagnostic Studies
None specific; cultures for evaluation of infection; consider pelvic ultrasound to rule out structural abnormalities.

### ▶ Diagnosis
Secondary dysmenorrhea, evaluate underlying condition.

### ▶ Clinical Therapeutics
***Primary:*** NSAIDs, mefenamic acid (Ponstel), diet, exercise, patient education, or oral contraceptives. Useful to start medications 24 hours prior to onset of menses.

***Secondary:*** Treat underlying condition.

### ▶ Health Maintenance Issues
***Primary:*** Reassurance and exercise are beneficial.

***Secondary:*** Routine follow-up and management of underlying cause.

## B. Premenstrual Syndrome

### ▶ Scientific Concepts
Premenstrual syndrome (PMS) is a group of physical, mood, and behavioral changes that occur in a regular cyclic relationship to the late luteal phase of the menstrual cycle. More than 75% of all menstruating women suffer from some premenstrual symptoms. Most prevalent in women in their 30s to 40s. Etiology unknown, but likely multifactorial with physiologic and psychological components. Proposed etiologies include abnormalities in the estrogen–progesterone balance, disturbance of the renin-angiotensin-aldosterone pathway, excess prostaglandin production, decreased endorphin production, or receptor sensitivity.

### ▶ History & Physical
Mood changes (depression, hostility, irritability, crying spells, etc.), somatic changes (appetite, bloating, fatigue, headache, hot flashes, mastalgia), cognitive changes (confusion, poor concentration), and behavioral changes (hyperphagia, social withdrawal).

### ▶ Diagnostic Studies
None specifically. Menstrual diary most useful. History and physical examination to rule out other disorders. *Diagnostic and Statistical Manual (DSM)* criteria: five or more symptoms; disturbance in the absence of other conditions; (timing) symptoms increase up to 14 days before menses, relieved within 4 days of the start of the menses, and do not recur until at least the 12th day of the cycle.

### ▶ Diagnosis
Rule out psychiatric syndromes. The history and physical may suggest other entities.

### ▶ Clinical Therapeutics
Pharmacologic interventions such as NSAIDs, trial of oral contraceptives, diuretics with severe edema, and more specific therapy (e.g., danazol, alprazolam, medroxyprogesterone) as indicated.

► Clinical Intervention

Therapy should be comprehensive, including education, lifestyle modification (exercise; relaxation therapy; diet; decrease salt, caffeine, alcohol, etc.). Dietary supplementation ($B_6$, calcium, primrose oil, multi-vitamins, magnesium, vitamin E) may be helpful.

► Health Maintenance Issues

Patient education and empowerment are important.

## VII. MENOPAUSE

► Scientific Concepts

Characterized as the sequelae of symptoms related to permanent cessation of menses; the period in which ovarian function declines and estrogen production is insufficient to produce proliferation of the endometrial lining. The estrogen receptors located throughout the body respond to diminishing circulating estrogens, hence the multisystemic impact of menopause experienced by most women. Mean age at menopause is 51; range, 40–58. Premature menopause is defined occurring before age 40. Menopause may also be surgically induced.

► History & Physical

Gradual decrease and ultimate cessation of menses; atrophy of estrogen-dependent tissue (skin, breast, uterus, bladder, pelvic floor, and vagina); vasomotor changes (hot flashes and sweating); psychological changes, including depression, nervousness, and anxiety; increased risk of arteriosclerosis and osteoporosis.

► Diagnostic Studies

Usually none are required. If diagnosis is questionable in a younger patient, an elevated serum FSH suggests ovarian failure, but can also be diagnostic of menopause in an older patient. Endometrial biopsy and/or D&C in patients who have intermenstrual or postmenopausal bleeding.

► Diagnosis

Rule out pregnancy.

► Clinical Therapeutics

General measures include adequate calcium intake (elemental calcium, 1,500 mg/d PO). Despite much observational evidence, the balance of risks and benefits for hormone use in healthy postmenopausal women remains uncertain. Short-term use of a conjugated estrogen, 0.625 mg PO, micronized estradiol, 1 mg, for the first 25 days of each month, a 4-cm estrogen patch, or estrogen-containing vaginal creams alone or in combination may be indicated for menopausal symptoms such as vasomotor symptoms and vaginal dryness. Estrogen replacement therapy (ERT) for prophylaxis against coronary heart disease or osteoporosis is no longer recommended.

► Clinical Intervention

Alternative therapeutic regimens include use of soy products (phyto-estrogens), B complex vitamins; exercise; and cessation of cigarette smoking.

► Health Maintenance Issues

During the perimenopausal period, women should be reminded to use contraception as ovulation and subsequent pregnancy remain a possibility. Regular Pap smears; annual pelvic and breast exams; mammography; and endometrial biopsy in patients with abnormal vaginal bleeding are recommended. Estrogen therapy is contraindicated if there is: preexisting or current estrogen-dependent neoplasm (breast, ovary, uterus, cervix, vagina), history of thromboembolic disease, evidence of cholestatic hepatic dysfunction, or undiagnosed vaginal bleeding.

# VIII. BREAST

## A. Inflammatory Breast Disease

► Scientific Concepts

Inflammatory changes and infection (mastitis) in the breast are more common in lactating women. Breast abscess can be associated with lactation, duct occlusion, or fistulous tracts secondary to squamous epithelial neoplasia. *Staphylococcus aureus* from the infant's nose or throat, abrasion of the nipple, and prolonged engorgement are common causes of breast infection or inflammation. Without treatment, mastitis may lead to breast abscess.

► History & Physical

Unilateral, focal, tender breast mass, and/or generalized breast tenderness, swelling, erythema, localized increased temperature, nipple drainage, and generalized malaise are common. An abscess is accompanied by fever and exquisite point tenderness in the breast.

► Diagnostic Studies

Diagnosed by history and physical. CBC, erythrocyte sedimentation rate (ESR), and, if drainage, culture with sensitivity of drainage to identify pathogen.

► Diagnosis

History most significant in making diagnosis. Rule out inflammatory carcinoma.

► Clinical Therapeutics

NSAIDs for inflammation and pain. If puerperal infection is present, cover for gram-positive organisms (e.g., dicloxacillin or cephalexin [Keflex]). Nonpuerperal mastitis require coverage for both gram-positive and anaerobic bacteria, such as amoxicillin and clavulanic acid potassium (Augmentin).

► Clinical Intervention

Warm soaks and emptying of the affected breast (breastfeeding or pumping) and careful nipple hygiene with hexachlorophene (pHisoHex) or providone-iodine (Betadine) provide symptomatic relief. Aspiration under ultrasound or incision and drainage may be indicated if abscess or duct ectasia.

► Health Maintenance Issues

Routine health measures include reassurance, especially to exclude carcinoma; regular expression of milk; and early treatment of inflammation or infections.

## B. Fibrocystic Breast Disease

▶ Scientific Concepts

A benign fibrocystic change of the breast involving a spectrum of clinical and physical findings. Clinical findings: breast swelling, pain, and tenderness; symptoms may vary with menstrual cycle. Physical findings: cystic change, nodularity, stromal proliferation, and epithelial hyperplasia. Usually varies with menstrual cycle as an exaggerated stromal response to hormonal factors. Not associated with increased cancer risk if no atypical hyperplasia. More common in women 30–40 years of age, but can persist lifelong. Etiology unknown.

▶ History & Physical

Family history of cystic breast is common. Cyclic, bilateral or unilateral tenderness, engorgement, fluctuant masses, breast thickening, which improve following menses, are common.

▶ Diagnostic Studies

Patient history is most helpful. Ultrasound and mammography may be first diagnostic interventions. Serum prolactin and TSH as well as fine-needle aspiration and biopsy or excisional biopsy may be indicated (rare).

▶ Diagnosis

Rule out breast cancer, inflammation of the chest wall.

▶ Clinical Therapeutics

Treatment is related to severity of symptoms. Vitamin E, 600 IU qd for 8 wks, progestins (e.g., norethynordrel and norethindrone acetate), and NSAIDs alone or in combination provide relief.

▶ Clinical Intervention

In severe cases, danazol, 200–400 mg qd × 4 to 6 months, may be indicated. Bromocriptine and tamoxifen are other possible choices for recalcitrant cases. Dietary restriction of caffeine, primrose oil, cessation of cigarette smoking (nicotine), and well-fitting supportive brassiere are recommended.

▶ Health Maintenance Issues

Reassurance and regular breast exams are encouraged.

## C. Fibroadenoma

▶ Scientific Concepts

The second most common form of benign breast disease. This solid, benign neoplasm is more common in young women but may occur at any age after menarche.

▶ History & Physical

Well-circumscribed, round, firm, mobile, nontender, rubbery nodule, average 2–3 cm in diameter. Usually solitary but can be multiple (in 15–20% of patients); occur bilaterally 25% of the time. They typically do not change during the menstrual cycle.

▶ Diagnostic Studies

Ultrasound, mammography, and aspiration cytology (fine-needle biopsy) are most useful in making diagnosis.

▶ **Diagnosis**
Rule out breast cancer.

▶ **Clinical Therapeutics**
Clinical examination, fine-needle biopsy to make diagnosis, radiologic studies, and observation or excision.

▶ **Clinical Intervention**
As above.

▶ **Health Maintenance Issues**
This condition is generally benign. Reassurance and routine, age-appropriate mammography.

## D. Nipple Discharge

▶ **Scientific Concepts**
Although considered one of the warning signs of breast cancer, 90% of women with nipple discharge have benign disease or no pathology. Nipple discharge with nipple discomfort, burning, or itching is suggestive of duct ectasia. Bloody discharge is suggestive of intraductal papilloma, but can also be found with duct ectasia and pregnancy.

▶ **History & Physical**
Unilateral, spontaneous nipple discharge of clear to milky fluid or sticky yellow-green, multicolored, or blood-tinged fluid requires further evaluation for endocrine or other pathology. The chance of a nipple discharge being associated with cancer increases with age.

▶ **Diagnostic Studies**
Milky discharge: rule out mechanical stimulation, medication; check prolactin. Opalescent discharge (single duct): hematest. Bloody or serous discharge: mammogram first, then may require galactogram. Yellow-green discharge: cytology and/or culture and sensitivity.

▶ **Diagnosis**
Rule out breast cancer, prolactinoma.

▶ **Clinical Therapeutics**
Clinical examination, radiologic studies, and/or fine-needle biopsy to make diagnosis. Observation or excision based on findings.

▶ **Clinical Intervention**
As above.

▶ **Health Maintenance Issues**
This condition is generally benign. Reassurance and routine, age-appropriate mammography.

## E. Breast Cancer

▶ **Scientific Concepts**
Malignant neoplasm in the breast. Most common nonskin malignancy in women in the United States, with one in nine women developing breast cancer in their lifetime. Classified as noninvasive (in situ) and invasive (infiltrating). Family history is the most important epidemiologic factor.

► **History & Physical**

After family history, a long history of unopposed estrogen, nulliparity, early menarche, and late menopause are considered risk factors for breast cancer. Inconclusive risks include high dietary fat and obesity. Signs include discrete breast mass, puckering of breast skin, dimpling, nipple retraction, discharge, lymphedema, and lymphadenopathy.

► **Diagnostic Studies**

Physical examination, mammography, fine-needle aspiration, ultrasound, and biopsy with cytologic confirmation are recommended.

► **Diagnosis**

Extensive, includes benign disorders such as abscesses, hematomas, or fibroadenomas; fibrocystic changes; hyperplasia; sarcomas and lymphomas.

► **Clinical Therapeutics**

Treatment range includes lumpectomy, surgical excision to mastectomy; hormonal therapy (most commonly tamoxifen); chemotherapy (cyclophosphamide, methotrexate, or fluorouracil); radiotherapy and/or chemotherapy are employed depending on staging and patient preference.

► **Clinical Intervention**

Surveillance for recurrent disease is critical. Staging is based on tumor size, palpable nodes, and metastasis (TMN classification) and are signified stages I to IV. The status of axillary lymph node involvement is an important indicator of disease prognosis and relapse.

► **Health Maintenance Issues**

Starting in puberty, all women are encouraged to perform monthly self breast exams (SBEs) to become familiar with normal tissue and to detect changes. In addition, women over 18 are advised to have yearly clinical breast exams. Screening mammography and clinical breast exams are controversial for women between age 40 and 50, with some recommending baseline mammograms and clinical breast exams for women over 50.

## IX. HEALTH MAINTENANCE

### A. Screening

► **Scientific Concepts**

The primary care provider has the opportunity to impact on women's health maintenance. An evaluation of reproductive health status should address general health status, with emphasis on health promotion and disease prevention, patient psychological and emotional health, as well as screening, early intervention, treatment, and management of the conditions common to the gynecological patient.

► **History & Physical**

Menstrual history, sexual history, obstetric history, fertility, contraception, and history of STDs should be considered. All women aged 14 years and older should be routinely screened for domestic violence. Routine physical examination includes a general screening physical exam with special focus on the breasts, abdomen, pelvic, rectal, rectovaginal, and bimanual exams.

▶ Diagnostic Studies

Age specific, including Pap smear, cultures, breast exam, and instructions on SBE, lipid profile, rubella status, and STD screening tests.

▶ Diagnosis

Not applicable.

▶ Clinical Therapeutics

The general gynecologic exam should be done annually along with counseling regarding tobacco, alcohol, caffeine, diet, exercise, adult immunizations, routine health screening, and safety.

▶ Clinical Intervention

Should be done as appropriate for the specific findings during the annual exam.

▶ Health Maintenance Issues

*Adolescent population (ages 13–18):* Health screening should include questions about potential violent behavior (suicide, homicide, domestic violence), high-risk sexual behavior, tobacco, alcohol, and drug use, family relations. Counseling should address healthy behaviors (exercise, diet, spiritual, social, and emotional health), prevention of unhealthy behaviors or their consequences (i.e., STD and pregnancy prevention, seat belt and helmet use).

*Adult population (ages 19–39):* In addition to the issues of the adolescent population, adult women should also be screened for risks of cardiovascular disease, cerebral vascular accidents, accidents, breast cancer, osteoporosis prevention (exercise, calcium, and vitamin D intake), and cervical cancer. This group must also be screened for pregnancy preparation (e.g., folate supplementation) and fertility issues.

*Middle-age population (ages 40–64):* In addition to the screening done for the two previous populations, this group must also be screened for menopausal changes, the development of osteoporosis, cardiovascular disease, specific cancers (breast, colon, uterine).

*Elderly population (ages 65 and over):* History and screening as above plus questions to address medication use, lifestyle, depression, hygiene, diet, and exercise.

*General preventive medicine lab studies:* Pap smears every 1–3 years, blood pressure check annually or more frequent if cardiovascular problem present, STD tests as indicated, lipid profile every 5 years or more frequent if indicated by history, baseline mammography at age 40 and annually after age 50, fecal occult blood, colonoscopy at age 50. Check for current recommendations at www.preventiveservices.ahrg.gov.

## B. Contraception

▶ Scientific Concepts

One of the most sensitive and intimate decisions made by an individual or by a couple is that of fertility control. This decision is affected by religious/philosophical convictions, patient age, long- and short-term goals of childbearing (now, later, never), patient's lifestyle and sexual patterns, patient's comfort level with her own body, cost, and existent medical conditions.

## Methods of Contraception

1. **Barrier methods**
   - **Latex condoms:** Cover penis during coitus and prevent deposition of semen in the vagina. *Advantages:* Highly effective when used properly and regularly, convenient, inexpensive, no prescription needed, provides major protection against STDs. *Disadvantages:* Both partners may experience some reduction of sensation; must be used properly; failure related to error in technique and/or timing of placement or removal. Cultural barriers to use of condoms and partner reluctance to use must be explored. Effectiveness is increased with concurrent use of spermicidal foam, jelly, or cream.
   - **Vaginal diaphragm/cervical cap:** Provides a mechanical barrier between vagina and cervical canal, to be used with spermicidal agent. *Advantages:* Use of device is limited to episodes of sexual activity. It is relatively inexpensive, concurrent use of spermicidal agent increases effectiveness, and offers limited protection against STDs. *Disadvantages:* Device must be "fit" by a health professional. Must be inserted properly, failure related to error in technique and/or timing of placement or removal. Patient must be able and willing to insert the device properly with every intercourse. Slight incidence of cervical dysplasia and toxic shock syndrome. Device must be kept in place at least 6 hours post coitus (24–48 hours for cervical cap). Slight incidence of reaction to spermicidal agent.
   - **Spermicidal preparations (contraceptive sponge, foams, jellies, and creams used alone):** Function to kill sperm cells and act as a mechanical barrier to entry of sperm into cervical canal. *Advantages:* Convenient, inexpensive, no prescription needed. *Disadvantages:* Unreliable due to displacement and incomplete coverage of cervical os. Slight incidence of reaction to spermicidal agent.

2. **Intrauterine device (IUD):** Plastic or metal device introduced into the endometrial cavity through the cervical canal. Mode of action unknown; theory suggests that the placement of a foreign body creates a hostile environment to the ovum and prevents implantation. *Advantages:* Long-term protection, requires a single decision, is reversible. *Disadvantages:* Requires insertion by a trained health professional. *Side effects and complications:* Pain or discomfort during insertion, uterine perforation (rare), uterine cramping reaction to material used and size of device; pregnancy (rate is ~0.4–2.8/100 women in 12 months of use); spontaneous expulsion (rate varies with size, shape, and stiffness of device); increased menstrual flow and dysmenorrhea; increased incidence of extrauterine pregnancy; increased incidence of pelvic infections/PID and related sequelae. Currently, the Copper T Cu 380 can be retained for up to 8 years; Progestasert must be replaced annually. The IUD is not recommended for women who have had multiple sexual partners, who have STDs, or who have not been pregnant.

3. **Hormonal contraceptives:** Synthetic steroids similar to natural female hormones (estrogens and progestins) that, when used in combination, inhibit ovulation. Combined pills (estrogen and progestin) are started on the 5th day of the cycle, continued 20–21 days; withdrawal

bleeding generally occurs 3–5 days after completion of cycle (menses like blood flow, slight shedding); cycle is then repeated. During a typical cycle, under combined oral contraceptive regimen, there is no rise in FSH and LH during the first half of the cycle; thus, follicular growth is not initiated, ovulation does not occur. New methods of delivering combined estrogen and progestin include the contraceptive patch and the vaginal ring. The patch is applied to one of four locations on the woman's body weekly for 3 weeks. Each patch is left in place for 7 days and then discarded; during the fourth week no patch is applied and the women has a withdrawal bleed (menses).

The contraceptive vaginal ring is inserted into the vagina by the patient and left in place for 3 weeks. At the end of the third week it is removed, discarded, and the women has a withdrawal bleed during the fourth week.

Hormonal implants consist of progestin capsules placed under the skin, slowly releasing hormones that block ovulation. Hormonal implants are effective for up to 5 years. Hormonal injections, most commonly medroxyprogesterone (Depo-Provera), also function to suppress ovulation but will function to alter the cervical mucus and inhibit implantation.

*Advantages:* Highly effective; regular and less painful menses; possible decrease in the incidence of ectopic pregnancy, ovarian cancer, endometrial cancer, and benign breast disease; decreased menstrual fluid loss; decreased incidence of dysmenorrhea; increased protection against osteoporosis.

*Disadvantages and side effects:* Increased incidence of thromboembolic disease, including pulmonary embolism, cerebral thrombosis, deep vein thrombosis, and coronary thrombosis; risk increases with age and with concurrent cigarette smoking; risk of endometrial and cervical cancers have been reduced with the introduction of triphasic oral contraceptives, which contain a lower dose of progestin and estrogen. None of the hormonal therapies offer protection against STDs, and all require administration or prescription from a health care provider. With Depo-Provera, some women may experience a significant delay to regular ovulation. Emergency contraception is also available for pregnancy prevention when unprotected sex occurs during midcycle. A combination of high-dose contraceptive pills is prescribed and taken within 72 hours of the unprotected intercourse. The mechanism of action is poorly understood, but it is theorized that the high dose of oral contraceptives may prevent ovulation, change the consistency of the cervical mucus making it less hospitable for the sperm, or prevent implantation of a fertilized egg. Emergency contraception does not cause the abortion of an established pregnancy.

4. **Rhythm or ovulation method:** Requires that coitus be avoided during the time of the cycle when a fertilized ovum and sperm could meet in the oviduct. Accurate prediction or indication of ovulation is essential to the success of the rhythm method. Means of predicting ovulation:
   - **Calendar method:** Based on a formula of menstrual pattern recorded over several months, coitus should be avoided on day 14 ± 3 days.
   - **Basal body temperature (BBT) method:** Temperature taken rectally or orally in morning before any physical activity is undertaken; slight drop in temperature 24–36 hours after ovulation, then rises

abruptly 0.3°–0.4°C or 0.5°–0.7°F. The third day after rise in temperature is considered to be the end of the fertility period.

- **Luteinizing hormone peak:** Most accurate method of determining ovulation time. Test is performed on serum and is costly and time consuming but is very useful in the treatment of infertility when the timing of coitus or artificial insemination is of great importance. *Advantages:* Considered natural method of contraception. *Disadvantages:* Unreliable, increased margin of error, and variability of menstrual cycle.

5. **Induced abortion:** Deliberate termination of pregnancy in a manner that ensures that the embryo or fetus will not survive. Very controversial; subject to social, legal, and religious pressures. Indication for induced abortion may be categorized as maternal, paternal, fetal, social, etc. Some of the more common indications include obstetric (prior major uterine injury or damage, increased maternal age, multiparity, recurrent preeclampsia, eclampsia, etc.) and medical complications (surgical, orthopedic, hematologic, cardiovascular pulmonary, urologic, immunologic, endocrine neurologic, oncologic, infectious, psychiatric disorders, maternal inability to care for child, etc.).

    Method of induced abortion is determined primarily by the duration of pregnancy, patient's health, and physical facilities. *Suction curettage* is the most efficient, rapid method; used to terminate pregnancies less than 12 weeks, can be performed on an outpatient basis, with local or light anesthesia, limited blood loss, and least likelihood of uterine perforation. Complications, although rare include infection, excessive bleeding (~2%), uterine perforation (under 1%). *Sharp curettage* must be performed during the first trimester and is performed as a standard D&C such as for the diagnosis and treatment of abnormal uterine bleeding. Blood loss, duration of surgery, and likelihood of damage to the cervix or uterus are greatly increased when surgical curettage is used. At least 5% of abortions in the United States are still performed by sharp curettage. *Induction of labor by intra-amniotic instillation of an oxytocic agent (saline abortion)* involves the aspiration of amniotic fluid and replacement with saline, urea, or, most commonly, one of the prostaglandins, generally during the second trimester. The patient must be monitored until the fetus and placenta are delivered. Complication rate can be high (up to 20%) and can include disseminated intravascular clotting, sepsis, retained placenta, hemorrhage due to uterine inertia, hypernatremia, cervical laceration resulting from tumultuous labor in an "unripe" cervix, and delivery of a live fetus. *Abortifacients* such as mifepristone (RU 486) in combination with a prostaglandin taken orally can be used up to 9 weeks gestation to induce abortion. Other abortifacients can be used parenterally, by intra-amniotic injection, or vaginally in the form of suppositories alone or in combination with a *Laminaria* tent to evoke labor (*Laminaria* tent placed in the cervix for a few hours to soften the "unripe" cervix). Side effects include severe nausea, vomiting, diarrhea, tachycardia, substernal pressure, and paralytic ileus.

6. **Sterilization:** A permanent method of contraception chosen increasingly by men and women. Sterilization is the most frequent reason for laparoscopy in the United States. Clear, comprehensive counseling is essential for women and men considering sterilization. Patients must

be informed of the risks, effectiveness, and chances of reversibility with this procedure. There are several procedures that may be performed and vary according to the portion of oviduct in women and vas deferens in men that are sutured or cut and the method employed. Complications are uncommon in men and women. Women may experience pain, menstrual disturbances, and psychological problems. Complications in men usually involve slight bleeding, skin infections, reactions to sutures or local anesthetics. Sterilization in men and women should be considered permanent.

▶ History & Physical

Complete history and physical examination are recommended prior to use of the vaginal diaphragm; cervical cap; hormonal contraceptives taken orally, vaginally, or transdermally, implanted, or injected; IUDs; surgical sterilization. Condoms, sponges, and spermicide do not require complete history and physical prior to use.

▶ Diagnostic Studies

Pap smear, cultures recommended prior to use.

▶ Diagnosis

Rule out pregnancy prior to use of any contraceptive.

▶ Clinical Therapeutics

Patient education and counseling are integral to effective use of any contraceptive. Risk factors, convenience, instruction on proper use, and protection from STDs and HIV should be discussed with patient prior to use.

▶ Clinical Intervention

As above.

▶ Health Maintenance Issues

Monitoring as appropriate for each method.

## X. OTHER DISEASES AND DISORDERS

### A. Infertility

▶ Scientific Concepts

Fertility is considered to be compromised if a couple fails to conceive after 1 year of unprotected intercourse. Sterility refers to an intrinsic inability to conceive. *Primary infertility:* never having conceived. *Secondary infertility* refers to previous history of conception but current inability to conceive after 1 year. Fertility challenges plague 10 to 15% of all couples. The incidence increases with age. Several factors contribute to infertility, including genital or pelvic factors (endometriosis, tubal occlusion, or cervical anomalies), endocrine dysfunction (hypothyroidism or hypogonadism), or ovulatory dysfunction. Male and female factors are equally contributory to incidence of infertility, with etiology unknown in ~10% of cases.

▶ History & Physical

Evaluation includes menstrual, sexual, and obstetric history; history of pelvic surgery, exposure; medication; drug use; and history of pelvic infections. Endometriosis is often associated with cyclic premenstrual pain and dysmenorrhea.

### ▶ Diagnostic Studies

Evaluation should follow in a logical, stepwise fashion, including complete history and physical on both partners, semen analysis, post-coital test, cervical mucus assessment, basal body temperature (BBT), serum progesterone, hysterosalpingogram, and endometrial sampling.

### ▶ Diagnosis

Identify underlying disorder, condition, or factor.

### ▶ Clinical Therapeutics

Therapeutics are targeted to the cause of infertility. Clomiphene citrate, 50 mg PO for 5 days to induce ovulation; surgery (in vitro fertilization or intrauterine insemination for tubal or cervical factor).

### ▶ Clinical Intervention

Treatment may be prolonged. Patient education, exploration of options, and limits of intervention should be discussed.

### ▶ Health Maintenance Issues

Prevention of STDs and subsequent pelvic infection. The emotional support of the patient and partner should be considered carefully. Infertility can cause great distress and stress for the patient and in the relationship between the patient and her partner.

## B. Endometriosis

### ▶ Scientific Concepts

Endometriosis typically occurs between the ages of 25 and 40 but may also affect those as young as 18. Over 2 million women in the United States are affected and incidence transcends all races. Endometrial tissue, normally found in the uterine epithelial lining, escapes the uterine cavity and grows outside the uterus. Exact etiology is unknown, yet theory suggests that retrograde menstruation flows through the fallopian tubes and outside into the pelvic cavity and wayward endometrial cells implant on the ovaries, fallopian tubes, cul-de-sac, uterosacral ligament, bladder, and intestines. The presence of extrapelvic sites suggests lymphatic or vascular metastases. Risk factors include short menstrual cycles (< 27 days), menstrual flow duration of 8 days or more, women with uninterrupted menstruation for more than 15–20 years, nulliparity (by choice or otherwise), and positive family history.

### ▶ History & Physical

Dysmenorrhea, menorrhagia, dyspareunia, infertility, abnormal bleeding, and cyclic pelvic pain are more typical symptoms. Also may have low back pain and/or rectal pain that increases 1 to 2 days before menses begins and persists throughout flow; premenstrual spotting; midcycle bleeding; irregular bleeding; menorrhagia, dyspareunia, and dysmenorrhea; urinary and bowel dysfunction and pain. Physical examination should be done at midcycle and again before or during menses (if endometrial nodules or implants are present, they should be larger during perimenstrual exam); retrovaginal palpation is best means to examine (common site for implants) and may demonstrate a thickened rectovaginal septum and an indurated cul-de-sac. Pelvic fullness and tenderness may be noted on pelvic exam. Fixed adnexal masses may be noted, or a laterally displaced cervix. Colored lesions may be present on umbilicus, vulva, vagina, or cervix.

▶ Diagnostic Studies

Direct visualization with laparoscopy or laparotomy is required for definitive diagnosis. Laparoscopy may be diagnostic and therapeutic, with laser vaporization of implants, drainage and lysis of pelvic lesions. Imaging tests and serum immunoassay markers are noninvasive methods but have limited sensitivity. Serum immunoassay CA-125 increases in ovarian cancer as well as endometriosis but may be useful if monitoring response to treatment.

▶ Diagnosis

Differential includes all causes of acute abdomen, intra- and extra-uterine pregnancy, ruptured ovarian cysts, as well as urinary and GI disorders.

▶ Clinical Therapeutics

Treatment must be individualized and guided by the age of the patient, future childbearing plans, and severity of symptoms. Medical options are temporizing and include: continuous oral contraceptives or medroxyprogesterone (30–50 mg daily) to suppress ovulation. GnRH agonists such as leuprolide acetate, androgen-derivative, danazol (400 to 800 mg/d IM × 9 months), or nafarelin 0.4–0.8 mg intranasally daily induce a reversible "pseudomenopause" and also treat pain in severe cases more effectively than oral contraceptives. Conservative therapy typically involves ablation and excision of visible endometriosis during laparoscopy preserving the reproductive organs to allow for future fertility. Definitive therapy includes total abdominal hysterectomy with bilateral salpingo-oophorectomy, lysis of adhesions, and removal of endometriosis lesions.

▶ Clinical Intervention

Close patient monitoring and additional diagnostic interventions may be indicated.

▶ Health Maintenance Issues

Endometriosis cannot be prevented or cured, but signs and symptoms generally regress with menopause.

## XI. COMPLICATED PREGNANCY

### A. Early Pregnancy Complications

#### 1. Extrauterine Pregnancy

▶ Scientific Concepts

Ectopic pregnancy causes 15% of all maternal deaths and risk for recurrence is 7- to 13-fold. Extrauterine pregnancy occurs most commonly in the ampulla or other portion of the fallopian tube, less often in the pelvis, ovary, or abdomen. Risk is increased with IUD for contraception, history of pelvic infection, adhesions, previous tubal pregnancy or surgery, history of endometriosis or endometritis.

### ▶ History & Physical

Early pregnancy symptoms, amenorrhea followed by irregular bleeding or spotting, pelvic pain, colicky abdominal pain and cramping. Shoulder pain, syncope, and peritoneal signs are associated with intraperitoneal bleeding. The uterus is softened, normal size or slightly enlarged, but smaller than expected for gestational dates.

### ▶ Diagnostic Studies

Urine pregnancy test, beta-hCG (quantitative and qualitative) to determine pregnancy; transvaginal ultrasound is the single most valuable modality in the workup; transabdominal ultrasound, culdocentesis, laparoscopy or laparotomy (especially with peritoneal findings), Rh status for Rh-negative mothers are all useful. Uterine curettage is performed only for nonviable pregnancies.

### ▶ Diagnosis

Rule out spontaneous abortion, acute abdomen, appendicitis, salpingitis, ruptured ovarian cyst.

### ▶ Clinical Therapeutics

Nonsurgical management for small, unruptured ectopic pregnancy may include methotrexate (50 mg/m$^2$). Laparoscopic surgery and segmental resection of the tube are indicated. Salpingectomy may be indicated in the treatment of a large ruptured ectopic pregnancy.

### ▶ Clinical Intervention

Early treatment (prior to rupture) is the goal. Complications include hemorrhage, hypovolemic shock, infection, infertility, and loss of reproductive organs.

### ▶ Health Maintenance Issues

Reliable contraception and reduction of risk factors recommended.

## 2. Spontaneous Abortion

### ▶ Scientific Concepts

A spontaneous abortion (SAB) refers to a pregnancy that ends naturally before 20 weeks gestation. SABs occur in approximately 15–25% of all pregnancies. It is estimated that 60–80% of all SABs during the first trimester are < 12 weeks and associated with chromosome abnormalities; infections, maternal anatomic defects, immune and endocrine factors are other associated factors. Second trimester SABs have various etiologies including: maternal infection, maternal anatomic defects, fetotoxic exposure, and trauma, but not usually chromosomal abnormalities. There are different classifications of SABs, depending on whether the products of conception (POC) have passed and depending on whether the cervix has dilated. *Complete abortion* is the complete expulsion of all POC before 20 weeks gestation; *incomplete abortion* is partial expulsion of some but not all POC; *inevitable abortion* means no POC expulsed, but bleeding and dilation of the cervix is such that a viable fetus is unlikely; *threatened abortion* refers to any extrauterine bleeding before 20 weeks without dilation of the cervix or POC expulsion; *missed abortion* is the death of an embryo or fetus before 20 weeks with complete retention of POC (these often proceed to complete abortions in 2–4 weeks).

▶ History & Physical

Vaginal bleeding or spotting with a pink, brownish discharge is common. Uterine cramping, pelvic pain, cervical dilatation, rupture of membranes, possible passage of clotted or other nonviable products, and decreased symptoms of pregnancy. Uterine enlargement, softening of the cervix, and adnexal tenderness may be noted on bimanual exam.

▶ Diagnostic Studies

Sterile speculum exam to determine bleeding source, cultures, beta-hCG (quantitative), CBC, blood type, antibody screen. Ultrasound examination for identification of gestational sac and to access fetal viability is most useful.

▶ Diagnosis

Rule out ectopic pregnancy, cervical polyp, molar pregnancy (hydatidiform mole), and membranous dysmenorrhea. In second trimester, preterm labor and incompetent cervix need to be ruled out.

▶ Clinical Therapeutics

Stabilization if bleeding and hypotensive. Observation, beta-agonists (isozuprine), bedrest, and nothing per vagina may effectively manage threatened abortion, but patients are at increased risk for preterm labor and preterm rupture of membranes. D&E (dilation and evacuation) is generally indicated for incomplete and inevitable abortions, with tissue sent to pathology; IV or PO antibiotic therapy for infected and septic abortions and analgesia as needed.

▶ Clinical Intervention

Bleeding following D&E may be effectively treated with oxytocin, 3–10 units IM, or methylergonovine, 0.2 mg IM. Karyotyping of products of conception, genetic screening, and special care for subsequent pregnancies including surgical reinforcement of the cervix (cerclage stitch) may be warranted for habitual abortion.

▶ Health Maintenance Issues

Prognosis for future pregnancies after threatened abortion and D&C for incomplete or inevitable abortion is good. Guilt and sadness are common; counseling and support recommended.

## B. Hisk-Risk Pregnancies

### 1. Adolescent Pregnancy

▶ Scientific Concepts

Pregnancy before the age of 19 poses added risk for mother and child. Incidence of ectopic pregnancy, spontaneous abortion, prematurity, intrauterine growth retardation, and newborns with low birth weight is greater in teen pregnancy. Risk also increased for fetal and neonatal deaths.

▶ History & Physical

Concurrent STDs; malnutrition; sexual, alcohol, and substance abuse; and late prenatal care complicate teen pregnancies.

► **Diagnostic Studies**

Complete history and physical examination, including Pap smear and cultures, beta-hCG, screening for STDs as per routine.

► **Diagnosis**

Early diagnosis of pregnancy and prompt initiation of prenatal care are recommended. Patients age 16 and younger have an increased risk of preeclampsia or eclampsia.

► **Clinical Therapeutics**

Prenatal vitamins that include iron and folate.

► **Clinical Intervention**

Routine prenatal care, screening, support services, and referral for interventions appropriate to pregnant teens.

► **Health Maintenance Issues**

Patient education and support as needed.

## 2. Other High-Risk Pregnancy

► **Scientific Concepts**

High-risk pregnancy is broadly defined as one in which the mother or fetus/newborn is or will be at risk for morbidity or mortality before or after birth. Maternal nutrition and exposures, prenatal care, preexisting medical conditions, genetic abnormalities, or obstetric disorders may impose higher risks for mother and fetus.

► **History & Physical**

Initial screening should include maternal age (higher risk with adolescent and advanced maternal age), obstetric history (history of habitual abortion, previous stillbirth, neonatal death, premature or small- or large-for-gestational-age infant, grand multiparity, previous Rh isoimmunization, previous preeclampsia or eclampsia, previous or known genetic anomaly), history of reproductive disorders, medical complications of pregnancy, or history of exposure to teratogens. Complete physical examination, including Pap smear and pelvic exam with special attention to thyroid, breast, heart, lungs, abdomen, and vasculature.

► **Diagnostic Studies**

Diagnostic studies specific to condition. Beta-hCG (qualitative and quantitative), serum alpha-fetoprotein, ABO and Rh, sickle cell prep, and pelvic sonogram as per routine. Amniocentesis may be indicated.

► **Diagnosis**

Identify underlying condition or risk.

► **Clinical Therapeutics**

Specific to condition.

► **Clinical Intervention**

As above.

► **Health Maintenance Issues**

Reassurance, close monitoring, patient education and counseling depending on diagnosis.

# C. Premature Rupture of Membranes/Prematurity

▶ **Scientific Concepts**

Premature labor is defined as uterine contractions and cervical changes before the 37th week of gestation. Premature labor may or may not progress to mature rupture of membranes. Prematurity is a common sequela of premature rupture of membranes (PROM). Risk factors for preterm labor and PROM include incompetent cervix, uterine surgery, uterine anomalies, multiple gestation, intrauterine and urinary tract infections, abnormal placental placement, dehydration, stress, and cigarette smoking. Dangerous fetal complications of PROM at any gestational age are prolapse of the umbilical cord and fetal bradycardia caused by cord compression.

▶ **History & Physical**

PROM most commonly presents as a gush of fluid from the vagina followed by persistent, uncontrolled leakage, though some patients report only intermittent leakage or perineal wetness. Premature labor signs may be subtle, including increased uterine activity, contractions, intestinal cramping, vaginal discharge or bleeding, and pressure or pain in the pelvis, back, or thighs. Digital examination of the cervix in women with possible preterm labor or preterm PROM should be avoided until the diagnosis of ruptured membranes has been excluded.

▶ **Diagnostic Studies**

Sterile speculum exam, fern test (assessment of pooled fluid, air dried on a slide, noting arborization, fern pattern), nitrazine test (positive test is 90–98% accurate for the presence of amniotic fluid), L/S ratio (assessment of fetal maturity), ultrasound, and, in some cases, amniocentesis. Cervical secretions should also be sent for culture and sensitivity. An ultrasound evaluation for amniotic fluid volume should be performed in women with preterm PROM to determine fetal presentation, fetal weight, and gestational age.

▶ **Diagnosis**

Monitor patient, rule out rupture of membranes.

▶ **Clinical Therapeutics**

Depending on severity. If no rupture of the membranes: monitoring, hydration, bedrest, tocolytics (terbutaline, 0.25 mg subcutaneously × 6 doses), and outpatient use of beta-sympathomimetics (ritodrine) may be employed. Other clinical therapeutics include magnesium sulfate, indomethacin, or calcium channel blockers. The goal is to sustain pregnancy to as close to 35 weeks as possible. If PROM, maternal and fetal indications for immediate delivery should be ruled out before considering other management options. The principal maternal indication for delivery is chorioamnionitis. If a firm diagnosis of chorioamnionitis can be made (maternal fever >101°F, uterine tenderness, and leukocytosis > 20,000), delivery should be undertaken promptly regardless of the gestational age. In the absence of indications for immediate delivery, gestational age should be carefully assessed to estimate the relative risks for the fetus of delivery versus expectant management. Clinical surveillance of expectantly managed patients with preterm PROM includes frequent examinations for maternal heart rate, contractions, uterine tenderness, fever greater than or equal to 38°C, and nonstress testing, looking for variable decelerations, tachycardia, and absent movement.

▶ Clinical Intervention

With no evidence of fetal distress or infection, and fetal pulmonary maturity cannot be confirmed, there are three management options: (1) expectant management, where patient is hospitalized for intensive surveillance for signs of fetal compromise or infection, at which time labor is allowed or induced if necessary (associated with a low cesarean rate, but requires at least daily fetal assessment and is not always accurate); (2) immediate delivery for pregnancies ≥ 32 weeks or estimated fetal weight ≥ 1,500–1,800 g (avoids need for ongoing surveillance, but high rate of cesarean delivery for failed induction, also commits to delivery pregnancies that might continue to allow fetal development and reduced neonatal morbidity); or (3) attempt to delay delivery in order to influence the relative risks of prematurity and infection (e.g., use of antibiotics to reduce morbidity and prolong pregnancy, corticosteroids for reducing fetal morbidity/mortality with PROM before 32 weeks). Management is individualized according to status of membranes (intact vs. ruptured) and gestational age. Risk to fetus is greatest in pregnancy < 24–26 weeks' gestation.

▶ Health Maintenance Issues

Identification of etiology is most important in minimizing recurrence. Patient and family support recommended.

## D. Antepartum Hemorrhage

### 1. Abruptio Placenta

▶ Scientific Concepts

Defined as premature separation of the placenta prior to delivery, may be graded as follows:

*Grade 1:* Slight vaginal bleeding and some uterine irritability are usually present. Maternal blood pressure is unaffected, and the maternal fibrinogen level is normal. The fetal heart rate pattern is normal.

*Grade 2:* External uterine bleeding is mild to moderate. The uterus is irritable, and tetanic or very frequent contractions may be present. Maternal blood pressure is maintained, but the pulse rate may be elevated and postural blood volume deficits may be present. The fibrinogen level may be decreased. The fetal heart rate often shows signs of fetal compromise.

*Grade 3:* Bleeding is moderate to severe but may be concealed. The uterus is tetanic and painful. Maternal hypotension is frequently present and fetal death has occurred. Fibrinogen levels are often reduced to less than 150 mg/dL; other coagulation abnormalities (thrombocytopenia, factor depletion) are present.

The etiology of placental abruption is unknown, but maternal hypertension (>140/90 mm Hg) seems to be the most consistently identified factor predisposing to placental abruption. Blunt external maternal trauma (e.g., secondary to motor vehicle accident or battering) is an increasingly important cause of placental abruption. Other risk factors include: multiple gestation, uterine decompression, acquired or inherited thrombophilias (e.g., factor V Leiden mutation), and previous history of abruption. Some studies have implicated advanced parity or age, maternal smoking, poor nutrition, cocaine use, and chorioamnionitis as additional risks.

► History & Physical

Acute-onset vaginal bleeding in the second or third trimester, painful contractions, moderate to severe abdominal or back pain, uterine tenderness, hypertonia, and fetal distress. Blood loss may be concealed; clinical signs of shock may not correlate with degree of vaginal bleeding.

► Diagnostic Studies

Diagnosis is made on clinical suspicion. CBC, platelet count, PT/PTT, and fibrinogen levels useful in management. Ultrasound has become the standard of care and though not definitive, more than 50% of patients with confirmed placental abruption demonstrate evidence of hemorrhage. Ultrasound can identify locations and size of placental abruption and is also used to establish prognosis, as well as help with external fetal monitoring and assessment of fetal well-being.

► Diagnosis

Uterine rupture, placenta previa, or labor.

► Clinical Therapeutics

Severe abruptio is best managed with rapid delivery via cesarean section. In patients remote from term, with both mother and fetus clinically stable, tocolytic agents have been used; magnesium sulfate has less adverse cardiovascular side effects than β-sympathomimetics.

► Clinical Intervention

Management depends on grading, with maternal and fetal hemodynamic stabilization of prime importance. If hemodynamically stable, mild abruptio may be monitored, with bedrest until fetus is mature, and vaginal delivery. Placental abruption frequently stimulates the clotting cascade, resulting in disseminated intravascular coagulation (DIC); serial measurements of plasma fibrinogen provide valuable information regarding the coagulation status of the patient and will help estimate the volume of blood loss that has occurred.

► Health Maintenance Issues

Abruptio placenta is a medical emergency that requires prompt intervention, maternal stabilization, and assessment of the fetus.

## 2. Placenta Previa

► Scientific Concepts

Characterized by placental implantation in the lower uterine segment, either partially covering the cervical os (partial previa and marginal previa), totally covering the cervical os (total previa), or low-lying placenta where the placental edge is in the lower uterine segment but does not encroach on the internal cervical os. Placenta previa is related to poor uterine vascularization or large placental mass (multiple gestation or hydrops). Incidence increases with previous uterine surgery, leiomyoma, previous placenta previa, multiparity, and advancing maternal age. The common practice of second-trimester ultrasound for detection of fetal anomalies has led to most cases of placenta previa being detected antenatally prior to the onset of significant bleeding.

▶ History & Physical

Patients present with bright red, painless vaginal bleeding in the second or third trimester. Placenta previa should be suspected in all patients presenting with bleeding after 24 weeks' gestation. Previa may be identified on routine, early sonogram that requires later confirmation because most cases of placenta previa diagnosed in the second trimester will resolve.

▶ Diagnostic Studies

In patients diagnosed prior to 24 weeks' gestation, a repeat ultrasound between 24 and 28 weeks' gestation should be done to confirm resolution of the radiographic diagnosis of placenta previa. Transabdominal and transvaginal ultrasound are most useful in locating placenta and degree of previa. A digital vaginal examination to document cervical dilatation is absolutely contraindicated, making it difficult to make a firm diagnosis of preterm labor.

▶ Diagnosis

Rule out abruptio placenta, vas previa, and infection.

▶ Clinical Therapeutics

Management decisions depend on the gestational age, amount of bleeding, fetal condition, and presentation. At 37 weeks' gestation with evidence of uterine activity or with persistent bleeding, delivery is the treatment of choice. For 24–36 weeks' gestation, expectant management is the treatment of choice: maintenance of the fetus in a healthy intrauterine environment, and maintenance of the maternal condition (e.g., keeping hematocrit 30–35%). Half of all patients require early delivery because of failed expectant management due to excessive bleeding with or without uterine contractions. If preterm labor is present, tocolytics may be indicated, with magnesium sulfate being the agent of choice. Observation, education, bedrest, coital restriction, and serial sonograms for placenta position and fetal assessment may be indicated for mild previa. Digital vaginal and/or rectal examination must be avoided so as to avoid digital separation of placenta and uncontrollable hemorrhage. Vaginal delivery may be attempted after 36 weeks' gestation in patients with marginal previa after fetal maturity assessment. Hemodynamic stabilization and fetal assessment are primary. Prompt delivery via cesarean section may be indicated if uncorrectable fetal compromise is evident.

▶ Clinical Intervention

Third-trimester vaginal bleeding is a medical emergency that requires prompt evaluation and management.

▶ Health Maintenance Issues

Minimization of risk factors.

## 3. Unspecified Antepartum Hemorrhage

▶ Scientific Concepts

Obstetric hemorrhage is one of the three leading causes of maternal death and a major cause of perinatal morbidity and mortality. Extrusion of cervical mucus (bloody show) is the most common cause of bleeding late in pregnancy. Most blood loss from placental challenge is maternal, yet fetal loss is also possible. Nonobstetric causes of third-trimester antepartum hemorrhage include cervicitis, cervical erosion, polyps, vaginal laceration, and neoplasia. Obstetric causes include placenta abruptio, placenta previa, uterine rupture, and abnormal clotting mechanisms. Uterine rupture may occur in a previously scarred uterus (particularly after a classical [vertical] uterine incision) or may result from uterine manipulation (forceps, uterine curettage), trauma, or overaggressive use of IV oxytocin. Other risk factors are uterine anomalies, tumors, and placenta percreta (invasion of the placenta through the uterine wall).

▶ History & Physical

There are no reliable signs of impending uterine rupture. Symptoms of shock related to acute blood loss include pallor, syncope, thirst, dyspnea, restlessness, agitation, anxiety, and confusion. Symptoms can be nonspecific and include maternal hemodynamic instability, fetal bradycardia, vaginal bleeding, and loss of function of uterine pressure monitors. Consider rupture of the uterus with complaints of increased suprapubic pain and tenderness with labor, sudden cessation of uterine contractions, "tearing" sensation, vaginal bleeding, regression of presenting part, and disappearance of fetal heart tones. The abdomen may be firm, painful, or expanding. Palpation may evoke contraction. Fetal heart tone may be muffled, and fetal heart rate may be increased or decreased.

▶ Diagnostic Studies

Antepartum hemorrhage is a medical emergency that requires prompt evaluation and immediate life support intervention. If patient condition permits, ultrasound is useful in assessing placental position, presence of retroplacental clot, and fetal well-being.

▶ Diagnosis

Differential includes obstetric and nonobstetric causes of late-pregnancy vaginal bleeding. Uterine rupture may be diagnosed following delivery.

▶ Clinical Therapeutics

Evaluation of vaginal bleeding in late pregnancy should take place in setting equipped to manage maternal hemorrhage and a compromised neonate. Digital rectal and vaginal exams must not be performed until placenta previa has been ruled out. Acute management efforts include airway management, fluid replacement and expansion and use of vasoactive drugs if indicated. Laparotomy, cesarean section, or hysterectomy may be indicated.

▶ Clinical Intervention

As above.

▶ Health Maintenance Issues

The complications of ruptured uterus and antepartum hemorrhage include shock, postoperative infection, uterine damage, thrombophlebitis, amniotic fluid embolus, disseminated intravascular coagulation, renal failure, pituitary failure, and death.

## E. Hypertension in Pregnancy

▶ Scientific Concepts

Hypertensive disorders are the most common medical complications of pregnancy, with a reported incidence between 5 and 10%, and are a major cause of maternal and perinatal mortality and morbidity worldwide. Hypertension in pregnancy is characterized by an increase in systolic and/or diastolic blood pressure, > 140/90 mm Hg. Hypertension in pregnancy is more common in women with a prior history of hypertension, women over 30, obesity, multiparity, and those with diabetes or renal disease. The classic triad of preeclampsia has included hypertension, proteinuria, and edema. However, there is now universal agreement that edema should *not* be considered as part of the diagnosis of preeclampsia due to its common occurrence in pregnancy and the fact that one third of preeclamptic women do not exhibit it. At present, preeclampsia is primarily defined as gestational hypertension plus proteinuria. In mild preeclampsia, diastolic blood pressure remains below 110 mm Hg and the systolic blood pressure remains below 160 mm Hg. Eclampsia is preeclampsia with tonic–clonic seizures of no other etiology. Risk factors for preeclampsia include teenage pregnancy, advanced age pregnancy, multiple fetuses, African American, chronic hypertension, and positive family history in a first-degree relative. Poor perinatal outcome is usually seen in patients who have hypertension plus proteinuria, including the following: placental infarct or abruption, intrapartum fetal distress, uteroplacental insufficiency, prematurity issues (if early delivery necessary), and intrauterine growth retardation. About 10% patients with severe preeclampsia go on to develop the HELLP Syndrome in which the patient presents with *h*emolytic anemia, *e*levated *l*iver enzymes, and *l*ow *p*latelets. This disorder is characterized by rapid deterioration of liver function and thrombocytopenia, with poor maternal and fetal outcomes. Hypertension may be minimal in these patients.

### ▶ History & Physical

In addition to elevated blood pressure, patients with preeclampsia as well as those with hypertension in pregnancy may complain of mild headache, visual disturbance, hyperreflexia, apprehension, papilledema, altered consciousness, oliguria, pulmonary edema or cyanosis, and epigastric pain. Eclampsia is characterized by worsening of the above symptoms, muscle twitching, seizures, and coma.

### ▶ Diagnostic Studies

Blood pressure readings (greater than 140 systolic or 90 diastolic on two occasions at least 6 hours apart), physical examination to assess for nondependent edema (face and/or hands), and 24-hour urine for protein are the primary diagnostic studies. Creatinine clearance, aspartate transaminase, bilirubin, and lactic dehydrogenase may also be elevated. Diagnosis of the HELLP Syndrome is presence of schistocytes on peripheral blood smear, elevated total bilirubin, and elevated lactate dehydrogenase, liver enzymes, and low platelets.

### ▶ Diagnosis

Rule out chronic hypertension, pregnancy-induced or worsening hypertension, and underlying renal or renovascular disease.

### ▶ Clinical Therapeutics

Methyldopa and hydralazine are the safest and most effective antihypertensives for use during pregnancy. Beta blockers, angiotensin-converting enzyme (ACE) inhibitors, calcium channel blockers, and thiazide diuretics are contraindicated in pregnancy. Low doses of aspirin in patients with chronic hypertension may decrease the risk of preeclampsia. Magnesium sulfate, 4 g IV over 20–30 minutes and a maintenance dose of 1–2 g IV, is standard therapy for inpatient management of preeclampsia and seizure prophylaxis. In eclampsia, magnesium sulfate is initiated at the time of diagnosis and continued for 12–24 hours after delivery, requiring careful monitoring for toxicity.

▶ Clinical Intervention

The primary treatment of preeclampsia and eclampsia is delivery. Induction of labor is the treatment of choice for term pregnancies, unstable preterm pregnancies, or pregnancies where there is evidence of fetal lung maturity. Bedrest, increased water intake, and regular blood pressure monitoring in mild preeclampsia may facilitate delay of delivery to more viable fetal age. In general, antihypertensive therapy for mild preeclampsia is not indicated.

▶ Health Maintenance Issues

Lower blood pressure is of benefit to the mother; there is no direct fetal benefit to blood pressure reduction. Maternal morbidity and mortality due to hypertension in pregnancy are rare in the United States but can cause hemorrhage, stroke, seizures, pulmonary edema, and renal failure.

## F. Diabetes in Pregnancy

▶ Scientific Concepts

Risk factors for developing gestational diabetes include: maternal age >25, obesity, family history, previous macrosomic infant, and history of unexplained or recurrent abortions.

▶ History & Physical

Family and personal history of diabetes mellitus, as well as risk factors above. Persistent glycosuria.

▶ Diagnostic Studies

Between 24 and 28 weeks gestation screening, all pregnant women should be screened using the 1-hour glucola test; if one or more risk factors, screening should be done at first prenatal visit and each trimester. If blood sugar > 140 mg/dL, then a 3-hour glucose tolerance test (GTT) is necessary to confirm. If GTT is positive, the White classification system is used to determine the patient's type for prognostic monitoring. Once diagnosis is made, further evaluation of fetus by ultrasound (to establish age, congenital abnormalities), screening for neural tube defects (16–22 weeks), fetal echocardiography should be offered.

▶ Diagnosis

Early diagnosis of diabetes and prompt management of blood glucose are critical. Close monitoring of mother and fetus throughout pregnancy with appropriate education.

▶ Clinical Therapeutics

Lifestyle modification for type 2 diabetes. Insulin should be prescribed for type 1 and type 2 patients who do not respond to lifestyle modifications; the safety of currently available oral antidiabetic agents is not yet assured during early pregnancy.

► Clinical Intervention

Thorough patient education, tight control of glucose, American Diabetes Association diet, and exercise management. Insulin therapy based on failure of diet and exercise (for gestational diabetics) or as required, with blood glucose monitoring. Close surveillance of fetal well-being beginning 28–32 weeks, with kick counts, serial ultrasonography for growth or polyhydramnios, nonstress testing and biophysical profiles after 32 weeks. Inducement of labor between 38 and 40 weeks with mature fetal lungs and tight glycemic control during delivery.

► Health Maintenance Issues

With the onset or recognition of glucose intolerance during pregnancy, the mother has a 15–20% chance of developing diabetes mellitus within the first year. Fifty percent of gestational diabetics will have diabetes during subsequent pregnancies. Infants of gestational diabetes have increased risk of obesity and type 2 diabetes later in life.

## G. Infections During Pregnancy

### 1. Infection of the Genitourinary Tract

► Scientific Concepts

Pregnant women have a greater risk of developing UTIs. Genitourinary tract infections as well as asymptomatic bacteriuria in pregnancy are associated with low birth weight and preterm labor and are the most common cause of miscarriage during the second trimester of pregnancy. Screening for asymptomatic bacteriuria in the 16th week of gestation is routinely performed. Risk increases with history of recurrent UTI in nonpregnant state and diabetes mellitus. Approximately one third of all pregnant women with asymptomatic bacteriuria progress to develop pyelonephritis. *Escherichia coli* accounts for > 70% of all UTIs.

► History & Physical

Patients may be asymptomatic or complain of urgency, frequency, dysuria without vaginal discharge. Back pain, fever, vomiting, and costovertebral angle tenderness may suggest pyelonephritis.

► Diagnostic Studies

Urine dipstick may be positive for leukocyte esterase, nitrite, and protein. Full culture and sensitivity of the urine are indicated, especially in cases of suspected pyelonephritis, even though the results are not likely to change the management plan. Screening for bacteriuria early in pregnancy may be indicated. The most common pathogens in pyelonephritis are *E. coli, Klebsiella, Enterobacter,* or *Proteus.* Staph, strep group B, and *Enterococcus* are less common.

► Diagnosis

Rule out vulvovaginitis and intrauterine infection.

► Clinical Therapeutics

If colony count is > 100,000 colonies/mL of a single pathogen, a 3-day treatment of amoxicillin, ampicillin, or cephalexin, 250 to 500 mg PO q 6–8 h, with a repeat colony count 10 days later. Positive bacteria after 3-day course of therapy or recurrent infection later in the pregnancy is indication for suppressive prophylaxis with a once-daily dose of antibiotics. Symptomatic cystitis should be treated for 7–10 days because shorter courses are associated with high failure rates.

▶ **Clinical Intervention**

Asymptomatic bacteriuria, lower UTI, and, in some cases, mild pyelonephritis early in pregnancy may be effectively treated on an outpatient basis. Outpatient management requires that the patient be able to take medications orally. Hospitalization is indicated for patients with moderate to severe pyelonephritis or > 24 weeks' gestation.

▶ **Health Maintenance Issues**

Preventive measures include increased water intake, frequent voiding, and proper hygienic practices (wiping from front to back, empty bladder before and after intercourse).

## 2. Other Infections

▶ **Scientific Concepts**

Infectious agents are classified according to whether they cross the placenta or cause serious problems for the fetus and the newborn. The following infectious agents place the pregnant mother and fetus at higher risk for morbidity and mortality: rubella, cytomegalovirus (CMV), HSV, hepatitis B (HBV), toxoplasmosis, parvovirus, HIV, varicella zoster virus, group B streptococcus, and bacterial vaginosis (BV). See Table 9–2 for risks to fetus and neonate as well as diagnosis and treatment of these infections.

# H. Fetal Complications of Pregnancy

## 1. Disorders of Fetal Growth

▶ **Scientific Concepts**

Fetal weight can be estimated by using ultrasound. If a fetal estimated weight is less than the 10th percentile, the fetus is considered small for gestational age (SGA); those greater than 90th percentile are considered large for gestational age (LGA). Screening for disorders of fetal growth is done during routine prenatal care.

SGA infants are associated with higher rates of morbidity and mortality for their gestational age. Risk factors include: genetic/chromosomal abnormalities, intrauterine infections, fetotoxins or exposures, high-altitude pregnancy, and intrauterine growth restriction (IUGR) secondary to either maternal (e.g., chronic disease) or placental factors.

LGA is less important than the diagnosis of fetal macrosomia (usually a birth weight greater than 4,000 g). Risk factors for macrosomia: maternal diabetes, obesity, postterm pregnancy, previous LGA infant, parental size, advance maternal age. Neonatal risks accompanying macrosomia include: birth trauma injuries, low Apgar scores, hypoglycemia, polycythemia, hypocalcemia, and jaundice.

▶ **History & Physical**

History may reveal risk factors that are associated with common causes of decreased or increased growth potential. Fundal height measurements to determine need for further evaluation. Leopold's examination may reveal a large infant in the third trimester.

▶ table 9-2

## INFECTIOUS DISEASES COMPLICATING PREGNANCY

| Agent | Risks | Diagnosis | Treatment |
|---|---|---|---|
| CMV | Subclinical or mild illness in the mother; congenital anomalies esp. CNS; neonatal death | Rare diagnosis in mother unless hepatitis or mono-like syndrome | None—antivirals unsuccessful |
| HSV | Fetal loss, prematurity in pregnancy; ophthalmologic or neurologic sequelae; neonatal disease fatal if disseminated; primary infection has higher fetal and neonatal attack rate | Viral culture and differentiation between primary and secondary infection | Cesarean section if lesions present; acyclovir prophylaxis if active lesions in final 4–6 weeks' gestation |
| HBV | Third-trimester infections increase; risk of prematurity, fulminant disease, chronic HBV carrier | HbsAg screen prenatally | Hep B immunoglobulin for exposure during pregnancy or neonatally to infants of HbsAg+ mothers |
| BV | PROM, preterm labor, chorioamnionitis, low birthweight | "Whiff" test, clue cells, culture | Metronidazole (vaginal gel, if nausea) or clindamycin |
| Toxoplasmosis | Depends on fetal age: first-trimester sequelae severe, abortion, stillbirth, congenital defects; avoid cat litter boxes | IgM and IgG titers in mother, targeted US, PUB sampling at birth | Spiramycin, after 14 weeks GA pyrimethamine plus sulfonamide; first- or second-trimester diagnosis may decide to terminate pregnancy |
| Rubella virus | Congenital rubella syndrome (deafness, cardiac abnormalities, cataracts, mental retardation) esp. during first trimester | IgM titers in infant, targeted US of fetus | None; prevention with screen and vaccine |
| Parvovirus | Hydrops fetalis if < 20 weeks' gestation, congenital anomalies, fetal death | IgM and IgG titers in mother, US of fetus to determine hydrops | Intrauterine transfusion for hydropic fetus |
| HIV | If no treatment, 20–30% transmission perinatally | HIV screen, HIV diagnostic algorithm | Zidovudine or AZT during after first trimester, intrapartum and neonatally; cesarian lowers transmission by two thirds |
| Varicella | Abortion, stillbirth; if congenital infection during first 20 weeks, possible limb hypoplasia, microcephaly, chorioretinitis; during neonatal period, mortality rate as high as 30% | VZV titers | VZIG within 72 hours of exposure or to mothers who develop varicella 5 days prior to delivery |
| Group B strep | Chorioamnionitis, endomyometritis; neonatal sepsis with severe implications (neonatal mortality 25–50%) | Rectovaginal culture screening at 36–37 weeks | Known infection treated with IV penicillin G while in labor; treat unknown status < 37 weeks GA with ROM > 18 hours, treat with IV penicillin G |

CMV, cytomegalovirus; CNS, central nervous system; HSV, herpes simplex virus; HBV, hepatitis B virus; HbsAg, hepatitis B surface antigen; Hep B, hepatitis B; BV, bacterial vaginosis; PROM, premature rupture of membranes; IgM, immunoglobulin M; IgG, immunoglobulin G; US, ultrasound; PUB, percutaneous umbilical blood; GA, gestational age; HIV, human immunodeficiency virus; AZT, zidovudine; VZV, varicella zoster virus; VZIG, varicella zoster immune globulin; IV, intravenous; ROM, rupture of membranes.

### ▶ Diagnostic Studies

Routine prenatal fundal height measurements (in cm) beginning at 20 weeks' gestation should equal the gestational age (GA) (e.g., 23 weeks GA = 23 cm). It is imperative to ensure accurate dating of the pregnancy. Ultrasound measurements should be done for any fundal height 3 cm less or 3 cm more than expected. For SGA infants near term that have fallen off the growth curve, further fetal testing (with nonstress tests [NSTs] or oxytocin challenge tests [OCTs]) should be done to assess stress and decisions about delivery made.

### ▶ Diagnosis

Ultrasound measurements use biparietal diameter, femur length, and abdominal circumference. Estimates are accurate usually within 10–15%. Lower fundal heights are also associated with oligohydramnios.

### ▶ Clinical Therapeutics

For SGA secondary to placental insufficiency, preeclampsia, collagen vascular disorders, or vascular disease may be treated with one baby aspirin per day.

### ▶ Clinical Intervention

Once SGA is established, infants at risk for IUGR need to be followed with serial ultrasound scans for growth. Underlying etiology should be determined and factors that are treatable should be instated (e.g., nutritional/substance abuse counseling). For SGA infants near term, further testing helps determine if delivery is necessary. For SGA infants remote from term, frequent antenatal testing with NSTs, OCTs, weekly ultrasounds for fetal growth, and possible hospital admission for monitoring.

Management of macrosomic infants includes prevention, monitoring. Diabetic mothers need tight blood glucose control. Other treatable factors include less maternal weight gain in obese patients with nutritional counseling. LGA pregnancies are often induced before macrosomia, which may increase the risk for cesarian delivery.

### ▶ Health Maintenance Issues

The risk of having an SGA or LGA baby increases with a previous SGA or LGA pregnancy. Subsequent fetuses should be monitored closely. In LGA/macrosomic infant of an obese mother, the mother should be counseled to lose weight before the next pregnancy.

## 2. Disorders of Amniotic Fluid

### ▶ Scientific Concepts

Amniotic fluid reaches its maximal volume (800 mL) at about 28 weeks gestation and is maintained until term, when it begins to fall to about 500 mL (40 weeks GA). Maintenance is due to production by fetal kidneys and lungs, by fetal swallowing, and the interface between the membranes and the placenta. Any disturbance of these functions will cause a pathologic change in the amniotic fluid. Ultrasound measures amniotic fluid volume by the amniotic fluid index (AFI). An AFI < 5 is considered *oligohydramnios*, > 20 is considered *polyhydramnios*. Oligohydramnios can be due to decreased production or increased withdrawal of fluid. Causes include: decreased placental perfusion, genitourinary (GU) tract congenital anomalies, and most commonly, rupture of membranes. Oligohydramnios has a 40-fold increase in perinatal mortality and is associated with anomalies (especially GU tract) and IUGR.

Polyhydramnios occurs in 2–3% of all pregnancies and is not considered as ominous as oligohydramnios. It is also associated with congenital abnormalities, hydrops, and is more common in pregnancies complicated by diabetes or multiple gestation.

#### ▶ History & Physical

Patients may measure size less than (oligohydramnios) or greater than (polyhydramnios) for dates. Patients with a history of ruptured membranes, postterm pregnancy, or suspected of IUGR should be screened for oligohydramnios.

#### ▶ Diagnostic Studies

An AFI < 5 as measured by ultrasound makes the diagnosis of oligohydramnios. Requires further study regarding etiology, especially if IUGR (e.g., cord Doppler flow). An AFI of > 20 makes the diagnosis of polyhydramnios.

#### ▶ Diagnosis

Diabetic mothers and those with multiple gestations should be routinely screened for polyhydramnios.

#### ▶ Clinical Therapeutics

Amnioinfusion for oligohydramnios may be utilized if meconium or frequent decelerations of the fetal heart rate are present.

#### ▶ Clinical Intervention

Management of either of these conditions depends on their etiology. If at term or post dates, labor is usually induced for oligohydramnios. The risks of cord prolapse and malpresentation are increased with polyhydramnios, requiring close monitoring and evaluation.

### 3. Rhesus Factor (Rh) Incompatibility

#### ▶ Scientific Concepts

Rh incompatibility or isoimmunization is characterized as incompatibility between the infant's blood type and that of its mother, resulting in destruction of the infant's red blood cells. After delivery, red blood cells of an Rh-positive fetus precipitate development of antibodies against the Rh-positive blood in an Rh-negative mother. In subsequent pregnancies, anti-Rh antibodies cross the placenta and may destroy fetal blood. The resulting anemia may be severe enough to cause fetal death (erythroblastosis fetalis).

#### ▶ History & Physical

The diagnosis is often made after delivery. Maternal signs during pregnancy include decreased fetal growth and/or movement. Signs in the infant include pallor, jaundice beginning 24 hours after delivery, unexplained bruising, swelling, poor reflex response, and lack of normal movement.

#### ▶ Diagnostic Studies

Parental history, maternal assessment of Rh factor, and antibody titering are most useful. Amniocentesis may be indicated if maternal antibodies are elevated.

► **Diagnosis**

Rule out minor group incompatibility.

► **Clinical Therapeutics**

Treatment generally involves serial measurement of indirect Coombs, antibody titering, fluid replacement, ultraviolet light, vitamin K, and transfusion.

► **Clinical Intervention**

Rh-negative patients who are not sensitized should be treated with antepartum anti-Rh gamma globulin (RhoGAM) to prevent sensitization. They should receive another shot postpartum, if the fetus is Rh positive. RhoGAM is given to the mother at 28 weeks' gestation and within 72 hours of delivery, abortion, ectopic pregnancy, or miscarriage to prevent formation of antibodies that might affect subsequent pregnancies. Antibody titers may be drawn anytime during the pregnancy. Rh-negative patients who are sensitized should be followed closely with serial ultrasounds and amniocentesis (to measure bilirubin in the fluid, an indicator of hemolysis).

► **Health Maintenance Issues**

Infant care, feeding, and prognosis are excellent.

## 4. Trisomy

► **Scientific Concepts**

It is now known that spontaneous abortions occurring in the first 8 weeks have an approximate 50% incidence of chromosome abnormalities. Translocation, deletions, and rearrangements during meiosis lead to the loss of chromatin material. Trisomy may occur with any chromosome, with 13, 18, and 21 being the most common trisomic conditions seen in living individuals. Trisomy 21 (Down syndrome) is the most frequent autosomal chromosomal syndrome, occurring in 1 of every 800 liveborn infants; trisomy 18 occurs in 1 per 8,000 live births; trisomy 13 occurs in about 1 per 20,000 live births.

► **History & Physical**

Advanced maternal age, previous history of genetic disorder, or low maternal serum alpha-fetoprotein (MS-AFP) on routine screening suggest further investigation. Diagnosis is often made after delivery.

► **Diagnostic Studies**

Fetal sampling via chorionic villus sampling, amniocentesis, or percutaneous umbilical blood sampling (PUBS) is definitive. Maternal serum beta-hCG in patients with Down syndrome pregnancies is on average two times the value of unaffected pregnancies.

► **Diagnosis**

Rule out CNS malformation. Elevated MS-AFP at 15–18 weeks' gestation (optimal time for assessment) suggests neural tube defect.

► **Clinical Therapeutics**

No specific treatment.

► **Clinical Intervention**

If identified during pregnancy, care should be nondirective and supportive of parental decisions within the legal, ethical, and professional framework.

► Health Maintenance Issues

Risk increases with maternal age. Support and individual as well as family counseling are recommended.

## 5. CNS Malformation in Fetus

► Scientific Concepts

Infants with disorders of the CNS, including spina bifida and neural tube defects, tend to have a positive family history, multifactorial inheritance, or recurrence risk. Anencephaly occurs in 50% of neural tube defects. Poor glycemic control increases risk in diabetic patients. Neural tube defects may be incidentally identified during routine sonogram. Maternal serum can be evaluated for neural tube defects, usually done between 15 and 18 weeks' gestation. Screening programs can detect 90% of anencephalic fetuses and 80% of fetuses with open spina bifida. Elevated MS-AFP is also seen with gastroschisis, omphalocele, multiple gestations, and large fetal hemorrhages, among other conditions.

► History & Physical

Degree of suspicion during pregnancy or by family/pregnancy history prompts further evaluation.

► Diagnostic Studies

Elevated MS-AFP warrants further evaluation by ultrasound and follow-up of any detected ultrasound abnormalities by amniotic fluid for acetylcholinesterase, which may also be elevated. Patients with increased risk (positive family history, advanced maternal age) should be counseled on the risks and benefits of screening, including potential of false–positive results. Ultrasonography is used in conjunction with laboratory testing, detecting both open spina bifida (71–100% detection rate) and anencephaly (100% detection rate).

► Diagnosis

Differentiate between nervous system malformations.

► Clinical Therapeutics

No specific treatment.

► Clinical Intervention

Diagnosis, nondirective genetic counseling, and consideration of options. Emergency care involves delivery via cesarean section. If pregnancy is maintained, monitoring for hydrocephalus is indicated.

► Health Maintenance Issues

Genetic and personal counseling are important in reaching future childbearing decisions. Dietary supplementation with folic acid and weight loss in obese patients may reduce the risk of neural tube defects.

## 6. Multiple Fetuses

► Scientific Concepts

The frequency of multiple gestation has increased in the past two decades, in part due to assisted reproductive technology, with 2% of all pregnancies being multiple gestations. The natural cause of multiple gestation is unknown in most cases. Women who have borne twins have a 10-fold increased chance of subsequent multiple births. Thirty percent of all twins are monozygotic (resulting from fertilization of a single ovum by a single sperm), and approximately 70% are dizygotic (fraternal twins produced from two separate fertilized ova). Risk factors for multiple gestation include: family history, late childbearing, African American ancestry, and use of ovulation induction. Complications of multiple gestation include growth retardation, cord compression, entanglement, abruptio and placenta previa, preeclampsia, prematurity, cord prolapse, abnormal presentation and position, and postpartum hemorrhage.

▶ History & Physical

Signs and symptoms include uterine enlargement greater than expected for dates, excessive maternal weight gain, multiplicity of body parts, polyhydramnios, and recording of multiple fetal heart tones.

▶ Diagnostic Studies

Most multiple gestations are identified by ultrasound. The level of hCG, human placental lactogen, and MS-AFP are elevated for gestational age. Early consideration of the possibility of multiple pregnancy aids in early diagnosis and early intervention, including glucose management and prevention of prematurity.

▶ Diagnosis

Multiple pregnancies must be distinguished from a large, single pregnancy; date calculation error; polyhydramnios; hydatidiform mole; and abdominal tumors.

▶ Clinical Therapeutics

No specific medication. Close monitoring of maternal and fetal well-being decreases morbidity and mortality associated with multiple gestation. Because of increased complications, multiple gestations are managed as high-risk pregnancies.

▶ Clinical Intervention

Iron supplementation; high-protein diet; less physical exercise; more bedrest; prompt evaluation of vaginal infections, preeclampsia, or glucose variability; and more frequent antenatal visits improve outcome.

▶ Health Maintenance Issues

Mortality rate of multiple pregnancy is only slightly higher than single gestation. Morbidity and complications (risk of hemorrhage, abnormal presentation, operative delivery, PROM, etc.) are increased. Reduction of the incidence of low-birth-weight infants is the goal in managing multiple gestation.

## I. Other Complications of Pregnancy

### 1. Hyperemesis Gravidarum

▶ Scientific Concepts

At least 75% of pregnant women experience some nausea or vomiting, especially during the first trimester of pregnancy (most resolve by 16 weeks). This is usually self-limiting, with pregnant patients maintaining adequate nutrition and hydration. Hyperemesis gravidarum is a condition where continual vomiting may cause dehydration and electrolyte disturbance.

► **History & Physical**

History of pernicious nausea and vomiting. Signs of dehydration, ketonuria, and electrolyte imbalance.

► **Diagnostic Studies**

Helpful laboratory tests include: urine specific gravity, urine acetones/ketones, serum acetone, serum electrolytes. May see a hypochloremic alkalosis. Large amounts of urine or serum acetone suggests lipolysis is supplying energy sources and need for subsequent IV therapy.

► **Diagnosis**

Rule out other conditions that may predispose to vomiting (e.g., viral gastroenteritis, UTI, multifetal gestation, gallbadder disease, hepatitis, migraine).

► **Clinical Therapeutics**

For hypochloremic alkalosis, normal saline with 5% dextrose is often used. Antiemetics such as Compazine (rectal suppository bid), Phenergan (rectally), or Tigan (200 mg q6h po) are commonly used. Although antiemetics may be given orally, this route is not always successful. They may need to be given by IV.

► **Clinical Intervention**

Rehydration for dehydrated patients and correction of electrolyte abnormalities. Goal is to maintain adequate nutrition and hydration. Antiemetics as noted to help relieve nausea and vomiting. Occasionally tube feeding or parenteral nutrition may be warranted. For mild to moderate nausea and vomiting, accupressure bands have been used in place of antiemetics.

► **Health Maintenance Issues**

Education regarding eating small frequent meals and avoiding food that may be unappealing. Prenatal vitamins (especially iron formulations) may increase GI symptoms, but adequate folic acid intake (0.4 mg/d) and iron store must be maintained.

## 2. Incompetent Cervix

► **Scientific Concepts**

Incompetent cervical os is characterized by passive and painless dilation of the cervix in the second trimester and may be a result of cervical instrumentation, surgery, laceration, or congenital anomaly. Increased incidence in multiple gestation, history of cervical conization, cervical amputation, and intrauterine exposure to diethylstilbestrol (DES).

► **History & Physical**

Clinical diagnosis is marked by gradual, painless dilatation and effacement of the cervix with membranes visible through the cervix. Symptoms include painless vaginal discharge of pink or bloody fluid, contractions, and pelvic pressure.

► **Diagnostic Studies**

Diagnosis is made on history of repeated second-trimester spontaneous abortions and physical examination.

► Diagnosis

Objective criteria in the absence of the typical history have been lacking. Dilators or balloons and digital examination of the cervix are highly subjective. Ultrasound provided characteristics of reduced competence are: a short cervix (< 20 mm before 24 weeks), and possible funneling of the internal os. Rule out other etiology of miscarriage.

► Clinical Therapeutics

No medical intervention.

► Clinical Intervention

Surgical intervention includes prophylactic placement of a transvaginal cerclage at 12–16 weeks' gestation or in a nonpregnant patient.

► Health Maintenance Issues

Education; counseling; and restriction of intercourse, prolonged (> 90 minutes) standing, and heavy lifting following cerclage are recommended. The cerclage is easily removed prior to delivery.

## 3. Fetotoxic Exposure

► Scientific Concepts

Drug-induced teratology accounts for 2–3% of all fetal congenital malformations; most result from genetic, environmental, and unknown causes. Drugs given during pregnancy may alter placental function, produce a lethal or toxic effect on the embryo, or change myometrial activity. From day 0 to day 11 of gestation, exposure to toxins may have the "all or none" effect with regard to major anomalies; from days 11–57, the fetus is most susceptible to the effect of teratogens; after 57 days' gestation, the organs are formed and increasing in size with a teratogenic effect manifesting in growth retardation, decrease in organ size, or derangement of organ systems.

► History & Physical

History, risk factors, degree of exposure relative to gestational age precipitate investigation. Known teratogens are to be avoided: viruses (rubella); parasites (toxoplasmosis); bacteria (syphilis); heavy metals (mercury); medications such as cancer chemotherapeutic agents, antiepileptics, anticoagulants, antibiotics (tetracycline); radiation.

► Diagnostic Studies

Intrauterine evaluation is limited to high-resolution sonogram.

► Diagnosis

The diagnosis is specific to the condition evaluated.

► Clinical Therapeutics

Specific to exposure and evaluation.

► Clinical Intervention

Patient education toward avoidance of potential toxin is best intervention.

► Health Maintenance Issues

See Clinical Intervention above.

## 4. Substance Abuse

▶ **Scientific Concepts**

The most commonly abused substances in pregnancy, alcohol and cigarettes, contribute to poorer outcomes: increased perinatal mortality, preterm delivery, growth restriction. Heavy alcohol use (> 3 oz/6 drinks per day) is associated with features of fetal alcohol syndrome (prenatal or postnatal growth retardation, CNS involvement, abnormal facies). Opiate abuse causes 3- to 7-fold increases in stillbirth, fetal growth restriction, preterm birth, and neonatal mortality: it creates more problems neonatally with acute withdrawal with an increased risk of fetal death (3 to 5%). Cocaine has been associated with placenta abruptio and CNS effects.

▶ **History & Physical**

All patients should be questioned about alcohol, tobacco, and substance abuse at their first and subsequent prenatal visits.

▶ **Diagnostic Studies**

Several screening questionnaires, such as CAGE and T-ACE, are useful in assessing alcohol consumption.

▶ **Diagnosis**

The diagnosis is specific to the history of substance abuse elicited.

▶ **Clinical Therapeutics**

Specific to exposure and evaluation, but of limited value due to teratogenic or other effects on pregnancy.

▶ **Clinical Intervention**

Patient education toward avoidance of particular substances is best intervention. Management of patients is compounded by multiple substance use, social circumstances, inadequate prenatal care, and poor nutrition. Aggressive counseling programs for alcohol abuse may decrease risk to participants. Tobacco shows a dose–response effect, and patients should be counseled to quit or at the minimum, decrease, cigarette use, with smoking cessation programs. Multidisciplinary programs are often necessary to manage social and psychiatric issues of drug-addicted patients.

▶ **Health Maintenance Issues**

Primary caregivers should begin counseling women of childbearing age on effects of various substances and programs for cessation prior to pregnancy.

## 5. Postterm Pregnancy

▶ **Scientific Concepts**

A postterm pregnancy is one that extends beyond 42 weeks (294 days after the last menstrual period). The incidence is between 5–10%, with postterm pregnancies at higher risk for fetal demise, oligohydramnios, macrosomia, growth restriction, meconium staining, and aspiration. Risk to the mother is cesarean delivery.

▶ **History & Physical**

A pregnancy beyond 42 weeks with accurate dates. At 41 weeks, review dates (up to 40% of women will be unsure of their last menstrual period [LMP]) and perform cervical digital exam to determine favorability of labor induction.

▶ **Diagnostic Studies**

With pregnancies that extend past 40 weeks, NSTs are done weekly in conjunction with cervical exams.

▶ **Diagnosis**

With accurate dating (firm LMP, first trimester ultrasound), a pregnancy beyond 42 weeks.

▶ **Clinical Therapeutics**

If at 41 weeks, the cervix is not favorable for induction, a cervical ripening agent such as Prostaglandin E2 gel (0.5 mg intracervically q6h 2–3 times), Prostaglandin E2 delayed release vaginal insert 12 hours prior to induction, or Mistoprolol (25- to 50-µg tablet in the posterior vaginal fornix q3h).

▶ **Clinical Intervention**

At 41 weeks, with reliable dates, a cervical digital examination is done to assess whether favorable for induction. If unfavorable, NSTs are done twice weekly or patient may have an NST at one visit and a biophysical profile at the other. If NST is nonreassuring, induction is indicated. After 42 weeks, the patient is usually induced regardless of cervical examination.

## 6. Postpartum Hemorrhage

▶ **Scientific Concepts**

Postpartum hemorrhage complicates about 10% of deliveries and is defined as a blood loss > 500 mL for vaginal delivery or > 1,000 mL for cesarean section. Causes may include: uterine atony (loss of tone and contractility), genital tract laceration, retained products of conception including placenta, placenta accreta, or uterine inversion. Predisposing factors include prolonged labor, infection, macrosomic infant, uterine overdistention (e.g., multiple gestation), grand multiparity, instrumentation, or use of drugs known to decrease uterine muscle contraction (halogenated inhaled anesthetics, beta-adrenergic agonists, and magnesium sulfate).

▶ **History & Physical**

If vaginal bleeding persists after delivery of the placenta, aggressive intervention should be employed. Signs and symptoms of acute blood loss should be monitored.

▶ **Diagnostic Studies**

Postpartum hemorrhage is a medical emergency that requires prompt evaluation and immediate life support intervention.

▶ **Diagnosis**

Cause of bleeding should be identified.

▶ **Clinical Therapeutics**

Fluid expansion and replacement should be initiated. Administration of uterotonic medications such as oxytocin, carboprost tromethamine, and ergot preparations. Oxytocin is often routinely given as a dilute infusion (20 U/L of IV fluid) after delivery to promote uterine contraction. Bolus doses are avoided because hypotension can result. Carboprost-tromethamine (Hemabate) is a potent uterotonic medication given IM (250 µg). The ergot derivatives ergonovine maleate and methylergonovine maleate are effective uterotonic medications with usual dose of 0.2 mg IM. Bimanual compression and massage of the uterus and careful exploration of the uterus, with immediate removal of any retained particles and repair of lacerations, should be initiated immediately. Curettage and uterine packing are no longer favorable interventions. Management of uterine inversion involves correction of the inversion manually and may require uterine muscle relaxation (e.g., nitroglycerine).

▶ Clinical Intervention
As above.

▶ Health Maintenance Issues
The complications of postpartum hemorrhage include shock, postoperative infection, uterine damage or loss, renal failure, and death.

## XII. ROUTINE PRENATAL CARE

▶ Scientific Concepts
The goal of antenatal care is to achieve the best possible maternal and fetal outcome. Diagnosis of pregnancy with accurate dating, confirmation of intrauterine implantation, and comprehensive data collection including history, physical examination, and appropriate laboratory tests are the first order. Danger signs include any vaginal bleeding, swelling of face or fingers, severe headache, dimness or blurring of vision, abdominal pain, persistent vomiting, fever or chills, dysuria, escape of fluid from the vagina, or marked changes in frequency or intensity of fetal movements.

▶ History & Physical
Patient may have a variety of common, nonspecific complaints, including nausea, vomiting, fatigue, breast tenderness, urinary changes, and, most commonly, amenorrhea. On physical examination, uterine softening and enlargement, bluish discoloration of the uterus (Chadwick's sign), and softening of the cervix (Hegar's sign) may be evident. Auscultation of fetal heart tone (audible at 10–12 weeks' gestation), monitored at each visit thereafter. Leopold maneuvers (checking the position of the fetus) can be done later in pregnancy. Quickening (the mother being able to feel fetal movement) usually happens between 16 and 20 weeks gestation.

▶ Diagnostic Studies
Documentation of a positive pregnancy test (serum beta-hCG), CBC, urinalysis, urine culture, blood group and Rh, antibody screen, rubella titer, serologic test for syphilis, hepatitis B surface antigen, sickle cell prep, Pap smear, and cultures for gonorrhea and chlamydia should be completed at the first visit. MS-AFP at 15–18 weeks and 50-g glucose screening at 24–28 weeks are also recommended. Fetal imaging via ultrasound early in pregnancy and in third trimester is most useful in assessing implantation, gestational age, and fetal growth.

▶ Diagnosis
Diagnosis of uncomplicated pregnancy versus high-risk pregnancy guides interventions and management.

▶ **Clinical Therapeutics**

Prenatal vitamins and iron supplementation are commonly prescribed throughout pregnancy and lactation. Folic acid consumption of no less than 0.4 mg per day is necessary to decrease the risks of neural tube defects, and more commonly the prescription strength is 1.0 mg per day.

▶ **Clinical Intervention**

Patient education; discussion of maternal nutrition, lifestyle adaptations, and exposure to medications, drugs, or other potential toxins; reassurance and surveillance for complications are the mainstay of routine prenatal care.

▶ **Health Maintenance Issues**

Uncomplicated pregnancy should be monitored every 4 weeks for the first 32 weeks, every 2 weeks from 32 to 36 weeks, and weekly from 36 weeks until delivery. Each prenatal visit should include assessment of maternal weight, blood pressure, measurement of fundal height, screening for peripheral edema, urinalysis, and assessment of fetal position, movement, and fetal heart tones. Intervention is specific to pathologic change.

*Prenatal visits 6–12 weeks:* Extensive prenatal history, pelvic exam to confirm uterine size and growth, document fetal heart tones, chorionic villus sampling between 10 and 12 weeks when necessary.

*Prenatal visits 12–18 weeks:* Genetic counseling should be offered to all women age 35 or older and those with a family history of inheritable diseases, or a former delivery with genetic disorder; offer screening tests for neural tube defects, MS-AFP, estriol, and hCG—"triple screen."

*Prenatal visits 12–24 weeks:* Fetal ultrasound exam to determine dating and evaluate fetal anatomy; ultrasound done between 18 and 20 weeks is most common, but earlier ultrasound is best for determining dates, and later ultrasound is best for assessing fetal development.

*Prenatal visits 20–24 weeks:* Patient education done on signs and symptoms of preterm labor, and premature rupture of membranes.

*Prenatal visits 24 weeks to delivery:* Ultrasound examination is performed as indicated.

*Prenatal visits 26–28 weeks:* Screening for gestational diabetes.

*Prenatal visits 28 weeks:* In Rh-negative patients, an antibody screen should be repeated if it was negative earlier in pregnancy. $Rh_o(D)$ immune globulin is administered at this time.

*Prenatal visits 28–32 weeks:* Check CBC to evaluate anemia.

*Prenatal visits 28 weeks to delivery:* Determine fetal position and presentation, assess for signs and symptoms of preterm labor or PROM, ask mother about fetal movement. Fetal assessment is performed as medically indicated.

*Prenatal visits 35–37 weeks:* Obtain culture for group B streptococcal colonization of the mother.

*Prenatal visits 36 weeks to delivery:* Patient education about birth plan (patient's preference for the management of labor and delivery, her options for analgesia and anesthesia, who she wants to be present at the delivery), indicators of the onset of labor, hospital or birthing center admission. Weekly cervical examinations are not necessary unless indicated by specific situation. Confirmation of fetal lung maturity is necessary for elective delivery prior to 39 weeks (induction or cesarean section).

*Prenatal visits 41 weeks and later ("postdates"):*  Monitor mother and fetus as needed—cervical exams and antepartum fetal testing.

## XIII.  NORMAL LABOR AND DELIVERY

### ▶ Scientific Concepts

After an adequate period of intrauterine development (approximately 280 days), the fetus is ready to begin life outside of the mother. The process of leaving the uterus is termed *labor.* It is important to understand the normal process of labor and delivery. Labor is commonly defined as the regular uterine contraction activity that results in the progressive effacement and dilatation of the uterine cervix. Labor may be caused by endogenous oxytocin production, prostaglandin release, progesterone withdrawal, or drop in fetal cortisol levels. It is characterized by progressive contractions that occur at decreasing intervals and at increasing intensity, associated with cervical dilatation and effacement. There are four stages of labor defined as:

*Stage I:*  0–10 cm dilation of the cervix. This stage usually lasts 12–18 hours. It is further divided into three phases: Latent phase—characterized by cervix dilation 0–3 cm; mild contractions; contractions are 5–30 minutes apart lasting 15 to 40 seconds. Active labor—characterized by cervix dilation 4–8 cm; stronger more uncomfortable contractions; 2–5 minutes apart lasting 45–90 seconds. Deceleration (also called "transition")—cervical dilation is 8–10 cm; contractions are every 2 minutes lasting 60–90 seconds. The contractions are strong and painful. Latent phase lasts 6–12 hours. Active labor lasts about 4–6 hours, and transition usually takes less than 2 hours.

*Stage II:*  Time from complete cervical dilation until the delivery of the infant. Nulliparas average 117 minutes; multiparas average 46 minutes. This is when the mother is "pushing."

*Stage III:*  Time from delivery of the infant until delivery of the placenta and membranes. Duration is about 30 minutes.

*Stage IV:*  The first hour of recovery.

Dystocia is any deviation from the normal process of labor that results in a prolonging of any phase or stage of labor. Arrest is labor dystocia that is so markedly slow that it does not appear that labor is able to progress any further.

### ▶ History & Physical

Patient may complain of progressive abdominal, back, pelvic, or thigh pain and nausea/vomiting associated with uterine contractions that may last for 30–90 seconds and occur every 1–3 minutes. Cervical effacement and dilatation may last up to 20 hours in primigravidas. Patients should not be delivered vaginally if an active herpes infection is suspected.

### ▶ Diagnostic Studies

Evaluation includes history and physical examination; fetal monitoring of heart rate; detection of ruptured membranes; and pelvic exam for staging, fetal presentation, engagement, descent, and assessment of amniotic fluid (meconium, nitrazine test, and ferning).

► Diagnosis

Diagnosis is made on serial examinations and assessment of normal progression of labor.

► Clinical Therapeutics

Interventions are supportive. Ineffective contractions and failure to progress may be treated with oxytocin. Cephalopelvic disproportion and maternal complications may be treated with cesarean section.

► Clinical Intervention

The benefit of episiotomy to mother or infant has not been proven. Supportive measures during labor such as ambulation, positioning, and deep breathing offer relief to some.

► Health Maintenance Issues

Pregnancy is a normal physiologic process. Efforts toward maintaining a well-balanced diet, moderate exercise, precautions against exposure to toxins, patient education, early and regular prenatal care, and attention to patient and family psychosocial needs improve fetal and maternal outcome and patient's sense of well-being.

## BIBLIOGRAPHY

Beckmann C, Ling F, Herbert W, et al. *Obstetrics and Gynecology*, 3rd ed. Philadelphia: Williams & Wilkins; 1998.

Burnett, AF. *Clinical Obstetrics and Gynecology, A Problem-Based Approach.* Malden, MA: Blackwell Science; 2001.

Callahan TL, Caughey AB, Heffner LJ, eds. *Blueprints in Obstetrics & Gynecology*, 2nd ed. Malden, MA: Blackwell Science; 2001.

Crump W. UTIs in pregnancy: A case-based report. *Family Practice Recertification* 21(10):45–52; 1999.

Dambro M. *Griffith's 5-Minute Clinical Consultant.* Philadelphia: Lippincott Williams & Wilkins; 1999.

DeCherney AM, Pernoll ML. *Current, Obstetric and Gynecologic Diagnosis and Treatment,* 8th ed. East Norwalk, CT: Appleton & Lange; 1994.

Dixon D, Rayz S, White G. Gestational diabetes mellitus: An update and review for primary care providers. *Physician Assistant* (March):28–35; 1999.

Goldberg J. *The Instant Exam Review for the USMLE Step 3*, 2nd ed. Stamford, CT: Appleton & Lange; 1997.

Goroll AH, Mulley AG, May LA, Mulley AG Jr, eds. *Primary Care Medicine: Office Evaluation and Management of the Adult Patient,* 4th ed. [online text]. Philadelphia: Lippincott Williams & Wilkins; 2000. Available from: http://mdconsult.com.

Gries-Griffin J. Abnormal Pap test results. *Advance/PA;* July 1995.

Hutchins FL Jr. Fibroids in primary care. *The Clinical Advisor;* September 1998.

Keene GF. Office gynecology, common reproductive disorders. *Clin Rev* 9(1):58–80; 1999.

Ling FW, Duff P, eds. *Pocket Guide for Obstetrics and Gynecology: Principles for Practice.* New York: McGraw-Hill; 2002.

Miller H, McEvers J, Griffith J. *Instructions for Obstetric and Gynecologic Patients,* 2nd ed. Philadelphia: WB Saunders; 1997.

Moyers-Scott P. Performing cervical polypectomy. *JAAPA* 12(6):81–91; 1999.

Rakel RE, Bope ET, eds. *Conn's Current Therapy 2002*, 54th ed. [online text]. Philadelphia: WB Saunders; 2002. Available from: http://mdconsult.com.

Raplin A, Laghlin D. Guidelines for diagnosis and treatment of premenstrual syndrome. *Family Practice Recertification* 21(1):41–68; 1999.

Ryan KJ, ed. *Kistner's Gynecology & Women's Health,* 7th ed. [online text]. St. Louis: Mosby; 1999. Available from: http://mdconsult.com.

Stoffey W. Using medications safely in pregnancy. *PA Today* (September 28):11–15; 1998.

Tierney LM Jr, McPhee SJ, Papadakis MA, eds. *Current Medical Diagnosis & Treatment,* 42nd ed. New York: Lange Medical Books/McGraw Hill; 2003.

# Endocrinology 10

*Dwight M. Deter, PA-C*

# I. DISEASES OF THE THYROID GLAND

## A. Hyperthyroidism

▶ Scientific Concepts

The cause may be autoimmune, idiopathic, infectious, or iatrogenic; 15% of patients have family members with same disorder. Peak age is 20–40 years. Female:male ratio is 5:1. Graves' disease is an autoimmune disorder found particularly in the young, which is responsible for 80% of hyperthyroidism cases. Toxic multinodular goiter is a more common cause of thyrotoxicosis in the elderly. Iodine-induced hyperthyroidism may be precipitated by medications containing large amounts of iodine. Subacute thyroiditis is characterized by a painful, tender goiter with transient hyperthyroidism. Antibodies (thyroid stimulating immunoglobulins or TSI) develop against thyroid-stimulating hormone (TSH) receptor sites in the thyroid cell membrane and stimulate the thyroid cell to increase growth and function. Pregnancy, iodide excess, lithium therapy, glucocorticoid withdrawal, bacterial or viral infections may trigger the acute episode. In thyroid storm, the number of catecholamine binding sites may be increased in heart and nerve tissues, causing increased sensitivity to circulating catecholamines. The level of catecholamines may be elevated secondary to severe illness.

▶ History & Physical

In hyperthyroidism, palpitations, nervousness, easy fatigability, hyperkinesia, diarrhea, excessive sweating, heat intolerance, weight loss, increased appetite, tachycardia, tremor, thyroid enlargement, muscle weakness and atrophy, proptosis, onycholysis, and pretibial myxedema may be present. In thyroid storm, there is acute exacerbation of all symptoms of thyrotoxicosis marked by hypermetabolism and excessive adrenergic response, which may culminate in hyperpyrexia, heart failure, shock, coma, or death. This commonly occurs after surgery, radioactive iodine therapy, or parturition in a patient with inadequately controlled thyrotoxicosis or during a severe illness such as uncontrolled diabetes, trauma, acute infection, severe drug reaction, or myocardial infarction.

▶ Diagnostic Studies

Elevated free thyroxine ($FT_4$) and suppressed TSH and clinical symptoms support the diagnosis of hyperthyroidism. Continue evaluation by obtaining radioiodine uptake. If the uptake is high, consider Graves' or toxic nodular goiter. If uptake is low, consider the hyperthyroid phase of subacute thyroiditis. The acute-phase Hashimoto's thyroiditis, Graves' disease, or toxic nodular goiter in iodine-loaded patient is also a possibility.

In thyroid storm, serum thyroxine ($T_4$), $FT_4$, and triiodothyronine ($T_3$) are elevated and the TSH is suppressed. Refer to Table 10–1 for further information concerning the diagnostic approach to the evaluation of hyperthyroidism.

▶ Diagnosis

Differential diagnosis of thyrotoxicosis:

***Toxic adenoma (Plummer's disease):*** Benign active nodules localized to one lobe of the thyroid. "Hot" nodule on thyroid scan is usually treated with radioactive iodine.

► table 10-1

DIAGNOSTIC APPROACH TO EVALUATION OF HYPERTHYROIDISM

| Condition | History or Physical Exam | Serum Free $T_4$ | Serum-Sensitive TSH | Further Evaluation |
|---|---|---|---|---|
| Normal | Normal | Normal | Normal | |
| Hyperthyroidism 2° severe illness | Clinically hyperthyroid | ↓ | Normal or ↓ | ↓ $T_3$ |
| $T_3$ thyrotoxicosis | Clinically hyperthyroid | ↓ | Normal or ↓ | ↑ $T_3$ and ↑ RAIU scan |
| Ingestion of liothyronine (Cytomel) | Clinically hyperthyroid | ↓ | Normal or ↓ | ↑ $T_3$ and ↓ RAIU scan |
| Hyperthyroidism | Thyroid gland enlarged or normal | ↑ | ↓ | |
| Thyrotoxicosis factitia | Thyroid gland not enlarged | ↑ | ↓ | ↓ RAIU scan ↓ Serum thyroglobulin |
| Subacute thyroiditis | Thyroid gland tender | ↑ | ↓ | ↓ RAIU scan ↑ Serum thyroglobulin |

$T_4$, thyroxine; TSH, thyroid-stimulating hormone; $T_3$, triiodothyronine; RAIU, radioactive iodine uptake; ↑, increased; ↓, decreased.

***Toxic multinodular goiter:*** Characteristically occurs in older patient with long-standing multinodular goiter and some stress or iodine load.

***Subacute or chronic thyroiditis:*** Tender, painful goiter is noted. Mild to severe thyrotoxicosis is caused by acute release of $T_3$ and $T_4$. Radioiodide uptake is diminished. The condition may spontaneously subside over several months.

***Thyrotoxicosis factitia:*** Caused by the ingestion of excessive amounts of thyroid hormone usually for weight control. Thyroid exam is normal except for symptoms of hyperthyroidism.

► Clinical Therapeutics

Antithyroid drugs propylthiouracil (PTU) or methimazole (tapazol) are most useful in pregnant women and the young with small glands and mild disease. Give until spontaneous remission of disease occurs. Relapse rate is 60–80% even after treatment for 1 year. Monitor course of therapy with regular $FT_4$, TSH, and complete blood count (CBC). Duration of therapy is 6 months to 1 year.

Subtotal thyroidectomy is rarely recommended. Complications of surgery may include recurrent laryngeal nerve injury or hypoparathyroidism (~1% of cases).

The use of radioactive iodine $I^{131}$ for those older than 21 and not pregnant is the preferred therapy. The patient usually becomes euthyroid in 2–4 months. Eighty percent will eventually develop hypothyroidism. Follow serum $FT_4$ and TSH levels every 4–6 weeks. Replacement therapy with levothyroxine is usually indicated. In pregnancy, radioactive iodine is contraindicated. May use propylthiouracil and rarely subtotal thyroidectomy. Beta-adrenergic blocking agents alleviate tachycardia, hypertension, and may prevent cardiac arrhythmia.

► Clinical Intervention

Thyroid storm: Administer beta blocker to control arrhythmias and tachycardia. Verapamil may be necessary for severe heart failure in the presence of asthma or arrhythmia. PTU or methimazole (tapazol) are the immediate drugs of choice to decrease thyroid hormone production. Acetaminophen, fluids, electrolytes, and nutritional support are also important. A cooling blanket may be necessary for hyperpyrexia. Treat underlying and/or precipitating disease.

► Health Maintenance Issues

Remission and exacerbations over time result in the need for definitive treatment by thyroidectomy or radioactive iodine. Thyroidectomy is rarely necessary. Afterwards, most remain euthyroid for a short time but eventually become hypothyroid and need thyroid replacement therapy. It is usually appropriate to begin thyroid replacement therapy when the TSH rises to high normal levels.

## B. Hypothyroidism

► Scientific Concepts

Hypometabolic state caused by decrease or lack of thyroid hormone. Hypothyroidism is divided according to the following classifications: primary (thyroid failure), secondary (pituitary TSH deficit), tertiary (deficient hypothalamic thyroid-releasing hormone [TRH]), or peripheral (resistance to the action of thyroid hormones). Primary hypothyroidism causes 90% of cases. Chronic autoimmune (Hashimoto's) thyroiditis is the most common cause in the United States and occurs with or without goiter. Other common causes include $I^{131}$ therapy and thyroid surgery. Congenital hypothyroidism occurs in 1:4,000 newborns. In adults > 65 years, the frequency is 2–4%. In the general population, the frequency is reportedly 0.5–1.0%, but may actually be higher.

► History & Physical

Fatigue, weakness, weight gain, hoarseness, constipation, depression, slowed mentation, muscle cramps, menstrual irregularities, and/or infertility may occur. Firm goiter with multiple nodules or a nonpalpable gland; bradycardia and distant heart sounds; myxedema; slow, hoarse, husky speech; cool, dry, thick, yellow-colored skin (carotenemia) and loss of scalp hair and eyebrows; puffy face and hands; dull facial expression; shallow, slow respirations; delayed relaxation of deep tendon reflexes; cerebellar ataxia; diminished memory; peripheral neuropathy and parasthesias; carpal tunnel syndrome are physical examination findings.

► Diagnostic Studies

Elevated TSH and decreased $FT_4$ indicate primary hypothyroidism. Elevated thyroid peroxidase antibodies (TPO) microsomal thyroid antibodies is confirmatory for Hashimoto's thyroiditis.

Refer to Table 10–2 for further information concerning the diagnostic approach to the evaluation of hypothyroidism.

► Clinical Therapeutics

Initiate low doses of levothyroxine and titrate dosage from 50 to 100 µg/d every 4–6 weeks according to TSH assay and clinical response. Use lower starting dose in cardiac disease since this may exacerbate

► table 10-2

**DIAGNOSTIC APPROACH TO EVALUATION OF HYPOTHYROIDISM**

| Condition | History or Physical Exam | Serum Free $T_4$ | Serum-Sensitive TSH | Further Evaluation |
|---|---|---|---|---|
| Normal | Normal | Normal | Normal | |
| Primary hypothyroidism | Commonly mild symptoms, frank myxedema occurs rarely | ↓ | ↑ | |
| Hashimoto's thyroiditis, postpartum thyroid dysfunction or recovery from severe illness | Goiter noted frequently in Hashimoto's thyroiditis | Normal or ↓ | ↑ | Antithyroglobulin antibodies detected in 90% of those with Hashimoto's thyroiditis |
| Secondary hypothyroidism (hypopituitarism) | Clinically hypothyroid | ↓ | Normal or ↓ | |
| TSH suppression 2° to dopamine or corticosteroids | Clinically hypothyroid or euthyroid | ↓ | Normal or ↓ | TRH test or serial monitoring of TSH and Free $T_4$ |

$T_4$, thyroxine; TSH thyroid-stimulating hormone; TRH, thyroid-releasing hormone; ↑, increased; ↓, decreased.

angina. Concomitant administration of cholestyramine, antacids, and/or iron supplements interfere with absorption of levothyroxine.

► Clinical Intervention

Be alert for altered mental status, compromised ventilation, hypothermia, cardiomyopathy, and/or ataxia perhaps even coma.

► Health Maintenance Issues

Repeat free $T_4$ and TSH every 4–6 weeks until therapeutic response of TSH is achieved and a maintenance dose of levothyroxine is established. Repeat free $T_4$ and TSH annually thereafter. Average maintenance dosage is 100–150 µg/d in adults. It may be necessary to increase dose of levothyroxine by 25% for pregnant and lactating patients based on TSH levels. Elderly patients may require a decrease of levothyroxine dosage based on TSH levels.

## C. Neoplasms of the Thyroid

► Scientific Concepts

Thyroid cancer is rare. Incidence is 0.004% in the United States. Most thyroid nodules are benign. Female:male ratio is 4:1. Common presentation is a single nodule of the thyroid or a dominant nodule increasing in size in a multinodular gland. The four major types of thyroid carcinomas are papillary, follicular, medullary, and anaplastic.

*Papillary carcinoma* is a slow-growing cancer that makes up 70% of cases and is more likely to be found in females in their second or third decade of life.

*Follicular carcinoma* comprises 15% of all thyroid malignancies. It is more aggressive than papillary carcinoma and has an increasing incidence with age.

***Medullary carcinoma*** comprises < 5% of all thyroid malignancies. In the elderly, it occurs as a sporadic unifocal lesion of the thyroid. It may also occur as part of a multiple endocrine neoplasia type II (MEN II) as an inherited autosomal dominant disorder of the thyroid with pheochromocytoma and hyperparathyroidism.

***Anaplastic carcinoma*** comprises 1% of all thyroid malignancies and is the most aggressive form of thyroid cancer. It is differentiated into two histologic types: giant cell and small cell. Patients with small cell have a 20% survival rate at 5 years. In those diagnosed with giant cell, death usually occurs within 6 months after diagnosis.

### ▶ History & Physical

The benign thyroid nodule is typically found in older females with a family history of goiter. On physical examination, soft thyroid nodules are noted in the presence of multinodular goiter. The typical malignant thyroid nodule is found in a patient with a family history of thyroid cancer, history of recent thyroid growth, and/or head and neck irradiation as a child. On physical examination, a palpable, solitary, firm, or dominant nodule that is inconsistent with the surrounding glandular tissue is noted. Late-stage findings include vocal cord paralysis, lymphadenopathy, and/ or metastasis to lung or bone.

### ▶ Diagnostic Studies

Evaluate with the following studies: Free $T_4$, TSH, and TPO microsomal thyroid antibodies are used to rule out the "lumpy" thyroid of Hashimoto's thyroiditis.

Ultrasound distinguishes cystic nodules (benign) from semicystic or solid (possibly malignant). Scanning techniques with $^{123}I$ or $^{99}m\ TcO_4$ differentiate "hot" nodules (benign) from "cold" nodules (malignant). Perform fine-needle aspiration. If cytology shows benign cells, no further evaluation is required. If tissue is malignant or suggestive of malignancy on histocytopathologic exam, surgical intervention is necessary. Suppression therapy with levothyroxine may result in regression of a benign nodule, while malignant nodules remain unchanged. Serum calcitonin is elevated in medullary thyroid cancer. Serum thyroglobulin is measured after therapy for thyroid cancer and if elevated, suggests metastatic disease.

### ▶ Diagnosis

The only definitive way to diagnose carcinoma of the thyroid is histologically.

### ▶ Clinical Therapeutics

Hashimoto's thyroiditis requires lifelong replacement of thyroid hormone. Use levothyroxine, 2–3 µg/kg/d (average dose 100–150 µg/d), to limit thyroid enlargement and prevent hypothyroidism.

### ▶ Clinical Intervention

For papillary or follicular thyroid carcinoma, a near complete thyroidectomy is necessary. Thyroidectomy is performed if nodule > 2 cm along with minimal neck dissection for lymph nodes if metastasis is suspected. Four to 8 weeks postoperative, need thyroid body scan when the TSH is elevated. If residual radioactive iodine uptake occurs, then radioactive iodine is an effective treatment. If the tumor fails to concentrate radioactive iodine, use local radiotherapy. Repeat thyroid body scan annually until no further uptake is observed. Maintain on levothyroxine, at a dose sufficient to suppress the TSH. Medullary cancer is treated similarly, but outcome is not as successful. Follow serum calcitonin or carcinoembryonic antigen (CEA) levels. Screen family members for receptor tyrosine kinase (RET) oncogene in an effort to predict risk of medullary carcinoma. Anaplastic cancer is treated with bulk removal and palliative radiotherapy. Staging predicts outcome.

► Health Maintenance Issues

Levothyroxine is given for TSH suppression. Evaluate supersensitive TSH to determine if the patient is receiving adequate thyroid replacement. Inquire about bone pain, headaches, and cough at 6-month to 1-year intervals. Examine for lymph node metastasis or recurrent thyroid mass. Monitor serum thyroglobulin level after thyroidectomy and rescan if increased levels are found since this may indicate recurrent cancer. Obtain a chest x-ray annually.

## II. PARATHYROID DISEASE

► Scientific Concepts

Primary hyperparathyroidism is caused by increased parathyroid hormone (PTH) secretion by single parathyroid adenoma (80%) or hyperplasia of all four glands (15%). Incidence is 42 per 100,000. Prevalence is 4 per 100 in females > 60 years of age. Female:male ratio is 4:1. Common feature of all hypercalcemic disorders (except for milk-alkali syndrome) is increased bone resorption of calcium. To a lesser extent, increased gastrointestinal (GI) absorption and decreased renal excretion of calcium contribute to disorders associated with hypercalcemia.

► History & Physical

Family history of hypercalcemia, early osteoporosis or renal stones, and multiple endocrine neoplasia (MEN type I or IIa). Patients are usually asymptomatic; however, they may present with central nervous system (CNS) complaints including fatigue, lethargy, difficulty concentrating, depression, personality changes, weakness, proximal neuropathy, psychosis, ataxia, or stupor. Renal complaints include nocturia, polyuria, polydipsia, or stones. GI complaints include nausea, vomiting, anorexia, or constipation. Be alert for cardiovascular complaints of bradycardia, which may lead to asystole. Mnemonic: stones, bones, abdominal groans, and psychiatric moans.

► Diagnostic Studies

Calcium (elevated), phosphorus (low to normal), alkaline phosphatase (increased or normal), renal function (decreased), 24-hour urinary calcium and PTH levels (increased in primary hyperparathyroidism). Glomerular filtration decreased. Electrocardiogram (ECG) shows shortened QT interval. Radiographs may show subperiosteal resorption of cortical bone in phalanges.

► Diagnosis

***Metastatic carcinoma:*** Second most common cause of hypercalcemia. Sources of metastatic cancers in decreasing frequency are lung, breast, and multiple myeloma. They account for > 50% of tumors that cause hypercalcemia. The PTH assay is suppressed.

***Familial benign hypocalciuric hypercalcemia:*** Autosomal dominant, lifelong asymptomatic hypercalcemia detectable in cord blood. Marked by hypocalciuria. Diagnosis is unequivocal because serum calcium, phosphate, alkaline phosphatase, urine calcium, and PTH levels overlap with those of primary hypoparathyroidism. Avoid unnecessary parathyroidectomy.

***Multiple endocrine neoplasia types I and IIa:*** May occur as part of three different familial (autosomal dominant) endocrinopathies: MEN I, which includes tumors of the pituitary and pancreas (insulinoma, gastrinoma); MEN IIa, which includes hyperparathyroidism, pheochromocytoma, and medullary thyroid cancer; and isolated familial hyperparathyroidism.

***Endocrine tumors:*** Uncomplicated pheochromocytoma produces parathyroid hormone-related peptide (PTHrp) from tumor. Tumors secreting vasoactive intestinal peptide (VIPoma) associated with hypercalcemia results from activation of PTH/PTHrp receptors.

***Endocrinopathies:***
- *Thyrotoxicosis:* Mild hypercalcemia occurs in 25% of thyrotoxic patients. PTH is suppressed.
- *Adrenal insufficiency:* Hypercalcemia is a feature of acute adrenal crisis.

***Lithium therapy:*** Limits the inhibition of PTH secretion and causes hypercalcemia and hypocalciuria. Levels of PTH detectable or elevated. May unmask primary hyperparathyroidism. Psychiatric condition is not alleviated by parathyroidectomy.

***Sarcoidosis and other granulomatous disorders:*** Ectopic production of 1,25 $(OH)_2D$ in macrophages of sarcoid tissue causes increased serum calcium. Serum phosphate, alkaline phosphatase, and urine calcium are normal or elevated. Level of PTH is suppressed. Other disorders include histoplasmosis, pulmonary eosinophilic granulomatosis, and untreated tuberculosis.

***Thiazide diuretic therapy:*** Chlorthalidone, metolazone, and indapamide produce mild transient hypercalcemia not explained by hemoconcentration. Underlying primary hyperparathyroidism becomes persistent when exacerbated by thiazides.

***Vitamin D and vitamin A excess:*** Vitamin D dosage > 50,000 IU daily causes increased calcium absorption and increased bone resorption. PTH is suppressed. Serum 25-hydroxyvitamin D levels are 5 to 10 times normal. Vitamin A, 50,000–200,000 IU qd, causes symptoms of headache, anorexia, glossitis, scaly pruritic rash, hepatomegaly and bone pain, elevated serum vitamin A and calcium.

***Milk-alkali syndrome:*** This pure absorptive hypercalcemia is caused by ingestion of excessive amounts of milk, calcium supplements, or absorptive antacids. The chronic condition is associated with soft tissue calcification of kidneys and nephrocalcinosis. Renal insufficiency may ultimately occur.

▶ Clinical Therapeutics

Suppress PTH secretion to reduce bone resorption with calcitonin. More aggressive therapy may be indicated with pamidronate or bisphosphonates that inhibit osteoclast bone resorption. Use plicamycin for refractory patients. Glucocorticoids are the first line for multiple myeloma, lymphoma, sarcoidosis, or intoxication with vitamin A or D. Medications for chronic hypercalcemia include glucocorticoids, oral phosphates, and indomethacin.

▶ Clinical Intervention

In all cases of very high calcium (>14), hydrate with intravenous (IV) normal saline and initiate diuresis with IV furosemide. Monitor and replace potassium and magnesium. Maintain a high daily intake of fluids (3–5 L/d) and of sodium chloride (>400 mEq/d) to increase renal calcium excretion unless contraindicated. Decrease or discontinue lanoxin dosage since hypercalcemia potentiates lanoxin toxicity. Discontinue vitamins A and D, estrogens, antiestrogens, and thiazide diuretics. Decrease dietary calcium and vitamin D.

Surgical parathyroidectomy is the definitive treatment of primary hyperparathyroidism. A parathyroid scan may localize an adenoma and make surgery more successful. In the presence of a single large parathyroid gland, remove the enlarged gland and, if in question, biopsy other glands. When multiple enlarged glands are present, suspect parathyroid hyperplasia and perform a 3½-gland parathyroidectomy (this leaves a sufficient remnant in the neck or allows transplantation to the forearm to prevent hypocalcemia). Complications include damaged recurrent laryngeal nerve and inadvertent removal and/or devitalization of all parathyroid tissue, resulting in hypocalcemia. Treat hypocalcemia with IV or PO calcium and vitamin D if necessary.

▶ Health Maintenance Issues

Prevent osteoporosis, kidney stones, and compromised kidney function. High recurrence rates of hypercalcemia are associated with parathyroid hyperplasia.

## III. DIABETES AND RELATED DISORDERS

### A. Diabetes Type 1 (Insulin-Dependent Diabetes Mellitus)

▶ Scientific Concepts

Primarily affects juveniles (<25 years of age), but occasionally adults. The majority of cases occur without genetic predisposition. A familial association is found in 10% of cases. There is a 30–50% concordance in monozygotic twins. Diabetes type 1 patients comprise 8% of all patients with diabetes in the United States. There is a lack of insulin secondary to failure of pancreatic beta cells. A virus or environmental insult triggers immune response that alters pancreatic beta cell antigens or molecules of the beta cell. Beta cell function is affected by mumps and coxsackie B4 virus, toxic chemical agents, cytotoxins, or antibodies released by sensitized immunocytes.

### ▶ History & Physical

Sudden onset (1–3 weeks). Commonly symptomatic with polyuria, polydypsia, weakness or fatigue, polyphagia with weight loss, and nocturnal enuresis. May also present with recent blurred vision, vulvovaginitis, or pruritus, other infections, peripheral neuropathy, or diabetic ketoacidosis (DKA).

### ▶ Diagnostic Studies

Fasting blood sugar ≥ 126 mg/dL on two occasions or 2-hour postprandial glucose ≥ 200 mg/dL after 75-g oral glucose load or a random glucose ≥ 200 with symptoms of diabetes (i.e., polydypsia, polyuria, nocturia, etc.). Serum insulin levels are low. Blood glucose is usually 300–500 mg/dL at presentation. Plasma glucagon levels are increased. Ketonemia and/or ketonuria is usually present.

### ▶ Diagnosis

Other causes of diabetes include hormonal excess (Cushing's syndrome, acromegaly, glucagonoma, pheochromocytoma), medications (glucocorticoids, diuretics, or oral contraceptives), insulin receptor unavailability, pancreatic disease (pancreatitis, pancreatectomy, hemochromatosis), genetic syndromes (hyperlipidemias, myotonic dystrophy, lipoatrophy), or gestational diabetes.

### ▶ Clinical Therapeutics

Insulin therapy with split doses of rapid-acting (lispro or regular) and intermediate-acting (NPH or Lente) insulin bid. Adjust dose according to home glucose monitored values.

### ▶ Clinical Intervention

Follow American Diabetes Association (ADA) diet, which allows calorie portion according to the following guidelines: 50% carbohydrates, 30% fat, and 20% protein. Maintain cholesterol intake at < 300 mg/d and sodium intake at < 3,000 mg/d. Reduce animal and saturated fats. Consume smaller portions more frequently. Achieve and maintain ideal weight. Increase exercise cautiously and exercise daily. Acceptable control:
60–120 mg/dL fasting blood sugar (FBS) and preprandial
< 140 mg/dL 2 hours postprandial
Hemoglobin $A_{1c}$ ($HbA_{1c}$) less than 7.0%.

### ▶ Health Maintenance Issues

End-organ damage results in coronary artery disease, hypertension, renal failure, blindness, autonomic and peripheral neuropathy, lower extremity amputations, myocardial infarction, cerebrovascular accidents, and early demise. Forty percent develop end-stage renal disease, a major cause of death. Dyslipidemia is common with goal of low-density lipoprotein (LDL) cholesterol < 100. Provide patient education concerning maintenance of ideal weight, annual ophthalmologic exams, podiatric exams, blood pressure evaluations, serum blood urea nitrogen (BUN) and creatinine, hemoglobin A1C (A1C), urinalysis, and urine microalbumin.

## B. Diabetes Type 2 (Non–Insulin-Dependent Diabetes Mellitus)

### ▶ Scientific Concepts

Type 2 diabetes accounts for 85–90% of the diabetic population. Resistance to insulin is accompanied by decreased beta cell function, causing diminished insulin production. Chronic hyperinsulinemic state exists to work against the peripheral resistance. Eventually, beta cells are unable to maintain this state and decrease in function leading to diabetic state. Endogenous insulin production is usually adequate to avoid ketoacidosis; however, DKA may accompany intense stress. Environmental factors include obesity, diet, physical activity, intrauterine environment, and stress.

### ▶ History & Physical

Onset occurs typically at age > 40 years but not uncommon in people younger than 20. Obesity is present in 80–90% of affected individuals. Strong familial genetic predisposition exists with 100% concordance in monozygotic twins. No association with autoimmune disease. In decreasing frequency, ethnic groups show a predisposition: Native American, Mexican American, African American, white. Usually has gradual onset over several years. Presenting symptoms include polyuria, polyphagia, polydypsia, and/or blurry vision, and one or more neurological or microvascular complications of the disease.

### ▶ Diagnostic Studies

Patients with type 2 diabetes are not ketosis prone under basal condition and do not require exogenous insulin for short-term survival. The following laboratory criteria must be met: FBS ≥ 126 mg/dL on two occasions or 2-hour postprandial glucose ≥ 200 mg/dL after 75-g oral glucose load or random glucose ≥ 200 mg/dL on two occasions with symptoms of diabetes. Random blood sugar at presentation is typically 300–500 mg/dL. Insulin levels may be low, normal, or high.

### ▶ Diagnosis

Other causes of diabetes include hormonal excess (Cushing's syndrome, acromegaly, glucagonoma, pheochromocytoma), medications (glucocorticoids, diuretics, or oral contraceptives), pancreatic disease (pancreatitis, pancreatectomy, hemochromatosis), genetic syndromes (hyperlipidemias, myotonic dystrophy, lipoatrophy), or gestational diabetes.

### ▶ Clinical Therapeutics

Initiate oral agents after failure of diet and exercise. Sulfonylureas stimulate insulin release from beta cells and may increase number of insulin receptors on hepatocytes, thus improving glucose uptake by skeletal muscle and adipose tissue. Expect reduction in blood glucose by 70–80 mg/dL. Side effects include severe hypoglycemia. Sulfonylureas are contraindicated in pregnancy. Biguanides (metformin) decrease hepatic gluconeogenesis. They are ideal for obese patients who have failed maximal sulfonylurea therapy. Fasting and postprandial hyperglycemia and hypertriglyceridemia are improved in the obese without the associated weight gain of insulin or sulfonylurea therapy. Side effects include GI upset, lactic acidosis, and decreased $B_{12}$ absorption. Biguanides (metformin) are contraindicated in type 1 diabetes (IDDM); lactic acidosis prone; renal, cardiorespiratory, or hepatic insufficiency; alcoholics; and elderly. Alpha-glucosidase inhibitors decrease postprandial hyperglycemia by decreasing the rate of absorption of most carbohydrates by binding more readily to intestinal disaccharidases than digested carbohydrate products. They are insulin sparing. Common side effect is flatulence. Thiazolidinediones (TZDs) improve insulin sensitivity in muscle and fat cells and may inhibit hepatic glucose output.

► Clinical Intervention

In crisis, insulin is used to treat severe hyperglycemia, hypertriglyceridemia, ketosis, or hyperosmolarity. If patients continually have elevated fasting and postprandial blood sugars or experience major trauma, stress, or surgery, insulin is often required. Insulin is indicated for all pregnant diabetics who are not diet controlled.

Lifestyle changes involve decreasing calorie intake in order to achieve and maintain ideal weight. Portion calories accordingly: 50% carbohydrates, 30% fat, 20% protein. Reduce cholesterol intake to < 300 mg/d and sodium intake to < 3,000 mg/d. Reduce animal and saturated fats. Exercise after meals or snacks with attention to blood glucose monitoring. Medications are second-line therapy after dietary changes and weight reduction fail to normalize blood glucose levels.

► Health Maintenance Issues

End-organ damage results in hypertension, renal failure, blindness, autonomic and peripheral neuropathy, atherosclerosis, and triglyceridemia. Dyslipidemia is common. Provide patient education concerning maintenance of ideal weight, annual ophthalmologic exams, podiatric exams, blood pressure evaluations, serum BUN and creatinine, urinalysis, and urine microalbumin. Follow $HbA_{1c}$ values for adequate glucose control.

## C. Hyperosmolar Hyperglycemic Nonketotic Coma

► Scientific Concepts

More commonly seen in middle-aged or elderly diabetics. Coexisting congestive heart failure or renal insufficiency is common. Episodes are precipitated by infection (pneumonia, urinary tract infection, or gram-negative sepsis), cerebrovascular accident, myocardial infarction, severe burns, subdural hematoma, acute pancreatitis, use of concentrated glucose solutions, or medications (furosemide, phenytoin, diazoxide, glucocorticoids). It is often associated with endocrine disorders (Cushing's disease, acromegaly, thyrotoxicosis).

Hyperglycemia, hyperglucagonemia, and increased hepatic glucose occur secondary to partial or relative insulin insufficiency. Glycosuria and osmotic diuresis with obligatory water loss ensues. Insulin levels are high enough to prevent lipolysis and ketogenesis but fail to prevent hyperglysuria. Fluid intake is inadequate. Renal insufficiency develops as plasma volume contracts, resulting in increased serum glucose and osmolarity leading to altered state of consciousness.

► History & Physical

Onset is insidious (days to weeks). Weakness, polydipsia, polyuria, weight loss, and progressively diminishing level of consciousness may occur along with evidence of dehydration.

► Diagnostic Studies

Blood glucose usually > 600 mg/dL; serum osmolality > 320 mOsm/L; elevated BUN; sodium and potassium normal, high, or low; ketones normal or mildly increased.

► Diagnosis

Distinguish from DKA, which generally occurs in younger, acidotic patients with type 1 diabetes. Those with hyperosmolar hyperglycemic nonketotic coma (HHNC) are almost always type 2 diabetics

► Clinical Therapeutics

Admit to intensive care unit (ICU); initial therapy is fluid replacement. Monitor clinical and laboratory response to therapy; record fluid type and amount, urine output, blood pressure, pulse, central venous pressure, and ECG.

*Fluid replacement:* Isotonic saline for circulatory collapse, then use 0.45% saline. When blood glucose falls to 250 mg/dL, use 5% dextrose in 0.45 or 0.9% saline.

*Insulin:* If fluid replacement alone is inadequate to decrease glucose, an IV insulin drip with 1–10 units of rapid-acting insulin (regular or lispro), may speed recovery. Then give rapid-acting insulin subcutaneously until oral hypoglycemics are tolerated.

► Clinical Intervention

Evaluate underlying cause with chest x-ray, cardiac enzymes, and serial ECGs. Perform a sepsis evaluation and provide empiric coverage.

► Health Maintenance Issues

Mortality in HHNC is higher than that of DKA since it primarily occurs in the elderly. Manage chronic diabetes and recognize and prevent predisposing factors and/or conditions.

## D. Hypoglycemia

► Scientific Concepts

*Hypoglycemic unawareness:* Chronic type 1 diabetic patients lose counterregulatory hormone secretion, especially glucagon and epinephrine, in response to hypoglycemia. Glucose levels at which a patient perceives symptoms can change. Patients under tight glucose control tend to experience symptoms at lower levels, which gives them less time to respond between onset of symptoms and loss of consciousness. Autonomic neuropathy leads to loss of sympathoadrenal response. *Fasting hypoglycemia* may result from increased insulin, sulfonylureas, or ethanol. It may also occur in the presence of nonbeta cell tumors, hepatic failure, chronic renal failure, adrenal insufficiency, renal failure, insulin autoantibodies, insulin receptor autoantibodies, hormonal deficiency (epinephrine, growth hormone, and glucocorticoids), and/or sepsis. *Postprandial hypo-*

*glycemia* occurs after gastrectomy with dumping syndrome and in some malabsorption syndromes.

▶ History & Physical

**Reactive hypoglycemia** occurs in response to a meal, specific nutrients, or a drug. It is the most common type of hypoglycemia. Symptoms occur 2–4 hours after a meal. The adrenergic response causes the typical symptoms of sweating, tremor, palpitations, anxiety, and hunger. The neuroglucogenic response causes symptoms of headache, dizziness, blurry vision, confusion, decreased fine motor skills, abnormal behavior, seizure, and loss of consciousness. **Spontaneous hypoglycemia** occurs in the fasting state. **Nocturnal hypoglycemia** may cause nightmares, vivid bizarre dreams, night sweats, and/or headache on awakening in morning, poor sleep, feeling unrested, seizure, and/or coma. **Hypoglycemic unawareness** in type I diabetics is particularly dangerous because it is asymptomatic.

▶ Diagnostic Studies

Hypoglycemia is diagnosed when the fasting plasma glucose is < 50 mg/dL and is accompanied by symptoms consistent with hypoglycemia that improve upon administration of IV glucose or ingestion of food (Whipple's triad).

▶ Diagnosis

Evaluate for hypothyroidism, adrenal insufficiency, nephropathy, and malabsorption syndrome. Insulinoma is likely when C peptide level is elevated or when episodes occur spontaneously in patients not taking hypoglycemic medication.

▶ Clinical Therapeutics

Carbohydrate ingestion alleviates symptoms. Frequent blood glucose self-monitoring is recommended.

▶ Clinical Intervention

Give IV glucose or oral carbohydrates immediately and recheck sugar in 15 minutes.

▶ Health Maintenance Issues

Permanent brain damage may result from prolonged severe hypoglycemia.

## IV. DISORDERS OF THE ADRENAL GLAND

### A. Adrenal Insufficiency

▶ Scientific Concepts

Primary adrenal insufficiency results from the destruction of adrenal gland through autoimmune, infiltration, or infectious process.

▶ History & Physical

Weakness, hypoglycemia, weight loss, GI discomfort, salt craving, mucocutaneous hyperpigmentation of lips and buccomucosal membranes, multiple freckles, generalized tan along with areas of vitiligo, decreased axillary and pubic hair, overt or orthostatic hypotension, and/or volume depletion occur.

► Diagnostic Studies

Adrenocorticotropic hormone (ACTH) stimulation test (Cortrosyn stimulation test) shows decreased morning serum cortisol, and increased ACTH. Metabolic acidosis, hyperkalemia, hyponatremia, hypercalcemia, and decreased glucose occur.

► Diagnosis

A normal response to administration of Cortrosyn (increase in plasma cortisol of at least 6 g/dL or a value greater than 20 g/dL) rules out primary adrenal insufficiency. Baseline levels of ACTH are high in primary adrenal insufficiency and low or normal in secondary adrenal insufficiency. Baseline aldosterone levels are low or normal in primary adrenal insufficiency, and there is no response to Cortrosyn.

► Clinical Therapeutics

Replace glucocorticoids using prednisone 5 mg in AM and 2.5 mg in PM or hydrocortisone 20 mg in AM and 10 mg in PM. Increase dose for obese or active persons and with concomitant use of barbiturates, phenytoin, and rifampin. Decrease dose in the elderly and those with liver disease, diabetes mellitus, peptic ulcer disease, and/or hypertension. Replace mineralocorticoids using fludrocortisone 0.05–0.30 mg/d. Increase dose if hypotension, orthostatic hypotension, and/or hyperkalemia occurs. Decrease dose if hypertension, hypokalemia, and/or edema occurs. Increase dose in case of any sudden increase of stress (e.g., accident, fracture, infection, or surgery)

► Clinical Intervention

Chronic adrenal insufficiency may evolve into acute adrenal crisis in the presence of severe infection, trauma, or surgery. Treat fever, dehydration, nausea, and vomiting. Avoid circulatory shock. Give hydrocortisone, 100 mg IV bolus, and repeat q8h. Taper daily dose during recovery by one third of daily dose until maintenance dosage is reached.

► Health Maintenance Issues

Medic Alert bracelets inform of steroid dependency. Adjust glucocorticoid dosage for mild illness or stress (double dose until resolved). Patients should not self-adjust mineralocorticoid dose.

## B. Cushing's Syndrome

► Scientific Concepts

Cushing's syndrome results from chronic glucocorticoid excess. Endogenous causes include disorders of the pituitary (68%), adrenal (17%), and ectopic sources (15%). **Pituitary adenoma (Cushing's disease)** causes increased random and episodic ACTH secretion, resulting in hypersecretion of cortisol and the absence of the normal circadian rhythm, primarily in women of childbearing age. Female:male ratio is 8:1. **Adrenal tumors** cause autonomous production of cortisol. Plasma ACTH levels are low. These tumors occur primarily in children. **Ectopic** causes result from autonomous ACTH production from extrapituitary malignancy (commonly bronchogenic carcinoma). Plasma ACTH levels are elevated. Adult males aged 40 to 60 years are primarily afflicted. **Exogenous** cause is steroid use.

▶ History & Physical

Common findings are central obesity (increased abdominal fat with relatively thin extremities), hypertension, glucose intolerance, plethoric moon facies, purple striae, hirsutism, menstrual dysfunction, sexual dysfunction, general and proximal muscle weakness, dorsocervical and supraclavicular fatty deposition, and/or osteoporosis.

▶ Diagnostic Studies

***Confirm hypercortisolism:*** Overnight dexamethasone suppression test or urinary steroid excretion tests (urinary free cortisol, 17-hydroxy-corticosteroids [17-OHCS]) are performed.

***Differentiate the form of Cushing's:*** Administer high-dose dexamethasone with concomitant measurement of 24-hour urinary 17-OHCS. Evaluate plasma ACTH level. Perform corticotropin-releasing factor (CRF) stimulation test.

***Localization of lesion:*** When pituitary lesion is suspected, perform magnetic resonance imaging (MRI). When adrenal lesion is suspected, perform ultrasound, computed tomography (CT) scan, or MRI. When ectopic lesion is suspected, perform chest x-ray and CT of the chest.

▶ Diagnosis

High-dose dexamethasone test: If urinary 17-OHCS is suppressed to > 50% of baseline, pituitary origin of Cushing's syndrome is likely. Failure to suppress 17-OHCS implies adrenal or ectopic Cushing's syndrome. Plasma ACTH levels measurable in a patient with hypercortisolemia implies ectopic or pituitary Cushing's. An undetectable ACTH level in the presence of hypercortisolemia establishes the diagnosis of adrenal Cushing's syndrome. Patients with pituitary Cushing's syndrome (90%) increase ACTH and cortisol levels upon administration of CRF, while those with ectopic and adrenal Cushing's syndrome have no ACTH or cortisol response. This test differentiates ACTH-dependent from ACTH-independent Cushing's syndrome; however, pituitary may not be distinguished from ectopic if the pituitary fails to respond. Further evaluation with inferior petrosal sinus sampling is warranted.

▶ Clinical Therapeutics

***Pituitary:*** Transphenoid resection of tumor followed by hydrocortisone replacement.

***Adrenal:*** Surgical removal of tumor.

***Ectopic:*** Use adrenal enzyme inhibitors (metyrapone, aminoglutethimide, ketoconazole).

▶ Clinical Intervention

***Pituitary:*** Pituitary microadenomas may be removed selectively; however, the remission rate is 85%. Consider pituitary x-irradiation for the young.

***Adrenal:*** Surgically remove adenomas or carcinoma.

***Ectopic:*** Surgically remove ACTH-secreting tumor if possible (usually not feasible). Consider adrenalectomy or adrenal enzyme inhibitors (metyrapone, aminoglutethimide, ketoconazole) or medical adrenalectomy with mitotane.

▶ **Health Maintenance Issues**

Failure to reduce hypercortisolism results in hypertension, cardiovascular disease, stroke, thromboembolism, susceptibility to infection, and ultimately death. While treatment of Cushing's disease (pituitary adenoma) improves survival, these patients experience increased mortality secondary to cardiovascular disease. There is excellent prognosis for adrenal adenomas but poor prognosis for adrenal carcinoma (life expectancy is 4 years). There is also poor prognosis for ectopic ACTH syndrome due to malignant tumor (life expectancy is days to weeks).

## C. Hirsutism

▶ **Scientific Concepts**

Overproduction of androgens (increased concentration of free testosterone) results from hyperplasia or tumor of adrenal glands and/or ovaries. Hypersensitivity of hair follicles to normal levels of androgens may occur. Increased 5-alpha-reductase activity results in increased conversion of androgens, especially testosterone from steroid precursors in peripheral tissues. Exogenous sources and certain drugs may induce terminal hair growth.

▶ **History & Physical**

Determine age of onset, rate of progression, and family history. Terminal hair growth occurs on upper lip, chin, neck, chest, lower abdomen, back, and inner thighs. Increased sebaceous gland activity causes acne. Anovulation, oligomenorrhea, and amenorrhea may occur. In severe cases, defeminization (breast atrophy, loss of body contours), virilization (frontal balding, increased muscularity, deepened voice, and clitoromegaly), and ovarian enlargement occur.

▶ **Diagnostic Studies**

Measure dehydroepiandrosterone sulfate (DHEA-S), testosterone (total or free), cortisol levels, prolactin level, luteinizing hormone (LH), follicle-stimulating hormone (FSH) levels, and thyroid function tests. Obtain CT of abdomen and ultrasound of ovaries.

▶ **Diagnosis**

***Polycystic ovary syndrome (Stein–Leventhal syndrome):*** Functional disorder of the ovaries that accounts for half the cases of clinical hirsutism. LH:FSH ratio is > 2.0. DHEA-S is normal or minimally elevated. Testosterone or androstenedione are moderately elevated. Serum free testosterone is elevated. Suppress testosterone with combination oral contraceptive.

***Idiopathic or familial:*** Strong familial predisposition with or without elevated androstanediol glucoronide, a metabolite of dihydrotestosterone, which is produced in skin. Hirsutism may be normal in view of genetic background. DHEA-S is normal or minimally elevated. Testosterone, serum free testosterone, and androstenedione are normal.

***Adrenal enzyme defects:*** Deficiency of 21-hydroxylase causes congenital genitalia ambiguity. Without corticosteroid replacement, virilization occurs. Salt wasting may occur. Adult onset of partial defect in 21-hydroxylase occurs without salt wasting. Evaluate serum 17-hydroxyprogesterone at baseline and after cosyntropin injection.

*Rare causes:* ACTH-induced Cushing's syndrome, acromegaly, and ovarian luteoma of pregnancy are rare. Adrenal carcinoma and ovarian tumors may result in elevated testosterone and androstenedione. If DHEA-S is elevated, consider adrenal source. Continue evaluation with pelvic exam and ultrasound and adrenal CT.

▶ Clinical Therapeutics
Suppress ovarian hormone production with oral contraceptives or progestins, glucocorticoids (dexamethasone), finasteride, flutamide, and spironolactone. Do not give antiandrogen therapy to pregnant women.

▶ Clinical Intervention
Laparoscopic bilateral oophorectomy is indicated for postmenopausal women with severe hyperandrogenism. Discontinue drugs that could potentially induce hair growth: androgens, cyclosporine, danazole, diazoxide, minoxidil, and phenytoin. Cosmetic treatment includes waxing, depilatories, shaving, bleaching, or electrolysis.

▶ Health Maintenance Issues
Evaluate and treat infertility.

## V. OTHER ENDOCRINE DISEASES

### A. Electrolyte Disorders

#### 1. Hypocalcemia

▶ Scientific Concepts
Most common cause is renal failure. Other causes include decreased intake or absorption (malabsorption, vitamin D deficit), increased loss (alcoholism, chronic renal insufficiency, diuretic therapy), endocrine causes (hypoparathyroidism, sepsis, pseudohypoparathyroidism, medullary thyroid carcinoma), and physiologic causes (decreased serum albumin, hyperphosphatemia, drug induced).

▶ History & Physical
Patients complain of paresthesias of lips and extremities, muscle cramps, and abdominal pain. Physical examination reveals laryngospasm with stridor, convulsions, ventricular arrhythmias, heart block, Chvostek's sign, and Trousseau's sign.

▶ Diagnostic Studies
Serum calcium is low. Correlate serum calcium with simultaneous concentration of serum albumin. Evaluate serum magnesium. ECG shows prolonged QT interval.

▶ Diagnosis
Renal failure causes decreased production of active vitamin $D_3$ and hyperphosphatemia.

▶ Clinical Therapeutics
Administer calcium gluconate, 10% (4.7 mEq/10 mL) IV 10 to 20 mL over 10–15 minutes, for tetany, arrhythmia, or seizures. Then decrease to 10–15 mg/kg over 4–6 hours. If asymptomatic, give oral calcium carbonate preparations and vitamin D.

▶ Clinical Intervention

Correct underlying defect.

▶ Health Maintenance Issues

Chronic hypocalcemia causes cataracts.

## 2. Gout

▶ Scientific Concepts

Excessive serum uric acid from underexcretion of uric acid by kidneys causes 90% of all gout. The remaining 10% of cases result from overproduction of uric acid. Deposition of monosodium urate crystals from supersaturated extracellular fluids occurs in soft tissue, causing gouty tophi. Deposition in joints causes inflammation known as *gouty arthritis.*

▶ History & Physical

Episodic attacks may be preceded by dehydration secondary to trauma, foods high in proteins and purines, alcohol, drugs (diuretics), surgery, acute medical illness, or renal failure. A monoarticular joint (usually first metatarsophalangeal joint) suddenly becomes severely painful. The midtarsal and ankle are also commonly affected. Other sites include the instep, knee, ankle, and elbow. Sudden onset of asymmetric polyarthritis is atypical for gout. A warm, tender, swollen erythematous joint is noted on physical exam. When multiple joints are affected, patient may be febrile.

▶ Diagnostic Studies

Serum uric acid level is usually elevated at onset of acute attack and may rise when symptoms resolve. If diagnosis is in question, aspirate synovial fluid of affected joint and observe joint fluid for birefringent crystals under polarized light microscopy.

▶ Diagnosis

Monosodium urate crystals (needle-shaped, strongly negative birefringent crystals) and therapeutic response to colchicine within 24–48 hours is pathognomonic for gout. Synovial fluid of pseudogout shows calcium pyrophosphate dihydrate crystals that are rhomboid or polymorphic shaped, weakly positive, and birefringent.

▶ Clinical Therapeutics

Gout prophylaxis agents include indomethacin, naproxen, sulindac, and other nonsteroidal anti-inflammatory drugs (NSAIDs). Allopurinol may be used alone or in combination with colchicine or probenecid as prophylactic therapy for patients with recurrent attacks.

▶ Clinical Intervention

For acute attacks, give colchicine, 1–2 mg diluted in 20 mL of 0.9% sodium chloride IV initially; followed by 0.5 mg IV q 6 to 12 h. IV administration should be slow to avoid extravasation. The maximum IV dose is 4 mg/24 h. Colchicine may also be administered, 0.5–1.2 mg PO initially, then 0.5–0.6 mg q 1–3 h until pain is relieved. The maximum total dose is 8–10 mg. For those who cannot tolerate colchicine or oral medications, consider glucocorticoids (IV or intramuscular [IM] ACTH). Those with monoarticular involvement may be treated with intra-articular administration of methylprednisone or betamethasone.

► Health Maintenance Issues

Avoid foods high in purines (anchovies, sweetbreads) as well as alcohol, aspirin, and diuretics. Evaluate for renal failure.

## B. Dyslipidemia

► Scientific Concepts

Cholesterol and triglycerides are not water-soluble and cannot be transported through the bloodstream as individual molecules. Lipoproteins serve as vehicles that transport cholesterol and triglycerides. The major lipoproteins are: (1) Chylomicrons that transport dietary triglycerides from the gut to adipose tissue and muscle. (2) Very-low-density lipoproteins (VLDL) transport endogenous triglycerides from the liver to adipose tissue and muscle. (3) Low-density lipoproteins (LDL) transport cholesterol from the liver to peripheral tissue. (4) High-density lipoproteins (HDL) transport cholesterol from peripheral tissues to the liver. Elevated LDL cholesterol is associated with an increase risk of heart disease and elevated HDL cholesterol is associated with a decreased risk. Elevated triglycerides are a risk factor for diabetes.

► History & Physical

Family history of dyslipidemia and/or arteriosclerosis, especially coronary artery disease (CAD) prior to age 55, may be present. Often patients are asymptomatic. Corneal arcus (juvenile) may be present. Tendinous xanthomas of the Achilles, patellar, and digital extensor tendons may occur in juveniles.

► Diagnostic Studies

Obtain total cholesterol, HDL, LDL, and triglycerides levels. Creatine phosphokinase (CPK) and hepatic panel should be obtained prior to treatment.

► Diagnosis

Familial hypercholesterolemia—markedly elevated cholesterol; familial combined hyperlipidemia—elevated cholesterol and triglycerides; familial dysbetalipoproteinemia—elevated cholesterol and triglycerides; polygenic hypercholesterolemia—elevated cholesterol; and familial hypertriglyceridemia—elevated triglycerides.

► Clinical Therapeutics

Hepatic hydroxymethyl glutaryl coenzyme A (HMG-CoA) reductase inhibitors (statins) inhibit rate-limiting enzyme in the formation of cholesterol. This class of medicine usually works best and is the first line of medication. These include atorvastatin, lovastatin, pravastatin, simvastatin, and fluvastatin. Most common side effect is myositis. Niacin is effective in mild lowering of cholesterol and raising the HDL, however may be poorly tolerated at full therapeutic doses due to flushing. Resins that bind bile acids lower cholesterol and include cholestyramine and colestipol. Fibric acid derivatives lower triglycerides and include gemfibrozil and clofibrate. Probucol is usually reserved for those patients with genetic disorders that have failed other treatment regimens.

► Clinical Intervention

Low-fat and low-cholesterol diet is recommended. Regular exercise should be encouraged. Achieve and maintain ideal body weight

► Health Maintenance Issues
National Cholesterol Education Program (NCEP) is based on CAD risk factors and the serum LDL cholesterol level:
No CAD or <2 risk factors—goal for LDL < 160
No CAD with 2 or more risk factors—goal for LDL < 130
Known CAD or diabetes—goal for LDL < 100

## BIBLIOGRAPHY

American Diabetes Association. Standards of Medical Care for Patients with Diabetes Mellitus. *Diabetes Care* 25:533–549; 2002.

Andreoli TE, Carpenter CCJ, Plum F, Smith LH, eds. *Cecil's Essentials of Medicine,* 2nd ed. Philadelphia: WB Saunders; 1990.

Begany T. When to screen, when to treat thyroid disease. *JAAPA* 11:72–87; 1998.

Carey CF, Lee HH, Woeltje KF, eds. *The Washington Manual of Medical Therapeutics,* 29th ed. Philadelphia: Lippincott-Raven; 1998.

Ferri FF, ed. *Practical Guide to the Care of the Medical Patient,* 2nd ed. St. Louis, MO: Mosby-Year Book; 1991.

Greenspan FS, Strewler GJ, eds. *Basic and Clinical Endocrinology,* 5th ed. Stamford, CT: Appleton & Lange; 1997.

Braunwald E, Fauci AS, Kasper DL, et al., eds. *Harrison's Principles of Internal Medicine,* 15th ed. New York: McGraw-Hill; 2001.

Largay J. Exercise recommendations for diabetic patients. *JAAPA* 11:22–36; 1998.

Lavin N, ed. *Manual of Endocrinology and Metabolism,* 2nd ed. Boston: Little, Brown and Company; 1994.

McDermott M., *Endocrine Secrets,* 3rd ed. Philadelphia, PA: Hanley & Belfus; 2002.

McTigue J. Cutaneous manifestation of thyroid disorders. *JAAPA* 11:12–17; 1998.

Sadler C, Einhorn D. Tailoring insulin regimens for type 2 diabetes mellitus. *JAAPA* 11:55–71; 1998.

Tierney LM Jr, McPhee SJ, Papadakis MA, eds. *Current Medical Diagnosis & Treatment,* 42nd ed. New York: Lange Medical Books/McGraw-Hill; 2003.

# Rheumatology and Orthopedics  11

*Donna L. Yeisley, MEd, PA-C*

## I. DISORDERS OF THE SHOULDER

### A. Fractures/Dislocations

▶ **Scientific Concepts**

The shoulder joint is one of the most complex in the body. Capable of a large amount of range of motion (ROM), it lacks stability, making it more prone to injury.

***Glenohumeral dislocations:*** The majority occur anteriorly as a result of a fall on an externally rotated, abducted arm.

***Fractures of clavicle:*** One of the most commonly fractured bones in the body, usually as a result of a direct fall against the shoulder or on an outstretched hand. The majority of fractures involve the middle third of the clavicle.

***Fractures of scapula:*** Less common and typically require a high-energy force to result in injury (motor vehicle crashes, falls, severe trauma). The mechanism of injury is a direct blow, trauma to the shoulder, or fall on an outstretched hand. Fractures are classified according to anatomic location, with fractures involving the glenohumeral joint being the most common, and fractures of the body of the scapula the least common.

***Fractures of proximal humerus:*** Minimally displaced or impacted fractures are common in elderly patients usually as a result of indirect trauma that consists of a fall on an outstretched hand with the elbow in extension.

▶ **History & Physical**

***Glenohumeral dislocations:*** Presents with severe pain and resisted attempts at moving the arm. In an anterior dislocation, the arm is held in external rotation with prominence of the acromion giving the shoulder a "squared off" appearance and limited internal rotation. Associated neurovascular injuries may occur, most commonly involving the axillary nerve. This produces decreased pinprick sensation over the deltoid muscle region. Posterior shoulder dislocations present with the arm adducted and internally rotated, a flat anterior and full posterior shoulder region with prominence of the coracoid process, and limited external rotation or abduction.

***Fractures of clavicle:*** Patients present with a history of trauma associated with an onset of swelling, deformity, and localized tenderness. The involved arm is usually held with the other upper extremity. Although there is rarely any neurovascular compromise, it is important to evaluate and document distal pulses, strength, and sensation.

***Fractures of scapula:*** Patients present with a history of trauma associated with tenderness overlying the scapula and the involved arm held in adduction. In more severe trauma cases, thorough evaluation for the presence of associated lung, thoracic cage, or shoulder girdle injury and neurovascular, abdominal, or spinal trauma should also be performed.

***Fractures of proximal humerus:*** Presentation includes a history of trauma, which may be mild especially in the elderly osteoporotic patient, and pain. Exam reveals tenderness and swelling involving the shoulder with or without associated crepitus and ecchymosis. The involved arm is usually held close to the body, and any movement of the arm increases complaints of pain. A thorough evaluation for associated neurovascular injuries should be performed. The most commonly injured nerve is the axillary nerve producing decreased sensation over the deltoid muscle region. The most common vascular injury is to the axillary artery suggested by the presence of paresthesia, pallor, pulselessness, or an enlarging hematoma.

► Diagnostic Studies

*Glenohumeral dislocations:* X-rays should be obtained prior to attempts at reduction. Anteroposterior (AP) views will reveal the dislocation, but the lateral or Y view will indicate whether the dislocation is anterior or posterior. Interpretation of the x-ray may be difficult especially in posterior dislocations.

*Fractures of clavicle:* X-rays of the clavicle will reveal most fractures; however, with fractures that involve the distal or proximal ends of the clavicle, tomograms or computed tomography (CT) scan may be needed.

*Fractures of scapula:* Most fractures are found on plain x-ray. Poorly visualized fractures and any fracture that involves the glenoid should be further evaluated with a CT scan.

*Fractures of proximal humerus:* The majority are diagnosed with plain x-rays of the shoulder. A CT scan can be ordered to further evaluate the bony anatomy or a magnetic resonance imaging (MRI) scan to evaluate soft-tissue injury to the rotator cuff.

► Diagnosis

*Glenohumeral dislocations:* Diagnosed by a thorough history, physical examination, and confirmatory x-rays. Anterior dislocations are common and usually easily diagnosed. Posterior dislocations may be missed and require a higher index of suspicion and more thorough evaluation.

*Fractures of clavicle:* Diagnosed by a history of compatible mechanism of injury and typical physical exam findings, and confirmed by x-ray or other imaging studies.

*Fractures of scapula:* Often diagnosis is missed or delayed due to other injuries sustained by the patient. With high-energy trauma to the thorax, this diagnosis should be considered once the patient is stabilized.

*Fractures of proximal humerus:* Diagnosed easily by history of injury, clinical presentation, and confirmatory imaging study.

► Clinical Therapeutics

After definitive treatment of the dislocation or fracture, analgesics may be prescribed based on the patient's level of pain.

► Clinical Intervention

*Glenohumeral dislocations:* Treated by reduction performed with adequate muscle relaxation and analgesia. Post reduction, the arm is immobilized in a sling for 1 to 2 weeks and then ROM is gradually allowed, avoiding motions that produce known instability.

***Fractures of clavicle:*** Simple fractures usually can be treated with a sling, displaced fractures with the figure-of-eight strap, and distal clavicle fractures with an acromioclavicular joint splint. Length of immobilization depends on patient age, with healing occurring as rapidly as 2 weeks in infants and 4–6 weeks for adults. After 2–3 weeks, the patient should start gentle ROM exercises as pain allows. Progression to strengthening exercises should occur once adequate healing has been documented.

***Fractures of scapula:*** The majority are treated with sling immobilization, ice, and appropriate analgesics. Early mobilization with ROM exercises is important to help prevent the onset of adhesive capsulitis. Any fracture involving articular surfaces, having significant displacement, or associated rotator cuff injury may require surgical repair. Hospital admission for patients with scapular body fractures may be indicated because of the risk of pulmonary contusion.

***Fractures of proximal humerus:*** Minimally displaced or impacted fractures are usually treated with sling or sling and swathe immobilization for 4 weeks with addition of pendulum ROM exercises performed in the sling once pain has subsided, usually about 2 weeks after injury. Full ROM exercises should be encouraged after 4 weeks. Displaced fractures may require closed manipulation and application of a hanging arm cast or open reduction, if closed management fails.

▶ Health Maintenance Issues

***Glenohumeral dislocations:*** The most common issue in anterior dislocations is recurrent dislocation, which is age related. Patients <30 have the highest rate of recurrences and may require corrective surgery. Patients >40 have fewer recurrences and primarily complain of shoulder stiffness that is best treated by brief immobilization with a sling and active ROM to avoid adhesive capsulitis. Older patients, especially those over 60, have an increased risk of an associated rotator cuff tear that requires surgical repair. Posterior dislocations are primarily associated with concomitant fractures. Rotator cuff tears and neurovascular injuries are less common than in anterior dislocations.

***Fractures of clavicle:*** Most fractures of the shaft of the clavicle heal without any complications. Rarely a serious neurovascular complication, such as tear of the subclavian artery or a brachial plexus injury, may occur. Distal clavicle fractures can have an associated tear of the coracoclavicular ligament especially in older adults, which may require surgical repair. Medial clavicle fractures can have associated intrathoracic injuries requiring treatment and may develop late complications of traumatic arthritis.

***Fractures of scapula:*** Isolated fractures heal without significant disability even though some malunion may be present. Associated injuries in more severe trauma may impact on the patient's long-term disability status.

***Fractures of proximal humerus:*** Patients should be encouraged to begin ROM exercises as soon as possible after the injury and sent to physical therapy, if needed. Any fracture involving the anatomic neck or articular surfaces may result in development of aseptic necrosis that may require shoulder arthroplasty in the future.

## B. Rotator Cuff Disorders

▶ Scientific Concepts

The rotator cuff is comprised of the tendons of the supraspinatus, infraspinatus, teres minor, and subscapularis muscles that attach at the humeral tuberosities, with the supraspinatus tendon most commonly involved. Rotator cuff disorders occur along a continuum of injury from mild inflammation to impingement syndrome to partial or full rupture of the rotator cuff. Mechanism of injury involves either acute trauma or is the result of chronic injury leading to degeneration.

▶ History & Physical

***Initial stage of rotator cuff disorders:*** Characterized by inflammation and edema causing presenting symptom of mild pain with activity. Exam reveals mild tenderness over the greater tuberosity without signs of limitation of motion (LOM) or weakness. Most often seen in patients <25 years of age and is completely reversible.

***Second stage of rotator cuff disorders:*** There is increasing tendonitis with symptoms of increasing pain, especially during the night, diffuse tenderness, and complaints of pain with overhead motion. LOM in abduction and external rotation occurs. Pain and crepitus are most severe between 60 and 120 degrees of abduction. Performance of the "impingement sign" by forced internal rotation of the abducted slightly flexed arm may cause impingement of the supraspinatus tendon against the coracoacromial ligament causing increasing complaints of pain.

***Third stage of rotator cuff disorders:*** Progressive degeneration of the rotator cuff and potential partial or complete tears. Majority of patients are >40 and have a chronic history of shoulder symptoms. Acute injury may involve a history of a fall onto an outstretched hand or an attempt to lift a heavy object. Patients have increased complaints of pain, often referred down the deltoid muscle; LOM, especially to abduction and external rotation; and weakness in abduction or flexion. Atrophy of cuff muscles is seen and the "drop-arm" test may be positive. If severe pain is present during the "drop-arm" test, a lidocaine injection into the tendon area can be utilized to relieve pain and the strength is then re-evaluated. Inability to actively maintain 90 degrees of passive shoulder abduction is suggestive of a rotator cuff tear.

▶ Diagnostic Studies

Clinically, it may be difficult to distinguish tendonitis from partial or complete tears of the rotator cuff. X-rays of the shoulder may be indicated in the first several weeks of symptoms, if a patient does not respond to initial treatment. Early findings include chronic changes in the tuberosity of the humerus and calcific deposits or the presence of degenerative arthritis in the acromioclavicular or glenohumeral joint. Plain films also rule out any other causes of shoulder pain. If a tear is suspected, several imaging options are available. An arthrogram helps distinguish between a partial or complete tear, however it is an invasive procedure. Ultrasound is a noninvasive alternative; however, it is most accurate with larger tears. MRI is the imaging test of choice and will reveal the presence of a tear and assess the operability.

► Diagnosis

The diagnosis is based on clinical findings. Imaging studies should be used to confirm the diagnosis, especially if surgery is contemplated.

► Clinical Therapeutics/Clinical Intervention

Treatment of early stage disease consists of rest, ice, sling immobilization, and nonsteroidal anti-inflammatory drugs (NSAIDs). If tendonitis is present, a corticosteroid injection alongside the tendon sheath is often curative. A physical therapy program should be instituted to restore normal motion followed by strengthening exercises to help prevent future recurrences. Partial or small rotator cuff tears may also respond to conservative treatment as outlined above. Surgery should be considered if patients do not respond to conservative treatment or in complete tears with loss of function and chronic pain.

► Health Maintenance Issues

ROM and strengthening exercises are important in the early stages of disease in an attempt to prevent further degeneration. Assessment of work activity and sports intensity with adaptation, if required, is helpful to reduce recurrences. Postoperatively, it is important to restore ROM prior to starting strengthening exercises.

## C. Separations

► Scientific Concepts

*Acromioclavicular separations:* Acromioclavicular (AC) dislocations or subluxations are commonly referred to as separations. Mechanism of injury involves a direct fall onto the tip of the shoulder. Most injuries occur in young, active males. A grade I separation involves a simple contusion or sprain; grade II a rupture of the AC ligaments; and grade III an associated rupture of the coracoclavicular ligaments. Less common and more severe grades ranging from grade IV to VI involve more significant displacement of the AC joint and associated muscle involvement.

*Sternoclavicular separations:* Sternoclavicular (SC) dislocations are rare due to the strong support of the surrounding ligamentous structures. Anterior dislocations are more common than posterior. Anterior dislocations occur as a result of a direct blow to the point of the shoulder, while posterior dislocations result from a direct blow to the clavicle or chest with the shoulder in extension.

► History & Physical

*AC separations:* History will reveal an injury consistent with the mechanism of injury, and patients often hold the arm close to the side of the body complaining of pain with any attempt at lifting the arm. Exam reveals tenderness and swelling over the AC joint with varying decreases in ROM depending on the extent of injury. Downward traction on the arm may increase the deformity.

*SC separations:* Patients present with an injury consistent with the mechanism of injury. Anterior dislocations produce a tender, visible prominence at the SC joint on exam. Although posterior dislocations are much less common, there is increased risk of injury to underlying structures, producing symptoms ranging from mild to moderate pain in the SC region to severe respiratory and vascular compression.

► Diagnostic Studies/Diagnosis

*AC separations:* While the diagnosis is made clinically, standard AC x-rays are ordered to determine the extent of the injury and to look for other fractures. An axillary view is also needed to identify posterior clavicle dislocation that is seen with grade IV dislocations. Differentiation of incomplete versus complete dislocations is routinely done by performing stress x-rays.

*SC separations:* This area is difficult to view with plain x-ray views, however an oblique view may be helpful. A CT scan is usually very sensitive and is the imaging procedure of choice.

► Clinical Therapeutics/Clinical Intervention

*AC separations:* Grade I and II injuries are treated with rest, ice, analgesics, and sling immobilization until acute pain subsides, usually within 2–4 weeks. A rehabilitative program to restore normal ROM and strength should be started as soon as possible. Treatment of grade III dislocations is controversial, especially in athletes and young manual laborers, and a decision between conservative or surgical repair requires thorough consideration of many factors. Any grade IV to VI injuries require evaluation for potential surgical repair.

*SC separations:* Anterior dislocations may be treated with a sling alone or an attempt at closed manipulation and reduction; however, the reduction is difficult to maintain. Pain usually subsides fairly quickly and, except for minor cosmetic deformity, function is not impaired. Even though open reduction is an option, it is rarely justified in an acute injury. Posterior dislocations often have associated life-threatening injuries that will require immediate attention. After stabilization, orthopedic consult for closed versus open reduction should be obtained.

► Health Maintenance Issues

*AC separations:* The majority of grade I or II AC injuries heal without further incidence; however, a small percent may develop late symptoms requiring excision of the distal clavicle. Athletes should be fully evaluated before return to sports is allowed.

*SC separations:* Anterior dislocations may result in some cosmetic deformity, but function is preserved. Posterior dislocations require immobilization after reduction followed by a simple exercise program to maintain strength in the upper extremity.

## D. Sprain/Strain

► Scientific Concepts

A sprain involves a joint and the stretching and tearing of ligaments, whereas a strain involves injury to the muscle or tendon. Sprains more specifically refer to the joint injury in which a dislocation has not taken place, but the ligaments are damaged. The most common location for shoulder sprain/strain involves the AC separations, grades I to III, as discussed above.

## II. DISORDERS OF THE FOREARM/WRIST/HAND

### A. Fractures/Dislocations

#### 1. Boxer's

▶ Scientific Concepts

This describes a fracture of the neck of the fifth metacarpal that results from a direct impaction force when a clenched fist strikes a hard object, such as occurs in fistfights, hence the name "boxer's fracture." It is the most common fracture involving the hand.

▶ History & Physical

Presents with a history consistent with the mechanism of injury, swelling and tenderness over the fracture site, a depression of the "knuckle" of the involved finger, and decreased ROM. The degree of dorsal angulation must be evaluated, as it will impact treatment decisions. The hand should also be assessed for the presence of rotational deformity by asking the patient to flex the fingers and noting any overlap of the fifth finger. Normally all the fingers should point to the navicular region. Distal sensation should also be assessed.

▶ Diagnostic Studies/Diagnosis

X-rays of the hand with posteroanterior (PA), lateral, and oblique views should be ordered.

▶ Clinical Intervention

Fractures with minimal displacement (<15 degrees) may be treated with a compression dressing or ulnar gutter splint for 1–2 weeks, followed by gradually increasing active exercises. Fractures with angulation between 15 and 40 degrees should be reduced prior to immobilization in an ulnar gutter splint for 3–4 weeks. Open reduction with percutaneous pin fixation may be indicated with angulation >40 degrees, if closed reduction is unsuccessful. In managing fractures of the hand, it is also important to recognize and treat any rotational as well as angular deformity to avoid resultant functional disability.

▶ Health Maintenance Issues

Fractures of the fifth metacarpal will not have any functional impairment if <40 degrees of angulation is present after healing. Fractures involving the other metacarpals tolerate smaller degrees of angulation and should be referred if any doubt of alignment is present.

#### 2. Colles'

▶ Scientific Concepts

This is the most common injury of the wrist and is seen in the elderly after a fall on the outstretched hand. The resultant fracture involves the distal radial metaphysis that is dorsally angulated and displaced, resulting in the typical "silver-fork" deformity. An associated fracture of the ulna styloid or injury to the ulnar collateral ligament of the wrist may be seen.

▶ History & Physical

Presents with history compatible with mechanism of injury. On exam, the wrist has a characteristic dorsiflexion or silver-fork deformity associated with pain, tenderness, and swelling. Palmar paresthesias may be present if there is associated compression of the median nerve. Assessment of distal neurovascular status should be performed. Examine the elbow for any signs of swelling or tenderness.

▶ Diagnostic Studies/Diagnosis

Based on clinical findings and confirmed by x-ray findings of a distal metaphyseal fracture of the radius with dorsal angulation and comminution. X-ray evaluation should include AP and lateral views of the forearm, including the wrist. X-rays of the elbow should also be ordered if there are any positive physical exam findings at the elbow region.

▶ Clinical Intervention

Treatment options include closed reduction with splinting and casting, percutaneous pin fixation, open reduction and internal fixation with plate and screws, and external fixation. The choice of treatment depends on many factors including the patient's age; fracture displacement, angulation, and degree of comminution; presence or absence of intra-articular involvement; and the desired level of functional ability post treatment.

▶ Health Maintenance Issues

Potential complications include malunion, joint instability, median nerve injury, and development of traumatic arthritis that can lead to a weak, stiff, and painful wrist.

3. Gamekeeper's Thumb

▶ Scientific Concepts

The most common injury to the metacarpophalangeal (MP) joint is sprain of the ulnar collateral ligament of the thumb, commonly referred to as *gamekeeper's thumb* or *skier's thumb*. Mechanism of injury involves the forceful abduction of the thumb away from the hand. Injury may include a tear of the ligament at the insertion into the proximal phalanx with the potential of associated dorsal capsule and volar plate injury.

▶ History & Physical

A history of an acutely sprained thumb, often from a fall on the hand or a chronic history of instability of the thumb associated with instability, weakness of the pincher grasp, and recurrent swelling of the MP joint are the usual presentations. Exam reveals local tenderness on the ulnar side of the MP joint and joint effusion. Once x-rays have been taken and a fracture is ruled out, clinical evaluation for joint instability by applying lateral and medial stresses to the joint is mandatory. If angulation of the finger occurs with stress, it indicates a tear of the collateral ligament; however if the patient has pain, but no instability, a sprain is diagnosed.

▶ Diagnostic Studies/Diagnosis

AP and lateral x-rays of the thumb are necessary to rule out fracture or fracture–dislocation prior to clinical assessment of stability. Stress views of the thumb may be ordered to accurately assess the degree of radial angulation, which indicates the severity of the tear of the ulnar collateral ligament.

▶ Clinical Intervention

Closed management involving application of a thumb spica splint or cast with immobilization for 3–5 weeks is usually sufficient for a sprain or partial ligamentous tear. Radial deviation of >30–40 degrees indicates a complete rupture of the ligament and requires surgical repair.

▶ Health Maintenance Issues

Patients may experience chronic symptomatic manifestations of ulnar collateral ligament injury. Surgical repair may be indicated to relieve these symptoms. In the presence of traumatic arthritis or if ligament repair is not possible, arthrodesis of the MP joint can be performed.

## 4. Humeral

▶ Scientific Concepts

Fractures involving the distal humerus are relatively uncommon in adults, but usually have a high risk for complications due to intra-articular involvement and the comminuted nature of most of the fractures involving the elbow region. Fracture types include supracondylar, transcondylar, intercondylar, T condylar, and lateral or medial condylar fractures. The most common elbow fracture found in children is the supracondylar fracture, which occurs as the result of an extension force causing posterior displacement.

▶ History & Physical

Patients present with a history of trauma and complaints of pain that increases with attempted flexion of the elbow. Exam reveals findings of edema, ecchymosis, and tenderness to palpation. Deformity will be present with any displaced fracture. Careful inspection should be done to look for any puncture wounds, indicating an open fracture. Evaluation of neurovascular integrity both proximally and distally is mandatory. The most common injury is to the ulnar nerve. Brachial artery occlusion, while not common, requires early recognition and treatment to avoid serious complications.

▶ Diagnostic Studies/Diagnosis

Minimal x-ray evaluation includes an AP and lateral view of the elbow. If there is no evidence of an obvious fracture, evaluate for the presence of a positive fat pad sign, indicating an occult fracture of the radial head. Further views of the elbow should be ordered as clinically indicated.

▶ Clinical Intervention

Treatment depends on several factors including the presence or absence of fracture displacement, intra-articular involvement, neurovascular compromise, and closed versus open fracture. The ultimate goal of treatment is to achieve and maintain reduction while allowing early range of motion of the joint. For simple nondisplaced fractures, closed management with some form of immobilization, splinting or casting, is sufficient. It is important to begin rehab with ROM, progressing to strengthening exercises as soon as possible. The majority of displaced fractures, markedly comminuted fractures, or fractures with any neurovascular compromise require surgical intervention.

▶ Health Maintenance Issues

The majority of adult patients with fractures involving the distal humerus will experience some degree of residual pain and stiffness. Other complications may include deformity, nonunion, ulnar neuropathy, and complications from vascular injury, such as ischemia of the forearm or compartment syndrome.

### 5. Nursemaid's Elbow

▶ **Scientific Concepts**

Subluxation of the radial head is often referred to as *nursemaid's elbow* or *pulled elbow*. It is the most common elbow injury in children under the age of 5 due to increased ligamentous laxity. Mechanism of injury is sudden traction on the hand while the elbow is in extension and the forearm is pronated, such as occurs when a child is lifted by the wrist or hand. This results in slippage of the annular ligament, which becomes entrapped between the radius and ulna.

▶ **History & Physical**

Initially the child may complain of pain, but this quickly subsides. The usual presentation is a complaint that the child refuses to use the arm and holds it in a slightly flexed and pronated position. Exam reveals tenderness over the radial head and resistance on attempted supination of the forearm.

▶ **Diagnostic Studies/Diagnosis**

Diagnosis is based on clinical findings. X-rays of the elbow are not necessarily indicated unless the history suggests another diagnosis or if reduction attempts are not successful.

▶ **Clinical Intervention**

Reduction should be carried out as soon as possible. Supinating and flexing the forearm while applying manual pressure over the radial head that is associated with a palpable click usually reduces this subluxation. If reduction is successful, the child should begin using the arm in a few minutes.

▶ **Health Maintenance Issues**

For a child with recurrent subluxations of the radial head, orthopedic consult is indicated. Recurrent subluxations often require some form of immobilization in a sling or possible cast.

### 6. Scaphoid

▶ **Scientific Concepts**

The scaphoid, or navicular, bone is the most common carpal bone to be fractured. Mechanism of injury involves a fall on an outstretched hand. The blood supply usually enters the distal portion of the bone and consequently fractures involving the mid-portion or proximal portion of the scaphoid are at increased risk for development of avascular (aseptic) necrosis.

▶ **History & Physical**

Patients may initially fail to seek medical attention at the time of injury thinking that they have only "sprained" the wrist. A history of trauma to the wrist should be asked about, and the patient usually complains of pain upon any attempted movement of the wrist. On exam, there is tenderness over the radial aspect of the wrist and the anatomical snuffbox. Other findings may include decreased wrist ROM and decreased grip strength. Neurovascular status should also be assessed.

▶ **Diagnostic Studies/Diagnosis**

Diagnosis is sometimes difficult, and a high degree of suspicion may be needed to appropriately diagnose and treat these fractures. Any patient who complains of chronic sprain signs and symptoms, especially with tenderness in the anatomical snuffbox region, should be treated for a suspected scaphoid fracture despite apparent negative x-rays. Initial x-rays of the wrist, including standard and scaphoid views, may fail to reveal evidence of fracture due to lack of displacement of the fracture fragments. Subsequent repeat x-rays in 2–3 weeks may reveal the presence of decalcification around the fracture. If this repeat x-ray is negative and the patient is still symptomatic, a bone scan or MRI should be considered.

► Clinical Intervention

Fractures of the scaphoid are best managed by orthopedic specialists. As mentioned above, even if initial x-rays are negative, the patient should be immobilized in a thumb spica splint or cast pending further evaluation. It is often difficult to determine the adequacy of fracture healing on routine x-ray evaluation. Length of immobilization can be generally dictated by the location of the fracture. Fractures of the distal pole should be immobilized for 6–8 weeks, mid-portion fractures for 8–12 weeks, and proximal fractures may require 12–24 weeks of immobilization or longer. If plain x-rays fail to reveal the amount of healing that has taken place, a tomogram should be considered. Displaced fractures or fractures that fail to heal may require surgical intervention.

► Health Maintenance Issues

These fractures are at high risk for development of nonunion, avascular necrosis and traumatic arthritis.

## B. Sprains/Strains

► Scientific Concepts

The majority of ligamentous injuries of the wrist involve the lunate due to its central location. Mechanism of injury involves forced dorsiflexion of the wrist usually sustained in a fall on the outstretched hand. The scapholunate ligament is the most commonly involved ligament. The extent of injury can vary from ligamentous injury to dislocation of the perilunate and lunate. Although ligamentous injuries of the wrist do occur, it is important to consider several other common wrist injuries that may present as "sprains," including navicular fractures as mentioned above.

► History & Physical

Patients present with a history of injury or chronic complaints of wrist pain. With scapholunate ligament involvement, pain and swelling on the radial aspect of the wrist sometimes associated with a clicking sensation upon movement of the wrist is found.

► Diagnostic Studies/Diagnosis

A simple sprain of the wrist should be a diagnosis of exclusion after consideration of other more serious conditions that may present with signs and symptoms of a "sprain." A routine wrist x-ray series is always indicated in evaluation to rule out any anatomical abnormality. Immobilization should be part of initial treatment even with an initial negative x-ray.

► Clinical Therapeutics/Clinical Intervention

Initial treatment consists of ice, elevation, and NSAIDs as necessary. The wrist should also be initially immobilized in a splint device during the acute phase until further evaluation can be performed in 1–2 weeks to rule out any more serious conditions, such as fracture or ligamentous rupture. An orthopedic consult is required for any evidence of joint instability, failed conservative treatment after 3 weeks, or ligamentous rupture.

#### ▶ Health Maintenance Issues

Osteonecrosis of the lunate bone (Kienbock disease) may occur secondary to an unrecognized fracture or with any injury that disrupts the blood supply. Initial x-rays are often negative for fracture, so a high index of suspicion is needed. The most appropriate imaging study for a suspected lunate fracture is an MRI. Progression of the disease eventually leads to end-stage arthritis of the wrist resulting in loss of motion, chronic pain, and decreased grip strength.

## C. Tenosynovitis

### 1. Carpal Tunnel Syndrome

#### ▶ Scientific Concepts

This is the most common entrapment neuropathy of the upper extremity involving the median nerve. Common precipitating factors include repetitive overuse trauma, pregnancy, rheumatoid arthritis, hypothyroidism, and associated neuritis from diabetes mellitus.

#### ▶ History & Physical

Patients present with initial complaints of intermittent pain, numbness, and tingling involving the thumb, index, and middle finger consistent with median nerve distribution. These symptoms are often greatest at night, waking the patient from sleep. They may also be precipitated by various repetitive activities performed with the wrist in flexion, such as typing and painting. An associated sense of weakness and clumsiness when attempting to use the hand may be seen. On exam, decreased sensation may be found along the sensory distribution of the median nerve. Reproduction of tingling or shooting pain upon volar wrist percussion (Tinel's sign) or when the patient flexes both wrists to 90 degrees with the dorsal aspects of the hands held in apposition for 60 seconds (Phalen's sign) are highly suggestive of carpal tunnel syndrome. A late finding is the presence of atrophy of the thenar muscles. Weakness of this muscle group can be evaluated by testing thumb opposition against resistance. A loss of two-point discrimination may also be found.

#### ▶ Diagnostic Studies/Diagnosis

Diagnosis is based on typical clinical findings. Further evaluation with electromyography (EMG) and/or nerve conduction velocity tests (NCV) is indicated in patients who fail conservative treatment and are being considered for surgical intervention.

#### ▶ Clinical Therapeutics/Clinical Intervention

Conservative treatment of early or mild carpal tunnel syndrome consists of rest; use of a cock-up splint, especially while sleeping; and a short course of anti-inflammatories, either NSAIDs or oral corticosteroids. An injection of corticosteroid into the carpal tunnel may also be helpful in relieving symptoms, but relief is usually temporary. Carpal tunnel syndrome associated with pregnancy should be treated conservatively, because complaints often resolve spontaneously after delivery. Patients who fail conservative measures, have presence of motor weakness, or have thenar atrophy should be evaluated for surgical intervention.

▶ Health Maintenance Issues

Carpal tunnel syndrome due to work-related repetitive activities may benefit from implementation of ergonomic modifications. In the presence of thenar atrophy, complete muscle strength, even after operative intervention, may not return. Permanent loss of sensation is also possible.

## 2. de Quervain's Tenosynovitis

▶ Scientific Concepts

A common condition involving the first dorsal extensor compartment of the wrist that occurs with overuse of the thumb resulting in inflammation involving the sheath that surrounds the abductor pollicis longus and extensor pollicis brevis tendons on the radial side of the wrist.

▶ History & Physical/Diagnosis

Patients present with complaints of pain involving the radial side of the wrist that is made worse with any lifting motion that requires the thumb to be in adduction and flexion and the wrist to be ulnarly deviated (picking a newborn up from a crib, making a fist, etc.). Patients with involvement of the radial sensory nerve may also complain of tingling or numbness. On exam, swelling and tenderness is noted over the distal radius. Active and passive ROM makes the pain worse and crepitus may be noted. Reproduction of pain upon ulnar deviation of the wrist with the thumb in full flexion within the palm of the hand (Finkelstein test) is considered diagnostic.

▶ Clinical Therapeutics/Clinical Intervention

Initial treatment of mild disease includes NSAIDs and immobilization with a thumb spica splint for 10–14 days. The splint should be periodically removed to apply moist heat and perform gentle ROM exercises to avoid joint stiffness. If symptoms continue despite immobilization, the tendon sheath may be injected with corticosteroid. Patients who fail to respond to conservative therapy should be evaluated for surgical intervention.

▶ Health Maintenance Issues

Recurrences may occur especially if the condition is work related and these cases should be referred for evaluation. Potential complications include chronic pain, loss of strength, or loss of thumb motion.

## 3. Elbow Tendonitis

Tendonitis is defined as an inflammatory condition of a tendon, which usually results from overuse. Elbow tendonitis is often considered synonymous with epicondylitis (see below), however the pathogenesis of epicondylitis involves degeneration of the tendinous unit and microtears, rather than inflammation.

## 4. Epicondylitis

▶ Scientific Concepts

*Lateral epicondylitis:* This condition is also referred to as *tennis elbow.* Symptoms are usually produced as a result of overuse causing degeneration of the tendinous attachments to the extensor muscles at the lateral epicondyle of the humerus. The most common site of involvement is the tendon of the extensor carpi radialis brevis. Repetitive wrist extension against resistance, such as occurs in tennis, is the primary mechanism of injury. Lateral epicondylitis is more common than medial.

***Medial epicondylitis:*** This condition also referred to as *golfer's elbow,* can be seen in any racquet or pitching sport. Symptoms occur as a result of overuse causing degeneration of the tendinous attachments to the flexor muscles at the medial epicondyle of the humerus.

▶ History & Physical

***Lateral epicondylitis:*** Patients present with gradual onset of pain aggravated by pronation of the forearm and concomitant dorsiflexion of the wrist (backhand serve in tennis, opening a jar or lifting). Exam reveals localized tenderness distal to the lateral condyle, reproduction of pain with resisted extension of the wrist while the elbow is in extension, and pain when lifting with the palm down.

***Medial epicondylitis:*** Symptoms of medial epicondylitis usually occur with active wrist flexion and forearm pronation involving the activities listed above. Exam findings include localized tenderness just distal to the medial condyle; reproduction of pain with resisted pronation of the forearm with the wrist in flexion and pain when lifting with the palm up. Associated ulnar nerve compression at the elbow may occur with medial epicondylitis. Acute rupture of the ulnar ligament may also occur, especially with throwing injuries. The patient usually complains of a "popping sensation" that occurred at the time of the throw.

▶ Diagnostic Studies/Diagnosis

Even though both lateral and medial epicondylitis are primarily diagnosed by clinical assessment, AP and lateral x-ray views of the elbow should be considered to evaluate for the presence of arthritis or osteochondral loose bodies.

▶ Clinical Therapeutics/Clinical Intervention

The majority of patients will respond to rest, especially from the offending activity; NSAIDs; and application of heat or ice. Use of a tennis elbow counter force strap may also be helpful. Once symptoms have subsided, stretching and strengthening exercises should be initiated. Local injections of corticosteroid in the area of maximum tenderness may also provide permanent relief. Surgery is reserved for severe cases that fail to respond to conservative treatment.

▶ Health Maintenance Issues

These conditions are usually self-limiting, but symptoms may continue for several months before full recovery. Some patients will have persistent pain and associated weakness with motions that involve forceful wrist extension or forearm supination.

## III. DISORDERS OF BACK/SPINE

### A. Ankylosing Spondylitis

▶ Scientific Concepts

Belongs to a group of disorders classified as seronegative spondyloarthropathies that also include psoriatic arthritis, reactive arthritis (Reiter's syndrome), and arthritis associated with inflammatory bowel disease. These disorders share many characteristics including inflammatory arthritis of the spine or large peripheral joints, presence of HLA-B27 antigen, and are seronegative for rheumatoid factor. HLA-B27 association is greatest with ankylosing spondylitis, being found in almost 90% of patients. The exact cause of the inflammation in ankylosing spondylitis is unknown. The inflammatory process usually starts in the sacroiliac joints and slowly progresses up the spine, eventually leading to bony fusion or ankylosis.

► **History & Physical**

Most common in young men aged 15–30. Onset is usually insidious with complaints of diffuse low back pain associated with morning stiffness that slowly progresses to loss of spinal movement and chest expansion. Some have associated complaints of peripheral arthritis and/or uveitis. Rarely aortitis and associated conduction defects are seen.

► **Diagnostic Studies/Diagnosis**

Early diagnosis is often difficult due to the insidious onset of the back symptoms and usual lack of systemic symptoms. Earliest x-ray changes involve sclerosis of the sacroiliac joints that eventually progress to ossification of the annulus fibrosis, calcification of spinal ligaments, and demineralized vertebral bodies that have a "squared off" appearance, often referred to as *bamboo spine*. HLA-B27 is usually positive, while rheumatoid factor is usually negative. An elevated sedimentation rate and findings consistent with mild anemia may be found.

► **Clinical Therapeutics/Clinical Intervention**

Initial treatment consists of the use of NSAIDs, usually indomethacin, and a physical therapy program that encourages mobilization and flexibility exercises to help maintain posture. Sulfasalazine has been shown to help with peripheral arthritis, but does not seem to benefit patients with primarily spinal symptoms. Some patients may develop severe bony changes that require surgical intervention.

► **Health Maintenance Issues**

The majority have persistent symptoms over decades. Progression of the disease is variable, and the importance of maintaining posture and avoiding thoracic kyphosis is paramount to prognosis. Patients who develop hip disease within the first 2 years of disease onset have the worst prognosis.

## B. Back Strain/Sprain

► **Scientific Concepts**

Low back pain due to muscular or ligamentous injury is very common. Primary causes include acute trauma or repetitive overload. Most acute injuries are self-limiting and heal well, but if an acute injury occurs in a patient with a chronic back condition, the course is more prolonged. Predisposing factors include increasing age (age 30–50 years); repetitive movements, such as lifting, pulling, bending, and twisting; and exposure to chronic vibration and prolonged sitting. Contributing factors include sedentary lifestyle, obesity, smoking, poor posture, and emotional stress.

► **History & Physical**

The majority of patients with acute back pain can relate a specific event that caused the onset of pain. The trauma may be as innocent as bending to pick something up from the floor. Patients often complain of radiation of the pain into the buttocks and/or radicular pain below the knee (sciatica), which suggests inflammation of the nerve roots or bulging of the nucleus pulposis (see below). The main focus of the history should be to determine if the patient has a more serious cause, such as infection, metastasis, inflammatory back disease, or a nonrheumatologic disorder, such as a leaking aortic aneurysm. Any history of urinary or bladder symptoms should be automatically referred for further evaluation. Exam reveals tenderness to palpation and spasm of the paravertebral muscles with a loss of the normal lumbar curve. There is decreased ROM in all planes, but especially in flexion. The neurologic exam, including sensory, motor, and reflexes, is usually within normal limits. Any evidence of significant or progressive neurologic deficits should be further evaluated.

▶ Diagnostic Studies

Lumbar x-rays are usually not indicated in the initial evaluation of acute low back pain, unless history suggests any of the more serious causes of low back pain. Any low back pain that fails to improve with conservative treatment of 4–6 weeks or begins to develop neurologic deficits should also be further evaluated with lumbar x-rays followed by MRI or CT scan, if indicated.

▶ Diagnosis

The diagnosis of low back strain/sprain is usually a clinical diagnosis; however, since muscle strain, ligament sprain, and mild early bulging of the nucleus pulposis all present with similar clinical signs and symptoms, the exact cause may not be determined. Regardless of cause, the initial treatment of each of these conditions is the same.

▶ Clinical Therapeutics/Clinical Intervention

The majority of patients will improve with conservative measures within 1–4 weeks. The most important focus of treatment should be treatment of acute symptoms with return to work as soon as possible, even in a limited capacity (light duty). Acute back strain/sprain usually responds to a short period of relative rest (3–5 days), NSAIDs or other non-narcotic analgesic (7–14 days), and gradual increase in activities as tolerated.

▶ Health Maintenance Issues

Education to help prevent recurrences is vital. This includes instruction in proper body mechanics, as well as muscle strengthening for the back and abdomen with a back flexibility program.

## C. Cauda Equina Syndrome

▶ Scientific Concepts

Cauda equina refers to the anatomical location of the spinal canal below the L1–L2 level, which contains the L2–S4 nerve roots. Sudden compression of these peripheral nerve roots causes the cauda equina syndrome. This may result from a large central disc herniation, epidural abscess or hematoma, and trauma, including fractures.

▶ History & Physical

Patients present with a history of trauma, preexisting spinal stenosis with a sudden increase in symptoms, or recent spine surgery with onset of fever/chills and increasing back and leg pain. The majority complain of difficulty with urination and/or bowel control associated with bilateral radicular pain and numbness. Exam reveals evidence of loss of motor and sensory function of the lower extremities, including poor anal sphincter tone and/or perianal numbness (saddle anesthesia).

▶ Diagnostic Studies/Diagnosis

Diagnosis is made on the clinical findings. Lumbar spine x-rays may be considered to rule out the presence of any structural problem such as a fracture or spondylolisthesis.

▶ Clinical Intervention

Cauda equina syndrome is a true surgical emergency and requires prompt surgical decompression.

▶ Health Maintenance Issues

Prognosis is considered good since peripheral nerves are able to regenerate; however, permanent paralysis and loss of sphincter tone are possible.

## D. Herniated Disk Pulposis

▶ Scientific Concepts

Disk herniations occur as the nucleus pulposis bulges, protrudes, or extrudes from the annulus fibrosis, usually posteriolaterally. Herniations most commonly involve the cervical regions of C5–C6 (C6 nerve root) or C6–C7 (C7 nerve root) and the lumber regions of L4–L5 (L5 nerve root) and L5–S1 (S1 nerve root). Although disc herniation may occur acutely with trauma, the more common cause is chronic degeneration secondary to increasing age (third and forth decades) and repetitive microtrauma.

▶ History & Physical

Pain in the cervical or lumbar region and radicular pain associated with numbness and paresthesias of the involved area are common. With lumbar involvement, coughing or sneezing may aggravate the pain. Exam reveals findings as outlined above with back strain/sprain; however, sensory changes along the involved dermatome, motor weakness of the involved muscle group, or reflex changes may be seen. Findings consistent with C6 nerve root involvement include decreased sensation on the dorsolateral aspect of the thumb and index finger, weakness in elbow flexion and wrist extension, and a decreased brachioradialis reflex. Findings consistent with C7 nerve root involvement include decreased sensation on the middle finger; weakness in elbow extension, wrist flexion, and finger extension; and a decreased triceps reflex. Findings consistent with L5 nerve root involvement include decreased sensation on the lateral aspect of the lower leg and dorsum of the foot, decreased dorsiflexion of the great toe, and trouble heel walking without any reflex involvement. Findings consistent with S1 nerve root involvement include decreased sensation on the lateral side of the ankle and plantar surface of the foot, trouble with toe walking, and a decreased Achilles reflex. With involvement of the lumbar area, straight-leg raising (SLR) is also usually positive. The additional presence of a positive contralateral SLR increases the probability of the presence of a herniated disk.

▶ Diagnostic Studies/Diagnosis

Most patients are diagnosed clinically and require no further diagnostic evaluation. Diagnostic evaluation is indicated in the presence of progressing neurologic deficits, failure to respond to conservative treatment (after 6–8 weeks), or if surgery is being considered. X-rays are usually performed first, and they may demonstrate disc space narrowing or may be normal. A MRI or CT scan with myelography will allow visualization of the disk and neural elements. One of these imaging studies should be obtained if surgical treatment is being considered. EMG studies will show changes after several weeks of symptoms and are especially helpful in defining the cause of cervical radiculopathy.

▶ Clinical Therapeutics/Clinical Intervention

The majority respond to conservative treatment as outlined above for low back strain/sprain. With cervical involvement, the use of a soft cervical collar during the acute phase may be of benefit. In patients with cervical or lumbar radicular pain, a short course of steroids may be indicated. Surgical intervention is reserved for patients who fail to respond to at least 6 weeks of conservative treatment or progressive neurologic signs.

▶ Health Maintenance Issues

Muscle paralysis, weakness, or chronic pain syndromes may develop. As previously discussed, a rare but serious complication of lumbar disk disease is cauda equina syndrome (see above). Prognosis postoperatively is better in patients whose leg pain is more severe than the back pain.

## E. Kyphosis/Scoliosis

▶ Scientific Concepts

**Kyphosis:** The normal contour of the spine includes cervical lordosis, thoracic kyphosis, and lumbar lordosis. Any change in the anteroposterior direction where the convexity is directed posteriorly is referred to as *kyphosis*. The most common causes include diseases of the discs and vertebral spaces. Congenital kyphosis may occur, but it is rare.

**Scoliosis:** Lateral curvature of the spine >10 degrees is considered scoliosis. Nonstructural scoliosis is due to a compensatory mechanism seen with leg length discrepancy or acute lumbar disc disease. The majority of structural scoliosis is due to idiopathic scoliosis with no known cause.

▶ History & Physical

**Kyphosis:** Relatively common in the elderly, especially in women, resulting from multiple areas of disc degeneration in the thoracic region. Patients may be symptomatic, often complaining of pain. On exam, the dorsal curve of the thoracic spine is accentuated, producing kyphosis and increasing the anteroposterior diameter of the chest.

**Scoliosis:** Idiopathic scoliosis is most commonly seen in preadolescent girls beginning between 8 and 10 years of age and progressing with growth. The patient is asymptomatic, and the presence of pain should indicate a need for diagnostic evaluation to rule out an underlying disorder. Check for vertebral and rotational deformities by having the patient bend forward and observe for the presence of a rib hump or abnormal paraspinal prominence of the muscles.

▶ Diagnostic Studies/Diagnosis

*Kyphosis:* X-rays of the thoracic spine reveal narrowing of the disc spaces, osteopenia, and an accentuated dorsal curve of the vertebral bodies.

*Scoliosis:* Diagnosis is confirmed by AP and lateral views of the spine with the patient standing. The degree of curvature is calculated by determining the Cobb angle. Indications for MRI include pain, neurologic deficit, or a left thoracic curve.

▶ Clinical Therapeutics/Clinical Intervention

*Kyphosis:* Exercises that strengthen the back and abdominal muscles help to maintain good posture. A light spinal support and use of mild analgesics may also help to relieve the symptomatic patient.

*Scoliosis:* Follow-up and treatment depend on multiple factors including the degree of curvature, skeletal maturity of the patient, and risk of progression. In general, curves <20 degrees are observed, progressive curves between 20 and 40 degrees are braced, and any curve >40–45 degrees should be evaluated for surgical correction.

▶ Health Maintenance Issues

*Kyphosis:* Respiratory function is usually not hampered unless the curvature is marked.

*Scoliosis:* Early detection, observation, and intervention as needed allow for the best outcome possible. Some curves will progress despite bracing, and referral for surgical correction should be made. Curves that progress to >60 degrees are associated with poor respiratory function in adulthood and a shortened life span.

## F. Low Back Pain

▶ Scientific Concepts

Even though the majority of low back pain is caused by lumbar strain/sprain or disk herniation (see above), more serious causes, such as infection, metastasis, inflammatory back disease, or a nonrheumatologic disorder, such as a leaking aortic aneurysm, must also be considered.

▶ History & Physical

Vertebral osteomyelitis should be suspected in a patient with a history of recurrent urinary tract infections and is especially seen in diabetic patients, intravenous (IV) drug users, and patients who are immunocompromised. Night pain, along with fever and weight loss, suggests the diagnosis of infection or malignancy. Vertebral body metastasis should be considered in a patient with a history of cancer and advanced age (over 50). Inflammatory back diseases include ankylosing spondylitis and other seronegative spondyloarthropathies (see above). Ankylosing spondylitis characteristically has back pain that worsens with rest and improves with activity.

Severe low back pain can be associated with renal nephrolithiasis, but it can also be seen with a leaking aortic aneurysm.

▶ Diagnostic Studies/Diagnosis

Diagnostic studies should be ordered according to the suspected diagnosis. A complete blood count (CBC), sedimentation rate, and C-reactive protein may reveal findings consistent with inflammation. A bone scan may be ordered to reveal findings consistent with osteomyelitis or malignancy. Lumbar x-rays, CT scan, or MRI should also be considered.

▶ **Clinical Therapeutics/Clinical Intervention**
Treatment will depend on the final diagnosis.

## G. Spinal Stenosis

▶ **Scientific Concepts**
Lumbar spinal stenosis is most commonly acquired; however, it may be congenital. It is characterized by narrowing of the spinal canal and nerve root foramina, resulting in compression of the neural elements. Most commonly this is due to degenerative changes that occur in older patients (over 60).

▶ **History & Physical**
Majority present with complaints of low back pain and/or trouble walking. Low back pain is usually vague and diffuse. Since flexion of the spine increases the spinal diameter, patients may state the pain is relieved somewhat by bending forward. Unsteadiness of gait is usually associated with "pseudoclaudication" defined as weakness and fatigue in the legs upon walking or prolonged standing. The occurrence while standing and failure to be shortly relieved when the patient stops walking help to differentiate this from true vascular claudication. Exam is unremarkable except for the presence of marked pain upon extension of the spine.

▶ **Diagnostic Studies/Diagnosis**
Evaluation may include lumbar spine x-rays, which reveal the presence of degenerative changes. CT scan or MRI will confirm the diagnosis.

▶ **Clinical Therapeutics/Clinical Intervention**
Initial therapy consists of analgesics, either NSAIDs or salicylates; a physical therapy exercise program that focuses on spinal flexion and abdominal muscle strengthening; and weight loss, if indicated. Narcotics should be avoided. Epidural corticosteroid injections may also be tried. Surgical decompression is reserved for patients who do not respond to conservative treatment measures.

▶ **Health Maintenance Issues**
Progression of the disease is variable. Some patients do well and require no intervention, whereas others develop severe limitation. Spinal stenosis can also be complicated by the development of cauda equina syndrome (see above).

## IV. DISORDERS OF THE HIP

### A. Aseptic Necrosis

▶ **Scientific Concepts**
Aseptic necrosis is also referred to as *avascular necrosis* or *osteonecrosis*. The most common cause of aseptic necrosis of the hip is trauma that results in disruption of blood supply to the femoral head. Leading causes of nontraumatic aseptic necrosis include alcoholism, idiopathic causes,

and systemic steroid use. Other risk factors include sickle cell disease, rheumatoid arthritis, and systemic lupus erythematosus.

### ▶ History & Physical

Majority present with complaints of a gradual onset of dull and aching or throbbing pain in the groin, lateral hip, or buttock. Acute pain may occur with sudden collapse of a necrotic femoral head. On exam, patients have an antalgic gait; pain with internal and external rotation; and decreased internal rotation, flexion, and abduction of the hip.

### ▶ Diagnostic Studies/Diagnosis

An MRI of the hip is best for evaluating changes in early stages of necrosis because x-rays may appear normal. Sclerosis of the femoral head as documented on AP and frog-lateral views of the pelvis is the earliest sign of aseptic necrosis on routine x-rays.

### ▶ Clinical Therapeutics/Clinical Intervention

Treatment is based on the extent of aseptic necrosis and its degree of involvement of weightbearing surfaces. The patient should be referred for orthopedic evaluation. Treatment of a hip that has not collapsed is controversial. Once the hip is collapsed, hip arthroplasty is the treatment of choice.

## B. Fractures/Dislocations

### ▶ Scientific Concepts

*Hip fractures:* Include femoral neck and intertrochanteric femoral fractures that are seen in elderly patients with osteoporosis. Femoral neck fractures result from a twisting injury, and intertrochanteric fractures result from a fall onto the hip. In the younger patient, hip fractures occur as a result of high-energy trauma.

*Hip dislocation:* Present when the femoral head is displaced from the acetabulum. Rarely occurs in adults and is usually the result of high-impact trauma, such as a motor vehicle crash. Majority are posterior and result from the knee being struck while the hip and knee are flexed. An associated fracture of the posterior acetabular wall is usually present.

### ▶ History & Physical

*Hip fractures:* Patients complain of pain, swelling of the hip region, and inability to ambulate after the fall. Affected leg is characterized by shortening and is held in external rotation and abduction.

*Hip dislocation:* Patients with posterior hip dislocations typically have severe pain and will not move the lower extremity. Paresthesis may be present. On exam, the affected leg is shortened and the hip is held in flexion, internal rotation, and adduction. Neurovascular assessment should be documented.

### ▶ Diagnostic Studies/Diagnosis

*Hip fractures:* Diagnosis confirmed by the presence of fracture on an AP pelvis and cross-lateral view of the involved hip. MRI imaging may reveal an acute occult hip fracture in a patient with negative x-rays and history supporting the presence of a fracture.

*Hip dislocation:* X-ray evaluation includes an AP of the pelvis, and AP and lateral views of the femur. The involved femoral head appears smaller than the uninvolved side in a posterior hip dislocation. The possible presence of an associated fracture of the acetabulum or femoral head should be looked for.

▶ Clinical Intervention

***Hip fractures:*** Treatment depends on the location, degree of displacement, and age/health of the patient. Surgical correction is required for most patients with a fractured hip. Nondisplaced femoral neck fractures and intertrochanteric fractures are usually treated by open reduction and internal fixation. Displaced femoral neck fractures are usually treated with hip arthroplasty. Nonsurgical treatment should be considered for any patient who was nonambulatory before the fracture.

***Hip dislocation:*** Once associated fractures have been ruled out, reduction of the dislocation should occur on an emergent basis to reduce the risk of aseptic necrosis. Reassessment of neurovascular status should be performed after reduction. Repeat x-rays and postreduction CT scan are ordered to confirm reduction and evaluate for any intra-articular bony fragments. Early ambulation with crutches and weight bearing as tolerated may occur after reduction of uncomplicated hip dislocations. Once the patient is pain-free, a physical therapy program including hip abduction and extension exercises should be started.

▶ Health Maintenance Issues

***Hip fractures:*** Elderly patients have a 20–30% mortality rate within the first year following fracture. Femoral neck fractures may disrupt the blood supply to the femoral head leading to nonunion of the fracture and aseptic necrosis (see above). Early stabilization of the fracture and mobilization of the patient is best to avoid the complications of pneumonia, deep venous thrombosis (DVT), and urinary tract infections.

***Hip dislocations:*** As mentioned above, aseptic necrosis may occur after dislocation of the hip. Additional risks include redislocation, a missed loose body or fracture, and the development of post-traumatic arthritis.

## C. Slipped Capital Femoral Epiphysis

▶ Scientific Concepts

This is a disorder of unknown cause involving displacement of the femoral head through the physis. Most common during the adolescent growth spurt, affecting boys more often than girls. Bilateral in about 25–30% of the patients.

▶ History & Physical

Most are obese with underdeveloped secondary sexual characteristics. Onset of symptoms is insidious and includes referred pain in the groin and/or knee associated with a painful limp. Hip pain may not be present, and any adolescent that presents with knee pain and has an unremarkable knee exam should have the hip evaluated. Exam reveals tenderness to palpation over the hip. Loss of internal rotation of the hip is the most reliable indication of slippage, however LOM in abduction is also seen. An external rotation deformity of the leg may be present.

▶ Diagnostic Studies/Diagnosis

Confirmed by abnormal findings on the AP and frog-lateral x-rays of the pelvis including widening of the epiphyseal plate and displacement of the femoral head. Severity of the displacement is classified according to the degree of posterior slippage. A displacement <30 degree is usually classified as mild, 30–50 degrees as moderate, and >50 degrees as severe.

▶ Clinical Intervention

Definitive treatment includes surgery. Once diagnosed, the patient is placed on crutches with nonweightbearing status and referred for orthopedic evaluation.

▶ Health Maintenance Issues

Severe cases are one of the most common causes of premature osteoarthritis in young adults. Appropriate stabilization of mild or moderate disease provides good long-term prognosis.

## V. DISORDERS OF THE KNEE

### A. Bursitis

▶ Scientific Concepts

Bursae form where skin travels over a bony protuberance or between tendons, ligaments, and bone. The prepatellar bursa is superficial and lies between the skin and the anterior patella. This bursa often becomes irritated from repetitive kneeling, leading to inflammation and formation of fluid. It may also fill with blood due to direct trauma or be involved with infection. Another bursa in the knee that is frequently symptomatic is the pes anserine bursa located along the anteromedial aspect of the knee that becomes inflamed in patients with associated medial joint arthritis.

▶ History & Physical

Initially, pain will be present only with activity or pressure. Localized swelling of the involved area, most noticeable with prepatellar bursitis (housemaid's knee) is usually present. Localized tenderness to palpation is present and, with pes anserine bursitis, is below the joint line. Assessment of gait and ROM of the knee is indicated.

▶ Diagnostic Studies/Diagnosis

Prepatellar and pes anserine bursitis are primarily diagnosed clinically. In patients with chronic knee pain, AP and lateral x-rays of the knee should be ordered to rule out any bony abnormality. If any signs of infection are present, arthrocentesis and subsequent culture of the fluid should be performed.

▶ Clinical Therapeutics/Clinical Intervention

Most patients respond to conservative treatment consisting of NSAIDs, ice, and activity modification. Treatment may also include aspiration of the bursae and injection of corticosteroid, if swelling and inflammation is marked and infection is not present. Infections are treated with aspiration or open drainage as well as oral or IV antibiotics depending on severity.

▶ Health Maintenance Issues

Chronic bursitis of the knee can lead to weakening of ligaments and/or tendons resulting in partial or complete ruptures of the involved structure.

## B. Fractures/Dislocations

▶ Scientific Concepts

***Fractures of the knee:*** Many knee fractures are intra-articular. Distal femur fractures occur through the femoral condyles or tibial plateaus. Femoral condyle fractures occur as a result of high-energy trauma in young patients and low-energy force in elderly patients with osteoporosis. Tibial plateau fractures result from valgus of varus stress applied to the joint. Fractures involving the patella are usually transverse and result from direct trauma to the knee.

***Knee dislocation:*** Acute traumatic dislocation is uncommon, but has a high incidence of associated neurovascular injuries. Complete dislocation occurs with high-energy trauma that disrupts the supporting ligaments and soft tissues. Most of the dislocations occur anteriorly.

▶ History & Physical

***Fractures of the knee:*** Patients present with a compatible history of injury and immediate onset of pain and swelling. Effusion is usually marked secondary to bleeding from intra-articular fractures. ROM is restricted due to pain and the presence of effusion. Assess neurovascular status of pulses and the function of the deep peroneal, superficial peroneal, and posterior tibial nerves. Inspect the skin for any break in integrity indicating an open fracture.

***Knee dislocation:*** Gross deformity is usually present associated with marked ligamentous instability. If spontaneous reduction of the dislocation occurred, gross deformity may be absent, but swelling should be evident. Careful evaluation of neurovascular status is warranted.

▶ Diagnostic Studies/Diagnosis

***Fractures of the knee:*** AP and lateral views of the knee demonstrate most fractures. Oblique views of the knee and CT of the knee may be indicated preoperatively. Doppler evaluation is helpful in suspected vascular injury.

***Knee dislocation:*** Angiography is performed post reduction, even in the presence of palpable distal pulses, to evaluate the patency of the popliteal artery.

▶ Clinical Intervention

***Fractures of the knee:*** Arthrocentesis is performed in marked knee effusions for pain relief. Most nondisplaced or minimally displaced fractures are treated conservatively with appropriate immobilization and subsequent active exercise program to restore strength and mobility. Displaced fractures and fractures with intra-articular involvement usually require surgical intervention. Open fractures require emergent surgical care.

***Knee dislocation:*** Reduction should be performed promptly in the emergency room. Neurovascular status is then reevaluated and angiography is usually performed. In young patients, surgical repair of ligamentous damage is usually performed, however older patients may be treated nonoperatively. Physical therapy to restore function is often required.

► Health Maintenance Issues

***Fractures of the knee:*** Nonunion or malunion is possible. Any fracture that disrupts the intra-articular surfaces, even with optimal care, is prone to development of traumatic arthritis.

***Knee dislocation:*** The severity of limb injury is the most predictive factor associated with the need for amputation versus salvage of the leg.

## C. Meniscal Injuries

► Scientific Concepts

Fibrocartilaginous menisci act as shock absorbers between the femoral condyles and tibial plateaus. Meniscal tears are the most common of all knee injuries. The medial meniscus is more frequently involved than the lateral. Injury to the meniscus may be isolated or associated with ligamentous ruptures. Tears occur acutely with a twisting injury while the foot is planted in a weight-bearing position, usually while playing sports. In older patients degeneration plays a role, often requiring little or no trauma, to produce a tear.

► History & Physical

Patients present with a history of injury involving twisting of the knee associated with a "popping" or "tearing" sensation followed by severe pain. Swelling and stiffness occurs over several hours with meniscal injuries, unlike the more immediate swelling of ligamentous injury. Restricted motion ("pseudolocking") after meniscal injury is most often due to hamstring tightness or effusion, but may be due to "true locking" of the knee when unstable meniscal fragments become trapped within the knee joint. Acute symptoms may subside over the first few days, but the patient will continue to experience intermittent episodes of pain, swelling, and sensation of the knee buckling or giving out. Exam reveals joint effusion, pain, and tenderness elicited over the affected joint line and LOM. McMurray's sign, indicative of meniscal injury, is positive when a painful click is felt with tibial torsion in a knee flexed at 90 degrees.

► Diagnostic Studies/Diagnosis

Diagnosis is made clinically and, except in cases of "true locking," conservative treatment is initiated. X-rays of the knee are indicated in patients with a history of trauma or an effusion to rule out any other disorders. MRI has replaced other more invasive methods of evaluating for meniscal injuries, however it should be reserved for patients who are not responding to conservative treatment after several weeks and for preoperative assessment. Knee aspiration may be performed to evaluate the joint fluid in suspected cases of infection or crystal arthropathy.

► Clinical Therapeutics/Clinical Intervention

Initial treatment consists of rest, ice, compression, and elevation (RICE). NSAIDs usually are prescribed for analgesia. Patients are instructed in use of crutches and started on quadriceps-strengthening exercises progressing to gentle ROM exercises in 2 to 3 days and weight-bearing activities as tolerated. Surgical repair, most often arthroscopically, is indicated in cases of true locking and is considered in younger patients with significant tears and older patients who do not respond to conservative treatment.

▶ Health Maintenance Issues

Recurrent episodes of stiffness, locking, or pain indicate a surgically significant tear. If not treated definitively, continued damage to the articular cartilage will occur and subsequent development of osteoarthritis is possible. Postoperatively, most patients do well and are able to return to normal activities within 3–6 weeks.

## D. Osgood–Schlatter Disease

▶ Scientific Concepts

The cause is unknown, but the condition affects the tibial tuberosity during adolescence. Most likely it is caused by repetitive microvascular injury that leads to avulsion at the patellar tendon insertion into the secondary ossification center of the tibial tuberosity. This explains the higher incidence in adolescents who are active in sports and the greater incidence seen in males.

▶ History & Physical

Patients present with complaints of localized pain, swelling, and tenderness over the tibial tubercle aggravated by activity. Exam reveals localized tenderness and swelling overlying the tibial tubercle, often bilaterally. During the acute phase, kneeling may be painful, but full ROM and stability are preserved.

▶ Diagnostic Studies/Diagnosis

While the diagnosis is primarily based on clinical findings, AP and lateral x-rays may be ordered. X-rays should be ordered in a patient with unilateral complaints to rule out other significant pathology, like tumor. X-rays of the knee in Osgood–Schlatter disease may be normal or show the characteristic fragmentation of the tibial tubercle apophysis.

▶ Clinical Therapeutics/Clinical Intervention

Treatment is conservative and includes stretching, NSAIDs, and ice after activity. Use of protective kneepads may also be beneficial. With severe symptoms, restriction of activity and intermittent immobilization may be necessary. Surgery is rarely indicated.

▶ Health Maintenance Issues

This is a self-limiting condition that ends with the closure of the upper tibial epiphyseal plate.

## E. Sprains/Strains

▶ Scientific Concepts

There is a wide range of ligamentous injury to the knee from a "simple" sprain to complete ligamentous rupture. Trauma may cause an isolated ligamentous injury or involve several ligaments and/or meniscal injury. Collateral ligament injury results from a varus or valgus stress overload applied to the knee. Cruciate ligament injury most commonly results from a twisting injury, hence the association with meniscal injury. Injuries to the anterior cruciate ligament are more common in females than in males.

▶ History & Physical

Patients present with a history of trauma consistent with the mechanism of injury. After injury, the majority of patients are unable to ambulate and immediate swelling occurs secondary to hemorrhage from the ligamentous or capsular tear. This is especially true in tears involving the anterior cruciate ligament. Incomplete tears or sprains are actually more painful than complete ligamentous rupture. A thorough knee exam is the cornerstone of diagnosis, but it may be difficult in the acutely swollen knee. Note the presence of any swelling, discoloration, or localized tenderness to palpation, which often denotes the anatomical location of the lesion. Knee stability must be evaluated and includes evaluation of valgus–varus stress to assess collateral ligaments and the drawer signs for cruciate ligament integrity. The Lachman test can also be utilized to evaluate the anterior cruciate and is more sensitive than the anterior drawer test. Clinical assessment includes grading the sprain according to the degree of severity. A first-degree sprain is characterized by minimal symptoms and no detectable joint instability. Second-degree sprains cause more severe pain and demonstrate minimal joint instability. Third-degree sprains cause severe pain at the time of injury, but minimal pain afterward, and are associated with marked instability of the joint.

### ▶ Diagnostic Studies/Diagnosis

Ligamentous injury is primarily diagnosed by clinical findings, but an AP and lateral knee x-ray are often performed to rule out any bony pathology. MRI has become the imaging study of choice for further evaluation of ligamentous injury should it be required.

### ▶ Clinical Therapeutics/Clinical Intervention

The majority of isolated collateral ligament injuries are treated with rest, ice, compression, and protection utilizing a hinged-knee brace and early rehabilitation. Treatment of cruciate ligament injuries depends on the patient's age and activity level as well as the presence of any additional injuries. Isolated injuries are most commonly treated conservatively. Reconstructive surgery may be required in the highly athletic patient or in one who continues with recurrent instability and/or experiences subsequent meniscal tears.

### ▶ Health Maintenance Issues

Recurrent instability, subsequent meniscal tears, and osteoarthritis of the knee are potential complications from ligamentous injury.

## VI. DISORDERS OF THE ANKLE/FOOT

### A. Fractures/Dislocations

#### ▶ Scientific Concepts

***Ankle fractures and dislocations:*** Ankle injuries are one of the most common injuries that present for evaluation. Most fractures result from eversion or lateral rotation forces applied to the talus. Ankle fractures are classified as stable or unstable. A stable fracture involves only one side of the joint, such as a nondisplaced fracture of the lateral malleolus. An unstable fracture involves both sides of the ankle joint and may be bimalleolar or trimalleolar. When posterior dislocation of the ankle occurs with a trimalleolar fracture, it is termed a *trimalleolar fracture-dislocation.*

***Fracture/dislocations of the foot:*** Fractures of the foot include fractures of the calcaneous, metatarsals, and phalanges. The calcaneus is the most commonly fractured tarsal bone, usually following a fall from a height. Ten percent are associated with vertebral compression fractures and 5% are bilateral. Fractures of the neck or shaft of the metatarsals commonly result from compression injury to the foot. Fractures involving the base or styloid of the fifth metatarsal are common and occur due to an inversion injury to the foot. Fractures involving the proximal shaft of the fifth metatarsal occur in a relatively avascular area and should be referred for treatment.

### ▶ History & Physical

***Ankle fractures and dislocations:*** Present with acute pain following the injury. Obvious deformity may be present dependent on the extent of displacement. Swelling and localized tenderness to palpation help to localize the fracture site. Assessment of stability, especially of the deltoid ligament, as well as neurovascular evaluation should be performed.

***Fracture/dislocations of the foot:*** Present with acute pain following injury and difficulty or inability to ambulate. Associated swelling, ecchymosis, and localized tenderness are present. Assessment of neurovascular status is mandatory.

### ▶ Diagnostic Studies/Diagnosis

***Ankle fractures and dislocations:*** X-ray evaluation includes the routine AP and lateral views as well as a mortise view of the ankle. These views document the majority of fracture/dislocations, however a CT scan may be necessary to evaluate complex fractures.

***Fracture/dislocations of the foot:*** Appropriate x-ray views will demonstrate the presence of fracture in the majority of cases. AP and lateral views of the spine should be ordered if there is any spinal tenderness present in a patient with a calcaneal fracture.

### ▶ Clinical Therapeutics/Clinical Intervention

***Ankle fractures and dislocations:*** Stable fractures are commonly treated with weight-bearing immobilization for 4–6 weeks followed by rehabilitation. Unstable nondisplaced fractures may be treated by non–weight-bearing immobilization for 6–8 weeks. All ankle fractures should be routinely reevaluated with x-ray 1–2 weeks following immobilization to determine if any displacement of the talus has occurred. Unstable displaced ankle fractures require either open or closed reduction; however, open reduction provides better joint restoration and resultant function. If dislocation of the talus is present, it should be reduced as soon as possible. Open fractures require immediate surgical treatment.

***Fracture/dislocations of the foot:*** Initial treatment of a calcaneal fracture involves application of a soft compression dressing, ice, and elevation due to the severe swelling that occurs. Treatment depends on the amount of displacement, however prolonged immobilization is not advised. ROM exercises should be started as soon as the fracture is stable, but weight bearing is not allowed for 6–8 weeks until fracture healing has occurred. Treatment of metatarsal fractures depends on the location and amount of displacement of the fracture. Undisplaced fractures of the neck or shaft of the metatarsals are usually treated with immobilization for 4–6 weeks and weight bearing as tolerated. Displaced fractures of the neck of the metatarsals often require reduction to avoid development of metatarsalgia. Avulsion fractures of the base of the fifth metatarsal are treated with immobilization until asymptomatic. Proximal fractures of the shaft of the fifth metatarsal heal slowly and require immobilization for a longer period of time and/or open reduction and internal fixation. Undisplaced fractures of the toes are usually treated by buddy taping the involved toe to an adjacent toe for 3–4 weeks until symptoms subside.

▶ Health Maintenance Issues

*Ankle fractures and dislocations:* Chronic instability, posttraumatic osteoarthritis, and complex regional pain syndrome may occur.

*Fracture/dislocations of the foot:* Posttraumatic arthritis occurs frequently in fractures involving the calcaneus. Malunion of a metatarsal shaft or neck fracture may result in metatarsalgia. Nonunion may occur in proximal fractures of the fifth metatarsal.

## B. Sprains/Strains

▶ Scientific Concepts

Ligamentous injury to the ankle represents the most common musculoskeletal injury. The most common mechanism of injury is an inversion injury resulting in ligamentous damage to the anterior talofibular ligament. More severe injury also involves the calcaneofibular ligament and, rarely, the posterior talofibular ligament. Ankle injuries are graded according to ligament involvement and degree of instability. A grade I sprain involves the anterior talofibular ligament and has no detectable instability. A grade II sprain involves injury to both the anterior talofibular ligament and calcaneofibular ligament with mild instability. A grade III sprain involves injury and significant instability caused by disruption of both ligaments.

▶ History & Physical

Pain, swelling, and loss of motion is common and dependent on the severity of the injury. Severe sprains often present with the patient describing a "pop" at the time of injury, with immediate onset of swelling and inability to ambulate. Exam reveals swelling, ecchymosis, and localized tenderness. Assessment of stability should be done by performing the anterior drawer and talar tilt tests. Motor and neurovascular function should be evaluated.

▶ Diagnostic Studies/Diagnosis

X-rays of the ankle should be performed to rule out the presence of fracture. Stress views of the ankle may be ordered to evaluate ligament stability.

▶ Clinical Therapeutics/Clinical Intervention

Treatment is aimed at preventing chronic pain and instability. Regardless of severity, most ankle sprains are treated conservatively. Initially a soft compressive dressing, elevation, ice, and NSAIDs are utilized. Protective bracing with weight bearing to tolerance followed by a progressive functional rehabilitation program is instituted. Mild sprains may respond in 2 weeks, but more severe injuries may require 6–8 weeks of treatment.

► Health Maintenance Issues

Untreated severe sprains as well as incomplete rehabilitation may result in chronic instability and pain.

## VII. INFECTIOUS DISEASES

### A. Acute/Chronic Osteomyelitis

► Scientific Concepts

Bone infection most commonly caused by bacteria, but may also be caused by fungal infections (*Blastomyces dermatitidis* or *Coccidioides immitis*) or tuberculosis in immunosuppressed patient. Acute osteomyelitis occurs within 2 weeks of disease onset. Chronic osteomyelitis is characterized by >1 month duration and presence of infected necrotic bone (sequestrum). Acute osteomyelitis is more common in children than adults. It usually results from hematogenous spread, but it may also be caused by direct contamination, such as occurs in trauma. *Staphylococcus aureus* is the most common organism involved in hematogenous spread. Other causes in infants and children include group B streptococci, gram-negative coliforms, and *Haemophilus influenzae*. Gram-negative infections (*Pseudomonas aeruginosa*) are an additional important cause in adults, especially involving the vertebral area secondary to IV drug abuse, diabetes mellitus, and indwelling urinary catheters. *Staphylococcus epidermidis* as well as *S. aureus* are most commonly involved after trauma and surgery. Most common site of involvement in children is the metaphyseal area of long bones; in patients > 50, it is the spine.

► History & Physical

Acute osteomyelitis presents with fever and chills associated with pain and localized tenderness of the involved bone. Exam reveals erythema, increased local warmth, and limitation of motion. Adult patients may have a less acute onset with absence of systemic symptoms. Chronic osteomyelitis is characterized by onset of inflammation and cellulitis after trauma or persistent drainage. May become latent and reactivate after minor trauma in the future.

► Diagnostic Studies/Diagnosis

Diagnosis confirmed by blood cultures or aspiration of involved bone. Labs reveal leukocytosis and an elevated sedimentation rate or C-reactive protein. X-rays may be normal early in disease. Initial change consists of soft-tissue swelling followed by periosteal elevation and finally bone infarct and collapse. MRI, CT scan, and bone scan are more sensitive than plain x-ray. Bone scans are particularly helpful in early osteomyelitis with unknown focus. MRI is best at detecting subtle changes. Chronic osteomyelitis reveals sclerotic changes, irregular areas of bone destruction, and sequestra on plain films.

► Clinical Therapeutics/Clinical Intervention

Give IV antibiotics as soon as cultures are obtained. Selection based on coverage of *S. aureus* and other most likely organisms. Traditionally, IV antibiotics are given for 4–6 weeks followed by oral agents (usually quinolone) for an additional 6–8 weeks. Surgical debridement is required in patients who fail to improve with antibiotics, have puncture wounds, or have necrotic bone. Urgent surgical intervention is needed with involvement of the spine. Immobilization (3–4 weeks) decreases pain and may prevent pathologic fracture. Follow C-reactive or sedimentation rate levels to monitor therapeutic response. It is important to prevent development of chronic osteomyelitis, which is difficult to treat and eradicate.

▶ Health Maintenance Issues

May be life-threatening especially in infants. Inadequate treatment or delay in diagnosis and treatment may lead to chronic infection. Pathological fractures, joint destruction, and bone defects may cause limb dysfunction.

## B. Septic Arthritis

▶ Scientific Concepts

Also known as *pyogenic arthritis*. Occurs due to introduction of bacteria into joint as result of hematogenous spread, direct penetration, or spread from adjacent tissue. Most common cause of infectious arthritis is secondary to disseminated gonococcal (*Neisseria gonorrhoeae*) infection. Seen in otherwise healthy adults, < age 40, more common in females compared to males (2:1 to 3:1) and male homosexuals. Nongonococcal septic arthritis has similar etiologic agents as cause osteomyelitis (see above). Risk factors for nongonococcal arthritis include bacteremia (IV drug use, endocarditis) and damaged joints (rheumatoid arthritis).

▶ History & Physical

Clinical picture depends on age of patient, offending organism, and host state. Gonococcal arthritis is usually seen in young sexually active patients with prodromal migratory polyarthritis followed by tenosynovitis (60%) or purulent monarthritis (40%), usually involving the knee. Characteristic dermatitis involving palms and soles present in most with absence of genitourinary (GU) symptoms. Nongonococcal arthritis is characterized by acute onset of monarticular involvement in large weight-bearing joints (knee and hip) and wrist. Pain is usual presenting complaint associated with fever and systemic symptoms. Exam reveals warm, edematous, diffusely tender joint with limitation and pain upon motion.

▶ Diagnostic Studies/Diagnosis

Diagnosis confirmed by positive cultures obtained from blood, joint, or GU system. Negative cultures do not necessarily exclude septic arthritis. White blood cell (WBC) count and sedimentation rate are usually elevated, but may be normal. X-rays may be normal or reveal soft-tissue swelling, but are helpful to rule out other joint pathology. If chronic infection is present, also obtain acid-fast and fungal testing. A rapid response to appropriate antibiotics is almost diagnostic of gonococcal infection.

▶ Clinical Therapeutics/Clinical Intervention

Begin broad-spectrum systemic antibiotic coverage as soon as cultures are obtained. Frequent repeat aspirations of joint may be required. Indications for surgical drainage include failure to respond to medical therapy in 2–4 days or presence of hip involvement. Rest, immobilization, and elevation of involved joint initially is followed by early active ROM exercises as tolerated. NSAIDs may be utilized for pain and inflammation.

Due to increasing gonococcal resistance to penicillin, initial inpatient treatment may be warranted to confirm diagnosis, start treatment, and rule out presence of endocarditis.

► **Health Maintenance Issues**

Early appropriate treatment helps avoid joint disruption or development of osteomyelitis. Most mortality occurs from polyarticular sepsis (30%) or respiratory complications (5–10%).

## VIII. NEOPLASTIC DISEASE

### A. Bone Cysts/Tumors

► **Scientific Concepts**

The most common lesion involving the bone is metastatic disease to the spine. Primary malignancies that commonly metastasize to the spine include lung, breast, prostate, kidney, and thyroid cancers. Primary malignant and benign tumors of the bone are uncommon. The most important factor in determining the type of bone tumor is the age of the patient.

► **History & Physical**

The initial complaint of metastatic lesions is pain that does not go away with rest and is present at night. Pathological fractures may occur and are suggested by a history of sudden worsening of pain after mild trauma. Systemic symptoms such as fever, malaise, and weight loss may also be seen with malignant tumors. Benign lesions may present as a painless mass. Exam may reveal the presence of a mass, localized tenderness, limited ROM, and regional lymphadenopathy. A limp may be present with lower extremity involvement. In older patients, careful examination of other systems should be included to search for signs of a possible primary tumor.

► **Diagnostic Studies/Diagnosis**

X-rays will usually identify the location of the lesion. Further evaluation by CT is best for benign bony lesions, because it documents bony changes and degree of calcification within the lesion. Malignant lesions are more appropriately evaluated with MRI, which documents soft-tissue extension of the lesion into the medullary canal or muscle. To evaluate for primary lesions or further spread of metastatic disease, a bone scan, chest x-ray, and a CT scan of the chest may be ordered. A biopsy is usually obtained to make a definitive diagnosis.

► **Clinical Therapeutics/Clinical Intervention**

Benign bony lesions may be simply observed or surgically excised depending on symptoms and potential for growth. Malignant lesions are usually surgically excised and adjunct treatment with chemotherapy and radiation may be indicated.

► **Health Maintenance Issues**

Pathological fractures may occur and malignant lesions may cause a decreased life span.

## B. Ganglion Cysts

▶ Scientific Concepts

Ganglions are the most common benign soft-tissue tumors of the hand and wrist. Their cause is unknown. The most common location is the dorsum of the wrist at the radiocarpal region, but ganglions may also be seen on the volar aspect.

▶ History & Physical

Patients present with a painless soft mass that is freely moveable. There is usually no associated history of trauma. Fluctuations in the size of the mass may occur with levels of activity.

▶ Diagnostic Studies/Diagnosis

Diagnosis is based on clinical findings. In a patient with local dorsal wrist pain and no palpable mass, a MRI may reveal the presence of a deep ganglion.

▶ Clinical Therapeutics/Clinical Intervention

Asymptomatic ganglions may simply be observed. Aspiration and steroid injection may provide temporary relief of symptoms, but recurrence is common. Surgical excision may be considered in symptomatic patients.

▶ Health Maintenance Issues

Ganglia may recur at the same site in 5–10% of patients.

## C. Osteosarcoma

▶ Scientific Concepts

Osteosarcoma is the most common primary bone malignancy. The metaphysis of the distal portion of the femur is the most frequent site (50–75%). Onset usually occurs during puberty with a greater incidence in boys compared to girls.

▶ History & Physical

Patients present with pain or swelling in or around a joint, especially the knee. Often a history of a sports-related injury is elicited. Exam reveals tenderness to palpation and may reveal a palpable mass.

▶ Diagnostic Studies/Diagnosis

X-rays of the involved area may reveal the presence of a lytic lesion or a mixed destructive and osteoclastic pattern with extensive soft-tissue involvement. MRI of the involved area is utilized to stage the lesion.

▶ Clinical Therapeutics/Clinical Intervention

Treatment consists of surgical resection and chemotherapy.

▶ Health Maintenance Issues

Prognosis with current therapy has improved to a 5-year survival rate of 60%.

## IX. OSTEOARTHRITIS

▶ Scientific Concepts

Osteoarthritis (OA), also referred to as *degenerative joint disease* or *osteoarthrosis,* is the most common type of noninflammatory arthritis. It is characterized by progressive loss of articular cartilage and bony overgrowth of the joint surface (osteophytes), most prominently in the weight-bearing hip and knee joints as well as the spine. Incidence increases with age, obesity, previous joint trauma, and repetitive occupational activity, such as seen in carpenters, coal miners, and jackhammer operators. Inflammation is usually minimal.

### ▶ History & Physical

Patients initially present with complaints of articular stiffness lasting less than a half hour, which is relieved by activity. Pain of the involved joints is made worse by activity, including weight bearing, and is relieved by rest. Exam reveals the presence of crepitus, swelling, and limited ROM. Joint enlargement results from presence of joint effusion, synovial hyperplasia, or osteophytes. Osteophytes involving the distal interphalangeal (DIP) joint are termed *Heberden's nodes* and those of the proximal interphalangeal (PIP) joint are called *Bouchard's nodes*. ROM is mildly decreased until severe changes are present. Disuse atrophy of surrounding musculature may develop quickly. Although considered non-inflammatory, mild inflammation with increased warmth of the joint may be present. In later stages of the disease, pain is often not relieved by rest.

### ▶ Diagnostic Studies/Diagnosis

X-rays of the involved joint reveal characteristic findings of joint space narrowing and osteophyte formation. Periarticular ossicles and subchondral bone cysts may also be present. No specific laboratory abnormalities are seen in primary OA and synovial fluid analysis is unremarkable.

### ▶ Clinical Therapeutics/Clinical Intervention

The primary goals of treatment include relief of pain and prevention of progression. Pain relief is usually obtained with use of acetaminophen or NSAIDs. Capsaicin cream may also be helpful in reducing pain. Intra-articular steroid injections may be beneficial in acute flare-ups, but should be limited to no more than two to three injections per year, especially in weightbearing joints. Relative rest of involved joints during acute flare-ups by use of removable splints or braces for upper extremity involvement and cane or crutch for lower extremity involvement will help reduce inflammation and pain. Stretching and low impact exercises help to maintain muscle tone and decrease stiffness. Advanced OA, especially of the hip and knees, usually requires joint replacement surgery. Indications for surgery include pain at rest, night pain, and/or severe limitation of motion. Alternative therapies for OA include the use of glucosamine, chondroitin sulfate, *S*-adenosyl-L-methionine (SAM), and viscosupplements. The first three substances are available as over-the-counter dietary supplements. Currently, the Food & Drug Administration (FDA) has approved the use of viscosupplements in patients with knee OA.

### ▶ Health Maintenance Issues

Weight reduction has been shown to be beneficial in reducing the risk of lower extremity OA, especially in the knee. Protection of joints from excessive force and overuse, as outlined above, may slow progression. Younger patients, who undergo arthroscopic joint debridement or osteotomy, may eventually require total joint replacement.

## X. OSTEOPOROSIS

▶ Scientific Concepts

This is a common metabolic bone disease that results in a loss of both bone matrix and mineral, resulting in bone fragility. It is multifactorial in etiology and is classified as primary (type I or II) or secondary. Type I osteoporosis is seen most commonly in postmenopausal women as a result of loss of estrogen that allows increased osteoclastic bone resorption. Affecting primarily trabecular bone, crush fractures of the vertebrae and distal radial fractures (Colles' fractures) are common. Type II, also known as *senile osteoporosis,* is associated with aging. It results from a gradual decline in osteoblastic activity without associated increase in osteoclastic activity. Affecting both trabecular and cortical bone, vertebral wedge fractures and hip fractures are common. Type II is mostly seen in persons over age 60–70 and affects both males and females. Elderly females often have elements of both type I and type II osteoporosis. Secondary osteoporosis is caused by certain medications (alcohol, steroids, heparin, anticonvulsants), disuse from prolonged immobilization, certain malignancies, and endocrine disorders. Common risk factors for osteoporosis include a small, thin body build; Caucasian or Asian race; cigarette smoking; sedentary lifestyle; low calcium intake; and strong family history.

▶ History & Physical

Osteoporosis is asymptomatic unless fractures occur. Patients present with back pain, fracture, progressive loss of height, and thoracic kyphosis. Vertebral fractures usually occur first with little or no history of trauma, and hip fractures occur later after age 65. Exam in the early stages may be normal. As the disease progresses, findings include localized tenderness over fracture areas, loss of body height (usually > 2 inches), dorsal kyphosis (Dowager's hump), and chronic pain.

▶ Diagnostic Studies/Diagnosis

Plain x-ray findings of osteopenia, especially in the spine and pelvis, are often the first indication of osteoporosis. The most common method of detecting bone loss and assessing fracture risk is through the use of dual-energy x-ray absorptiometry (DEXA). Considered the gold standard, it is also utilized to monitor the effectiveness of treatment. Some protocols call for the use of quantitative ultrasound as a screening test. CT densitometry of the vertebrae is also highly accurate. Laboratory screening should consider the secondary causes of osteoporosis and include evaluation for thyroid, hematological, and malignancy disorders.

▶ Clinical Therapeutics/Clinical Intervention/
   Health Maintenance Issues

The best treatment is prevention with the goal of maximizing peak bone mass in the young and minimizing bone loss after menopause. Weightbearing physical activity, adequate dietary intake of calcium/vitamin D, and reducing the fall risk of elderly patients are important general prevention measures. Current FDA-approved medications for the prevention and treatment of osteoporosis are all antiresorptive agents, including calcium, vitamin D, hormone replacement therapy, alendronate, calcitonin, and raloxifene.

## XI. RHEUMATOLOGIC CONDITIONS

### A. Fibromyalgia

▶ Scientific Concepts

Etiology is unknown. Proposed theories include sleep disorders, depression, viral infections, and abnormal sensory processing.

▶ History & Physical

Most frequently seen in women aged 20–50 years who present with diffuse achiness, stiffness, headache, and fatigue associated with multiple trigger areas of clinical tenderness. Minor exertion may aggravate the pain and increase fatigue. Objective signs of inflammation are not present.

▶ Diagnostic Studies/Diagnosis

Fibromyalgia is a diagnosis of exclusion. Diagnostic criteria established by the American College of Rheumatology include widespread pain present for 3 months; presence of axial skeletal pain with distribution on the right and left sides as well as above and below the waist; and pain and tenderness at 11 or more of the 18 trigger points. Thyroid testing should be done to rule out hypothyroidism, which may produce a secondary fibromyalgia syndrome. Any additional laboratory or x-ray diagnostics are always normal and should be limited by a thorough history and physical examination.

▶ Clinical Therapeutics/Clinical Intervention

Patient education and reassurance that this is neither an inflammatory disease nor the prodrome of a more serious debilitating disease is warranted. Although no cure is available, symptom relief may be obtained. A combination of stretching and aerobic exercise is helpful to increase flexibility and conditioning. Pain management measures may include the use of NSAIDs, tricyclic antidepressants, trazadone, and topical capsaicin cream. Use of corticosteroids and narcotics should be avoided.

▶ Health Maintenance Issues

Support groups are often helpful to aid the patient in dealing with social and environmental factors. The chronic pain associated with fibromyalgia may lead to depression, anxiety, and inactivity.

### B. Gout/Pseudogout

▶ Scientific Concepts

Classified as crystalline deposition diseases, gout and pseudogout are characterized by crystal deposits in the synovium and other tissues, which leads to development of inflammation. Gout is caused by monosodium urate crystals and pseudogout by calcium pyrophosphate dihydrate crystals. The majority of gout is caused by underexcretion of serum uric acid (90%) and in the remaining cases by overproduction of serum uric acid. Primary gouty arthritis is an inherited metabolic disorder involving a disturbance of purine metabolism leading to hyperuricemia. Secondary gout may be associated with many causes, including leukemia and hemolytic anemia, or may be drug-induced, especially with thiazide diuretic use. Risk factors for gout include obesity, excessive alcohol intake, trauma/surgery, and high-purine diet. The etiology of pseudogout, also known as *chondrocalcinosis* and *calcium pyrophosphate dehydrate deposition* (CPDD), is unknown.

### ▶ History & Physical

*Gout:* Patients present with acute onset of an intensely painful, swollen, erythematous joint, often with fever. The MP joint of the great toe (podagra) is most commonly involved (50%), but the ankle, tarsal joints, and knee may also be affected. Precipitating events include exercise, excessive alcohol intake, surgery, and physical or emotional stress. Polyarticular attacks, soft-tissue tophus formation, joint destruction, and associated renal failure are indications of disease severity.

*Pseudogout:* Usually seen in patients age 60 or older. Patients present similarly to acute gout, but the initial clinical presentation is less severe and more commonly involves the knee. Other involved joints may include the elbows, wrists, ankles, hips, and shoulders.

### ▶ Diagnostic Studies/Diagnosis

*Gout:* Definitive diagnosis is made by aspiration of the joint, which reveals needle-shaped, negatively birefringent crystals. Single serum uric acid levels may be normal, but serial determinations usually reveal an increased level.

Mild leukocytosis and an elevated sedimentation rate may be seen during acute attacks. A 24-hour urine uric acid determination may be helpful for treatment options. Initial x-rays are often normal, but later may reveal multiple punched-out lesions.

*Pseudogout:* Definitive diagnosis is made by aspiration of the joint, which reveals weakly positive, birefringent rhomboid-shaped crystals. X-ray changes include calcification noted primarily in the knee meniscus, annulus fibrosis, radioulnar disc, and symphysis pubis. Although there are no specific blood abnormalities, diagnostic tests to rule out hypothyroidism, hyperparathyroidism, hemochromatosis, and hypophosphatasia may be indicated.

### ▶ Clinical Therapeutics/Clinical Intervention

*Gout:* Acute gout is primarily treated with NSAIDs, indomethacin 25–50 mg tid. Colchicine may also be used, but it has a higher side effect profile. Adjunctive treatment of the acute attack includes rest, elevation, moist heat, and possibly short-term narcotic pain relief. Prophylactic long-term therapy includes dietary modifications, weight loss, avoidance of hyperuricemic medications, and reduction of serum uric acid. Undersecretion of uric acid (24-hour uric acid level < 800 mg/d) is treated with uricosuric drugs (probenecid or sulfinpyrazone). Overproducers of uric acid (> 800 mg/d) are treated with allopurinol.

*Pseudogout:* Acute episodes are treated with aspiration and cortisone injections as well as NSAIDs for acute pain.

### ▶ Health Maintenance Issues

*Gout:* Chronic hyperuricemia may lead to the development of nephropathy and renal stones.

*Pseudogout:* Structural joint damage in CPDD is rare.

## C. Juvenile Rheumatoid Arthritis (JRA)

▶ Scientific Concepts

Etiology is unclear, but it appears to be related to genetic predisposition and environmental triggers. HLA-DR4 and HLA-DR5 play a role in the type and progression of disease. Pathogenesis includes the interaction of T cells and cytokines, including tumor necrosis factor producing inflammation. Three types of JRA are seen. The most common is pauciarticular (40–50%) followed by polyarticular and systemic.

▶ History & Physical

Clinical presentation depends on the type of JRA. Early-onset pauciarticular JRA is seen in girls more frequently than boys (4:1) with onset before age 4 years. Late-onset disease (age 10–12) is more frequent in males. Pauciarticular JRA is characterized by synovitis in < four joints, primarily the knee, ankle, and elbow. Asymptomatic uveitis may occur. Systemic signs are less frequent to absent. Polyarticular JRA is seen primarily in girls with symmetrical joint involvement of > five joints, including small and large joints. It is associated with low-grade fever, fatigue, rheumatoid nodules, and anemia. Systemic JRA occurs at any age equally in boys and girls. Findings include synovitis in one to two joints, high spiking fevers, and a classic rash.

▶ Diagnostic Studies/Diagnosis

No single diagnostic test will confirm the diagnosis. The American Rheumatic Association established four criteria for diagnosis including chronic synovial inflammation of unknown cause, onset before age 16, objective signs of arthritis in one or more joints for 6 consecutive weeks, and exclusion of other diseases. A positive antinuclear antibody (ANA) found in pauciarticular JRA patients is considered a risk factor for development of uveitis. Rheumatoid factor is only positive in about 15% of patients, primarily in polyarticular JRA. Sedimentation rate is often normal. X-ray findings are similar to adult rheumatoid arthritis except that joint destruction is not as frequent.

▶ Clinical Therapeutics/Clinical Intervention

NSAIDs are treatment of choice along with ROM and muscle strengthening exercises. Regular ophthalmologic slit lamp exams are indicated. Referral for consideration of disease-modifying antirheumatic drugs (DMARDs) is appropriate with persistent synovitis.

▶ Health Maintenance Issues

Prognosis depends on the type of JRA, rheumatoid factor status, the course of the disease, and the response to and side effects of treatment. Eye involvement in pauciarticular JRA may lead to permanent loss of vision.

## D. Polyarteritis Nodosa

▶ Scientific Concepts

Classified as a vasculitis syndrome. The etiology is unknown. Associated with hepatitis B or C and hypertension. Characterized by pathological features of inflammation and necrosis of blood vessels, primarily involving medium-sized vessels (peripheral nerves, mesenteric vessels, heart, and brain).

▶ History & Physical

Gradual onset over weeks to months. Presents as combination mononeuritis multiplex and systemic signs of fever, malaise, and weight loss. Specific findings depend on arteries involved. Classically includes skin findings of livedo reticularis, subcutaneous nodules, skin ulcers, and possibly digital gangrene. Renal artery involvement leads to renin-mediated hypertension. Abdominal angina associated with nausea and vomiting and infarction. There is asymptomatic cardiac involvement, but lung involvement is rare.

▶ Diagnostic Studies/Diagnosis

Diagnosis is confirmed by angiogram (aneurysmal dilations) or biopsy of involved tissue. Sedimentation rate is markedly elevated with slight anemia and leukocytosis. Positive serologic tests for hepatitis B or C in 10–30% patients.

▶ Clinical Therapeutics/Clinical Intervention

Usually responds to high-dose steroids (up to 60 mg prednisone daily). Severe cases may require IV steroids and immunosuppressive agents. In hepatitis cases, follow steroids with antiviral treatment and plasmapheresis.

▶ Health Maintenance Issues

Five-year survival rate with treatment has improved to 60–90%. Associated renal insufficiency, proteinuria, gastrointestinal (GI) ischemia, and central nervous system (CNS) or cardiac involvement decreases prognosis. Relapse after remission may occur. Incidence of chronic disease is greater in patients with hepatitis B or C.

## E. Polymyositis

▶ Scientific Concepts

Systemic disorder of unknown etiology associated with a cellular-mediated immune response against muscle. Peak incidence in elderly (5th and 6th decade) and in women twice as often as men.

▶ History & Physical

Gradual and progressive painless proximal muscle weakness with difficulty ascending stairs, getting up from sitting position, or rising from hands and knees. Fever, malaise, and weight loss may occur. Dysphagia and dyspnea may occur. Muscle atrophy and contractures are late complications.

▶ Diagnostic Studies/Diagnosis

Diagnosis confirmed by muscle biopsy. Creatine kinase (CK) and lactate dehydrogenase (LDH) usually elevated. ANA may be present. Myopathic EMG abnormalities are present.

▶ Clinical Therapeutics/Clinical Intervention

Moderate- to high-dose corticosteroids (40–60 mg/d) are initial treatment. Addition of methotrexate or azathioprine in patients who fail to respond to steroids. Physical and occupational therapy to increase strength and ROM.

► Health Maintenance Issues

Pulmonary involvement increases the patient's morbidity and mortality.

## F. Polymyalgia Rheumatica (PMR)

► Scientific Concepts

Systemic inflammatory disorder associated with HLA-DR4 and infectious environmental agents. Ten percent of patients develop giant cell (temporal) arteritis. More common in female (60%) patients, with a peak incidence between 60 and 80 years of age.

► History & Physical

Presents as chronic, symmetrical pain and stiffness of the proximal muscles, notably the shoulder and pelvic girdle. It is most severe in the morning and with exertion. Associated low-grade fever, malaise, fatigue, anorexia, and weight loss. Exam reveals poorly localized tenderness and limitation of motion due to pain. Muscle atrophy and contractures may occur.

► Diagnostic Studies/Diagnosis

Clinical diagnosis based on above findings with an elevated sedimentation rate (> 50–100 mm/h) in the majority (90%) of patients. Associated mild normochromic, normocytic anemia (50% patients), thrombocytosis, and leukocytosis (12,000–16,000). Order thyroid-stimulating hormone (TSH) to rule out hypothyroidism and immunoelectrophoresis to rule out multiple myeloma. Bone scan reveals increased uptake involved regions. Diagnosis should be questioned if patient fails to respond to treatment within 1 week.

► Clinical Therapeutics/Clinical Intervention

Isolated PMR is treated with low-dose (10–20 mg/d) prednisone. Most respond rapidly with resolution of symptoms within 48–72 hours and normalization of laboratory abnormalities after 7–10 days. Once controlled, slowly taper steroids to lowest level that still controls symptoms. Monitor with serial sedimentation rates and CBC. Most need to be treated for 1–2 years.

► Health Maintenance Issues

Must consider long-term effects of systemic corticosteroid use, especially osteoporosis in the elderly female population.

## G. Reiter's Syndrome (Reactive Arthritis)

► Scientific Concepts

Seronegative arthropathy of unknown etiology that develops after enteric or sexually transmitted infections (STIs). The reactive arthritis that develops is sterile. Incidence is equal following enteric infections and is greater in males compared to females (9:1) following STIs. Associated with HLA-B27 in > 85% of cases.

► History & Physical

Patients are usually young, and symptoms appear within days to weeks following infection. Presents as acute asymmetric oligoarthritis, usually involving the knee or ankle associated with fever and weight loss. Eye involvement (uveitis, conjunctivitis), low back pain, and heel pain are common. Mucocutaneous lesions include balanitis, stomatitis, and keratoderma blennorrhagicum. Sacroiliitis occurs in 20% of patients.

► **Diagnostic Studies/Diagnosis**

Clinical diagnosis supported by the presence of urethritis, conjunctivitis/uveitis, mucocutaneous lesions, and aseptic arthritis. Supported by the presence of HLA-B27 and an elevated sedimentation rate. Cultures rarely show initial precipitating infectious cause.

► **Clinical Therapeutics/Clinical Intervention**

Treat symptomatically with NSAIDs. Arthritis is often self-limited and resolves within a few months. The role of antibiotics is controversial, but treatment with tetracycline may be beneficial in males with urethritis. Sulfasalazine may be used in patients who fail to respond to NSAIDs and antibiotics.

► **Health Maintenance Issues**

Chronic recurrent episodes of arthritis may occur, leading to more permanent or progressive joint disease.

## H. Rheumatoid Arthritis

► **Scientific Concepts**

Chronic systemic disorder of unknown etiology felt to be autoimmune in nature. Process is characterized by cell-mediated immune response (T cells) involving cytokines (interleukin and tumor necrosis factor) and loss of normal apoptosis function. Response is initially an inflammatory one against soft tissue and later cartilage, with eventual erosion and destruction of the articular surface. Most common in females (3:1) with prevalence increasing with age and peaking between ages 40–50. Evidence of HLA-DR haplotype involvement.

► **History & Physical**

Characterized by symmetric polyarticular pain, swelling, and morning stiffness (> 1 hour) involving the wrists, metacarpals (MCPs), and PIP joints, but sparing the DIP joints. Prodromal systemic symptoms including weakness, anorexia, malaise, and fatigue are common. Onset is gradual with remissions and exacerbations of symptoms. Exam of acutely involved joints reveals effusion, warmth, tenderness, and limitation of motion. Later findings include progressive changes of joint deformities involving subluxations, dislocations, and contractures. Extra-articular manifestations include rheumatoid nodules, pulmonary fibrosis, pericarditis, and vasculitis.

► **Diagnostic Studies/Diagnosis**

Clinical diagnosis based on American Rheumatology Classification involving characteristic symptoms, signs, laboratory data, and radiologic findings. No one specific test confirms diagnosis. Rheumatoid factor is positive in 70–80% of patients, but also may be positive in other disease states or apparently healthy person. Sedimentation rate is usually elevated, and a moderate normocytic normochromic anemia is present. ANA is positive in 20% of patients. Early x-rays are often normal. First x-ray change is presence of soft-tissue swelling and juxta-articular demineralization most commonly seen in wrist or feet. Later findings include joint space narrowing, erosions, and deformity.

▶ Clinical Therapeutics/Clinical Intervention

Goals of treatment include reducing inflammation and pain, preventing deformities, and preserving function. Salicylates, NSAIDs, splinting, and corticosteroids (oral or intra-articular injections) are used to decrease inflammation and pain. Early consideration should be given to initiation of disease-modifying agents, such as methotrexate or newer tumor necrosis factor inhibitors (etanercept or infliximab). Antimalarials (hydroxychloroquine), gold salts, sulfasalazine, azathioprine, and leflunomide may also be considered. A physical therapy program and exercise to preserve joint function, muscular strength, and endurance is of paramount importance. End-stage disease may require joint replacement surgery.

▶ Health Maintenance Issues

Complications of significant disability within 10–20 years of diagnosis. May cause premature death.

## I. Systemic Lupus Erythematosus (SLE)

▶ Scientific Concepts

An inflammatory autoimmune disorder characterized by production of autoantibodies to components of the cell nucleus. Inflammation, vasculitis, and immune complex deposition affecting multiple organ systems. Most common in females (85% patients) in the childbearing years, especially Caucasians. Genetic association with HLA haplotypes (DR2 and DR3).

▶ History & Physical

Clinical presentation and progression varies widely from a benign disease with characteristic malar rash ("butterfly" rash), arthritis, and fatigue to a more severe and life-threatening form involving progressive nephritis with resultant renal failure and neurologic complications. Joint symptoms are seen in 90% and are usually the first complaint. Arthritis is systemic and similar to rheumatoid arthritis, but rarely is destructive or deforming. Ocular findings, oral ulcers, and photosensitivity may be seen. Cardiopulmonary involvement includes findings compatible with pleurisy and pericarditis.

▶ Diagnostic Studies/Diagnosis

Consider drug-induced "lupus-like syndrome" before making diagnosis of SLE (chlorpromazine, hydralazine, isoniazid, methyldopa, procainamide, and quinidine). SLE diagnosed by presence of multisystem clinical features and positive serologic testing (4 or more of 11 criteria for classification of SLE by American College of Rheumatology). ANA positive in majority (95–100%) of patients, but may also be seen in healthy patients. Antibodies to double-stranded DNA (50%) and to Smith (Sm) (20%) are more specific, but not always positive. Hematologically may have findings of anemia, leukopenia, or thrombocytopenia. Monitor serum blood urea nitrogen (BUN) and creatinine for renal involvement. Renal biopsy may be required.

▶ Clinical Therapeutics/Clinical Intervention

Mild form of the disease treated supportively with rest, NSAIDs, topical corticosteroids, and sunscreen. Rashes and joint symptoms unresponsive to initial measures may be treated with antimalarials (hydroxychloroquine). Serious complications are treated with systemic corticosteroids and may require immunosuppressive agents, such as cyclophosphamide or methotrexate.

### ▶ Health Maintenance Issues

Course marked by spontaneous remission and relapses. Monitor patients with CBC, platelet count, serum creatinine, and urinalysis on regular basis. More intense monitoring required for patients with known renal involvement. Increasing survival rates (10 year rate > 85%), with infection the most common cause of death.

## J. Scleroderma/Sjogren's Syndrome

### ▶ Scientific Concepts

**Scleroderma:** Connective tissue disease also known as *systemic sclerosis*. Chronic disorder characterized by degenerative, inflammatory, and fibrotic changes of the skin and internal organs. Limited scleroderma (CREST syndrome; 80%) more common than diffuse (20%).

**Sjogren's syndrome:** Chronic autoimmune disorder involving the exocrine glands. Characterized by immune-mediated inflammatory process. Primarily female (90%) with average age of onset at 50 years old.

### ▶ History & Physical

**Scleroderma:** Presents with polyarthralgia and Raynaud's phenomenon (> 90%) associated with subcutaneous edema, fever, and malaise. Eventually, there is thickening of skin with telangiectasia and pigment changes. Most patients develop dysphagia and hypomotility of GI tract. Diffuse scleroderma patients may have findings of pulmonary fibrosis, cardiac abnormalities, or renal involvement.

**Sjogren's syndrome:** Most commonly present with dry mouth (xerostomia) and dry eyes (xerophthalmia). May develop keratoconjunctivitis sicca, dysphagia, Raynaud's phenomenon, arthralgias/arthritis, and myalgias. Systemic and major organ involvement less common.

### ▶ Diagnostic Studies/Diagnosis

**Scleroderma:** Clinical diagnosis aided by pattern of involvement. Skin involvement limited to distal extremities and face in CREST syndrome. Diffuse skin thickening associated with internal organ involvement in diffuse scleroderma. Majority with positive ANA. May have positive scleroderma antibody (SCL-70). CREST patients are also positive for anti-centromere antibody (50%).

**Sjogren's syndrome:** Based on clinical findings of xerostomia and xerophthalmia associated with presence of autoantibodies, primarily rheumatoid factor (70%), ANA, and antibodies to extractable nuclear antigens of Ro (SS-A) and La (SS-B). Biopsy of involved glands, usually salivary, confirms diagnosis.

### ▶ Clinical Therapeutics/Clinical Intervention

**Scleroderma:** Supportive treatment measures of symptoms and monitoring for organ involvement are the primary management goals.

**Sjogren's syndrome:** Symptomatic treatment involves artificial tears, sipping water, sugar-free gums, and candy for sicca components. Emphasize need for careful dental hygiene. Avoid smoking and use of decongestants or anticolinergics. Muscarinic agonists may be helpful in treating dry mouth, but have limited use due to side effects. Corticosteroids and immunosuppressive agents may be needed in severe progressive disease.

▶ Health Maintenance Issues

***Scleroderma:*** Prognosis worse in patients with diffuse disease, males, elderly, and African Americans. Death usually from renal, cardiac, or pulmonary failure. Increased association with breast and lung cancer.

***Sjogren's syndrome:*** Usually benign course with normal life span. May be affected by associated disease manifestations. Increased risk of developing lymphoma.

## BIBLIOGRAPHY

Greene WB, ed. *Essentials of Musculoskeletal Care,* 2nd ed. Chicago, IL: American Academy of Orthopedic Surgeons/American Academy of Pediatrics; 2001.

Hay WW, et al., eds. *Current Pediatric Diagnosis and Treatment,* 15th ed. New York: Lange Medical Books/McGraw-Hill; 2001.

Mercier LR. *Practical Orthopedics,* 5th ed. St. Louis, MO: Mosby; 2000.

Robbins L, ed. *Clinical Care in the Rheumatic Diseases,* 2nd ed. Atlanta: Association of Rheumatology Health Professionals; 2001.

Skinner HB. *Current Diagnosis and Treatment in Orthopedics,* 3rd ed. New York: Lange Medical Books/McGraw-Hill; 2003.

Tierney LM Jr, McPhee SJ, Papadakis MA, eds. *Current Medical Diagnosis & Treatment,* 42nd ed. New York: Lange Medical Books/McGraw-Hill; 2003.

Tintinalli JE, et al., eds. *Emergency Medicine: A Comprehensive Study Guide,* 5th ed. New York: Health Professions Division/McGraw-Hill; 2000.

# Neurology 12

*William H. Marquardt, MA, PA-C*

## I. ALZHEIMER'S DISEASE

► Scientific Concepts

The single most common cause of progressive dementia. Incidence is directly related to advancing age and affects both genders equally. Life expectancy is about 5–10 years from the onset of symptoms, with infection or inanition as the cause of death.

► History & Physical

In the initial or *mild stage,* impairment of recent memory is typical. Slowly progresses, with patients becoming disoriented to time and then to place. The *moderate stage* is characterized by increasing confusion, with belligerence and restlessness often replacing the depression noted earlier. Difficulty naming and doing calculations causes the patient to quit working or managing family finances. Personal grooming habits deteriorate, hallucinations or delusions occur, and full-time supervision is needed. In the *severe stage,* patients cannot function independently, cannot recognize themselves or their family, cannot use or understand language, and have no capacity for self-care. Paranoid psychosis, hallucinations, or delusions may be prominent. Incontinence and a bedridden state are terminal manifestations, with susceptibility to malnutrition and infections.

► Investigative Studies

There are no diagnostic laboratory findings. Nonspecific enlargement of the lateral ventricles or cortical atrophy may be noted on computed tomography/magnetic resonance imaging (CT/MRI). Stereotaxic brain biopsy or postmortem samples indicating senile plaques and neurofibrillary tangles provide the definitive diagnosis.

► Diagnosis

Dementia established by neuropsychometric examination, deficits in two or more areas of cognition, progressive worsening of memory, no disturbance of consciousness, onset between ages of 40 and 90, and absence of other disease. Other considerations include depression, cerebrovascular dementias, Parkinson's, Huntington's, Pick's, or pure memory disorders such as Korsakoff's amnesic disorder associated with chronic alcoholism.

► Clinical Therapeutics

Since cholinergic neuronal pathways degenerate and choline acetyltransferase is depleted, cholinesterase inhibitors such as tacrine and donepezil may provide subjective responses in improved behavior and amelioration of forgetfulness in the early stages.

► Clinical Intervention

None.

► Health Maintenance Issues

Appropriate family support is vital. Social services, day care programs, elder care, psychoactive medications, and institutionalization are eventually necessary.

## II. CEREBRAL PALSY

▶ **Scientific Concepts**

Nonhereditary and nonprogressive impairment of movement and posture since birth or in infancy (termed *static encephalopathy*). Etiology is often obscure and multifactorial. Higher incidence in small-for-gestational-age babies. Frequently, the cause is intrauterine hypoxia, but also may be secondary to intrauterine bleeding, infections, toxins, congenital malformations, or obstetric complications. Affects about 0.2% of neonatal survivors in the United States.

▶ **History and Physical**

Seventy-five percent of cases are spastic motor deficits in some combination (quadra, hemi, para, mono). Associated deficits include seizures (50%), mental retardation, and sensory and speech deficits. Clinical findings include muscular hypertonicity, hyperreflexia (clonus may be present), and extensor plantar reflexes. May see microcephaly (2 standard deviations [*SD*] below average), and ataxia may be prominent.

▶ **Diagnostic Studies**

There is no standard laboratory workup. Routine screening may be conducted for metabolic and genetic conditions.

▶ **Diagnosis**

If a progressive deterioration is noted early (3 months), a metabolic disorder is more likely. Subsequent deterioration may implicate one of a number of central nervous system (CNS) degenerative disorders.

▶ **Clinical Therapeutics**

Spasticity may be relieved with diazepam or baclofen. Symptoms of hyperactivity may also be treated with appropriate doses of methylphenidate or pemoline. Seizure management may be necessary.

▶ **Clinical Intervention**

A variety of surgical procedures for amelioration of moderate to severe spasticity have been devised.

▶ **Health Maintenance Issues**

The goal is to achieve maximal potential for the child, instead of "normality." Psychological counseling and support for both patient and family are vital. In about 30% of patients with mild disease, motor deficits will resolve by age 7 and many are able to lead fairly normal lives.

## III. DISEASES OF THE PERIPHERAL NERVES

### A. Diabetic Neuropathy

▶ **Scientific Concepts**

Common complication of diabetes, which may be characterized by a mixed polyneuropathy (sensory, motor, and autonomic) in 70% of cases, the remainder being predominantly sensory. May also present as mononeuropathies affecting various peripheral or cranial nerves individually.

Usually related to duration and severity of hyperglycemia, and may be the presenting symptom of occult diabetes. Symptoms are likely secondary to vascular insufficiency or infarction of nerve.

▶ **History & Physical**

Numbness, paresthesias, dysesthesias (burning), hyperesthesias, and pain, more common in the legs than the arms. May present as diminished reflexes or reduced vibratory sensation in the legs before other symptoms of decreased sensation to light touch, pinprick, temperature, and proprioception are evident. Other late findings include postural hypotension; cardiac rhythm abnormalities; and bowel, bladder, gastric, and sexual dysfunction.

▶ **Diagnostic Studies**

Nerve conduction studies can assess severity of involvement. Further workup is done primarily to rule out other causes of polyneuropathy.

▶ **Diagnosis**

Uremia; alcoholic/nutritional deficiencies; connective tissue vasculitis; $B_{12}$ deficiency; hypothyroidism; toxic, paraneoplastic amyloidosis must be ruled out.

▶ **Clinical Therapeutics**

Optimal control of diabetes is key, but there are no specific therapies for peripheral nerve involvement. Phenytoin, carbamazepine, tricyclic antidepressants, and mexiletine may be helpful for neuropathic pain.

▶ **Clinical Intervention**

Surgical decompression may be necessary for an entrapment neuropathy.

▶ **Health Maintenance Issues**

Tight control of diabetes needed, maintaining the lowest levels of glucose that can be safely achieved. Routine, aggressive foot care is important.

## B. Bell's Palsy

▶ **Scientific Concepts**

Mononeuropathy exclusively involving the facial nerve (7th cranial nerve [CN]) and without evidence of other neurologic disease. Pathology is related to facial nerve axonal degeneration, but the cause is unknown. Seen in all ages, but more common in pregnant women and diabetics. Eighty percent of cases recover spontaneously.

▶ **History and Physical**

Unilateral weakness of facial muscles generally occurs abruptly, but may take hours or up to a day. Ipsilateral ear pain may precede the weakness or occur concurrently. Patient may also note impaired taste sensation, lacrimation, or hyperacusis.

▶ **Diagnostic Studies**

All studies are normal

▶ **Diagnosis**

Other causes of facial palsy include tumors, herpes zoster infection (Ramsay Hunt syndrome), Lyme disease, acquired immunodeficiency syndrome (AIDS), and sarcoidosis.

▶ **Clinical Therapeutics**

A course of oral corticosteroids (prednisone, 60 mg/d × 3 days and tapering over 1 week), if begun within 5 days of onset, may increase the number of patients who fully recover.

▶ **Clinical Intervention**

Electrical stimulation of the nerve may be helpful. If stimulation produces movement, the prognosis is good.

▶ **Health Maintenance Issues**

Eye protection is crucial

## C. Guillain-Barré Syndrome

▶ **Scientific Concepts**

Acute idiopathic polyneuropathy; most common cause of acute flaccid paralysis since the eradication of polio. In 60% of cases, the condition follows an event such as an infection (herpes, *Campylobacter jejuni*), inoculations, childbirth, surgery, or immune suppression.

▶ **History & Physical**

May begin as minor back or leg pain with paresthesias, but usually presents as symmetrical weakness, typically in the legs first, and more marked proximally than distally. Exam may reveal decreased or absent reflexes. Weakness may be severe, and may be a life-threatening emergency if involving the muscles of respiration or swallowing. Sensory abnormalities are common, but they are generally less prominent than the motor symptoms. May also involve marked autonomic dysfunction including tachycardia and other cardiac irregularities, labile blood pressure, respiratory distress, sphincter disturbances, or paralytic ileus.

▶ **Diagnostic Studies**

Cerebrospinal fluid (CSF) analysis may reveal dramatic elevations of protein but a normal cell count. Electrophysiologic studies may show decreased conduction velocities, both sensory and motor, or evidence of denervation or axonal loss.

▶ **Clinical Therapeutics**

Plasmapheresis and intravenous (IV) immunoglobulin are remarkably beneficial and increase extent of recovery, shorten time on a respirator, and shorten the time to being able to walk independently.

▶ **Clinical Intervention**

Patients should be hospitalized and their respiratory status monitored as autonomic involvement may quickly lead to complications and death from orthostatic hypotension or arrhythmias.

▶ **Health Maintenance Issues**

The clinical picture ceases to progress at about 4 weeks and then resolves completely in weeks to months in 70–75% of patients. One fourth of patients will be left with a mild neurologic deficit, and about 5% will die as a result of respiratory failure.

## D. Myasthenia Gravis

▶ **Scientific Concepts**

Postsynaptic neuromuscular junction disease in which antibodies to the acetylcholine receptors reduce the number of functioning receptors and lead to muscle weakness. Can occur at any age and is more common in younger women and older men.

▶ **History & Physical**

Typically an insidious onset, often following or concurrent with an infection. Presenting complaints commonly include diplopia, difficulty in chewing or swallowing, nasal speech, respiratory difficulties, or limb weakness. Symptoms often fluctuate in intensity secondary to activity, with recovery following rest.

▶ **Diagnostic Studies**

Administration of anticholinesterase drugs, such as edrophonium (Tensilon test) or neostigmine, produces an increase in the strength of weak muscles for several minutes. Electrophysiologic testing involving repetitive stimulation of the motor nerve may detect impaired transmission. Single-fiber electromyography is also helpful. Eighty to 90% of generalized myasthenia patients can be found to have serum acetylcholine receptor antibodies. Chest x-ray or CT may reveal a coexisting thymoma.

▶ **Clinical Therapeutics**

Anticholinesterase drugs, typically oral pyridostigmine, provide symptomatic benefit but do not change the course of the disease. Corticosteroids or immunosuppressive agents such as azathiopine are typically reserved for patients who have had a thymectomy and who respond poorly to anticholinesterase drugs.

▶ **Clinical Intervention**

Thymectomy leads to symptomatic relief of generalized symptoms but is not fully understood. Plasmapheresis may be necessary for patients in myasthenic crisis, those with a rapidly progressive disease course, or prior to surgery that is likely to produce postoperative respiratory compromise.

▶ **Health Maintenance Issues**

Care should be taken during concurrent infection, surgical procedures, pregnancy, or other conditions of stress. Extreme care must be taken to avoid medications known to impair neuromuscular transmission (quinine, quinidine, procainamide, propranolol, phenytoin, lithium, tetracycline, and aminoglycoside antibiotics).

## IV. PRIMARY HEADACHES

### A. Tension Headache

▶ **Scientific Concepts**

The most common benign headache disorder, accounting for up to 60% of primary headaches. There is no specific underlying pathophysiologic mechanism, and the classic description of neck and scalp muscle contraction may well be secondary. Women are more commonly affected than men.

▶ **History & Physical**

A detailed history and physical assessment is necessary to rule out evidence of a more ominous diagnosis or to determine an underlying condition causing the headaches. Tension headaches are typically described as steady ("bandlike"), nonthrobbing, bilateral, or global head pain that is not associated with a prodrome, neurologic signs or symptoms, and nausea or vomiting. History must carefully address prior efforts at medical management, as many chronic tension headaches are secondary to analgesic overuse.

▶ **Diagnostic Studies**

Erythrocyte sedimentation rate (ESR) may be significantly increased in arteritis; CT or MRI for mass or sinusitis.

▶ **Differential Diagnosis**

Consider migraine, posttraumatic, facial pain, depression, tumors, arteritis, postherpetic, intracranial mass, infections, drug withdrawal, visual problems, menstrual, temporomandibular joint (TMJ) dysfunction.

▶ **Clinical Therapeutics**

For management of acute, episodic headaches, aspirin, acetaminophen, and nonsteroidal anti-inflammatory drugs (NSAIDs) are generally effective, but tension headaches also respond to ergotamines and other migraine drugs. A significant number of patients develop secondary analgesic rebound headaches, so careful monitoring, including use of over-the-counter and alternative therapies, is vital.

▶ **Clinical Intervention**

Psychotherapy, physical therapy, and relaxation techniques may provide relief in selected patients.

▶ **Health Maintenance Issues**

Close management of underlying medical problems possibly responsible for headache, including cervical spondylosis, TMJ dysfunction, sinus disease, and hypertension.

## B. Migraine Headache

▶ **Scientific Concepts**

Two thirds to three quarters of patients are women, with an overall lifetime prevalence of ~16%. Tends to be early onset, in second and third decades; a family history of migraine is common. Several specific classifications, but the most basic is migraine either with, or without, aura. Aura and headache phases have classically been thought to be related to intracranial vasoconstriction and extracranial vasodilation. Recent studies surround the role of serotonin and have led to many newer and specific antimigraine drugs.

▶ **History & Physical**

It is important to try and elicit history of potential triggering factors, including tyramine-containing foods, meats preserved with nitrites, chocolate, MSG, fasting, menses, sleep deprivation, strong odors, or unusual stress. Physical examination is done to exclude other concurrent conditions.

***Without aura:*** Unilateral headaches 4–72 hours in length; moderate severity; aggravated with activity; associated with nausea, vomiting, photophobia, and phonophobia.

***With aura:*** Aura may be visual (scintillations [flashing lights], photopsias [flashes of light], or fortifications [jagged lines]) or sensory (tingling or numbness in the hand/mouth distribution). Headaches with throbbing pain, usually unilateral, photophobia, nausea but seldom vomiting. Headache severe lasting 4–72 hours, aggravated by physical activity, often relieved with sleep.

▶ **Diagnosis**

Consider cerebrovascular disease such as transient ischemic attacks (TIAs), cerebrovascular accident (CVA), subarachnoid hemorrhage, vasculitis; brain tumors or other mass lesions; posttraumatic headache; use of vasodilators; hypoxia or hypercarbia; hypoglycemia; fever; sinusitis; glaucoma; withdrawal from drugs including caffeine.

▶ **Clinical Therapeutics**

***Mild-moderate:*** Aspirin, acetaminophen, NSAIDs, Midrin.

***Severe:*** Dihydroergotamine, sumatriptan, or one of the newer triptans available in various dose forms, butorphanol nasal spray. With the advent of specific therapies for migraine, opioids and other potentially habituating medications such as butorphanol nasal spray should be avoided or used with caution.

***Prophylaxis:*** Propranolol, timolol, methysergide, calcium channel blockers, amitriptyline, valproate.

▶ **Health Maintenance Issues**

Avoidance of possible precipitating factors such as caffeine, chocolate, red wine, cheese, nuts, yogurts, stress, smoking, inadequate sleep, hunger, and some oral contraceptives.

## C. Cluster Headache

▶ **Scientific Concepts**

Seen much more frequently in men than in women, and typically begins at a later age than migraine. Usually no family history.

▶ **History and Physical**

Stereotypical clusters of brief, severe, constant nonthrobbing headaches lasting from 10 minutes to less than 2 hours. Headaches are consistently unilateral and tend to recur on the same side, beginning as a burning sensation behind the eye and associated with conjunctival injection, tearing, nasal stuffiness, and a Horner's syndrome (miosis, ptosis) ipsilaterally. Episodes may be precipitated by use of alcohol or vasodilating drugs. Headaches commonly occur at night and awaken the patient and then recur daily for a "cluster" period of weeks to months. Patients may then go without another cluster for months or even years.

▶ **Diagnostic Studies**

Thorough history and physical exam to exclude other causes of significant headache. Routine studies are of no value after stereotypical pattern establishes the diagnosis.

▶ **Clinical Therapeutics**

Oral medications are generally ineffective owing to the short duration of the headache. Abortive therapies include 100% oxygen via mask at 8–10 L/min for 10–15 minutes, sumatriptan (injection or nasal spray), dihydroergotamine.

▶ **Clinical Intervention**
None.

▶ **Health Maintenance Issues**
None.

## V. INFECTIOUS DISEASES

### A. Bacterial Meningitis

▶ **Scientific Concepts**

Inflammation of the meninges typically caused by bacteria that had colonized the mucous membranes of the nasopharynx, paranasal sinuses, or the middle ear. This is followed by local tissue invasion, bacteremia, and hematogenous seeding of the subarachnoid space and a secondary inflammatory response due to release of cytokines such as interleukin-1, interleukin-6, and tumor necrosis factor (TNF) leading to secondary brain edema, increased intracranial pressure, and altered cerebral blood flow. Etiologic agents are generally relative to the age of the patient and/or predisposing condition. *Escherichia coli, Streptococcus agalactiae,* and *Listeria monocytogenes* are more common in neonates and infants. *Streptococcus pneumoniae* and *Neisseria meningitidis* predominate from age 3 months to about 50 years, with *Haemophilus influenzae* also commonly presenting in those up to 18 years. In those over 50 years, *S. pneumoniae, L. monocytogenes,* and the gram-negative bacilli, with the latter two seen most frequently in those immune compromised. Those with a history of head trauma or neurosurgery or having a CSF shunt are susceptible to staphylococci, as well as the gram-negative bacilli and *S. pneumoniae.*

▶ **History & Physical**

Most patients have 1–7 days of symptoms prior to presentation. Fever, headache, vomiting, neck stiffness, and confusion are common, but many will not present with the complete syndrome. Examination may reveal signs of systemic or parameningeal infection such as skin abscess or otitis. Petechial rash is seen in the majority of those with *N. meningitidis.* Evidence of meningeal irritation is seen in ~80% of cases but is often absent at the extremes of age or with profoundly impaired consciousness. Focal neurologic signs, seizures, and/or cranial nerve palsies may also be observed.

▶ **Diagnostic Studies**

The essential investigation is prompt lumbar puncture and CSF analysis, after observing for focal neurologic deficits or evidence of increased pressure (e.g., vomiting or papilledema). If these are present, imaging should be accomplished prior to lumbar puncture. Blood cultures will identify the causative organism in up to 90% of cases. Complete blood count (CBC) with differential may provide evidence of systemic disease. X-rays of the chest, sinuses, or mastoids may reveal the primary site of infection.

► **Diagnosis**

CSF may appear turbid to grossly purulent, with the pressure being elevated in ~90% of cases. CSF white cell count may range from 1,000 to 10,000 in bacterial disease with predominant neutrophils. CSF glucose may be markedly decreased, and protein may range from 100 to 500 mg/dL. CSF cultures are positive in ~80%. CSF Gram stain may also identify the organism in as many as 80% of cases.

► **Clinical Therapeutics**

Antibiotics must penetrate blood–brain barrier. Culture-specific treatment preferred but often must treat empirically, particularly if the CSF is not clear and colorless. Neonates and infants are started on ampicillin (100 mg/kg IV q8h) *plus* cefotaxime (50 mg/kg IV q6h) or ceftriaxone (50–100 mg/kg IV q12h), while children up to 18 can be started on only one of the latter two at the same dose. Those age 18–50 empirically receive ceftaxamime (2 g IV q6h) or ceftriaxone (2 g IV q12h). Older adults should receive either ceftaxamine or ceftriaxone plus ampicillin (2 g IV q4h). Those with head trauma or a history of neurosurgery receive vancomycin (15 mg/kg IV q6h up to 2 g/d) *plus* ceftazidime (50–100 mg/kg IV q8h up to 2 g q8h). Duration of treatment is generally 10–21 days.

► **Clinical Intervention**

May need to remove hardware (shunt, ventriculostomy, etc.) in neurosurgery patient if possible.

► **Health Maintenance Issues**

Children should be routinely immunized against *H. influenzae*. A vaccine is available for travelers to areas where *N. meningitidis* may be endemic, and household or close contacts of affected patients may be treated prophylactically with rifampin (20 mg/kg/d as two divided doses for 2 days). Those in similar contact with *H. influenzae* patients take rifampin 20 mg/kg/day as a single daily dose for 4 days.

## B. Viral Meningitis/Encephalitis

► **Scientific Concepts**

Viral infections of the meninges (meningitis) or brain parenchyma (encephalitis). Children and young adults are most frequently affected, with symptoms secondary to enteric viruses (echovirus, coxsackie A, and coxsackie B). Uncommonly associated with mumps, herpes simplex type 1, and Epstein-Barr. Pathologic changes consist of an inflammatory reaction mediated by lymphocytes.

► **History & Physical**

Often presents as an acute confusional state. May present with fever, headache, neck stiffness, photophobia, and pain with eye movement, but patient generally does not appear as ill as in bacterial meningitis. Accompanying viral infection may be reflected by rash, pharyngitis, adenopathy, pleuritis, carditis, jaundice, organomegaly, diarrhea, or orchitis suggestive of a particular etiologic agent. If involving the brain (encephalitis or meningioencephalitis), may see marked alteration of consciousness, seizures, or other focal neurologic signs.

► **Diagnostic Studies**

Prompt analysis of the CSF is the most important investigation after imaging, if there are signs of increased intracranial pressure. CBC and differential may be helpful, and blood cultures should be drawn. Liver functions and serum amylase may be helpful relative to presenting signs and symptoms.

► **Diagnosis**

CSF pressure is generally normal or only slightly increased, as is the CSF protein. CSF cells are generally lymphocytes or monocytes, and number < 1,000. May see atypical lymphocytes and/or increased amylase if associated with mumps. Blood counts may be normal, leucopenia, or a mild leukocytosis.

► **Differential Diagnosis**

In the setting of a mononuclear cell pleocytosis, must consider: partially treated bacterial meningitis, syphilitic, tuberculosis (TB), fungal, parasitic, neoplastic etiologies. CSF wet mounts, stained smears, and appropriate cultures will distinguish these.

► **Clinical Therapeutics**

With the exception of herpes meningitis, there is no specific therapy required other than support care. Aspirin or Tylenol may be taken for headache, but low-grade fever requires no treatment as fever may contribute to the host response. Phenytoin or phenobarbital may be required if seizures are present.

► **Clinical Intervention**

In severe cases with coma, ventilator support with IV or nasogastric (NG) feeding may be required.

► **Health Maintenance Issues**

Generally none, with spontaneous resolution of all symptoms within 2 weeks regardless of etiology.

## VI. MOVEMENT DISORDERS

### A. Parkinson's Disease

► **Scientific Concepts**

Prevalence is 1–2 per 1,000 in the United States, with an equal gender distribution. Incidence increases with age and begins most often between ages 45 and 65. In Parkinson's disease, the etiology is undetermined, but several drugs or toxins can produce a reversible Parkinsonism syndrome. Dopamine depletion due to degeneration of the dopaminergic neurons in the substantia nigra produces an imbalance of dopamine and acetylcholine, and the goal of treatment is to restore that balance by replacing dopamine or blocking the effect of acetylcholine.

► **History & Physical**

The principal features are bradykinesia, rigidity, and tremor. Bradykinesia (slowness of movement) is often the presenting sign. Patients lose dexterity for fine motor movements and have difficulty getting up from a chair. Rigidity is of a cog wheeling nature. Tremor is 3–5 cycles/s and is known as *pill rolling*. Other findings include masked facies with infrequent blinking, micrographia, shuffling gait, flexed posture, dysarthria, or drooling. There is no muscle weakness, the deep tendon reflexes are normal, and patients have a normal plantar response.

► Diagnostic Studies

No routine investigations will confirm the diagnosis.

► Differential Diagnosis

Similar symptoms may be seen with depression, essential tremor, vascular disease, hydrocephalus, Creutzfeldt–Jakob disease, Shy-Drager syndrome, and Wilson's disease.

► Clinical Therapeutics

Amantadine, with mild anticholinergic activity, is a frequent first choice for early symptoms. Anticholinergics such as trihexyphenidyl or benztropine are generally prescribed for tremor and rigidity. Levodopa, alone or in combination with carbidopa, reduces all symptoms including bradykinesia. Bromocriptine and other ergot derivatives have a direct stimulant effect on dopamine receptors. Selegiline, an monoamine oxidase (MAO) inhibitor, inhibits the breakdown of dopamine and enhances the effect of levodopa.

► Clinical Intervention

Surgery is rarely necessary, as medications are almost universally effective. Stereotaxic thalamotomy may reduce or eliminate tremor and rigidity but not bradykinesia. Fetal or autologous adrenal medullary tissue or fetal substantia nigra transplanted to the caudate nucleus has also been performed.

► Health Maintenance Issues

Physical and speech therapy may be helpful early in the disease. Several aids to daily living may allow the patient to be more functional including: rails or banisters for support, eating utensils with large handles, nonslip rub matting rather than loose carpets or rugs, devices to amplify the voice, and chairs that will gently assist the patient to stand from a seated position.

## B. Huntington's Disease

► Scientific Concepts

The protypic choreiform disorder is inherited in an autosomal dominant manner, so the offspring of affected patients have a 50% chance of developing the disorder. Patients typically present in the fourth or fifth decade with chorea or dementia and live an average of 15 years after onset.

► History & Physical

Initial symptoms may be either abnormal movements or intellectual changes, and both will ultimately be prominent. Early mental changes may be irritability, moodiness, and antisocial behavior, but a more obvious dementia subsequently develops. Initial movement symptoms may be only a minor restlessness, but the rapid, nonrhythmic, nonstereotype movements that flow inconsistently from one body area to another (chorea) eventually surface. These may coexist with slow, writhing movements known as athetosis, producing coreoathetosis.

▶ **Diagnostic Studies**
Genetic testing provides a definitive diagnosis and permits the asymptomatic detection of the disease.

▶ **Differential Diagnosis**
A number of drugs may induce chorea, including dopaminergic drugs, antipsychotic drugs, lithium, phenytoin, and oral contraceptives. Other hereditary disorders featuring chorea include benign hereditary chorea, paroxysmal choreoathetosis, and Wilson's disease.

▶ **Clinical Therapeutics**
There is no treatment for the dementia, but the movement disorder may respond to dopamine receptor–blocking drugs, such as haloperidol or chlorpromazine, and drugs that deplete dopamine from nerve terminals, such as reserpine.

▶ **Health Maintenance Issues**
There is no cure, and life expectancy is 10–20 years after clinical onset.

## C. Essential Tremor

▶ **Scientific Concepts**
Postural tremor of unknown cause in otherwise normal patients. May develop in teen and early adult years, but often much later. Often has a familial basis with an autosomal dominant pattern, and two genes have been implicated.

▶ **History & Physical**
Usually presents as 5- to 9-Hz oscillation of the hands and forearms impairing fine motor tasks. May be accompanied by head tremor, termed *titubation*. The legs tend to be spared, and the remainder of the physical exam is normal. Occasionally speech may be affected when laryngeal muscles are affected. Patients commonly report that small quantities of alcohol may transiently suppress the tremor. They may also report that stress, caffeine, or sleep deprivation may aggravate.

▶ **Diagnostic Studies**
None.

▶ **Clinical Therapeutics**
If necessary, propranolol may be prescribed but will have to be taken indefinitely. If the patient has predictable circumstances where tremor is troublesome or embarrassing, propranolol can be administered in a single oral dose prior to the event. Primidone may also be effective.

▶ **Clinical Intervention**
In the case of disabling tremor that is unresponsive to medications, thalamotomy or high-frequency thalamic stimulation by an implanted electrode may be effective.

## VII.  MULTIPLE SCLEROSIS

▶ Scientific Concepts

One of the most common neurologic disorders, thought to have an autoimmune basis. Initial symptoms generally appear in young adults ages 20–40, especially Caucasians and those living in northern latitudes. A number of studies with twins suggest a genetic predisposition, and a familial incidence is noted on occasion. Often classified as *relapsing–remitting* indicating episodic episodes with periods of relative recovery, or *chronic progressive* in which the course is slowly progressive without periods of remission. Another segment of patients start as the former and become progressive, termed *secondary progressive*. Prognosis is better with females and an onset prior to age 40 with visual and somatosensory symptoms only. Some degree of disability will eventually result, but only half of all patients will be mildly or moderately disabled after 10 years.

▶ History & Physical

Most common presenting complaints are weakness, numbness, or unsteadiness in one limb; sudden loss or blurring of vision in one eye; dysequilibrium; diplopia; or bladder dysfunction. Symptoms may occur abruptly and then disappear after days to weeks. Subsequent attacks may follow after an interval of months to years and may be the same as previous attacks or a new constellation of symptoms. History may reveal an association between attacks and stress, systemic infection, fever, childbirth, and hot weather. Lhermitte's sign (electrical sensations that spread down the body with flexion of the neck) present with multiple sclerosis (MS) and with cervical spinal cord lesions. Examination during later attacks may reveal optic atrophy; nystagmus; dysarthria; and upper motor neuron, sensory, or cerebellar deficits in some or all limbs.

▶ Diagnostic Studies

MRI may detect subclinical as well as symptomatic demyelinating lesions in the periventricular white matter of the brain and the spinal cord. CSF is abnormal in ~90% of patients, with elevations of myelin basic protein, a mild lymphocytosis, and slightly increased protein, especially after an acute relapse. Electrophoresis reveals discrete bands in the immunoglobulin G (IgG) region (oligoclonal bands) in ~90% of patients. Visual, auditory, or somatosensory evoked potentials may assist in the diagnosis and in detection of subclinical disease.

▶ Diagnosis

Diagnostic criteria: two separate CNS lesions; two or more separate episodes; involvement of the white matter; objective findings on exam; patient between 10 and 50 years old; no other disease accounting for symptoms. Also may have two attacks with one lesion and abnormal CSF or one attack with two lesions and abnormal CSF. The course is one of remission–relapse. Differential includes hysteria, encephalomyelitis, vasculitis, Lyme disease, syphilis, sarcoidosis, AIDS, stroke, tumors, and syringomyelia (cavitation of the spinal cord).

▶ Clinical Therapeutics

Corticosteroids (prednisone 60–80 mg qd for 10 to 14 days for mild symptoms; methylprednisolone 1 g IV daily for 3–5 days for more severe symptoms) hasten recovery from acute relapses but do not prevent further episodes. For patients with relapsing–remitting disease, beta-interferon (given intramuscularly [IM] once/week) decreases the frequency of the attacks, as does glatiramer acetate (copolymer-1) given subcutaneously, daily. Baclofen, diazepam, and dantrolene may be helpful for spasticity.

▶ Clinical Intervention

No surgical intervention.

▶ Health Maintenance Issues

Physical therapy is useful to prevent contractions, and routine supportive measures for neurogenic bladder or constipation. Psychological support may be required.

## VIII. CENTRAL NERVOUS SYSTEM TRAUMA

▶ Scientific Concepts

*Epidural hematoma:* Collection of arterial blood between the inner table of the skull and the dura. Generally arises from the middle meningeal artery after a skull fracture. Rare in the very young and old secondary to dural adhesion to the skull.

*Subdural hematoma:* Collection of venous blood between the dura and arachnoid. An asymptomatic small clot may lyse and form membrane—a chronic subdural. May be from an insignificant head injury in the elderly, especially if they are on warfarin.

▶ History & Physical

*Epidural hematoma:* Expanding mass that may lead to transtentorial herniation. *Triphasic* injury with an initial loss of consciousness, followed by a "lucid interval" in which patient promptly regains consciousness. Several hours later, the patient begins a rapid deterioration as the hematoma expands and intracranial pressure increases.

*Subdural hematoma:* Varied presentation—may be dramatic, life-threatening neurologic deficits if large and fast growing, or only subtle neurologic changes if small. Presentations include cognitive deficits, focal neurologic deficits, or seizures secondary to the mass effect.

▶ Diagnostic Studies

*Epidural hematoma* and *subdural hematoma* both diagnosed with CT. MRI may be used but takes longer and is more expensive. Suspect either if a fracture is present on skull x-ray.

▶ Clinical Therapeutics

No pharmacological treatment for either.

▶ Clinical Intervention

Surgical removal after radiographic localization for epidural or subdural. If the patient has a unilaterally enlarged pupil, most often the lesion is on the same side as the pupillary abnormality. A burr hole done at the bedside may be all that is needed for a chronic *subdural hematoma* since it is liquefied.

► Health Maintenance Issues

Generalized safety measures to prevent head injury, especially for those on anticoagulants.

## IX. SEIZURE DISORDERS

► Scientific Concepts

A seizure is caused by a transient disturbance of cerebral function secondary to an abnormal paroxysmal neuronal discharge in the brain. Epilepsy is the condition characterized by recurrent seizures. In *idiopathic* epilepsy no specific cause is identified. Numerous causes for secondary seizure include: head trauma (especially if the dura was penetrated), congenital abnormalities and perinatal injuries, tumors, vascular disease, and degenerative disorders such as Alzheimer's. Seizures may also occur with CNS infection (meningitis, encephalitis, brain abscess); withdrawal of alcohol, barbiturates, benzodiazepines, or anticonvulsants; or in metabolic disorders such as hypocalcemia, hyponatremia, uremia, hypoglycemia, and hyperosmolar states. *Febrile seizures* are brief generalized tonic–clonic seizures in children < 5 years, associated with a febrile episode but with a normal exam and negative family history.

► History & Physical

*Generalized Seizures:* In generalized, tonic–clonic seizures, there is sudden loss of consciousness, either without warning or sometimes with nonspecific symptoms or aura. In the tonic phase, lasting 10–30 seconds, there is loss of consciousness and tonic contractures of the limb muscles that cause the patient to fall. This is followed by clonic (alternating contracting and relaxation) symmetric limb jerking that may last 30 to 60 seconds or more. Unconsciousness may extend for several minutes. In the recovery phase, the patient exhibits postictal confusion and often headache with full recovery in 10–30 minutes. Physical exam is essentially normal. *Absence* (petit mal) seizures are much shorter generalized seizures, lasting 5–10 seconds, without loss of postural tone and with no postictal period.

*Partial Seizures:* *Simple* partial seizures are brief (5–180 seconds) focal motor seizures involving a single muscle group in the face or limb and may spread to contiguous areas of the cortex. Other types include *somatosensory* simple partial seizures characterized by brief paresthesias or tingling, light flashes, or buzzing; *autonomic,* involving epigastric sensations, sweating, or flushing; and *psychic,* with déjà vu, illusions or hallucinations, and affective disturbances.

*Partial complex* seizures (psychomotor or temporal lobe) last 20–180 seconds and may involve any of the above either prior to, during, or following an impairment of consciousness and may be followed by a brief postictal period.

► Diagnosis

Electrolytes to assess metabolic abnormalities such as hypoglycemia, hypocalcemia, hyponatremia, and hypernatremia. Imaging is usually limited to new onset seizure to rule out neoplasm. EEG may support the clinical diagnosis, may provide a guide to prognosis, and may help to classify, thereby aiding in medication selection.

### ▶ Clinical Therapeutics

If recurrent seizures require medical management, the goal is to attain control with monotherapy with a specifically indicated drug, carefully individualizing doses with close follow-up. Proper management is directed toward treating the seizures and not the serum drug levels.

Phenytoin, carbamazine, or valproate are drugs of choice for adults with generalized tonic–clonic or partial complex seizures. Phenobarbital may also be useful for tonic–clonic seizures but is less so for complex partial seizures. Valproic acid or carbamazine are preferred for children with these disorders. A number of newer anticonvulsants (gabapentin, lamotrigine, topiramate, vigabatrin, and tiagabine) may be utilized if the more conventional medications do not produce optimal control of seizures. Valproic acid and ethosuximide are generally preferred for absence (petit mal) seizures.

### ▶ Clinical Intervention

Status epilepticus is a prolonged seizure, either convulsive or nonconvulsive, lasting >15–30 minutes. After drawing glucose, electrolytes, magnesium, blood urea nitrogen (BUN), give 50 mL of 50% dextrose and 100 mg thiamine IV. Then IV diazepam, 0.2 mg/kg, or lorazepam, 0.1–0.2 mg/kg, repeatedly until seizures stop plus loading dose of phenytoin (in saline as it precipitates in glucose solutions) or phenobarbital. When controlled, may start other anticonvulsants such as carbamazepine.

### ▶ Health Maintenance Issues

Routine clinical follow up to observe for medication-related effects such as gingival hyperplasia and hirsutism in patients taking phenytoin. Also monitor CBC in patients on carbamazepine to rule out agranulocytosis or aplastic anemia or check liver function tests in those on valproic acid to rule out hepatic dysfunction. Driving restrictions after a seizure vary from state to state. Titrate patient off anticonvulsants to prevent rebound seizures.

## X. VASCULAR DISEASE

## A. Transient Ischemic Attacks

### ▶ Scientific Concepts

Sudden onset of characteristic neurologic deficit reflecting focal involvement of the CNS secondary to disturbance of cerebral circulation. Occurs most frequently in older patients and those at risk for vascular disease. Most last a few minutes but may be symptomatic for over an hour. TIAs usually correspond to a vascular distribution, either carotid or vertebral. Cardiogenic activity may produce emboli. By definition, they resolve completely. Some patients will have a neurologic deficit that persists >24 hours but resolves completely within a few days; this is termed *reversible ischemic neurological deficit.* Important to note that one third of those with TIA will have a stroke within 5 years.

▶ History & Physical

***Carotid artery TIAs:*** Contralateral hand/arm weakness with sensory loss; face and leg symptoms are less severe; may be ipsilateral visual symptoms or aphasia, amaurosis fugax; no carotid bruits if stenosis is >95% secondary to low turbulence.

***Vertebrobasilar TIAs:*** Diplopia, ataxia, vertigo, dysarthria, either unilateral or bilateral visual loss, CN palsies, leg weakness on either side, perioral numbness, hemiparesis and even quadriparesis, drop attacks. Fundoscopy may reveal cholesterol plaques.

▶ Diagnostic Studies

Cardiac workup to exclude arrhythmias and new murmurs; hematologic workup to exclude coagulopathies; ESR to rule out temporal arteritis. Cholesterol, prothrombin time/partial thromboplastin time (PT/PTT), antiphospholipid antibodies, echocardiogram (ECG), transthoracic two-dimensional echocardiogram, CBC and differential, carotid Dopplers, magnetic resonance angiography. Arteriogram is the gold standard.

▶ Differential Diagnosis

Seizures with loss of consciousness, migraine, transient global amnesia, syncope, mass lesions, multiple sclerosis.

▶ Clinical Therapeutics

Admission for IV heparin beginning at 1,000 U/h adjusted to keep PTT 1.5 × normal, aspirin (recommended dose not established), sulfinpyrazone, dipyridamole by mouth for long-term prophylaxis. Ticlopidine in women and in cases of aspirin failure.

▶ Clinical Intervention

Carotid endarterectomy for those with a proven > 70% stenosis.

▶ Health Maintenance Issues

Control hypertension, serum cholesterol, and atrial fibrillation. Patient education regarding cessation of cigarette smoking and excessive alcohol use.

## B. Cerebrovascular Accidents

▶ Scientific Concepts

There are 500,000 new cerebrovascular accidents (CVAs) each year. They increase with age and are higher in African Americans. Risk factors include hypertension, elevated blood lipids, diabetes, obesity, family history, elevated fibrinogen, high hematocrit, coronary artery disease, congestive heart failure, atrial fibrillation, left ventricular hypertrophy, smoking, oral contraceptives, alcohol abuse, and physical inactivity. If secondary to atherothrombosis of a major vessel, then termed *ischemic;* these often occur during sleep, the patient waking with a new neurological deficit. *Lacunar* infarcts are small infarcts of the branches of the major cerebral arteries with etiologies of lipohyalinosis (deposition of a hyaline substance within the arterial wall leading to occlusion and seen secondary to hypertension) or embolism. *Intracerebral hemorrhage* occurs with direct bleeding into the brain and primarily secondary to hypertension; these often occur with the patient awake. *Subarachnoid hemorrhage* from arteries/veins bleeding into subarachnoid space. Illicit drug use, especially cocaine and amphetamines, must be considered.

▶ History & Physical
*Ischemic:* Varies with location of the lesion.
- *Internal carotid:* Ipsilateral blindness, contralateral hemiparesis, hemianopia, aphasia.
- *Middle cerebral:* Main trunk; hemiplegia, hemianesthesia, hemianopia, aphasia. *Upper division:* hemiparesis and sensory loss with arm affected more than leg, Broca's aphasia. *Lower trunk:* Wernicke's aphasia.
- *Anterior cerebral:* Hemiparesis and sensory loss affecting leg more than arm, impaired responsiveness, tactile anomia.
- *Posterior cerebral:* Hemianopia, hemiballism (involuntary throwing or flinging movements of the limbs), amnesia, oculomotor palsy.

*Hemorrhagic:*
- *Putamenal:* Severe hemiparesis/hemiplegia, hemianopsia, and aphasia.
- *Caudate:* Abrupt headache, vomiting, nuchal rigidity, and less frequently hemiparesis/gaze palsy.
- *Thalamic:* Hemiparesis/hemiplegia immediately; conjugate horizontal gaze deviation toward the lesion; upward gaze palsy with miotic, unreactive pupils with larger lesions. Lobar varies with hemiparesis of arm in frontal, sensorimotor and visual deficit in parietal, homonymous hemianopsia in occipital, Wernicke's aphasia in dominant temporal.
- *Cerebellar:* Sudden onset of nausea, vomiting, dizziness, inability to stand, headache but rarely loss of consciousness, limb or gait ataxia, facial palsy, ipsilateral gaze palsy. These strokes often worsen after initial presentation.
- *Pontine:* Generally leads to deep coma within minutes and decerebrate rigidity, bilateral pinpoint pupils, ocular motility disorders, abnormal respirations.

*Subarachnoid hemorrhage:* "Worst headache of life," 30% with change in level of consciousness, CN III palsy, nuchal rigidity, subhyaloid hemorrhages on fundoscopy in 25%.

▶ Diagnostic Studies
Carotid Dopplers, CT, MRI; arteriogram is gold standard. *Ischemic stroke* with hypodensity on CT that follows vascular pattern. *Hemorrhagic* with hyperdensity that may be parenchymal, subarachnoid, intraventricular, subdural, or a combination of these. Ischemic stroke on MRI with hypointensity in T1 and hyperintensity in T2. Hemorrhagic varies with date—if less than 24 hours, may not be visible, thereafter hyperintense on T1 images. Arteriogram is optimal for evaluating arterial lesions such as aneurysms and arteriovenous malformations. Magnetic resonance angiography rapidly replacing standard arteriograms. *Subarachnoid* with blood in basal cisterns and sylvian fissures on CT acutely, intraparenchymal blood and hydrocephalus later; MRI not useful acutely but excellent after a few days for detecting aneurysms, etc. Angiography is gold standard. Nontraumatic lumbar puncture 6–12 hours after headache with xanthochromic CSF.

► Diagnosis

Embolism, hemorrhage, trauma, migraine, seizure, epidural or subdural hematoma, neoplasm, abscess.

► Clinical Therapeutics

Carotid endarterectomy for prevention of *ischemic stroke,* also antiplatelet drugs such as aspirin, ticlopidine. *Hemorrhagic* with intensive care unit (ICU) management, hyperventilation, mannitol and steroids now controversial, surgery usually ineffective. *Subarachnoid* with nimodipine and hypertension to prevent vasospasm, general ICU management as this is an emergency.

► Clinical Intervention

Angioplasty for ischemic.

► Health Maintenance Issues

Control hypertension, treat bacterial endocarditis, resect atrial myxoma, treat atrial fibrillation, cessation of smoking, increase physical activity.

## C. Cerebral Aneurysm

► Scientific Concepts

Leakage from a congenital (berry) aneurysm is the most common and important cause of nontraumatic subarachnoid (SAH) hemorrhage. Most common in fifth and sixth decades, with an equal sex distribution. It is fatal in 50% of cases.

► History & Physical

Up to 40% of SAH patients have a small, self-limiting "herald bleed" causing atypical headache. Examination may reveal focal neurologic signs (e.g., ptosis, mydriasis, ophthalmoplegia) prior to rupture by compression of the brain or cranial nerves. With rupture, virtually every patient describes an abrupt "worst headache of his/her life."

► Diagnostic Studies

CT is done initially, will generally confirm hemorrhage, and may identify a focal source. MRI may detect brain stem atriovenous malformation (AVM) not seen on CT. Lumbar puncture reveals markedly elevated pressure and grossly bloody CSF. Cerebral angiography should be performed when appropriate, since multiple aneurysms occur in 20% of patients and will assist in planning for surgical treatment.

► Differential Diagnosis

Hypertensive intracerebral hemorrhage must be considered, but will present with prominent focal neurologic deficits. Acute bacterial meningitis is excluded following CSF examination.

► Clinical Therapeutics

Medical treatment is directed toward preventing rerupture by controlling arterial or intracranial pressure elevation. Medications impairing platelet function must be avoided.

► Clinical Intervention

Strict bed rest with the head elevated 15–20 degrees, mild sedation. Definitive surgical management involves clipping the neck of the aneurysm or the endovascular placement of a coil to induce clotting. An AVM may be removed by resection, or obliterated by ligation of feeding vessels or embolization via intra-arterial catheter.

▶ **Health Maintenance Issues**

Mortality rate from a ruptured cerebral aneurysm is high, with 50% dying from the initial hemorrhage or its consequences. Another 20% die from rebleeding if the aneurysm is not surgically corrected.

## XI. BRAIN TUMORS

▶ **Scientific Concepts**

Gliomas are most common at 60% of primary tumors followed by meningiomas at 20%. More than 100 types of tumors are known. Tumors are second only to stroke as neurological cause of death in adults. Etiologies varied: inherited with neurofibromatosis I, tuberous sclerosis, and bilateral retinoblastomas; environmental with ionizing radiation exposure possibly predisposing to meningiomas and gliomas.

▶ **History & Physical**

Headache in 40%. Frontal headaches are nonspecific, intermittent, dull, ipsilateral, supratentorial. Occipital headaches occur with tumors in the posterior fossa. Brain tumor headaches tend to wake the patient at night, improve during the day, and are worsened with coughing or exercise. Examination findings may include papilledema; seizures, especially in adults without a prior history; and an altered mental status. Tumors have signs/symptoms related to their location:

***Frontal lobe:*** Personality changes, especially disinhibition, irritability, impaired judgment, abulia (lack of initiative); exam showing gaze preference, forced grasping, snout reflex, anosmia, hemiparesis, seizures, aphasia, urinary frequency, gait difficulties.

***Temporal lobe:*** Varied seizures, aphasia, and superior quadrantanopsia.

***Parietal lobe:*** Contralateral sensory loss in proprioception, stereognosis, graphesthesia, aphasia, hemiparesis, homonymous field defects, agnosias, apraxias.

***Occipital lobe:*** Homonymous hemianopsia, visual seizures.

▶ **Diagnostic Studies**

Contrast-enhanced CT or MRI is the appropriate diagnostic study. Angiography occasionally useful. Other study modalities include visual fields, electroencephalogram (EEG), audiometry, CSF analysis, and endocrine evaluation depending on the clinical picture.

▶ **Differential Diagnosis**

An acute onset of symptoms, CVA, or intracranial hemorrhage. An evolving symptom picture with focal neurologic symptoms; fever and headache suggests an abscess. Changes in mental status may occur with various metabolic conditions, meningioencephalitis, and either primary or metastatic neoplasms.

► Clinical Therapeutics

Anticonvulsants, usually phenytoin, if seizures are present. Anticonvulsants not needed if tumor is small and infratentorial. Corticosteroids may decrease edema. May need head elevation, fluid restriction, diuretics, and/or hyperventilation if corticosteroids are not effective.

► Clinical Intervention

Observation if tumor "benign" on radiographic studies. Surgical resection or debulking to allow adjunct therapies to work better. Radiotherapy as either conventional beam therapy, stereotactic brachytherapy, stereotactic radiotherapy. Chemotherapy with varied agents. Being reviewed are immunotherapy, hormonal therapy, antiangiogenic agents, and gene therapy.

► Health Maintenance Issues

After diagnosis, physical therapy and rehabilitation, emotional and psychological support, hospice.

## BIBLIOGRAPHY

Devinsky O, Feldmann E, Weinreb HJ, Wilterdink JL, eds. *The Resident's Neurology Book.* Philadelphia: F.A. Davis; 1997.

Simon RP, Aminoff MJ, Greenberg DA, eds. *Clinical Neurology,* 4th ed. New York: Lange Medical Book/McGraw-Hill; 1999.

Stobo JD, Hellman DB, Ladeson PW, Petty BG, Traill TA, eds. *The Principles and Practice of Medicine.* Stamford, CT: Appleton & Lange; 1996.

# Psychiatry 13

*Anita Duhl Glicken, MSW, and Douglas R. Southard, PhD, MPH, PA-C*

## I. PSYCHOSES

### A. Affective Psychosis: Mania and Psychotic Depression

▶ Scientific Concepts

Tend to cluster in families. Incidence increases with age.

▶ History & Physical

Family history; clinical features of mood disorder precede psychotic state. Illness generally episodic rather than continuous. Symptoms include: *Mania*—hyperactivity, pressured and rapid speech, labile affect with elation or irritability, flight of ideas, distractibility, impulsivity, grandiosity, paranoia. *Depression*—psychomotor retardation, agitation, slowed speech, changes in appetite or weight, poor self-care, somatic delusions, guilt, derogatory hallucinations, suicidal ideation. Alcohol abuse common.

▶ Diagnostic Studies

No pathognomonic signs or studies; rule out medical etiology through history and lab work (i.e., thyroid and adrenal dysfunction).

▶ Diagnosis

Differentiate from other psychiatric disorders including personality disorders (schizophrenia), attention deficit hyperactivity disorder (ADHD), substance abuse, and/or intoxication. Rule out medical etiologies (thyroid, adrenal dysfunction, medications, Parkinson's disease, multiple sclerosis, pancreatic and other malignancies, lupus, central nervous system [CNS] tumors, cerebrovascular accidents [CVAs], viral illness).

▶ Clinical Therapeutics

*Acute mania:* Neuroleptics or benzodiazepines to control agitation. Lithium titrated to serum levels of 1.0 to 1.5. Anticonvulsants (valproic acid, carbamazepine) effective. Electroconvulsive therapy (ECT) may be used for rapid control.

*Psychotic depression:* ECT most effective; antidepressants combined with neuroleptic also effective. Poor response from antidepressants alone.

▶ Clinical Intervention

Hospitalization for protection of self and others and diagnosis. Therapeutics as above. Ongoing low-dose neuroleptics; antidepressants for depression; supportive therapies; family support.

▶ Health Maintenance Issues

Monitor improvement in target symptoms. Maintenance doses of medications should be closely monitored. For mania and bipolar, mood stabilizers should be continued on an outpatient basis for at least 4–6 months, at dose required for control of acute symptoms. Indefinite continuation should be considered after three or more manic episodes. Discontinuation of antipsychotics should be considered following symptom resolution. For psychotic depression, there is a 50% chance of relapse if antidepressants are discontinued before 6 months, so therapy should be continued for at least 6–12 months. Discontinuation should occur gradually and with longer prophylaxis considered if there is a history of recurrence, greater severity, long depressive episodes, and older age at onset. Support groups and therapy. Monitor possible alcohol and substance use.

## B. Paranoid States

### ▶ Scientific Concepts

Paranoia is a nonspecific symptom that can be present in personality disorders, delusional disorder, schizophrenia, mania or depression with psychotic features, brief psychotic disorder, and substance-related disorders.

### ▶ History & Physical

Course and severity of paranoid ideation varies.

### ▶ Diagnostic Studies

Laboratory screening should include complete blood count (CBC); complete chemistry profile, including electrolytes, liver function tests, renal function tests, and tests for calcium and magnesium; urine drug test; thyroid function tests; blood concentrations for any medications being taken. Once substance-related disorders and general medical conditions are ruled out, complete psychiatric evaluation will reveal diagnosis. Neuropsychological testing, electroencephalogram (EEG), computed tomography (CT), and/or magnetic resonance imaging (MRI) may help identify underlying organic conditions.

### ▶ Diagnosis

Differential may include paranoid personality disorder and delusional disorder of the persecutory type, typically with paranoid ideation that has been constant over long periods. Absence of delusions in paranoid personality disorder; prominent delusions in delusional disorder. Paranoia in mania or depression is present only during acute episodes. Schizophrenia usually identified by presence of other symptoms, such as thought disorders or hallucinations.

### ▶ Clinical Therapeutics

If patient is already taking antipsychotic medications, give another dose of that medication. In general, psychotic paranoid patients can be given haloperidol, thiothixene, fluphenazine, or trifluoperazine, all at doses of 2–5 mg by mouth (PO) or intramuscularly (IM) as needed. Paranoid conditions caused by intoxication or withdrawal from drugs can be managed with lorazepam, 1–2 mg PO or IM. Severely anxious paranoid patients can be treated with lorazepam. Paranoia with agitation caused by delirium or dementia can be managed with haloperidol, 1–5 mg PO or IM.

### ▶ Clinical Intervention

History, lab work, clinical therapeutics as described above. Treat in emergency room or office according to diagnosis. Dangerous patient may need hospitalization, even involuntary commitment. Question regarding suicide or homicidal ideation. Directly ask patient what he or she would do to those perceived against him or her. Ask about previous acts of violence and suicide attempts.

### ▶ Health Maintenance Issues

Follow-up related to diagnosis. Monitor improvement in target symptoms and long-term medication use. Psychiatric referral and support groups.

## C. Delusional Disorder (Formerly Paranoid Disorder)

▶ **Scientific Concepts**

Etiology unknown; genetically unrelated to schizophrenia and affective disorders; formerly called paranoia or paranoid disorder.

▶ **History & Physical**

Primary manifestation fixed, nonbizarre, systematized delusion; typically midlife onset; functioning variable; mental status exam typically normal except for delusional system; mood consistent with delusions.

▶ **Diagnostic Studies**

Toxicology screening, routine laboratory work, neuropsychological testing, EEG or CT scan for differential diagnosis.

▶ **Diagnosis**

Symptoms as above; the *Diagnostic and Statistical Manual,* 4th edition (*DSM-IV*) specifies seven subtypes based on predominant content of delusions; persecutory and jealous types most common, erotomanic and somatic types most unusual; also grandiose, mixed, and unspecified. Delusion can accompany many neurological and medical illnesses, including basal ganglia disorders, endocrinopathies, limbic system disorders, systemic disorders; differential diagnosis also to rule out malingering and factitious disorder with predominantly psychological signs and symptoms; delirium, dementia, substance-related disorders, schizophrenia, mood disorders, obsessive–compulsive disorder, somatoform disorders, and paranoid personality disorder.

▶ **Clinical Therapeutics**

In emergency, antipsychotic drug IM, followed by antipsychotic drugs like low-dose haloperidol, pimozide; maintenance doses typically low; some patients may receive no benefit; unresponsive patients to antipsychotic drugs may try antidepressants like lithium or anticonvulsants, particularly with family history of mood disorder; most common cause of drug failure is noncompliance.

▶ **Clinical Intervention**

Can generally be treated as outpatient; hospitalization for evaluation and differential; evaluation of patient's control over violent impulses; legal commitment may be necessary; individual psychotherapy, insight-oriented, cognitive, behavioral, and family therapy may be helpful. Stimulate continued motivation to receive help, emphasizing patient's management of anxiety and irritability. Do not support reality of delusions, but avoid making disparaging remarks about delusions.

▶ **Health Maintenance Issues**

Successful treatment may be satisfactory social adjustment rather than disappearance of delusions; continue to promote positive therapeutic alliance with patient; overgratification may increase patient's hostility and suspiciousness because not all demands can be met; emphasize that preoccupation with delusions interferes with daily life.

## D. Psychosis Originating in Childhood

▶ **Scientific Concepts**

Developmental factors relevant to treatment and diagnosis. Nature of psychological and neurobiological processes underlying psychotic phenomena in children and adolescents remains largely unknown. Before the *Diagnostic and Statistical Manual,* 3rd edition (*DSM-III*), all severe childhood disturbance was equated with schizophrenia. Epidemiology of psychotic depression in children is very limited, may be due to chemical factors, psychological factors, or both. Bipolar disorder develops in a sizeable minority of children and adolescents who initially present with depression.

▶ History & Physical

*Schizophrenia: Childhood:* Early-onset (EOS) and very-early-onset (VEOS) frequency increases after 11 years. *Adolescence:* Conditions as above with increasing frequency, develops gradually over weeks or months; symptoms often denied until situation becomes emergent. Emergent constellation of symptoms consistent with adult disorder includes at least two characteristic symptoms (delusions, hallucinations, disorganized speech, grossly disorganized or catatonic behavior) as well as social–occupational dysfunction and duration of at least 6 months.

*Mood disorders (major depression with psychosis and bipolar disorder):* Source of greatest diagnostic confusion. Longitudinal information clarifies nature of disorder underlying initial psychotic presentation. Manic symptoms vary with age. Children < 9 more likely to present with aggressiveness, emotional lability, and irritability. Older children with euphoria, grandiosity, or paranoid ideation and flight of ideas. Pressured speech, overactivity, and distractibility noted in all ages. Mania in adolescence similar to adults with psychotic features more common.

▶ Diagnostic Studies

No pathognomonic signs or lab studies. Symptoms as described above. Psychological testing (IQ), communication assessments, projective testing, and adaptive behavior. Physical and neurological examinations; evaluate potential substance abuse.

▶ Diagnosis

Schizophrenia—EOS after 13 years; VEOS before 13 years, quite rare. Difficulties in diagnosis in younger children. Delusions and hallucinations are often less elaborate in childhood. Disorganized speech and behavior may characterize a number of other conditions. For schizophrenia and mood disorders, rule out substance-induced psychotic reaction; medical illness that produces delirium; coexisting antisocial behavior disorder; ADHD; brief psychotic disorder. Major depression with psychotic features must be differentiated from manic phase of bipolar disorder.

▶ Clinical Therapeutics

*Schizophrenia:* Major tranquilizers effective during the active psychotic phase; lower doses during maintenance phase. Therapeutic effect may not be apparent for some time after treatment is initiated. Some patients fail to respond; for those patients, atypical antipsychotics should be considered.

*Mood disorders:* Pharmacologic treatments of adult mood disorders generally appropriate for children. Lithium in bipolar disorders and tricyclic antidepressants in treatment of major depression associated with psychosis. Selective serotonin reuptake inhibitors (SSRIs) and electroconvulsive therapy also considered.

► Clinical Intervention

*Acute:* Treatment of child with psychosis will depend on nature of disorder, characteristics of the individual, stage of illness, and developmental level of the child. Often, multiple treatment modalities, including pharmacotherapy (haloperidol, clozapine, risperidone, olanzapine, quetiapine), educational and family interventions, and supportive psychotherapy. Inpatient treatment may be needed during acute phase. *Follow-up:* Excessive medication is common. Possible short- and long-term side effects (sedation, weight gain) should be monitored with planned reevaluation. Baseline weight, lipid profile, and blood and glucose levels should be monitored. Family intervention programs may help reduce relapse rates. Supportive psychotherapy, educational interventions, and social skills training may be indicated. Cognitive behavior therapy (CBT) administered in school settings. Efficacy of transcranial magnetic stimulation (TMS) is under investigation. Long-term treatment program should be flexible and well integrated.

► Health Maintenance Issues

Ongoing flexible and integrated treatment program as above. Monitor medication use for possible side effects; potential substance abuse; comorbid conditions (e.g., depression). Adolescents with bipolar conditions are more likely than adults to relapse. Family programs may reduce relapse.

## E. Schizophrenia

► Scientific Concepts

Evidence that it runs in some families, path of transmission is unclear. Pathogenesis through stress diathesis model; constitutional factors determined by heredity (diathesis) interacting with environmental influences (stress) that precipitate overt expression of clinical symptoms. Pathological findings include nonspecific gliosis, cellular loss, and disordered orientation of the pyramidal cells in the hippocampus, suggesting developmental rather than degenerative disturbance.

► History & Physical

Family history; onset typically late teens through 20s; precipitated by stress. Often have premorbid schizoid features; begins gradually, duration of symptoms at least 6 months with at least two psychotic symptoms for at least 1 month. Constellation of symptoms rather than a single symptom; formal thought disorder; content of thought, perceptual disturbances, and alterations in emotions and behavior; loose associations, tangentiality, incoherence; mood-congruent and -incongruent delusions, paranoia, being controlled, thought broadcasting, grandiosity, religion and somatic delusions; visual and auditory hallucinations; bizarre and catatonic behavior; psychotic depression; may have soft neurologic signs, motor abnormalities.

► Diagnostic Studies

No pathognomonic signs or lab studies; typically, patient must exhibit two or more of following symptoms for a significant portion of time during a 1-month period: delusions, hallucinations, disorganized speech, grossly disorganized or catatonic behavior, negative symptoms; impaired functioning during active phase. Symptoms for at least 6 months; schizo-affective and mood disorder exclusion.

▶ Diagnosis

Symptoms as above; *DSM-IV* subtypes; paranoid, disorganized, cata-tonic, undifferentiated, and residual based on clinical presentation. Pos-itive and negative symptom classification. Positive: productive symptoms including delusions, hallucinations, and bizarre behaviors. Negative symp-toms marked by absence of functioning including affective flattening, avolition, social withdrawal. Differential diagnosis includes a wide range of nonpsychiatric medical conditions and a variety of substances that induce symptoms of psychosis and catatonia, including psychotic or cata-tonic disorder due to general medical condition and substance-induced psychotic disorder.

▶ Clinical Therapeutics

Neuroleptic agents for controlling active symptoms of psychosis and prophylactic effect to prevent relapse; two major classes of dopamine receptor antagonists (i.e., chlorpromazine, haloperidol, sulpiride) and serotonin–dopamine antagonists (i.e., clozapine, risperidone, olanza-pine); dopamine receptor antagonists appear to help only a small per-centage of patients (25%) with annoying and serious adverse effects. Serotonin–dopamine antagonists appear to be effective with broader range of patients and cause few extrapyramidal symptoms; however, clozapine carries a 1 to 2% risk of agranulocytosis. Recent research sug-gests olanzapine be considered as a first-line treatment of patients in acute episode.

▶ Clinical Intervention

Hospitalization to contain disruptive and dangerous behavior. Med-ical evaluation for presence of medical, neurological, or substance dis-orders that may be etiologically related. Neuroleptic agents as described above. Psychosocial intervention to complement the use of medication; connecting patient with appropriate aftercare treatment. After acute psy-chotic episode, goal should be to prevent relapse while adjusting med-ication to maintenance level. Continued use of neuroleptics reduces relapse rate. Reintegration of patient into community; home environ-ment major treatment milieu. Family treatment shown to reduce relapse in the first year. Day hospital programs for transition may be helpful for patients without support. Social skills training, supportive psychotherapy, and vocational rehabilitation may be indicated.

▶ Health Maintenance Issues

Designated case manager to coordinate multifaceted treatment plans. Continued monitoring of neuroleptic drug use and side effects. Suicide is common (50% of schizophrenic patients attempt suicide at least once); associated substance abuse; 75% smoke cigarettes; about 30 to 50% may meet diagnostic criteria for alcohol abuse or alcohol dependence; home-lessness related to deinstitutionalization of patients (estimates that one third to two thirds of homeless people are schizophrenic). Long-term prognosis is variable based on onset; precipitating factors; premorbid social, sexual, and work history; support systems; and presence of positive or negative symptoms. Late and acute onset, obvious precipitating factors, good premorbid history, social support, and positive symptoms indicate good prognosis.

## F. Other Nonorganic Psychoses

▶ **Scientific Concepts**
Various psychoses of nonorganic origin.

▶ **History & Physical**
*Schizoaffective disorder:* Concurrent symptoms of schizophrenia and depression or mania, with at least 2 weeks of psychotic symptoms alone.

*Schizophreniform disorder:* Same symptoms, history as schizophrenia but duration of < 6 months.

*Brief psychotic disorder:* Acute-onset psychosis with emotional upset and confusion often following stress. Duration < 1 month. Full return to premorbid functioning. Often seen in young adults.

*Shared psychotic disorder:* Patient delusional, develops in conjunction with submissive, dependent, isolated relationship with delusional person. Suicide or homicide pacts.

*Psychotic disorder not otherwise specified:* Psychotic symptoms that do not meet criteria for other disorders. Includes postpartum psychosis (occurs 2–3 weeks postpartum, usually primipara, risk of infanticide or suicide), culture-bound syndromes.

▶ **Diagnostic Studies**
Lab tests to rule out organic etiology or substance use.

▶ **Diagnosis**
Symptoms as specified above.

▶ **Clinical Therapeutics**
*Schizoaffective disorder:* Bipolar type; neuroleptic discontinued or reduced after stabilization; other options include carbamazepine, valproic acid, maintenance electroconvulsive treatment (M-ECT), lithium for maintenance, clozapine for refractory symptoms. Recent research suggests ziprasidone for short-term treatment with low side effects, or risperidone. Depressive type; neuroleptic with or without antidepressant, ECT, lithium also used.

*Schizophreniform disorder:* Neuroleptics for at least 6 months.

*Brief psychotic disorder:* Neuroleptic or antianxiety agent.

*Shared psychotic disorder:* Neuroleptics, olanzapine.

▶ **Clinical Intervention**
Clinical therapeutics as above with psychotherapy. Hospitalization as needed for patient safety and stabilization.

▶ **Health Maintenance Issues**
Follow-up as needed based on diagnosis. Supportive psychotherapy and family support.

## II. ANXIETY/MOOD/PERSONALITY DISORDERS

### A. Acute Stress Reactions

▶ Scientific Concepts

Intensity of the trauma (i.e., motor vehicle accident, military combat, rape, etc.) may be strongest predisposing factor. A history of personality disorder, major psychopathology, or low social support may also predict poor psychological adjustment to acute stressor. Expression of dissociation may be culturally influenced.

▶ History & Physical

Exposure to traumatic event within 4 weeks. Symptoms of anxiety, fear, dissociation (e.g., derealization, numbing detachment, reduced awareness of surroundings, depersonalization), reexperiencing event (images, thoughts, dreams, flashbacks). Avoidance of reminders of event. Impaired ability to perform necessary tasks.

▶ Diagnostic Studies

None required.

▶ Diagnosis

Lasts minimum of 2 days; if lasts more than 4 weeks, diagnose posttraumatic stress disorder (PTSD). Symptoms not due to drug effects or other medical condition. Impact of Event Scale useful for diagnosis.

▶ Clinical Therapeutics

Benzodiazepines or buspirone may be used for short-term treatment.

▶ Clinical Intervention

Psychotherapy to reduce dissociation, acknowledge trauma.

▶ Health Maintenance Issues

May have impaired ability to care for self. At risk for PTSD.

### B. Adjustment Disorders

▶ Scientific Concepts

Vulnerability to stress may be related to temperament, constitution, experiences, personality, severity of stressor.

▶ History & Physical

Identifiable stressor within range of normal experience (acute or chronic illness, employment problems, etc.) within 3 months. Distress in excess of what would be expected. Impaired social or occupational functioning.

▶ Diagnostic Studies

None required.

▶ Diagnosis

Emotional disturbance and impaired functioning greater than would be expected from identifiable psychosocial stressor. Stressors include school, divorce, job loss, illness. Onset within 3 months but no longer than 6 months unless stressor is chronic (e.g., chronic illness). If overreaction is part of pattern, diagnose personality disorder. Distress not due to bereavement. Rule out substance abuse. May be classified by predominant symptoms: depressed mood, anxiety, mixed anxiety and depressed mood, disturbance of conduct, mixed disturbance of emotions and conduct, or unspecified. Behavioral symptoms in adolescents; mood, anxiety symptoms in adults. If stressor outside normal range of experiences, diagnose PTSD.

▶ Clinical Therapeutics

Short-term medication for relief of anxiety, insomnia, and depressive mood.

▶ Clinical Intervention

Clarify barriers to problem resolution and develop therapeutic plan. Reduce stress (exercise, social support, cognitive restructuring, relaxation techniques, self-care, short-term therapy, group support). Treat substance abuse, underlying psychopathology if present.

## C. Anxiety/Panic Disorders

### 1. Panic Disorder

▶ Scientific Concepts

Significant evidence for genetic component; biological basis related to disturbances in norepinephrine and gamma-aminobutyric acid (GABA) neurotransmission. One-year prevalence is 1–2%; onset in third decade of life; more common in women. Often associated with mitral valve prolapse though no causal relationship has been established.

▶ History & Physical

Recurring, unexpected, sudden "panic attacks" involving intense fear or discomfort to include four or more of the following symptoms: sweating, shortness of breath, trembling/shaking, palpitations, chest pain, choking, dizziness/faintness, nausea/abdominal distress, fear of dying, fear of losing control, chills/hot flashes, paresthesias, derealization/depersonalization. Can be precipitated by stressful event but often occurs unexpectedly without identifiable stressor. Severity and frequency of panic attacks may vary considerably. Persistent concern (>1 month) regarding occurrence and consequences of recurrent panic attacks often leads to anticipatory anxiety. May be present with or without agoraphobia (avoidance of leaving the home alone or being in a confined social or physical environment that causes significant anxiety). Primary care provider or cardiologist typically consulted first for somatic complaints. Evaluate for excessive caffeine intake, positive family history, and comorbid depression; childhood anxiety disorder may be a predisposing factor. Physical exam may reveal tachycardia, elevated systolic blood pressure, hyperventilation, sweating, trembling, cold hands. Finding characteristics of mitral valve prolapse may be present.

▶ Diagnostic Studies

None are diagnostic; carbon dioxide and sodium lactate can precipitate panic.

▶ Diagnosis

Rule out other anxiety disorders and medical conditions including substance abuse (caffeinism, stimulants, alcohol, or sedative withdrawal), cardiac disorders, hypoglycemia, hyperparathyroidism, hyperthyroidism, hypoxia, pheochromocytoma, seizure disorders, and vestibular disease. Avoid excessive medical workups. Coded as with or without agoraphobia.

► **Clinical Therapeutics**
Tricyclic antidepressants, SSRIs, and high-potency benzodiazepines are effective.

► **Clinical Intervention**
Reassurance and relaxation training to manage acute panic attack. Rebreathing into paper bag may be helpful. Prompt referral to psychiatry/psychology for cognitive-behavioral intervention to include relaxation training for panic attacks and systematic desensitization if agoraphobia present. Eliminate caffeine and other stimulants.

## 2. Generalized Anxiety Disorder

► **Scientific Concepts**
Familial patterns, possible genetic component.

► **History & Physical**
Anxiety and worry on most days lasting more than 6 months. Inability to control apprehensive expectations. Anxiety frequency, duration, and intensity is excessive for current life stressors. Associated with three or more of following symptoms: easy to fatigue, sleep disturbance, difficulty concentrating, irritability, restlessness, and muscle tension. Muscle tension, aches, and soreness along with other symptoms of autonomic arousal are common. Significant impairment in occupational, interpersonal, and activities of daily living (ADL) functioning. Often associated with major depression.

► **Diagnostic Studies**
None required.

► **Diagnosis**
Not diagnosed if anxiety due to specific anxiety disorders, substance use, or other psychiatric or medical condition.

► **Clinical Therapeutics**
Although immediately effective, benzodiazepines should be used sparingly and only for up to several months due to potential for abuse. Buspirone is an effective initial treatment, although it does not provide as immediate relief as benzodiazepines. SSRIs, tricyclic antidepressants, and monoamine oxidase inhibitors (MAOIs) may be useful in selected patients. May need prolonged or intermittent treatment.

► **Clinical Intervention**
Cognitive–behavioral therapy. May be at increased risk for panic disorders.

## 3. Obsessive–Compulsive Disorder

► **Scientific Concepts**
Affects 2–3% of the population. Possible genetic contribution; probable serotonin system abnormality. Often present first to the family care practitioner.

► History & Physical

Persistent and consuming recurrent images, thoughts, and impulses; may be inappropriate and/or intrusive. Perceived as product of own mind (versus delusion or thought insertion). Typical obsessions include a preoccupation with aggression, order, sin, contamination, loss of control, doubt. Obsessions cause significant distress or anxiety that is excessive in respect to current life events. May feel driven to perform ritualistic behaviors (compulsions) to reduce anxiety. Typical compulsions (i.e., repeating words silently, repetitive touching, checking, washing, etc.) are time consuming and interrupt interpersonal, vocational, and ADL functioning. Onset generally by early adulthood; 75% have both obsessions and compulsions. Depressive feelings and major affective disorder very common. May have other anxiety disorders, anorexia nervosa, alcoholism, Tourette's syndrome. Dermatologic complaints may be present secondary to excessive washing.

► Diagnostic Studies

None required.

► Diagnosis

Differentiate excessive pleasure-seeking (i.e., eating, sexual activity, etc.) as opposed to anxiety-reducing (i.e., hand washing, checking, etc.) behaviors. Differentiate from obsessive–compulsive symptoms presenting in depression and schizophrenia that respond to specific treatments.

► Clinical Therapeutics

Fluoxetine (SSRI) and clomipramine (tricyclic antidepressant) effective in 60%; may require higher doses for several weeks to several months. Observe for agitation, sexual dysfunction (fluoxetine), and anticholinergic effects (clomipramine). Most effective when combined with cognitive–behavioral intervention.

► Clinical Intervention

Cognitive–behavioral therapy based on exposure to feared situation, thought stopping, and compulsive behavior blocking. Relapse common.

## 4. Posttraumatic Stress Disorder

► Scientific Concepts

Disorder is common in individuals exposed to extreme stressors, with some prevalence estimates exceeding 50%. Biological basis includes heightened sympathetic nervous system arousal.

► History & Physical

History of exposure to traumatic event threatening or causing serious injury to self or others. Typical events: criminal violence, combat, natural disaster, sexual abuse. Symptoms include intense fear and helplessness; recurrent nightmares, flashbacks, reliving of event; avoidance of event-related stimuli; emotional detachment and loss of interest; emotional distress and/or physiologic arousal on exposure to stimuli resembling or symbolizing traumatic event; persistent hyperarousal (insomnia, hypervigilance, decreased concentration, irritability). Onset usually within 3 months postevent but may be delayed for many months. Often associated with depression and substance abuse; other anxiety disorders may also be present. Lasts 1 month or more and impairs interpersonal, vocational, or ADL functioning.

► Diagnostic Studies

Increased autonomic arousal (i.e., galvanic skin response, electro-myogram, heart rate, blood pressure).

► Diagnosis

PTSD symptoms lasting < 1 month represent acute stress disorder; PTSD symptoms following less severe stressor (i.e., divorce, job loss) diagnosed as adjustment disorder.

► Clinical Therapeutics

Benzodiazepines for mild sedation should be used with caution secondary to abuse potential. Antidepressants often useful in those with and without comorbid depression.

► Clinical Intervention

Referral for psychiatric evaluation indicated. Some patients respond to the opportunity to express their feelings (ventilation) and to cognitive–behavioral approaches. Support groups and family education. Treatment for substance abuse and any concurrent disorders. Symptoms often refractory to treatment and accentuated during subsequent stressful periods.

## III. ATTENTION DEFICIT HYPERACTIVITY DISORDER

► Scientific Concepts

Familial aggregation; probable genetic contribution in some cases. Probable dysregulation in noradrenergic and dopaminergic neurotransmission. Associated with CNS abnormalities (i.e., Tourette's syndrome, seizure disorders). Greater prevalence in males. Most common mental health diagnosis in children.

► History & Physical

Classic triad involves age-inappropriate impulsivity, hyperactivity, or inattentiveness lasting 6 months or more. Symptom onset must begin before 7 years old. May exhibit careless mistakes, does not follow instructions or appear to listen, easily distracted, forgetful, fidgety, does not sit still, talks excessively, accident prone, difficulty awaiting turn during play, often interrupts others. Significant impairment in academic and interpersonal functioning; may be marked by presence of underachievement, substance abuse, suicide attempts, more frequent accidents, low frustration tolerance, and temper outbursts. Physical examination may demonstrate neuromaturational delays, poor psychomotor coordination, or speech and hearing problems including chronic otitis media, associated tic disorder in 10%.

► Diagnostic Studies

Behavioral rating scales are useful in describing classroom and home activities; common scales include the Conner's Parent Rating Scale and the Child Behavior Check List (CBCL), the latter of which assesses for a broader range of psychopathology. Neuropsychological testing may be indicated to detect specific learning disabilities. EEG if seizures are suspected; thyroid function tests if hyperthyroidism is suspected; hematocrit and lead level. Hearing, speech, or vision assessment as indicated by exam.

► Diagnosis

A comprehensive evaluation should be completed before making the diagnosis of ADHD as it may be misdiagnosed if based solely upon limited observation. Classic triad not present in all children; need at least hyperactivity/impulsivity or inattention/distractibility for diagnosis. Commonly associated with oppositional defiant disorder and conduct disorder, specific learning disorders, anxiety/mood disorders. Rule out schizophrenia, other psychotic disorders, pervasive developmental disorder, or other mental disorders.

► Clinical Therapeutics

Stimulants (e.g., methylphenidate, dextroamphetamine, methamphetamine, magnesium pemoline); side effects include insomnia and appetite suppression; long-term therapy may inhibit growth; 25 to 30% do not respond. Antidepressants (imipramine, desipramine, nortriptyline, bupropion) useful for children with associated tics and those experiencing side effects to stimulants; less effective than stimulants. Tricyclic antidepressants and SSRIs have generally not been useful in adults in absence of comorbid depression or dysthymia. Clonidine for marked aggression or hyperactivity; side effect is sedation, which may assist insomnia associated with stimulants.

► Clinical Intervention

Correction of hearing or vision impairments; specific educational interventions for learning disabilities. Family and individual psychotherapy/education. Environmental/behavioral management at home and school. Poorer prognosis associated with coexisting conduct disorder, low IQ, more severe symptoms. Higher risk for child abuse. Of the 3–10% of children diagnosed with ADHD, one third to two thirds (between 1 and 6% of the general population) continue to manifest symptoms into adulthood.

## IV. DEPRESSIVE DISORDERS

### A. Major (Unipolar) Depression

► Scientific Concepts

Complex psychobiological syndrome involving neurotransmitter dysregulation (primarily decreases in serotonin and norepinephrine) often precipitated by environmental stress, particularly the initial episodes. Probable genetic predisposition. Five to 10% prevalence in primary care settings; greater prevalence in females. Antidepressant medications increase neurotransmitter availability.

► History & Physical

Depressed mood (dysphoria) or loss of interest or pleasure for ≥ 2 continuous weeks. Four or more of the following: insomnia or hypersomnia, change in appetite, change in weight not due to dieting, psychomotor agitation or retardation, fatigue, feelings of worthlessness or guilt, difficulty concentrating, recurrent thoughts of death or suicide. Often associated with loss of libido, social withdrawal, indecisiveness, obsessive rumination, tearfulness, agitation. Significant impairment in interpersonal, vocational, or ADL functioning. Individuals with "masked depression" may initially present with physical complaints. Children and adolescents may have anxiety, social withdrawal, irritability, behavioral problems, or somatic complaints. Cognitive impairments often prominent in elderly patients. Increased prevalence in those with previous personal episodes or family history. Accentuated in some women during premenstrual period. May demonstrate seasonal pattern. May be precipitated by chronic medical or psychiatric illness. Associated with substance abuse. Increased risk of suicide. Factors influencing outcome in severe depression include duration of illness before treatment, severity of the index episode, treatment modality used, dosage and duration of and compliance with treatment, self-mutilation, refusal to eat, and treatment resistance.

► Diagnostic Studies

None diagnostic, though evidence of neuroendocrine dysfunction may be present on dexamethasone suppression test and sleep EEGs. Self-rating instruments (i.e., Beck Depression Inventory) can be of assistance in assessing depressive symptomatology.

► Diagnosis

Rule out bipolar depression and cyclothymia (mania/hypomania), dysthymia (less severe but chronic), self-limited bereavement after personal loss, lifelong pattern of mood instability representing a personality disorder, dementia, or mood disorder caused by medical illness or drugs.

► Clinical Therapeutics

As antidepressants tend to be relatively equal in their effectiveness in resolving acute depressive episodes, selection of initial medication often based on a favorable side-effect profile. The medication should have few effects hindering patient compliance (i.e., sexual dysfunction), address atypical depression features (i.e., hypersomnia), consider comorbid conditions (i.e., hypertension, cardiac disease), avoid interactions with other drugs (i.e., warfarin), and be consistent with patient preferences and financial resources. SSRIs (fluoxetine, sertraline, paroxetine) as well as nefazodone and venlafaxine are recommended first-line agents. Compared to other antidepressants, SSRIs generally have lower toxicity, fewer side effects, and once-per-day dosing. Side effects include sedation, insomnia, agitation, sexual dysfunction, weight gain, and dry mouth. Non-SSRIs include nefazodone, which is helpful for those with insomnia, and venlafaxine, which is less prone to produce sexual dysfunction. Additional agents include bupropion, which is less frequently associated with sexual dysfunction and fatigue and may facilitate weight loss, and trazodone, which is often coadministered to treat insomnia. Antidepressants should be given for 4–6 weeks at a full therapeutic level before assessing response. If necessary, alternative second-line agents include tricyclic antidepressants, which have a higher frequency of side effects (i.e., dry mouth, constipation, sedation, arrhythmia, weight gain, etc.) but cost less. Other medications, including MAOIs, which require a tyramine-free diet, and lithium, are perhaps best administered under a specialist's care.

► Clinical Intervention

Mild depression may be treated with psychotherapy alone; however, moderately to severely depressed patients (as well as those mildly depressed but with significant impairment in daily functioning) should be considered for antidepressant medications as well. Psychotherapy enhances pharmacotherapy effectiveness. Exercise and phototherapy may be of value in those with a seasonal pattern (typical of seasonal affective disorder). Individuals not responsive to initial therapy, having suicidal tendencies, or presenting with comorbid psychiatric or medical conditions may require referral for psychiatric evaluation and treatment. Individuals with significant suicidal risk or major impairment in daily functioning may require hospitalization. ECT is effective for those not responding to antidepressants, who present with psychosis, or who have significant suicidal risk.

### ▶ Health Maintenance Issues

Those with a history of recurrent episodes are at increased risk for continued occurrences; hence, long-term maintenance psychotherapy and treatment with antidepressant medication may be needed.

## B. Dysthymia

### ▶ Scientific Concepts

Complex psychobiological syndrome involving neurotransmitter dysregulation (primarily decreases in serotonin and norepinephrine) often precipitated by environmental stress. Possible genetic predisposition. Greater prevalence in females. Antidepressant medications increase neurotransmitter availability.

### ▶ History & Physical

Mood is chronically depressed for a minimum of 2 years (1 year for children/adolescents) with no lapse in symptoms > 2 months' duration. Symptoms must include two of the following: sleep disturbance, appetite disturbance, low self-esteem, fatigue, difficulty concentrating, hopelessness. Symptoms must cause significant impairment in social/occupational functioning or ADL. Onset is insidious and develops in childhood through early adulthood. No history of major depression or manic episode within first 2 years. Greater prevalence in women and in those with a family history of depression. Children with dysthymia often exhibit irritability, poor social skills, and impaired school performance.

### ▶ Diagnostic Studies
None required.

### ▶ Diagnosis

Rule out chronic psychotic disorder, substance-induced mood disorder, personality disorder (may coexist), or general medical disorder (i.e., hypothyroidism, neurodegenerative or autoimmune conditions, cerebral infarcts). Major depression can be coexisting condition.

### ▶ Clinical Therapeutics

As noted for major (unipolar) depression, SSRIs (fluoxetine, sertraline, paroxetine) as well as non-SSRIs such as venlafaxine are recommended first-line agents.

### ▶ Clinical Intervention

Psychotherapy and physical exercise are generally recommended. Group therapy may provide additional benefit to medication particularly in interpersonal and psychosocial functioning.

▶ **Health Maintenance Issues**

Individuals with dysthymia are at significantly increased risk of developing major depression.

## C. Bipolar Disorders

▶ **Scientific Concepts**

Complex psychobiological syndrome involving neurotransmitter dysregulation. Probable genetic component. Prevalence in females equals males in bipolar I disorder; females greater than males in bipolar II disorder.

▶ **History & Physical**

***Bipolar I disorder:*** Essential feature is the presence of one or more manic episodes. Distinct period of an abnormally expansive, elated, or irritable mood lasting ≥1 week, including three or more of the following: inflated self-esteem, distractibility, talkativeness, decreased need for sleep, flight of ideas, agitation or increased goal-directed activity, or engagement in excessive spending sprees or promiscuity having potentially negative consequences. Onset generally in adolescence or young adulthood. Symptoms lead to impairment in social or occupational functioning or ADL. Manic episode preceded or succeeded by one or more major depressive episodes; may be precipitated by stress. Associated with increased risk of suicide as well as impulsive and violent behavior, which may lead to marital conflict or criminal activity.

***Bipolar II disorder:*** History of one or more hypomanic episodes and one or more depressive periods. Hypomania represents a significant change in functioning involving a milder form of mania both in terms of symptoms and level of impairment. There is no history of mania or a mixed episode of major depression and mania. Associated with a significant risk of suicide, anxiety disorders, substance abuse, and borderline personality disorder.

▶ **Diagnostic Studies**

None required.

▶ **Diagnosis**

Rule out other mood disorders, including those due to a general medical condition or substance-induced, schizoaffective disorder, or another psychotic disorder. Bipolar I and II subtypes are categorized according to more recent episode: manic, hypomanic, depressive, or mixed. An increased cycling rate may be seen as the patient ages.

▶ **Clinical Therapeutics**

Approximately 70% respond to lithium after 2–3 weeks of therapy for mania, hypomania, and mixed episodes. Lithium has a small therapeutic range; hence, close monitoring of plasma lithium levels is necessary. Significant dose-related toxicity exists at plasma lithium levels > 1.5 mEq/L; symptoms include nausea, vomiting, diarrhea, tremor, and delirium; also closely monitor renal and thyroid function. Other adverse effects include polyuria, hypothyroidism, acne, and weight gain. Teratogenic and cardiac conduction effects require baseline pregnancy test and electrocardiogram (ECG). Anticonvulsants (i.e., valproic acid, carbamazepine) can be used when lithium is difficult to monitor or contraindicated. New antiepileptic drugs lamotrigine and topiramate also useful. Antipsychotic olanzapine 5 to 50 mg/d efficacious in bipolar I; other antipsychotics also useful, clozapine and risperidone. SSRIs may be initiated to treat depressive symptomatology unresponsive to lithium, although there is some risk of precipitating mania. ECT may also be initiated.

▶ Clinical Intervention

Psychotherapy, education, and family support may increase medication compliance and overall adaptation. Significant risk of suicide continues. Monitoring for key predictors of relapse and anticipation of high-risk situations; participation in support groups may be helpful. Those with rapid cycling have poorer prognosis and greater risk of suicide. Therapeutic drug monitoring (TDM) of psychotropic medications minimizes limitations of genetic variability in metabolism, toxicity, and poor compliance.

▶ Health Maintenance Issues

Majority of patients will relapse without prophylaxis; lithium generally provided for months or indefinitely in those exhibiting rapid cycling. Women at risk for postpartum episodes.

## D. Cyclothymia

▶ Scientific Concepts

Complex psychobiological syndrome involving neurotransmitter dysregulation. Probable genetic component. Prevalence in females equals males. Often exhibit a family history of affective and substance-related disorders.

▶ History & Physical

Recurrent, vacillating mood disturbance of at least 2 years' duration (1 year for children/adolescents) with symptoms of depression and hypomania and not pervasive or severe enough to be diagnosed as major depression or bipolar disorder; no lapse in symptoms > 2 months' duration. Symptoms must cause clinically significant impairment in occupation or social functioning or ADL. No history of manic, major depressive, or mixed episode within first 2 years. Disorder onset is generally adolescence, early adulthood. Often associated with a sleep disorder.

▶ Diagnostic Studies

None required.

▶ Diagnosis

Rule out schizoaffective disorder, schizophrenia or other psychotic disorder, borderline personality disorder, substance-induced disorder, or disorder due to general medical condition (i.e., hyperthyroidism).

▶ Clinical Therapeutics

May respond to lithium and anticonvulsant medications as noted under Bipolar Disorders.

▶ Clinical Intervention

Individual and group psychotherapy may be useful in facilitating adaptation to effects of mood swings on self-esteem and interpersonal functioning.

▶ Health Maintenance Issues

Substantial risk (15–50%) of progression to bipolar I or II disorder.

# V. PERSONALITY DISORDERS

▶ Scientific Concepts

Enduring maladaptive patterns of inner experience (cognition, affectivity) and behavior (impulse control, interpersonal functioning) that substantially deviate from the individual's cultural patterns. Maladaptive pattern is inflexible, pervasive across personal and interpersonal experiences; onset can be traced to adolescence or early adulthood, and causes clinically significant distress or impairment in occupational/interpersonal functioning. Genetic contribution suspected in some (e.g., schizotypal, antisocial, borderline); CNS serotonin dysregulation may be associated with aggressive, impulsive behavior. Symptoms/signs of personality disorders are often precipitated or exacerbated by stress. Most are ego-syntonic in that patients are comfortable with their personality traits even though their behavior may be dysfunctional.

▶ History & Physical

*Cluster A Disorders:*

- *Paranoid:* Pervasive suspiciousness and four of the following characteristics: preoccupied with the trustworthiness of (or reluctance to confide in) others, holds unjustified suspicions regarding sexual partner's fidelity, suspects others of malicious intent, perceives a threatening hidden meaning in benign remarks, or is hypersensitive to criticisms or perceives criticisms where none are apparent.
- *Schizoid:* Significant and pervasive pattern of social isolation and lack of joy in interpersonal/family relationships; demonstrates emotional coldness and poor response to social praise.
- *Schizotypal:* Cognitive distortions, eccentric behaviors, and social deficits, including altered perceptual experiences, magical thinking, ideas of reference, unusual speech patterns (stereotyped, vague, etc.), paranoid ideation, extreme social anxiety, few close friends, constricted or inappropriate affect, unusual behavior. Onset by early adulthood.

*Cluster B Disorders:*

- *Antisocial:* Onset at ≥ 18 years of age, with three or more of the following characteristics since age 15: disregard for social/lawful norms, pervasive lying/conning, physical aggressiveness, impulsivity, irresponsibility, disregard for safety of others, lack of remorse. Evidence of conduct disorder prior to age 15.
- *Borderline:* Pervasive pattern of impulsivity, unstable relationships, and altered affect with onset in early adulthood. Indicated by potentially self-damaging impulsivity, unstable self-image, marked mood swings, emptiness, suicidal or self-mutilating behavior, instability in social relationships (vacillates between devaluation and idealization), perceptions of abandonment, paranoidal ideation, and difficulty with anger control.

- *Histrionic:* Excessive self-centered orientation characterized by shallow yet rapidly changing emotions, stylized speech, self-dramatization, sexually seductive/provocative dress or behavior, attention seeking, highly susceptible to social influence, exaggerates level of interpersonal intimacy.
- *Narcissistic:* Pervasive preoccupation with self as indicated by fantasies of success, perceptions of self-importance or uniqueness, arrogance, feelings of entitlement, seeks admiration, exploitative, demanding, lacking in empathy.

### Cluster C Disorders:

- *Avoidant:* Pervasive social inhibition characterized by preoccupation with social criticism, avoidance of interpersonal situations that risk embarrassment, fear of being intimate, inhibition in new social contexts or when unclear of social acceptance.
- *Dependent:* Requires extensive social support as characterized by inability to perform independent tasks, difficulty making independent decisions, excessive fear of abandonment, attempts to immediately develop new supportive relationship upon cessation of old one; passive, submissive, and clingy behavior. May be exacerbated by chronic medical illness.
- *Obsessive–compulsive:* Rigid, perfectionistic, productivity oriented, preoccupied with rules, reluctance to delegate, excessive hoarding of valuable (i.e., money) as well as invaluable objects, stubbornness.

#### ▶ Diagnostic Studies

Standardized testing (e.g., Wechsler Adult Intelligence Scale–Revised [WAIS-R], Minnesota Multiphasic Personality Inventory [MMPI]) and projective testing (e.g., Rorschach) may facilitate diagnosis.

#### ▶ Diagnosis

Maladaptive pattern must lead to significant impairment in interpersonal functioning or ADL. Rule out other mental health disorders (i.e., mood disorders, psychosis [particularly with schizotypal]), substance abuse, adult attention deficit disorder, or medical illness (i.e., delirium, CNS trauma or tumor, temporal lobe epilepsy). Mixed personality disorders and atypical presentations are common.

#### ▶ Clinical Therapeutics

In general, medications are of limited value. Patients exhibiting psychotic decompensation may require major tranquilizers; schizotypal and borderline disorders may respond to low-dose neuroleptics; borderline disorders may also respond to SSRIs, MAOIs, or lithium. Those with anxiety may respond to anxiolytic or antidepressant medications.

#### ▶ Clinical Intervention

Treatment of comorbid conditions (i.e., alcohol or other drug abuse, depression); hospitalization if at risk of harm to self and others. Individual and group psychotherapy may be useful for patients and their families.

#### ▶ Health Maintenance Issues

Often resistant to therapy, personality disorders tend to be chronic.

# VI. PHYSICAL DISORDERS WITH PSYCHOGENIC ORIGIN

## A. Psychological Factor Affecting Medical Condition (Psychosomatic Disorders)

▶ **Scientific Concepts**

Psychological variables have the potential to influence the development, presentation, and progression of a wide variety of medical illnesses. This diagnostic category is reserved for cases in which psychological/ behavioral factors have a clinically significant impact.

▶ **History & Physical**

Clear evidence (generally including a temporal relationship) between psychological factors (coping styles, emotional state, maladaptive health behavior, psychophysiological stress response) and the development or exacerbation of symptoms of a known medical condition (e.g., asthma, headaches, angina, low back pain). Psychological factors may also increase risk of medical complications (e.g., continued smoking in the asthmatic patient).

▶ **Diagnostic Studies**

Temporal linkage between mental stress, excessive psychophysiological arousal, and medical symptoms may be demonstrated (e.g., interpersonal conflict, ambulatory monitoring revealing elevated blood pressure, and angina).

▶ **Diagnosis**

Establish temporal relationship. Rule out a general medical disorder or substance abuse causing the psychological symptoms, somatoform disorders in which there is no diagnosable medical illness, or the more specific case of pain disorder.

▶ **Clinical Therapeutics**

Limit addictive analgesics. Antidepressants may be helpful. Pharmacological/surgical therapy for the medical condition should be instituted as appropriate.

▶ **Clinical Intervention**

Stress management, including biofeedback, relaxation therapy, hypnosis, breathing exercises. Psychotherapy to facilitate identification and control of psychophysiological responses to stressful situations, enhance and extend range of problem-solving skills.

▶ **Health Maintenance Issues**

If limited response to isolated therapies noted above, may respond to intensive, comprehensive interdisciplinary intervention.

## B. Factitious Disorder (Munchausen Syndrome)

▶ **Scientific Concepts**

Intentional effort to gain benefit from sick role through report of symptoms or behavior suggesting medical disorder. True medical problems may coexist. Onset generally in early adulthood.

► **History & Physical**

Feigning of symptoms or intentionally inducing signs of disease (e.g., use of medications, thermometer manipulation, self-induced bruises) without obvious external incentives (e.g., avoidance of legal responsibility or work). Often complex or vague medical problems. May present history of repeated hospitalizations and signing out against medical advice. At risk of injury due to attempts to produce signs of medical disease.

► **Diagnostic Studies**

Studies as appropriate to symptoms to rule out true medical disorder.

► **Diagnosis**

Rule out true medical or another mental disorder including malingering and somatoform disorders. May have comorbid substance abuse or personality disorder.

► **Clinical Therapeutics**

None indicated.

► **Clinical Intervention**

Psychotherapy may be of assistance, particularly in conjunction with confrontation regarding the nature of the disorder.

► **Health Maintenance Issues**

Often reluctant to accept the diagnosis despite clear evidence; the disorder is generally chronic. Careful monitoring may assist in preventing iatrogenic complications.

## C. Malingering

► **Scientific Concepts**

Intentional effort to gain benefit from sick role through report of symptoms or behavior suggesting medical disorder. True medical problems may coexist. Onset associated with external need for medical illness.

► **History & Physical**

Symptoms intentionally produced for obvious reasons (e.g., to avoid occupational, military, legal, or financial responsibilities; obtain drugs; or gain clear secondary social support from sick role). Uncooperative, exaggerated disability claims. May, in some circumstances, represent non-pathologic, adaptive behavior.

► **Diagnostic Studies**

Rule out true medical or another mental disorder including Munchausen syndrome and somatoform disorders. Comorbid antisocial personality disorder is common.

► **Diagnosis**

No objective finding to substantiate symptoms.

► **Clinical Therapeutics**

None indicated.

► **Clinical Intervention**

Eliminate external secondary gain motivating symptoms; confront regarding appropriate diagnosis; supportive psychotherapy.

► Health Maintenance Issues

Resolution of conflict with external motivating forces may produce reduction or elimination of symptoms.

## VII. SOMATOFORM DISORDERS

### A. Somatization Disorder

► Scientific Concepts

A broad-ranging pattern of physical complaints causing clinically significant impairment, beginning before 30 years of age and lasting several years. Symptoms inconsistent with medical findings. Onset in adolescence or early adulthood. Some familial association. Occurs primarily in women.

► History & Physical

Somatic complaints are not intentionally produced and include at least four pain symptoms, one sexual symptom, two gastrointestinal symptoms, and one pseudoneurological symptom. Symptoms are often vague and presented in a dramatic fashion. Symptoms cannot be explained by a known medical condition, or if a medical condition is present, the impairment or degree of complaint is clearly excessive. History of treatment by numerous practitioners with potential for extensive evaluations and multiple surgeries. Substance abuse, depression, anxiety, and personality disorders are common comorbid conditions.

► Diagnostic Studies

Laboratory studies generally do not support symptoms.

► Diagnosis

Rule out general medical conditions and other mental disorders, particularly pain disorder, schizophrenia, or other somatoform disorder.

► Clinical Therapeutics

Avoid addictive medications (opiates, benzodiazepines). Antidepressants (nefazodone) may be helpful. Gabapentin may be effective for patients where pain is predominant symptom.

► Clinical Intervention

Psychotherapy particularly for depression, suicidal ideation, or substance abuse. Develop primary care provider rapport with patient and determine appropriate utilization of medical consultative services. Cognitive behavior therapy may benefit some patients.

► Health Maintenance Issues

Therapeutic course is generally chronic over many years; focus on satisfactory management rather than cure.

### B. Conversion Disorder

► Scientific Concepts

Evidence of sensory or voluntary motor dysfunction not well explained by a general medical condition. More common in low socioeconomic status or rural populations; more frequent in women. Thought to represent expression of an unconscious mental conflict or to elicit secondary gain. Onset generally between 10 and 35 years of age.

▶ History & Physical

Sensory or voluntary motor function deficits or symptoms suggesting a neurological or other general medical condition. Deficits/symptoms not intentionally induced but may be precipitated or exacerbated by stress. May exhibit lack of concern regarding the symptoms despite clinically significant distress or occupational/interpersonal impairment. Deficits/symptoms include seizures, unconsciousness, paralysis, ataxia, loss of sensation, and blindness; not limited to sexual dysfunction or pain complaints. May have comorbid personality disorder.

▶ Diagnostic Studies

Neurological studies show an absence of expected neurological findings given symptoms/signs.

▶ Diagnosis

Symptoms/deficits are not consistent with known neuroanatomy and physiology. Attempt to rule out neurologic or general medical condition recognizing that some patients (~25%) may subsequently develop symptoms/signs of a known medical illness. Also rule out drug-induced or culturally sanctioned behavior as cause of symptoms, malingering, major depression, schizophrenia, and other somatoform disorders.

▶ Clinical Therapeutics

Minor tranquilizers may be helpful for anxiety.

▶ Clinical Intervention

Psychoanalysis and cognitive–behavioral therapy helpful for some. Supportive therapy for family; identification and removal of potential for secondary gain. Patients without comorbid psychiatric disorders and who have identifiable stressors precipitating onset of symptoms may have best prognosis.

## C. Pain Disorder

▶ Scientific Concepts

Pain is a subjective experience influenced by the patient's cognitive and affective state. The perception of pain and the experience of suffering can occur both with and without recognizable organic pathology. The experience of pain can be reduced through cognitive–behavioral therapy as well as by analgesics and antidepressants intervening in the neurochemical pathways. Onset is generally 30–50 years of age; musculoskeletal pain may be more prevalent in women.

▶ History & Physical

Pain causing clinically significant distress and functional impairment is the predominant symptom. No evidence of intent to produce symptoms; but psychological factors appear to precipitate or exacerbate the pain. Physical findings consistent with the development of pain may or may not be present; however, findings are not judged to be sufficient to explain intensity of pain or level of disability. Complaints may be diffuse or vague; excessive analgesic usage and high likelihood of extensive medical care/surgery. Comorbid depression, substance abuse, social isolation, anxiety, and insomnia are common.

► **Diagnostic Studies**
Laboratory studies may identify organic pathology or be negative.

► **Diagnosis**
Psychological factors must have significant influence in precipitating, exacerbating, or maintaining the pain experience. Symptoms must not meet criteria for dyspareunia. Rule out malingering, factitious disorder, or major depression, anxiety, or psychotic disorder as primary diagnosis. Pain disorders classified as associated with psychological factors or associated with psychological factors and a general medical condition.

► **Clinical Therapeutics**
Analgesics (in moderation) and antidepressants for pain; nonsteroidal anti-inflammatory agents (NSAIDs).

► **Clinical Intervention**
If addicted to analgesics, hospitalization for detoxification may be needed. Pain management training using cognitive–behavioral techniques including physical activity is generally indicated. Self-hypnosis may be useful for functional abdominal pain in children and adolescents.

► **Health Maintenance Issues**
Assessment for suicide potential in those with severe depression. Careful review of medical/surgical utilization.

## D. Hypochondriasis

► **Scientific Concepts**
Psychodynamic explanations for this preoccupation with fear of having a serious disease focus on displaced anxiety. Behavioral analyses find that secondary gain may or may not be present. Development and maintenance may depend on misinterpretation of somatic symptoms and signs. Past experience with serious illness, anxiety, and depression are often present. Onset in young adulthood.

► **History & Physical**
Pervasive fear of having serious disease based on selective attention to, and preoccupation with, somatic signs/symptoms. Fear exists for at least 6 months despite extensive medical evaluation and appropriate reassurance. Anxiety/fear causes clinically significant distress as well as interpersonal or occupational impairment. May or may not recognize that fear is excessive or unreasonable. Reluctant to explore psychiatric basis; excessive utilization of medical resources. Symptoms may exacerbate in response to stress.

► **Diagnostic Studies**
No evidence of pathophysiology warranting patient's concerns.

► **Diagnosis**
Rule out body dysmorphic disorder (fears restricted to concern about appearance), delusional disorder, obsessive–compulsive disorder, generalized anxiety disorder, panic disorder, separation anxiety, a major depressive disorder, or another somatoform disorder.

▶ Clinical Therapeutics
Antidepressant and/or anxiolytic therapy for comorbid depression and anxiety as indicated.

▶ Clinical Intervention
Psychotherapy may be of some value.

▶ Health Maintenance Issues
Careful review of medical utilization. Generally chronic course, although remission can occur particularly in those with sudden onset.

## E. Body Dysmorphic Disorder

▶ Scientific Concepts
Excessive concern with perceived defect in physical appearance, may be symbolic for perceived personal inadequacies. Onset in adolescence.

▶ History & Physical
Preoccupation with portion of physical appearance, generally the face, which contains an imagined or slight defect. Preoccupation exceeds culturally appropriate expectations, causes clinically significant distress, and/or impairment in occupational or interpersonal functioning (social isolation). Excessive grooming may be present; repeated cosmetic surgery is common. Physical examination does not reveal evidence of anatomical defect warranting severity of patient's concerns.

▶ Diagnostic Studies
None required.

▶ Diagnosis
Rule out normal concerns regarding appearance, anorexia nervosa, major depressive disorder. Comorbid major depressive disorder, social phobia, obsessive–compulsive disorder, and delusional disorder may be present.

▶ Clinical Therapeutics
Antidepressants (SSRIs) may be helpful.

▶ Clinical Intervention
Psychological assessment with particular focus on interpersonal skills proficiency; psychotherapy may be helpful.

▶ Health Maintenance Issues
Severity of preoccupation may wax and wane over time; focus of preoccupation may change. Evaluation for suicidal potential is appropriate, particularly if depression is present.

## VIII. EATING DISORDERS

### A. Anorexia Nervosa

▶ Scientific Concepts
Occurs in 0.5–1% of adolescent girls; 10–20 times more often in females. Most frequent in developed countries. Biological, social, and psychological factors implicated. Familiar mood disorders common. Neuro-

chemically diminished norepinephrine and activity suggested. Inverse relationship between 3-methoxy-4-hydroxyphenylglycol (MHPG) and depression; endogenous opioids may contribute to hunger denial.

▶ History & Physical

Weight loss or lack of weight gain leading to body weight at least 15% below normal expected weight for age and height. Profound body image disturbance, pursuit of thinness often to the point of starvation. Symptoms of bulimia may occur. Postmenarcheal women have absence of at least three consecutive menstrual cycles.

▶ Diagnostic Studies

As weight loss grows profound, signs include hypothermia, dependent edema, lanugo, and metabolic changes; amenorrhea; impaired water diuresis. ECG changes; endocrinological and medical problems secondary to starvation. Screening lab tests include serum electrolytes with renal function tests; thyroid function tests; glucose amylase and hematological tests; ECG; cholesterol level; dexamethasone suppression test; carotene level. May find decreased thyroid hormone and serum glucose levels. Nonsuppression of cortisol after dexamethasone; hypokalemia, increased blood urea nitrogen; hypercholesterolemia; cardiovascular; hypotension and bradycardia.

▶ Diagnosis

Symptoms as above. Subtypes:

**Restricting type:** Has not engaged in binge eating or purging behavior during current episode.

**Binge eating/purging type:** Regularly engages in binge eating or purging behavior during current episode.

Complicated by denial of symptoms, secrecy around eating rituals, and resistance to treatment; rule out medical illness and various mental disorders, including depressive disorder, somatization disorder, schizophrenia, and bulimia nervosa.

▶ Clinical Therapeutics

Cyproheptadine, up to 32 mg/d, shows some benefit for nonbulimic patients; cyproheptadine may be helpful due to weight gain side effect; treatment of comorbid depression with antidepressants; serotonergic antidepressants such as fluoxetine, sertraline, and paroxetine may be useful.

▶ Clinical Intervention

Hospitalization may be necessary due to medical complications and suicidal risk. Treat medical complications; intravenous (IV) fluids or nasogastric feedings may be mandated. Evaluate for depression. Supportive, cognitive–behavioral, family therapy with goal of weight maintenance and eating behavior normalization, symptom reduction.

▶ Health Maintenance Issues

Course varies greatly: spontaneous recovery without treatment, recovery after a variety of treatments, fluctuating and deteriorating course resulting in death caused by complications of starvation; overall mortality rate 5 to 18%; restricting type may be less likely to recover; short-term response to hospital treatment is good; important to monitor medical complications; social relationships often poor; and depression often present.

## B. Bulimia Nervosa

▶ Scientific Concepts

Estimates range from 1 to 3% of young women. More common in women than men, onset often late adolescence. High achievers, decreased serotonin and/or norepinephrine have been implicated; familial depression.

▶ History & Physical

Recurrent episodes of binge eating; a sense of lack of control over eating. Self-induced vomiting, misuse of laxatives or diuretics, fasting, or excessive exercise to prevent weight gain. Behaviors occur, on average, at least twice a week for 3 months. Self-evaluation unduly influenced by body shape and weight. Does not occur exclusively during episodes of anorexia nervosa. May show dehydration, menstrual disturbance, hypotension, and bradycardia. Check oral cavity for dental enamel erosion and hands for signs of abrasion secondary to self-induced vomiting. Family relationships generally distant and conflictual.

▶ Diagnostic Studies

Lab studies of electrolytes and metabolism may show abnormalities due to purging and various degrees of starvation (particularly hypokalemia and hypochloremia). May show nonsuppression on dexamethasone suppression test. May show dehydration and hypomagnesemia and hyperamylasemia. Complete psychiatric evaluation for comorbid depression, anorexia nervosa, substance abuse, and personality disorders.

▶ Diagnosis

Symptoms as above; *DSM-IV* subtypes:

*Purging type:* Regularly engages in self-induced vomiting or misuse of laxatives, diuretics, or enemas.

*Nonpurging type:* Uses other inappropriate compensatory behaviors, such as fasting or excessive exercise but not those in purging type.

Seizure disorders; CNS tumors; Kleine–Levin syndrome; Kluver–Bucy syndrome; coexisting borderline personality disorder; anorexia nervosa, binge eating/purging type.

▶ Clinical Therapeutics

Antidepressant medications including SSRIs such as fluoxetine may be higher than dose typical for treatment of depression (60 to 80 mg/d). Imipramine, desipramine, trazodone, MAOIs helpful at dosages usually given for treatment of depressive disorders. Cognitive–behavioral therapy or interpersonal psychotherapy often more effective than antidepressants.

▶ Clinical Intervention

Correct medical complications such as electrolyte imbalance. Most treated as outpatients. Individual cognitive–behavioral, group, and family therapy helpful in reducing bingeing. Hospitalization with suicidality, substance abuse, or when extreme purging results in electrolyte and metabolic disturbance. Chronic disorder with waxing and waning course; therapy may be prolonged; after 5–10 years, about half recover fully, 20% continue to meet full criteria.

### ▶ Health Maintenance Issues

Some patients with mild course may have long spontaneous remissions; often secretive about problem; many have concurrent major depression, anxiety disorder, chemical dependency. Monitor medical complications and long-term medication use. Prognosis dependent on severity of purging sequelae, frequency of vomiting resulting in electrolyte imbalance, esophagitis, salivary gland enlargement, and dental caries.

## C. Obesity

### ▶ Scientific Concepts

No specific genetic marker; central feedback regulation loop involving the leptin and melano cortinergic pathways has provided therapeutic targets; multicausal factors; 80% have family history; metabolic differences, decreased activity, eating behaviors; > 50% of general population, one third or more of children and adolescents in the United States; six times more common in women of low socioeconomic status than higher status; prevalence increases threefold between ages 20 and 50.

### ▶ History & Physical

Family history; often childhood onset; body weight exceeds by 20% standard weight listed in usual height–weight tables; body mass index (BMI—body weight in kilograms divided by height in square meters) correlates with morbidity and mortality (normal range, 20–25). Overweight classified as BMI = 25 to 29.9 kg/m²; obese classified as BMI ≥ 30 kg/m².

### ▶ Diagnostic Studies

Lab studies for medical complications; correlation with cardiovascular disorders, hypertension, and hypercholesterolemia twice as common; diabetes, gout, hyperlipidemias; proteinuria, nephrosis, and renal vein thrombosis; osteoarthritis; higher-than-normal mortality rate from colon, rectal, and prostate cancer in men; higher-than-normal mortality rate in women from cancer of gallbladder, biliary passages, breast, uterus, and ovaries.

### ▶ Diagnosis

Symptoms as above; genetic, developmental, physical activity, brain damage, clinical and psychological factors; close to 50% develop mild anxiety and depression. Night-eating syndrome, in which people eat excessively after evening meal; bulimia; Pickwickian syndrome, 100% over desirable weight with associated respiratory and cardiovascular pathology. Associated clinical disorders include Cushing's disease; myxedema; adiposogenital dystrophy; prolonged use of serotonergic agonists may be associated with weight gain.

### ▶ Clinical Therapeutics

Sibutramine and orlistat (Xenical) inhibit fat absorption; must be used in conjunction with a mildly hypocaloric, low-fat diet; contribute to modest weight loss and maintenance; and reduce obesity-associated risk factors. Pharmacotherapy most effective when used in combination with modification of eating and exercise behavior.

▶ Clinical Intervention

Greater potential for success with treatment plan with four components: pre-evaluation, exercise, behavioral plan, and maintenance plan.

*Diet and exercise:* Best method, balanced diet of 1,100 to 1,200 calories supplemented with vitamins, particularly iron, folic acid, zinc, and vitamin $B_6$; total unmodified fasts for short-term weight loss, but have associated morbidity including orthostatic hypotension, sodium diuresis, and impaired nitrogen balance; ketogenic diets, high protein and fat associated with nausea, hypotension, and lethargy; increased physical activity. Energy deficit of 500 to 1,000 kcal/d; reductions in total energy intake recommended; dietary fat intake to less than 30% of total energy intake. Benefit from 150 minutes of moderate intensity exercise per week, progressively increase to goal. Exercise of 200–300 minutes per week facilitates long-term weight maintenance.

*Surgery:* Gastric bypass, stomach transecting or stapling; gastroplasty, size of stomach stoma is reduced yielding successful results although vomiting, electrolyte imbalance, and obstruction may occur; lipectomy for cosmetic reasons with no effect on long-term weight loss.

*Counseling:* Behavior modification somewhat successful; new eating patterns, operant conditioning through rewards; group therapy for support; nutrition education.

*Follow-up:* Ongoing evaluations of goal achievement, negative effects of treatment.

▶ Health Maintenance Issues

Treatment presented within perspective of risk factors; obesity has adverse effects on health, cardiovascular disorders; hypertension and hypercholesterolemia; diabetes, especially type II, can be reduced by weight reduction; may have comorbid depression, anxiety disorder; higher mortality from colon, rectal, prostate, gallbladder, biliary passages, breast, uterine, and ovarian cancer; mortality correlated with degree of obesity; prognosis for weight reduction is poor; of patients who lose significant amounts of weight, 90% regain; particularly poor prognosis for those who had childhood obesity.

## IX. SUBSTANCE ABUSE DISORDERS

### A. Alcoholism

▶ Scientific Concepts

Recent work has identified specific effects of alcohol on neurotransmitter systems including gamma-aminobutyric and serotonin, dopamine, and opioid receptors.

*Type 1:* Onset in adulthood; gradually increasing consumption; both males and females; characteristics of perfectionism, dependency, introversion; some family history; amenable to treatment; 75% of all alcoholics.

*Type 2:* Onset in adolescence and early adulthood; antisocial, risk-taking, impulsive, aggressive characteristics; strong family history; predominantly males; treatment resistant; 25% of all alcoholics.

Some biological features may be inherited: resistance to intoxication, below normal rise in cortisol after drinking, below normal epinephrine release after stress. No typical alcoholic personality identified. Cultural patterns and genetics associated with patterns of drinking and risk of alcohol abuse.

► History & Physical

If not intoxicated, may present with anxiety, tension, insomnia, depression, headache, blackout, nausea/vomiting or other gastrointestinal symptoms, tachycardia, palpitations, minor injuries due to falls; may attempt to conceal alcohol use. Screen with CAGE (four questions: annoyance with Criticism to drinking; Attempts to cut down; Guilt about drinking; morning Eye-opener); 95% certain diagnosis if three "yes" answers. If intoxicated, may present with alcohol on breath, be lively, emotionally labile, irritable, uncoordinated, have slurred speech and/or ataxia; may be uncooperative, assaultive, dangerous. If in withdrawal, may present with tachycardia, tremulousness, weakness, malaise, nausea/vomiting, diaphoresis, orthostatic hypotension, hyperreflexia, insomnia, hypervigilance, anxiety, irritability, tinnitus, mild illusions and hallucinations, and/or blurred vision worse in the first 12 to 18 hours of the day without drinking. May have convulsions, particularly in the first 2 days of withdrawal. Life-threatening delirium tremens (DTs) in 5% of alcoholics: disorientation, agitation, hallucinations, delusions, sweating, tachycardia, hypertension, tremor, fever, ataxia; increased risk if malnourished or other illness present; 10–15% mortality rate, usually due to secondary infection or acute heart failure. Alcohol-induced psychotic disorder presents with intense auditory hallucinations and other symptoms of withdrawal but usually not disoriented; usually self-limited but can become chronic. May have vertebral or rib fractures.

► Diagnostic Studies

Urine drug screen; breath or blood alcohol level. Blood level of 80–110 mg/dL associated with legal intoxication; > 150 mg/dL without intoxication suggests tolerance. May have increased mean corpuscular volume and abnormal liver function tests. Additional studies to consider: folate, vitamin $B_{12}$, electrolytes (include calcium and magnesium), CBC, ECG, urinalysis, and chest x-ray and CT of head.

► Diagnosis

Presence of impaired social and occupational functioning due to alcohol over 1-year period; inability to stop drinking once started; persistent desire and/or repeated attempts to decrease intake without success; continued drinking despite obviously serious negative consequences (i.e., health, marriage, job); tolerance to alcohol (increased amounts needed for effect); symptoms of withdrawal and/or compulsive and continuous use. Rule out schizophrenia, bipolar disorder, anxiety, attention deficit disorder, antisocial disorders. If intoxicated, rule out hypoglycemia, CNS infection, other drug toxicities, subdural hematoma.

► Clinical Therapeutics

Naltrexone and acamprosate may be useful for prolonging abstinence; use of tricyclic antidepressants and SSRIs in depressed alcoholics. Disulfiram may be useful as deterrent in cooperative patients.

*Intoxicated:* May require sedation (e.g., diazepam, 5–20 mg).

*Withdrawal:* Benzodiazepines preferred for sleep, reduce agitation, conserve energy, induce calm; taper off over 4 to 8 days. Barbiturates, chloral hydrate, carbamazepine may also be used; avoid oversedation. Diazepam and carbamazepine for seizures. Thiamine, 100 mg IM, then 50 mg PO tid × 4 days. Chlordiazepoxide for tremulousness, delirium. Clonidine for sweating, tachycardia, tremor. Antianxiety agents may be useful in 1–2 weeks following withdrawal.

▶ Clinical Intervention

Help patient to confront denial; discuss drinking in open, matter-of-fact, nonjudgmental manner. Insist on total abstinence; provide support and encouragement. Expect relapses; encourage patient to continue working and stay socially active. Family therapy/marital therapy may be useful. Group therapy most effective (i.e., 12-step AA).

*Intoxicated:* Interact in nonthreatening, respectful, patient manner but be ready to use restraints. Consider hospitalization if at risk for withdrawal or becoming comatose; otherwise, consider sending home, jail for observation.

*Withdrawal:* Hospitalize if severe. Include family/familiar people, lighted room, clear directions and explanations, supportive environment. Use restraints if needed; constant observation. Provide good nutrition, multivitamins, high-carbohydrate diet; correct fluid/electrolyte imbalances. Measure pulse, blood pressure, and temperature every half hour initially; treat shock with fluids, vasopressors, whole blood. Monitor for hypoglycemia, prolonged prothrombin time, fever. Treat injuries due to falls and/or withdrawal from other substances if present. Possible complications include pneumonia, tuberculosis, urinary tract infection, hypoglycemia, anemia, gastritis with hematemesis, hemorrhagic pancreatitis, cirrhosis, hepatic failure, meningitis. Insomnia, depression, anxiety, irritability may continue for weeks.

▶ Health Maintenance Issues

Counsel patients and follow up for complications including hypertension, gastritis, gastric ulcer, diarrhea, anemia, pancreatitis, cirrhosis, impotence, insomnia, esophageal and rectal varices, Wernicke's encephalopathy. Patients are prone to drug abuse, motor vehicle and other accidents, suicide, poisonings, drownings, assaults, job loss.

## B. Caffeine/Tobacco Disorders

▶ Scientific Concepts

*Tobacco (nicotine):* Conditioned response; some association with other psychiatric, substance use disorders.

▶ History & Physical

*Caffeine:* Presents with symptoms of agitation, muscle twitching, restlessness, insomnia, diuresis, anxiety, excitement, gastrointestinal disturbance, cardiac arrhythmia. Flushing with intake of two cups of coffee. *Withdrawal symptoms:* headache, fatigue over 4–5 days.

*Tobacco (nicotine):* Assess by number of cigarettes smoked per day, how soon lights up in morning. *Withdrawal symptoms:* irritability, malaise, craving, weight gain, increased appetite, restlessness, anxiety, headache, difficulty concentrating, gastrointestinal distress, bradycardia, cough, insomnia, depression.

▶ Diagnostic Studies
None.

▶ Diagnosis
By history.

▶ Clinical Therapeutics
*Tobacco (nicotine):* Nicotine patch or gum particularly effective when combined with behavior therapy. Continued smoking with nicotine patch/gum may cause cardiac death. Bupropion (Zyban) may facilitate ability to achieve and maintain smoking cessation. Clonidine may help decrease withdrawal symptoms; side effect is hypotension. Among patients who failed treatment, consider buproprion SR alone or in combination with nicotine patch.

▶ Clinical Intervention
*Caffeine:* Gradual decrease in consumption may be better tolerated than abrupt cessation.

*Tobacco (nicotine):* Smoking cessation groups, self-help literature, counseling, behavior modification interventions. Residential treatment for tobacco dependence may be superior to outpatient treatment in some smokers moderately to severely nicotine dependent.

▶ Health Maintenance Issues
*Tobacco (nicotine):* Discuss complications of continued use: pulmonary, cardiac, peripheral vascular, neoplastic diseases.

## C. Drug Dependence

▶ Scientific Concepts
*Stimulants (amphetamines, cocaine, antiobesity drugs, crack, others):* May be swallowed, snorted, injected, smoked (crack). Highly addictive. Amphetamines used medically for attention deficit disorder, narcolepsy, depression in elderly. Cocaine used medically in the treatment of nosebleeds and as local anesthetic in ears, nose, throat. Antiobesity drugs usually unsuccessful due to tolerance. No tolerance to tendency to develop psychotic symptoms indistinguishable from schizophrenia although tolerance to other effects develop.

*Opioids (heroin, codeine, meperidine, methadone, pentazocine):* Street preparation may be tainted with quinine, procaine, lidocaine, lactose, mannitol, and may be contaminated with bacteria, viruses, or fungi. High mortality rate associated with street preparations. Users predominantly in urban areas; more common in males, health care professionals, chronic pain patients, African Americans. Can be snorted (heroin), smoked (opium), injected IV or subcutaneously, ingested (pharmaceutic opioids). Associated with depression and antisocial personality disorder.

*Sedatives, hypnotics, anxiolytics (benzodiazepines, methaqualone, barbiturates, chloral compounds, others):* Effects include euphoria, sedation, psychomotor impairment, amnesia, fatigue, headache, depression, gastrointestinal disturbance. Users often include young drug abusers who combine these with other agents, or patients who become dependent iatrogenically. Short-acting drugs (e.g., amobarbital) are more lethal at lower doses than long-acting compounds (e.g., phenobarbital). Death from overdose of benzodiazepines alone is rare.

***Hallucinogens (LSD, psilocybin, mescaline, methylenedioxymethamphetamine [MDMA], others):*** May be taken orally or smoked.

***Phencyclidine (PCP, angel dust):*** Injected intravenously, snorted, smoked, or eaten to produce hallucinogenic effects.

***Inhalants (gasoline, volatile glues, solvents, nitrates, cleaners, others):*** Often used by adolescents to induce euphoria. Possible death by accidental asphyxiation.

***Anabolic steroids:*** Taken orally or intramuscularly, usually in adolescents and/or athletes.

***Cannabis (marijuana, hashish, tetrahydrocannabinol [THC]):*** Most commonly used illicit drug; smoked or eaten.

▶ **History & Physical**
See Table 13–1.

▶ **Diagnostic Studies**
See Table 13–1.

▶ **Diagnosis**
Substance dependence when three or more of the following are present: tolerance (increased amounts required to achieve same effect, or decrease effect with continued use of same amount of substance); withdrawal (substance-specific withdrawal syndrome, or other substance taken to relieve or avoid withdrawal syndrome); increased amounts used or longer time of use than originally intended; inability to decrease use or control substance use; significant amounts of time spent to obtain, use, or recover from substance; discontinuing important social, occupational, or recreational activities due to substance; continuing use despite knowledge/awareness that it is exacerbating or causing physical or mental problems.

▶ **Clinical Therapeutics**
***Amphetamines, cocaine:*** *Intoxication:* If symptoms are severe, benzodiazepines for agitation. May need to treat dysrhythmias. *Withdrawal:* Antidepressants for depression after thorough detox. Caution should be exercised with haloperidol and phenothiazines as they may lower the seizure threshold.

***Opioids:*** *Intoxication/overdose:* Naloxone administration can be lifesaving in cases of respiratory depression. *Withdrawal:* Be prepared for abstinence syndrome in narcotic-dependent patients. Severe abstinence syndrome may require methadone until symptoms are controlled. Clonidine may be useful for anxiety and craving during the detox phase.

***Sedatives, hypnotics, anxiolytics:*** For acute overdose of benzodiazepines, IV flumazenil. Otherwise, long-acting benzodiazepine taper.

## ▶ table 13-1

### SUBSTANCE ABUSE: DIAGNOSTICS

| | Mild–Moderate Intoxication | Severe Intoxication | Withdrawal |
|---|---|---|---|
| Stimulants | Euphoria, increased energy and alertness, talkativeness, sexual arousal, insomnia, increased ability to perform repetitive tasks, decreased appetite, anxiety, irritability, pupillary dilatation, hypertension, increased heart rate, psychomotor agitation, hyperthermia, weight loss, nausea and vomiting. Often associated with sexually transmitted diseases, depression, sexual dysfunction, social isolation. Urinalysis positive for 1–3 days. | *Toxic psychosis:* visual, auditory, lactile hallucinations, delusions, mania, paranoia, aggression, hypervigilance, pupillary dilatation, elevated blood pressure and heart rate, arrhythmias, seizures, exhaustion, coma, intracranial hemorrhage; may progress to delirium or sudden cardiac death. | Dysphoria, hypersomnia or insomnia, increased appetite, fatigue, agitation, anxiety, suicidal ideation, unpleasant dreams; may self-medicate with alcohol or other substances during withdrawal. |
| Opioids | Euphoria; apathy; analgesia without loss of consciousness; drowsiness; mental clouding; lethargy; dysphoria; hypoactivity; anorexia; constipation; itching; nausea and vomiting; slurred speech; hypotension; bradycardia; constricted pupils; needle tracks; flushed, warm skin (cutaneous vasodilation); dysarthria; impaired attention and memory; illusions.<br>*Dependency:* weight loss, hyposexuality, amenorrhea, criminal involvement, suicide attempts, accidents, other health problems. Urinalysis positive for 1–2 days. | Respiratory depression (may recur up to 24–72 hrs after apparent recovery), depressed reflexes, hypotension, shock, pulmonary edema, pupillary dilation, seizures, coma. | Dysphoria, myalgias, rhinorrhea, fever, nausea and vomiting, diarrhea, dilated pupils, restlessness, sweating, insomnia, yawning, piloerection, anxiety, craving, hypertension, tachycardia. |
| Sedatives/<br>Hypnotics/<br>Anxiolytics | Slurred speech, mood lability, drowsiness, incoordination, unsteady gait, impaired judgment, impaired attention and memory, nystagmus. Blood and urine tests positive for 1–2 days. | Respiratory depression, depressed reflexes, hypotension, hypoxemia, decreased cardiac output, bullous skin lesions and necrosis of sweat glands, hypothermia, coma, death (usually pneumonia or renal failure). | Insomnia, anxiety, autonomic hyperactivity, psychomotor agitation, anorexia, headache, dizziness, nausea and vomiting, malaise, tremor, transient hallucinations, seizures, death. |
| Hallucinogens | Depends on substance but, in general, hallucinations, anxiety and panic reactions, dilated pupils, blurred vision, perceptual changes, emotional intensity and lability, increased heart rate and blood pressure, paranoia, sweating, depersonalization, distortion of time sense, inappropriate affect; belief that perceptions, although disturbed, are real; depression. Laboratory evaluation rarely helpful. | Confused, psychotic individuals may be at increased risk for accidents that result in harm to self or others. | No specific withdrawal symptoms; may have flashbacks postcessation. |
| Phencyclidine | Euphoria, unpredictable violent behavior, paranoia, agitation, nystagmus, dysarthria, hypertension, tachycardia, analgesia, muscle rigidity, hyperreflexia, illogical thinking, ataxia, hyperacusis, hyperthermia, seizures; creatine phosphokinase and serum glutamic oxaloacetic transaminase may be elevated, urinalysis positive for up to several weeks. | Seizures, coma, death. | Agitation, seizures, muscle spasms, flashbacks. |

*(continued)*

► table 13-1 (continued)

### SUBSTANCE ABUSE: DIAGNOSTICS

| | Mild–Moderate Intoxication | Severe Intoxication | Withdrawal |
|---|---|---|---|
| Inhalants | Euphoria, dizziness, impaired judgment, altered states of consciousness, lethargy, psychomotor retardation, tremor, muscular weakness, blurred vision, perceptual disturbances, delusions, ataxia, disorientation, slurred speech, hyporeflexia, nystagmus. Laboratory analyses for inhalants are not generally available. | Dysarthria, aggression, blurred vision, lethargy, weakness. Can progress to delirium, seizures, coma. | Some sleep disturbance, disorientation, irritability, muscle spasms may be noted. |
| Anabolic steroids | Enhanced sense of well-being, increased muscle-mass, aggressiveness, impulsivity, irritability, mania, psychosis, depression, acne. | Chronic use may lead to hepatic damage, testicular atrophy, hirsutism in females. | Irritability, depression, anxiety. |
| Cannabis | Euphoria, impaired motor coordination, increased humorousness, distortion of time and space, dry mouth, impaired judgment, increased appetite, pupillary dilation, conjunctival erythema, suspiciousness, dysphoria, anxiety, depersonalization, social withdrawal, tachycardia, impaired memory, decreased libido. Urine positive up to 4 weeks. | *High doses:* psychosis (auditory and visual hallucinations), panic, delirium. *Chronic use:* possible amotivational syndrome. | Irritability and insomnia may be noted. |

Phenobarbital with a gradual taper is a second choice. For alcohol, use a long-acting benzodiazepine, multivitamins, thiamine, and magnesium.

***Hallucinogens:*** *Intoxication:* Benzodiazepines for anxiety; use haloperidol only if additional sedation needed.

***Phencyclidine:*** Benzodiazepines for agitation; haloperidol with caution for psychotic symptoms. Dantrolene for hyperthermia, and sodium nitroprusside for severe hypertension.

***Cannabis:*** Oral diazepam sometimes helpful for anxiety.

***Inhalants:*** Anxiolytics may be useful after detox. Propranolol for dysrhythmias. Oxygen by mask may be useful.

► Clinical Intervention

***Amphetamines:*** Supportive therapy, drug-free environment. Treat depression if present following withdrawal; be alert for suicidal ideation. Refer if persistent psychosis.

***Opioids:*** *Intoxication:* Support vital functions; provide supportive care. *Withdrawal:* Not medical emergency but very uncomfortable.

***Sedatives, hypnotics, anxiolytics:*** *Overdose:* Emesis if gag reflex is intact and ingestion within 30 minutes; otherwise, gastric lavage. Decrease intestinal absorption with cathartic agent. Close monitoring, maintenance of airway and blood pressure.

***Hallucinogens:*** *Intoxication:* Reassurance; ensure safe, quiet environment; supervision of behavior. *Flashbacks:* Reassurance if mild; referral if severe or persistent.

***Phencyclidine:*** Ensure safe, quiet, nonstimulating environment. If violent behavior develops, may require physical restraints.

***Cannabis:*** Treatment rarely needed; reassurance in quiet environment; evaluate for polydrug use.

***Inhalants:*** Close supervision, possible restraints may be necessary for acute intoxication. Long-term monitoring to identify relapse and prevent further access to substance.

***Anabolic steroids:*** Evaluate for depression.

▶ Health Maintenance Issues

Important to identify problem early and institute remedial therapy.

## X. OTHER BEHAVIORAL/EMOTIONAL DISORDERS

### A. Altered Mental Status/Confusional States

▶ Scientific Concepts

Confusion is a disturbance in clarity or coherence of thinking. Often considered a nonspecific sign of organic disorder; but can also occur in schizophrenia and psychotic mood disorders. Several causes of acute confusional state and/or delirium, including metabolic disorders (e.g., hypoglycemia, hyperglycemia, hyponatremia, hypoxia), systemic illness (e.g., anemia, febrile illness, hypertension), CNS disorders (e.g., subdural or epidural hematoma, seizure, stroke, infection, tumor), and drugs and medications (e.g., alcohol, barbiturates, antidepressants). May also indicate dementia; syndrome of the elderly most often caused by Alzheimer's disease.

▶ History & Physical

Cognitive impairment may include reduced attention, disorganized thought with rambling or incoherent speech, shifting levels of consciousness, sensory misinterpretations, illusions, hallucinations, disorientations, memory disturbances. History of delirium is acute with rapid onset of days or weeks in duration. Course and level of consciousness fluctuates, with orientation impaired periodically. Affect is typically anxious, irritable, with disordered thinking; recent memory is markedly impaired. Hallucinations are common; psychomotor skills often retarded, agitated, or mixed. Attention and awareness prominently impaired; symptoms are often reversible. History of dementia is chronic with insidious onset over months or years, progressive. Level of consciousness and psychomotor skills normal. Orientation is intact initially; affect labile but not anxious. Recent and remote memory impaired. Hallucinations less common; attention and awareness less impaired. Majority of symptoms not reversible.

▶ Diagnostic Studies

History, physical, lab studies to diagnose underlying problems. Mental Status Examination (MSE) to screen for wide range of cognitive functions. Workup to include neurological exam, CBC, chemistry profile, thyroid function tests, urinalysis, urine drug screen, blood concentrations of drugs being taken, venereal disease test, ECG, CT, MRI, and EEG as indicated.

### ▶ Diagnosis

Important to differentiate acute confusional state from dementia as identified by symptoms in history and physical. Acute loss of orientation to one or more of the parameters of person, place, and time may be related to acute cognitive impairment and/or decrease in level of consciousness. Delirium represents a medical emergency that mandates aggressive medical evaluation and treatment. Dementia is the progressive and chronic development of multiple cognitive deficits manifested in both memory impairment and one (or more) of the following: aphasia, apraxia, agnosia, executive functions. These deficits do not occur exclusively during the course of delirium.

### ▶ Clinical Therapeutics

*Delirium:* Goal is to treat underlying condition. High-potency antipsychotics for psychosis (haloperidol, 2–10 mg IM, may be repeated after 1 hour if first dose ineffective). Antipsychotics are less likely than benzodiazepines to worsen cognitive function; however, patients in alcohol or sedative–hypnotic withdrawal are best treated with benzodiazepine.

*Dementia:* Low dosages of all psychotropic medication in elderly. Antipsychotics such as haloperidol (0.5–5 mg/d) for behavior control, but elderly clear drugs more slowly than do young patients due to decreased hepatic and renal function. May have acute side effects including dystonia, parkinsonism, and hypotension. Tacrine (initially 40 mg/d up to a maximum of 160 mg/d in divided doses) for Alzheimer's disease; clinically significant improvement in 20–25% of patients who take it. Use with caution in patients with liver dysfunction.

### ▶ Clinical Intervention

*Delirium:* Immediately assess patient's condition; orient and reassure. All cases require hospitalization unless due to rapidly reversible process (e.g., insulin-induced hypoglycemia corrected with glucose infusion). Environmental control of impulsive or unpredictable patient to prevent violence. See Clinical Therapeutics above for acute state. Identify rate of onset of confusion and physical or psychological stressors. Conduct MSE, laboratory tests. Correct any metabolic, nutritional, electrolyte, or fluid abnormalities. Obtain neurological consult. Follow up with treatment when a definitive diagnosis has been made.

*Dementia:* Discontinue any medications that exacerbate dementia if possible (e.g., the $H_2$ antagonist cimetidine). Screen for depression and refer to mental health provider. Family support, including development of management plan for long-term care. Some evidence that cholinergic analogs (e.g., tacrine, 80 mg PO qd) may delay the manifestations of Alzheimer's disease.

### ▶ Health Maintenance Issues

*Delirium:* Monitor and follow up for underlying condition.

*Dementia:* Correct any nutritional and metabolic deficiencies. Preventive measures (changes in diet, exercise, and control of diabetes and hypertension) important in vascular dementia. Continued reassessment of treatment and options for care. Counsel family regarding prognosis, possible need for placement, syndromes that develop in caretakers (burnout, depression, anxiety).

## B. Elder/Child Abuse

▶ Scientific Concepts

***Elder abuse:*** Each year, over 1 million cases of elder abuse occur, with as few as 1 in every 14 victimizations reported. Majority of victims are white, widowed women, usually older than 75, living dependently; cognitive impairment and incontinence, nocturnal shouting, wandering, or manifestations of paranoia. Abuser is often a relative in the same household.

***Child abuse:*** There are 500,000 new cases of physical and sexual abuse reported each year, and 2,000–4,000 abused children die. An estimated 2–4 million children have been abused. Typical child abuser is single, unemployed mother under age 30, although may also be another caretaker such as father, babysitter, or friend. Many victims of physical abuse are also abused sexually. Physical abuse is also called *battered child syndrome.*

▶ History & Physical

***Elder abuse:*** Caregiver often under stress, suffering from alcoholism, marital problems, unemployment, financial difficulties, social isolation, drug abuse. Family history of violence or presence of mental illness or retardation. Key findings:
- *Physical abuse:* Lesions, alopecia, and hemorrhaging at nape of scalp; bruises, burns, and human bite marks; sexual assault.
- *Neglect:* Pallor, wasting, dehydration, decubitus ulcers, untreated injuries, poor hygiene.
- *Psychological abuse:* Depression, withdrawal, anger, agitation, or expression of ambivalent feelings.

***Child abuse:*** Obvious cases present with bruises, fractures (particularly those in several stages of healing), dislocations, burns, lacerations, focal neurological deficits, signs of intracranial bleeding, abdominal injury, malnutrition, or dehydration. If infant presents with retinal hemorrhages, must rule out "shaken baby syndrome." Munchausen syndrome by proxy occurs when caretaker brings child with fabricated illness, reporting nonexistent symptoms, altered lab tests, or induced illness. Sexual abuse presents with genital injury or irritation, foreign bodies in the vagina or rectum, excessive masturbation, venereal disease, or pregnancy. May also see PTSD as evidenced by sleep disorder or somatic complaints, regressive behaviors, hypersexuality, generalized low self-esteem, and sense of isolation. Emotional abuse presents as failure to thrive with hypokinesis, apathy, delayed responsiveness, malnutrition, and fearfulness. History of injury may be inconsistent with clinical findings or developmental level; delay in seeking care.

▶ Diagnostic Studies

***Elder abuse:*** Key findings as above. In addition to physical examination and in-depth interview, radiological and metabolic screening, toxicological and drug-level screen, hematological screening, CT.

*Child abuse:* Key findings as above; in addition to physical examination and in-depth interview, skeletal series, serologies, bleeding screening battery, CBC, creatine kinase as indicated.

▶ Diagnosis

*Elder abuse:* Seldom reported by its victims. Occurs in three basic categories: domestic, institutional, and self-neglect. Important to rule out normal changes in physical, emotional, and cognitive behaviors due to aging and medical conditions.

*Child abuse:* Rule out unintentional trauma, bleeding diathesis, dermatologic conditions, vitamin deficiencies, osteogenesis imperfecta, self-inflicted injuries, other medical or metabolic causes for failure to thrive.

▶ Clinical Therapeutics
N/A.

▶ Clinical Intervention

*Elder abuse:* First priority is to ensure safety while respecting autonomy. Hospitalization; competent patient must first provide consent. Mandatory reporting in most states to Adult Protective Services. Home visit upon discharge by visiting nurse or social worker. Continued mobilization of community, social, and health services.

*Child abuse:* Interview child alone, expert may be needed to elicit history, separate interview of parents. Treatment of injury or neglect. Hospitalization as needed. Ensure safety of child. Mandatory reporting of suspected abuse; documentation of findings, including pictures. Follow-up. Treatment of child for physical, emotional sequelae. Individual or group psychotherapy indicated. Treatment for abuser ranges from support to mandated therapy, removal of parent abuser or child, legal prosecution.

▶ Health Maintenance Issues

*Elder abuse:* Education, early intervention with supportive services in high-risk situations. Clear documentation of abuse. Referral and follow-up legal, social, psychiatric, community service including support groups for caregivers.

*Child abuse:* Follow-up legal, social, psychiatric, and community services. Support group for child and/or parents.

## C. Adult Domestic Violence

▶ Scientific Concepts

Battering in 20% of women seeking medical care; 22–35% of women presenting to emergency departments; 23% of prenatal patients; 25% of women who attempt suicide; 45–58% of mothers of abused children. Risk factors include pregnancy, social isolation, history of child abuse, substance abuse, criminal record.

▶ History & Physical

History may be incompatible with injury. Repeated trauma common. No diagnostic injury pattern, but injuries common in face, head, neck, breast, abdomen.

▶ Diagnostic Studies

Key findings as above. Physical examination and in-depth interview.

▶ Diagnosis

Positive findings on the physical examination and history. Sequelae include PTSD symptoms, low self-esteem, somatic complaints, depression, anxiety, substance abuse, suicide attempts.

▶ Clinical Therapeutics

N/A.

▶ Clinical Intervention

Treatment of injuries; evaluation for suicide risk. Ensure safety of victim and children. Respect victim's judgment regarding safety; increased risk of abuse when abused partner leaves. Assessment of continued risk and resources. Refer for medical, legal, psychiatric, and community services (battered women's shelter). Documentation including photos of injury. Follow-up plan in place.

▶ Health Maintenance Issues

Barriers to leaving abusive relationship should be addressed, including self-blame, feelings of helplessness, financial dependency, fear of retaliation. Continued sensitive questioning on the part of provider to reveal ongoing abuse.

## D. Rape/Crisis Adjustment

▶ Scientific Concepts

Rape is the forceful coercion of an unwilling victim to engage in a sexual act. Usually, this act is sexual intercourse; anal intercourse and fellatio also constitute rape. Male rape legally defined in most states as sodomy. Homosexual rape more frequent among men and occurs frequently in closed institutions. Rapist discharges aggression and aggrandizes self. PTSD resulting from aggravated assault, rape, or noncrime trauma affects over 4 million women in the United States. Female victims of aggravated assault are five times more likely to develop PTSD than female victims of noncrime trauma.

▶ History & Physical

Clinicians need high degree of suspicion for unreported rape; 50% are not reported. History and physical should take place in private with patient consent. Rape and sexual abuse victims are often confused after assault. History and physical reveals patient victim of act of violent humiliation, physical trauma. Often occurs in accompaniment to another crime.

▶ Diagnostic Studies

Prior to physical examination and data collection, obtain patient's permission due to possibility of repeated trauma through "medical rape." Physical examination, photographs, specimen collection from vaginal pool for police laboratory. Cervical and rectal cultures for gonorrhea and serology for syphilis, human immunodeficiency virus (HIV) testing. The practitioner must ensure that proper medical and legal protocols are followed to protect the patient as well as evidence for forensic purposes. Proper collection, labeling, and preservation of the chain of custody for samples is essential.

► Diagnosis

Establishing that a rape has occurred is a legal decision, not a medical diagnosis.

► Clinical Therapeutics

Usually no drug treatment after trauma is indicated. Some patients may experience overwhelming anxiety; short-term treatment with benzodiazepine such as alprazolam (0.5 to 1 mg PO tid), lorazepam (1–2 mg PO tid), or oxazepam (10 to 30 mg PO tid) may be needed. Insomnia may also respond to treatment above or with temazepam (15–30 mg PO hs) or flurazepam (15–30 mg PO hs). To prevent pregnancy, a 5-day course of medroxyprogesterone or diethylstilbestrol may be offered. To protect patient against sexual transmitted diseases and hepatitis, prophylaxis should be offered. HIV prophylaxis is controversial.

► Clinical Intervention

*Rape:* Offer appropriate medical, gynecological, and police services. Immediately treat patient for injuries sustained in the assault. Treat with clinical therapeutics as above.

*Crisis adjustment, general:* Evaluate victim for possible PTSD, which may not develop immediately; inform patient about possible sequelae. Offer crisis intervention–oriented therapy. Objective is to minimize psychological sequelae of trauma. Refer for ongoing psychotherapy, which should focus on reestablishing sense of control over environment, reducing feelings of helplessness and dependence, and addressing obsessional thoughts and other symptoms of PTSD. Refer to group therapy for trauma victims. Evaluate patient for underlying psychiatric conditions (e.g., substance dependence, schizophrenia) that may cause impaired judgment and place patient in danger of rape or trauma; if present, refer for treatment of underlying psychiatric disorder.

► Health Maintenance Issues

Many trauma victims have symptoms that continue for years, including reliving experience (flashbacks), preoccupation with experience, fear of being alone, nightmares, insomnia, and altered eating patterns. Somatic symptoms include headaches, nausea and vomiting, and malaise. Patient may avoid future sexual relationships or experience sexual symptoms such as vaginismus. Follow-up should include evaluation for PTSD and referral to support groups or mental health provider for symptom resolution.

## E. Sudden Infant Death Syndrome (Family)

► Scientific Concepts

Most common cause of death between 7 days and 365 days of age; 5,200–5,500 infant deaths per year in the United States; 1.4 sudden infant death syndrome (SIDS) deaths/1,000 live births.

► History & Physical

Most deaths between 1 and 3 months of age, peaking at 3 months. Males have higher incidence.

► Diagnosis

Diagnosis of exclusion after postmortem examination fails to reveal a cause of death.

▶ Clinical Therapeutics
N/A.

▶ Clinical Intervention
Intense, severe grief reactions common in parents; guilt, anger, somatic symptoms; overactivity, social isolation, psychosis, agitated depression. May lead to health problems, marital difficulties, behavior problems, and fears in siblings. Contact with dead baby, pictures, quick autopsy results; education regarding guilt and blame. Parent support groups; sibling and extended family support; social support; counseling. Look for delayed grief reaction.

▶ Health Maintenance Issues
Association of SIDS with prone sleeping has led to recommendation that all infants be placed in supine position or positioning baby alternating sides and back to help prevent molding.

## F. Uncomplicated Bereavement

▶ Scientific Concepts
Not considered a mental disorder; self-limited psychological process; about one third of bereaved spouses do meet criteria for major depressive disorder.

▶ History & Physical
Intense emotional distress, somatic symptoms, dissociation, preoccupation with deceased, anger, loss of habitual patterns of conduct, mourning; major depressive syndrome with anorexia, crying, loss of concentration, fatigue, anxiety, sleep disturbance; duration up to 1–2 years; anniversary reactions common.

▶ Diagnostic Studies
As above.

▶ Diagnosis
As above; rule out major depressive disorder based on symptoms' severity and length, lack of resolution; include preoccupation with worthlessness, hopelessness, suicidal ideation, blame for the death, psychomotor retardation.

▶ Clinical Therapeutics
Medication generally contraindicated unless used to treat an underlying depressive disorder. Preliminary data indicate major depressive symptoms occurring shortly after loss appear to respond to buproprion SR.

▶ Clinical Intervention
Encourage open grieving, expression of feelings; recognition of variability among family members; anticipatory guidance around anniversary events; referral to support groups, psychotherapy as needed.

▶ Health Maintenance Issues
Follow-up essential to monitor resolution of grieving process, uncover suicidal ideation, marital and family difficulties; support and reassure around normalcy of uncomplicated grief symptoms and reactions; refer if condition evolves into pathological grieving process or major depressive disorder.

## BIBLIOGRAPHY

American Psychiatric Association. *Diagnostic and Statistical Manual of Mental Disorders,* 4th ed. Washington, DC: American Psychiatric Association; 2000.

Berg DD. *Handbook of Primary Care Medicine,* 2nd ed. Philadelphia, PA: Lippincott-Raven; 1998.

Feldman MD, Christensen JF, Feldman W. *Behavioral Medicine in Primary Care: A Practical Guide.* Blacklick, OH: McGraw-Hill Professional Publishing; 1998.

Goldberg JS. *The Instant Exam Review for the USMLE Step 3,* 2nd ed. Stamford, CT: Appleton & Lange; 1997.

Kaplan HI, Sadock BJ. *Synopsis of Psychiatry,* 8th ed. Baltimore, MD: Lippincott, Williams & Wilkins; 1998.

Knesper DJ, Riba MB, Schwenk TL. *Primary Care Psychiatry.* Philadelphia, PA: W.B. Saunders Company; 1997.

Stoudemire, A. *Clinical Psychiatry for Medical Students,* 3rd ed. Philadelphia, PA: Lippincott-Raven; 1998.

# Hematology and Oncology 14

*Maura Polansky, MS, PA-C, and Kathryn Boyer, MS, PA-C*

## I. ANEMIAS

▶ Scientific Concepts

Anemia is defined by the concentration of plasma to red blood cells. It can result from decreased production, increased destruction, or both.

▶ History & Physical

Common symptoms include fatigue, weakness, dizziness, shortness of breath, chest pain, and pallor. The finding of koilonychia (flattened, spooned nails) can be seen in chronic anemic states. Many patients suffer from mild to moderate anemia but are asymptomatic.

▶ Diagnostic Studies

A complete blood count (CBC), mean corpuscular volume (MCV), and a peripheral smear will determine the presence and severity of anemia and help in distinguishing the type of anemia.

▶ Diagnosis

Normal laboratory values of hemoglobin and hematocrit depend on age and gender. The differential diagnosis of anemia includes pseudo-anemia secondary to increased blood volume (e.g., pregnancy, excess intravascular fluid, hyperproteinemia).

▶ Clinical Therapeutics

Treatment should be directed at the underlying etiology. Except for transfusion when necessary, no therapy should be initiated until the specific etiology has been established.

▶ Clinical Intervention

There is no absolute laboratory threshold to determine the need for blood transfusion. The decision to transfuse depends on the degree of anemia, rapidity of onset, comorbid illnesses, and symptomatology. Risks of transfusing blood products, including the risk of infections and transfusion reactions, must be considered.

▶ Health Maintenance Issues

Adequate dietary intake of iron, $B_{12}$, and folate are essential to avoid anemia. Dietary screening should be performed for individuals at increased risk of anemia.

## A. Iron Deficiency Anemia

▶ Scientific Concepts

Iron deficiency anemia may be an acute or chronic condition. Causes of frank or occult bleeding often include gastrointestinal (GI) bleeding, trauma, and excessive menstrual bleeding. Inadequate dietary intake (e.g., in childhood and pregnancy) can occur, but this is a less common cause of iron deficiency.

▶ History & Physical

General symptoms and signs of anemia may be present. With acute blood loss, symptoms and signs of intravascular hypovolemia should be identified, including orthostatic dizziness and orthostatic hypotension. Since anemia depends on the concentration of red blood cells in plasma, time after acute blood loss is required for fluid shifts to occur and anemia to be noted on laboratory analysis.

► **Diagnostic Studies**

Serum iron, ferritin, total iron-binding capacity (TIBC), and transferrin should be checked as these are typically abnormal in iron deficiency. The earliest stage of iron deficiency is depletion of iron stores in the bone marrow. However, marrow analysis of iron stores is rarely needed to establish the diagnosis of iron deficiency.

► **Diagnosis**

Iron deficiency anemia is one of the microcytic, hypochromic anemias; low serum iron, ferritin, and transferrin with high TIBC establishes the diagnosis. Once diagnosed, the etiology must be determined.

► **Clinical Therapeutics**

Oral iron replacement will usually take 2–3 months, and an additional 6–8 months of iron is recommended to fully replace iron stores. Follow-up is necessary to determine the adequacy of replacement and to ensure no continued blood loss. Supplemental iron should be discontinued once hemoglobin normalizes, as excessive iron use will mask continued or new blood loss and excess iron can be harmful to organs such as the heart, liver, and pancreas.

► **Clinical Intervention**

Identifying iron deficiency anemia is an important factor in diagnosing serious medical problems such as GI malignancies. Treatment of the underlying disorder may be the most important intervention for these patients.

► **Health Maintenance Issues**

Adequate dietary intake of iron is essential. This is of particular concern for infants and pregnant women. Infants receiving bottle feedings should be fed with an iron-fortified milk.

## B. Thalassemia

► **Scientific Concepts**

Thalassemias are a diverse group of genetic disorders leading to reduced globin chain production (quantitative abnormality with normal structure) of one or more subunits of hemoglobin, which may include alpha, beta, gamma, or delta. Those at highest risk of inheritance are ethnic groups from malaria-affected regions. However, the disorder can occur sporadically.

Alpha- and beta-globin deficiencies are the most common; these are the primary globins present after the first year of life. Manifestation of the disorder ranges from subtle abnormalities to severe disease.

Alpha-globin is determined by four genes. Therefore, alpha-thalassemia manifests as a spectrum depending on the number of genes involved from silent carriers with no hematologic abnormalities to Hb Barts with all four genes involved, which is incompatible with life. Approximately 1–3% of the African American population is homozygous for alpha-thalassemia-2, which typically results in a microcytosis without anemia.

Beta-globin is determined by only two genes; therefore, beta-thalassemia is divided into thalassemia minor (one gene) and thalassemia major (two genes). Thalassemia minor (thalassemia trait) is usually asymptomatic and often goes undiagnosed. It may manifest with mild anemia and requires no treatment. Thalassemia major results in severe anemia and usually manifests by 6 months of life.

### ▶ History & Physical

Symptoms and signs of anemia should be noted. Splenomegaly may be present.

### ▶ Diagnostic Studies

CBC, peripheral smear, reticulocyte count, and iron studies should be obtained initially. If thalassemia is suspected by these initial studies, hemoglobin (Hb) electrophoresis and alpha/beta-globin chain ratios should be ordered.

### ▶ Diagnosis

Microcytic, hypochromic anemia with characteristic target cells, poikilocytosis, elliptocytes, basophilic stippling on Wright stain may be present, and elevated reticulocyte count will be present. Normal iron studies will differentiate from iron deficiency anemia. Hb electrophoresis is necessary to confirm the diagnosis.

### ▶ Clinical Therapeutics

Most individuals with thalassemia require no treatment. Those with severe disease usually present early in life and may become transfusion dependent. Iron chelation therapy is then necessary to prevent iron overload.

### ▶ Clinical Intervention

Bone marrow transplantation is the definitive therapy for thalassemia major. Some may benefit from splenectomy if splenomegaly is present.

### ▶ Health Maintenance Issues

Genetic counseling is necessary for those at high risk. For individuals with the disease, folic acid supplementation may be needed due to the high bone marrow demands. Iron overload can occur in transfusion-dependent patients and should be tested for and treated. Iron overload may result in organ dysfunction.

## C. Lead Poisoning

### ▶ Scientific Concepts

Lead toxicity results in anemia by inhibiting the activity of enzymes in heme synthesis and by injuring red cell membranes, resulting in hemolysis. Exposures are common through ingested lead-containing paint and improperly glazed pottery for cooking or eating. Both children and adults can be affected.

### ▶ History & Physical

Abdominal pain, constipation, vomiting, and muscle weakness are common symptoms of lead toxicity. Neurological and psychological symptoms occur less commonly, but do occur more frequently in children than adults. A lead line (linear blue-black deposit of lead sulfide in gums near teeth) may be seen, as well as dental caries and motor disturbances.

### ▶ Diagnostic Studies

The evaluation should include a CBC, peripheral smear, reticulocyte count, and serum lead level.

► Diagnosis

Lead toxicity leads to a mild to moderate anemia with mild to moderate hypochromia and microcytic/normocytic erythrocytes. Basophilic stippling on Wright stain may or may not be present. The reticulocyte count is typically elevated and leukocyte count normal or slightly increased. Normal ferritin, marrow iron, and TIBC differentiates from iron deficiency anemia. Increased transferrin saturation and urinary aminolevulinic acid (ALA) with normal porphobilinogen will help to establish the diagnosis. The differential diagnosis includes acute intermittent porphyria.

► Clinical Therapeutics

Lead levels guide therapy: Acceptable levels are 15 to 40 µg/dL. Patients typically become symptomatic and require treatment when levels reach 80 µg/dL or more, although children may be symptomatic at lower levels. Lead poisoning is treated with ethylenediaminetetraacetic acid (EDTA) to chelate lead and allow urinary excretion. Small amounts should be given as encephalopathy can occur secondary to lead chelation. Lead levels should return to normal in a few weeks.

► Clinical Intervention

Identify and remove the source of lead.

► Health Maintenance Issues

Screening is recommended for those at high risk (e.g., children, especially those with behavioral problems).

## D. Anemia of Chronic Illness

► Scientific Concepts

Secondary to infectious (tuberculosis, pneumonia, chronic fungal disease, osteomyelitis, meningitis), inflammatory (rheumatoid arthritis, systemic lupus erythematosus, myocardial infarction), or malignant disease of more than 1 to 2 months duration. The primary cause is thought to be due to the effect of cytokines released by these tissues. The mechanisms include:

1. Decreased iron release from storage in macrophages. *↓ iron release*
2. Shortened erythrocyte survival. *↓ erythrocyte survival*
3. Impaired marrow response to shortened red cell life span resulting in no or inadequate elevation of the erythropoietin level. *↓ marrow response*

► History & Physical

Often patients may be asymptomatic, except for symptoms and signs of underlying disease. Symptoms often develop when the anemia is associated with certain underlying diseases such as cardiac or pulmonary disease.

► Diagnostic Studies

CBC, peripheral smear, and reticulocyte count should be initially obtained. Iron studies are needed if hypochromic erythrocytes are present.

► Diagnosis

Typically a mild to moderate anemia, but hematocrit levels within normal range that are decreased from the patient's baseline may be noted.

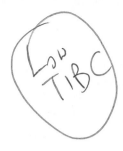

Usually the anemia is normochromic and normocytic, but may be hypochromic or microcytic. Moderate anisocytosis and minimal poikilocytosis is often present. The corrected reticulocyte count is normal to slightly increased. Serum iron is low with a low TIBC (in contrast to iron deficiency with increased TIBC).

### ► Clinical Therapeutics

Erythropoietin administration can be extremely effective, especially in anemia of chronic renal disease. Iron supplementation may be needed along with erythropoietin use to prevent inducing iron deficiency.

### ► Clinical Intervention

Directed at underlying illness; transfusion rarely needed.

## E. Sickle Cell Anemia

### ► Scientific Concepts

This is an autosomal dominant disorder resulting in sickling of erythrocytes. (Heterozygous (AS) = sickle cell trait; homozygous (SS) = sickle cell anemia.) Among those of African American decent, 8% are AS and 0.1 to 0.2% are SS. Sickling occurs when oxygen decreases at the tissue level, while sickled cells impede blood flow to tissue and organs. Hemolysis is also common.

### ► History & Physical

Pain, fatigue, weakness, and pallor are hallmark signs of this disease. Growth and sexual maturation are typically delayed. Cardiomegaly, hepatomegaly, and splenomegaly can result. Sickle cell crisis occurs with excessive deoxygenation of red cells, often precipitated by infection, dehydration, and high altitude. Complications of the disease include splenic infarction, renal papillary necrosis, aseptic necrosis, and cerebrovascular accident (CVA).

### ► Diagnostic Studies

CBC, peripheral smear, Hb electrophoresis, and sickle cell prep are needed to establish the diagnosis. Prenatal diagnosis can be made by amniotic fluid analysis.

### ► Diagnosis

Normocytic, normochromic anemia, which may be mild to severe, occurs after 6 months of life. Sickled cells are seen with SS, not AS (trait). Anisocytosis, elliptocytes, target cells, ovalocytes, and schistocytes are present on peripheral smears. Reticulocytosis, leukocytosis, and thrombocytosis may all be present. Hb electrophoresis is necessary to confirm the diagnosis.

### ► Clinical Therapeutics

No specific treatment for the disease has been established. Avoidance of triggers of sickle cell crises should be emphasized. Sickle cell crises should be treated with hydration, analgesics, and antibiotics when infection is suspected. Transfusion may be necessary but is not routinely indicated for affected individuals.

### ► Clinical Intervention

Bone marrow transplant is sometimes implemented with the potential for cure.

▶ Health Maintenance Issues

The prevention of sickle cell crises is important, as crises precipitated by infection are the primary cause of death in these patients. Vaccines, especially Pneumovax, play a critical role in preventing life-threatening infections. Folate supplementation is usually necessary to maintain adequate erythrocyte production. After a CVA, transfusions should continue for years to prevent another stroke. Genetic screening and counseling should be offered to women who are known carriers of the sickle cell gene.

## F. Aplastic Anemia

▶ Scientific Concepts

Aplastic anemia refers to a condition of pancytopenia due to severely hypoplastic or aplastic bone marrow. The most serious complications are typically due to neutropenia and thrombocytopenia. Underlying causes include congenital, acquired idiopathic, drug effects, radiation, and infections, including hepatitis, miliary tuberculosis, and parasites.

▶ History & Physical

Initial presentation may reflect an insidious or acute onset. Symptoms and signs are suggestive of anemia, thrombocytopenia, and neutropenia, such as bacterial infection (not viral) and hemorrhage. Usually no splenomegaly or lymphadenopathy is noted and the presence of either may suggest an alternative diagnosis.

▶ Diagnostic Studies

After a CBC, peripheral blood smear and reticulocyte count are obtained, bone marrow aspirate and biopsy are required to establish the diagnosis and exclude other potential illnesses. The differential diagnosis should include multiple myeloma, idiopathic thrombocytopenic purpura (ITP), acute leukemia, lymphoma, myelofibrosis, and myelodysplastic syndrome.

▶ Diagnosis

The peripheral blood will reveal decreased white blood cells (WBCs) with normal or mildly decreased lymphocytes and normocytic or slight macrocytic, normochromic red cells with a normal morphology. No immature cells are typically seen in the peripheral blood. The corrected reticulocyte count will be decreased. The bone marrow aspirate and biopsy reveals hypoplastic or aplastic marrow with increased fat and decreased hematopoietic cells, although patchy areas of normal cellularity may be noted. Lymphocytes and plasma cells are primarily seen but megakaryocytes are generally absent.

▶ Clinical Therapeutics

Supportive care alone can be provided for patients with mild disease. Blood products, immunosuppressive therapy, and androgens, which stimulate erythropoiesis, granulopoiesis, and thrombopoiesis, may benefit some patients. For those with severe disease, bone marrow transplantation is indicated and offers the best potential for cure. If patients are more than 40 years of age, immunosuppressive therapy is recommended over bone marrow transplantation (BMT).

► Clinical Intervention

For patients < 40 years of age, BMT results in higher survival when performed early in the disease, before any blood product transfusions. If BMT is considered, the patient should not be transfused with blood products from family members who may act as potential donors as this may sensitize the patient to minor antigens, increasing the risk of bone marrow rejection. Occasionally spontaneous remission occurs, especially if the precipitating cause is a drug that is discontinued.

► Health Maintenance Issues

Aplastic anemia can progress to acute leukemia. For BMT recipients, graft-versus-host (an immune reaction in which donor lymphocytes act against the host tissues) disease may occur. BMT requires cyclophosphamide or other intensive chemotherapeutic agents with or without irradiation. Irradiation increases risk of developing a secondary malignancy.

## G. Megaloblastic Anemia

► Scientific Concepts

Megaloblastic anemia is caused by impaired deoxyribonucleic acid (DNA) synthesis that results in slow cell division so erythrocytes become large. Causes include cobalamin ($B_{12}$) deficiency, folic acid (folate) deficiency, and drugs. The cause may be idiopathic.

$B_{12}$ is derived from consumption of meat and dairy products. Intrinsic factor (IF) is produced in the stomach and is required for intestinal absorption of $B_{12}$. Dietary deficiency occurs, but is uncommon. Pernicious anemia (i.e., lack of IF) is the most common cause of $B_{12}$ deficiency and is often the result of atrophy of gastric mucosa.

Folate is derived from fruits and vegetables. Folate deficiency can be the result of dietary deficiency, poor intestinal absorption, or increased demand (e.g., pregnancy). Dietary deficiency is most common, particularly in alcoholics and others with poor nutrition.

► History & Physical

***$B_{12}$ deficiency:*** Pale; mildly icteric; beefy, red, sore tongue; anorexia, weight loss, and diarrhea occur late due to malabsorption; neurologic manifestations (including numbness, paresthesia, weakness, ataxia, and disturbances in mentation) occur secondary to demyelination ("megaloblastic madness").

***Folate deficiency:*** May appear malnourished; diarrhea, cheilosis, glossitis, no neurologic manifestations.

► Diagnostic Studies

CBC, peripheral smear, folate and $B_{12}$ levels should be ordered in all patients suspected of megaloblastic anemia. In $B_{12}$ deficiency, Schilling test determines whether pernicious anemia is present. Serum folate levels reflect recent dietary intact of folate (i.e., preceding 2–3 days). Red blood cell folate is a more accurate measurement of folic acid levels and should be done if folate deficiency is suspected. However, red cell folate levels may also be diminished with $B_{12}$ deficiency.

► Diagnosis

Macrocytic anemia (MCV > 100 fL); anisocytosis; decreased levels of $B_{12}$ or folate diagnostic for etiology. Schilling test should be performed when $B_{12}$ deficiency is identified to diagnose IF deficiency. Labeled $B_{12}$ is given orally; unlabeled $B_{12}$ is given intramuscularly (IM). $B_{12}$ levels in the urine are then measured. If excretion of radiolabeled $B_{12}$ is low, the test is then repeated after a wash-out period. This time along with oral and IM $B_{12}$, IF is also given orally and levels measured in the urine. If there is a deficiency of IF, labeled $B_{12}$ will be excreted only when given without IF. The differential diagnosis of megaloblastic anemia includes liver disease, alcoholism, and hypothyroidism.

▶ Clinical Therapeutics

IM $B_{12}$ replacement should be given daily for the first 2 weeks, weekly until replaced, and then lifelong replacement given monthly is usually required. Folate 1 mg orally is given daily (parenteral is rarely needed). *Caution:* Folate can correct megaloblastic anemia even if caused by $B_{12}$ deficiency without correcting or by even aggravating neurologic manifestations (which can be permanent). Therefore, the $B_{12}$ level must be checked to rule out $B_{12}$ deficiency before folate is administered. Otherwise, both vitamins should be administered concurrently.

## H. Hemolytic Anemias

▶ Scientific Concepts

These are a group of hereditary or acquired disorders with an accelerated rate of erythrocyte destruction. The bone marrow is normal but incapable of keeping up with the accelerated destruction. Hereditary conditions include glucose-6-phosphate dehydrogenase (G6PD) deficiency, pyruvate kinase deficiency, and hemoglobinopathies. Acquired disorders include infections, hypersplenism, liver and renal disease, and microangiopathic disorders (e.g., disseminated intravascular coagulation). Hemolysis can occur either intravascularly or extravascularly.

▶ History & Physical

In addition to signs and symptoms of anemia, jaundice can be present. Splenomegaly may be present if the condition is chronic.

▶ Diagnostic Studies

CBC, peripheral smear, reticulocyte count, Coombs' test, serum chemistries, haptoglobin, and urinalysis are all generally indicated in the evaluation of a patient with suspected hemolysis.

▶ Diagnosis

Normocytic, normochromic anemia is typically present although a mildly increased MCV is sometimes noted. An appropriate elevation of the reticulocyte count should be seen. Microspherocytes and schistocytes on peripheral smear are often identified. Elevated lactic dehydrogenase (LDH) and indirect bilirubin are important indicators of hemolysis in an anemic patient.

▶ Clinical Therapeutics

Corticosteroids are often useful. Oral therapy can typically be used, although intravenous (IV) steroids may be necessary in critically ill patients. Once the disease has been stabilized, a gradual tapering course of the medication can be given over 1 to 2 months with close monitoring for commonly occurring relapses.

▶ Clinical Intervention

Transfusion of RBCs is complicated by the increased risk of further hemolysis. Patients should be observed closely for signs of transfusion reaction. Of course, treatment of the underlying disorder should be initiated whenever possible. Splenectomy may be necessary in patients who require chronic steroid administration to prevent relapse. Alternatively, immunosuppresive drugs such as cyclophosphamide have been used in those who do not respond to steroid therapy and splenectomy.

▶ Health Maintenance Issues

Avoidance of oxidative states is advised in patients with G6PD deficiency.

## I. Transfusion Reactions

▶ Scientific Concepts

Hemolytic reactions after a blood transfusion may be immediate or delayed. Life-threatening immediate reactions are associated with intravascular hemolysis and result from incompatible ABO antibodies (complement activating antibodies of immunoglobulin G or M [IgG or IgM]). The severity depends on the recipient's titer of antibodies. Extravascular hemolytic transfusion reactions result from a problem with the Rh system and are less severe, although they may also be life threatening. If these are mild, the only sign may be progressive unexplained anemia and/or jaundice.

▶ History & Physical

Clinical features include a hemolytic shock phase and may occur after a few milliliters of blood have been transfused or up to 2 hours after transfusion is completed. The patient may have urticaria, pain in the lumbar region, flushing, headache, precordial pain, shortness of breath, vomiting, rigors, pyrexia, or hypotension. Jaundice and/or disseminated intravascular coagulopathy (DIC) may even occur. Moderate leukocytosis is frequent. The oliguric phase is next, and renal tubular necrosis and acute renal failure may ensue. The diuretic phase occurs during recovery from acute renal failure.

▶ Clinical Intervention

The best treatment is prevention of reactions by ensuring compatible transfusions only. If one should occur, management consists of maintaining blood pressure and renal perfusion; administering furosemide, corticosteroids, antihistamines as necessary; and even using epinephrine for severe shock should it occur. Other transfusion reactions include the following:

*Febrile reactions:* May occur due to white cell antibodies. Clinical manifestations are rigors, fever, possible pulmonary infiltrates. These can be avoided by transfusing only leukocyte-poor packed red blood cells (RBCs; filtered).

*Nonhemolytic allergic reactions:* May occur if there is a hypersensitivity to donor plasma proteins and may result in anaphylactic shock, urticaria, fever, dyspnea, facial edema, rigors. Treatment is the immediate administration of hydrocortisone and antihistamines with or without epinephrine. Transfusing only washed red cells can prevent hypersensitivity reactions.

***Posttransfusion circulatory overload:*** Similar to pulmonary edema; can occur if large amounts of blood products are transfused rapidly, especially in patients with some degree of cardiac decompensation. The first clinical manifestations are usually a dry cough, fullness in head/neck; jugular venous distention may occur. Management is the same as that for congestive heart failure. Slow transfusion with diuretic use can prevent these reactions from occurring.

***Posttransfusion hepatitis:*** Rare with current screening methods, but may still occur.

***Transmission of cytomegalovirus (CMV) and Epstein–Barr virus (EBV):*** Hepatitis C may manifest itself 3 months after transfusion. Other known infectious agents that can be transmitted via transfusion include human immunodeficiency virus (HIV), mononucleosis, toxoplasmosis, malaria, syphilis, and CMV. Filtered products will reduce the risk of transfusion-acquired cytomegalovirus infection.

***Posttransfusion iron overload:*** May develop after repeated transfusions over several years without any blood loss, and may cause damage to the liver, myocardium, and endocrine glands.

## II. COAGULATION DISORDERS

### A. Factor VIII Disorders

#### 1. Hemophilia A

▶ Scientific Concepts

Deficiency of factor VIII is best known as hemophilia A; it is the most common severe bleeding disorder and the second most common congenital bleeding disorder. Approximately 1:10,000 males are affected. It is a hereditary disorder with X-linked recessive transmission, so only males are affected. Bleeding is due to a deficiency of factor VIII:C (factor VIII coagulant). The protein can be either quantitatively reduced (in the majority) or functionally defective.

▶ History & Physical

Bleeding may occur anywhere, most commonly seen as bleeding into joints (knees, ankles, elbows), into muscles, from the GI tract, or intracranially. Spontaneous hemarthroses are very characteristic of this disorder. Bleeding worsens with more severe disease, and those most affected may bleed spontaneously. Many hemophiliacs are HIV positive, most acquired via factor VIII concentrate transfusions. HIV-associated thrombocytopenia may aggravate bleeding.

▶ Diagnostic Studies

Activated partial thromboplastin time (aPTT) is prolonged, while prothrombin time (PT) and fibrinogen are normal. Platelet count should be normal, unless HIV-associated thrombocytopenia is present. Factor VIII:C levels are reduced while von Willebrand's factor and factor IX are normal.

▶ Diagnosis

Clinically indistinguishable from factor IX hemophilia (hemophilia B); only specific assays can distinguish the two. In contrast to von Willebrand's disease, the hemophiliac will have normal levels of factor VIII:A (factor VIII antigen). Variable degrees of severity exist depending on levels of factor VIII:C. The disease is classified as severe if levels are <1%; moderate if 1–5%; mild if >5%. Female carriers will have normal levels of factor VIII antigen.

▶ Clinical Therapeutics

The mainstay of therapy includes infusion of factor VIII concentrates, which are now heat treated to decrease possible HIV transmission. More severe bleeding requires more concentrate. The half-life of factor VIII:C is approximately 12 hours, which is important in determining amount of plasma to transfuse, especially during and after major surgery. If bleeding persists, EACA (epsilon-aminocaproic acid; Amicar) 4 gm orally every 4 hours for several days may help.

▶ Clinical Intervention

Intracranial hemorrhage is the most severe complication and the second most frequent cause of death in those with hemophilia. Aspirin should always be avoided. For mild hemophilia, DDAVP (esmopressin acetate) 0.3 µg/kg every 24 hours may be useful to prevent excessive bleeding during and after minor surgical procedures. DDAVP causes release of factor VIII:C and increases the level two to three times for several hours.

▶ Health Maintenance Issues

Major problem is disability due to recurrent hemarthroses. Another problem is the development of inhibitors (antibodies) to factor VIII in approximately 15% of patients. These patients cannot be supported by factor VIII concentrates. Overall prognosis is improving with increased availability of factor VIII concentrates.

## 2. Acquired Factor VIII Antibodies

▶ Scientific Concepts

Antibodies to factor VIII may develop postpartum or idiopathically and may produce a severe bleeding disorder.

▶ History & Physical

Spontaneous bruising or excessive bleeding with no prior history or family history of bleeding diatheses.

▶ Diagnostic Studies

Prolonged PTT, normal PT, platelets, and fibrinogen. Specific assays must be done to definitively diagnose.

▶ Clinical Therapeutics

Conservative hemostatic measures should be used to combat a hemorrhage. These include immobilization, compression, and EACA. Desmopressin may be given immediately. Transfusions of porcine-derived factor VIII concentrates may be necessary. Aspirin and nonsteroidal anti-inflammatory drugs (NSAIDs) should be avoided.

► Clinical Intervention

Immunosuppression of the antibody production may be effective with IV gamma-globulin initially, to be followed by administration of prednisone with or without cyclophosphamide. Other immunosuppressants that may be necessary include azathioprine, cyclosporin, or interferon-alpha.

► Health Maintenance Issues

Should be suspected in any acquired severe bleeding disorder with prolonged PTT.

## B. Factor IX Disorders

### 1. Hemophilia B

► Scientific Concepts

Factor IX is an intrinsic pathway coagulation factor synthesized in the liver and requiring vitamin K for biologic activity. Hereditary deficiency of this factor is hemophilia B, or Christmas disease, a sex-linked recessive disorder occurring in approximately 1 in 100,000 male births. Most often due to quantitative reduction in factor IX, but in up to one third of patients the defect is functional. Clinically, it is indistinguishable from factor VIII deficiency, but requires different treatment.

► History & Physical

Spontaneous hemarthroses, epistaxis, GI bleeding, intracranial hemorrhage, and excessive bleeding after trauma or surgery are characteristic. Hematuria and muscle hematomas are also relatively common.

► Diagnostic Studies

Prolonged PTT; normal PT and platelet count. Factor IX levels are decreased; factor VIII levels are normal.

► Diagnosis

Must be distinguished from hemophilia A and von Willebrand's disease by performing specific factor assays. Deficiency should be distinguished from an inhibitor.

► Clinical Therapeutics

Factor VIII concentrates are ineffective; rather these patients are treated and managed with factor IX concentrates or fresh frozen plasma. Infusion of recombinant or purified factor IX preparations should be given immediately after trauma to the head or face to prevent intracranial hemorrhage. In general, therapy is directed at rapid and effective infusion of the defective or deficient factor.

► Clinical Intervention

Aspirin should be avoided. DDAVP is not effective in this patient population. Half-life of factor IX is approximately 18 hours, so may prevent spontaneous hemarthroses if given approximately 3 times a week.

► Health Maintenance Issues

Families of individuals affected by hemophilia should maintain an ongoing relationship with a comprehensive hemophilia center.

## C. Factor XI Disorders

▶ Scientific Concepts

Factor XI is activated to XIa by XIIa in conjunction with kallikrein and kininogen. Rosenthal's disease is a deficiency of factor IX, occurring most often in Ashkanazi Jews. It is inherited as an autosomal XI recessive trait, therefore affecting males and females equally.

▶ History & Physical

Affected patients may have minor or major deficiency, with variations in presentation dependent on classification. Patients often present with posttraumatic bleeding or bleeding in the perioperative period. In contrast to those with hemophilia, spontaneous bleeding and hemarthroses are rare.

▶ Diagnostic Studies

Prolonged PTT; normal PT, platelets, and thrombin time. A factor XI assay is necessary to confirm the diagnosis. Other factor deficiencies must be excluded.

▶ Diagnosis

Factor XI deficiency should be suspected in any patient with a prolonged PTT or any family history or personal history of excessive bleeding. Acquired factor XI deficiency may occur.

▶ Clinical Therapeutics

Minor soft-tissue bleeding may not require treatment. If therapy is required, fresh frozen plasma or cryoprecipitate may be used. Plasma exchange may be necessary for refractory bleeding. Occasionally women who are deficient in factor XI have menorrhagia.

▶ Clinical Intervention

Aspirin should be avoided. Minor and major surgery has been safely accomplished with the adjunct utilization of antifibrinolytics, such as EACA or tranexamic acid. Plasma exchange may be necessary if bleeding persists or prior to major surgery.

## D. Thrombocytopenias

### 1. Idiopathic Thrombocytopenic Purpura

▶ Scientific Concepts

This is an acquired disease of isolated thrombocytopenia with no specific identifiable cause. The disorder is a result of immune complexes binding to platelets resulting in severe thrombocytopenia. Idiopathic thrombocytopenic purpura (ITP) typically is acute in onset. In children, it is often associated with viral infection. Other associated disorders include lupus, hematologic malignancies, and other infections.

▶ History & Physical

Symptoms and signs of bleeding predominate the clinical presentation including the presence of easy bruising, epistaxis, and frank bleeding. At times, the diagnosis may be made incidentally in an asymptomatic patient.

▶ Diagnostic Studies

CBC, peripheral smear, and coagulation studies should be obtained to establish the presence of thrombocytopenia and differentiate from other conditions, such as pancytopenia and disseminated intravascular coagulopathy. Bone marrow studies are at times indicated, such as in the elderly patient to rule out myelodysplastic syndrome.

▶ Diagnosis

Severe thrombocytopenia is the hallmark finding with the peripheral smear revealing large platelets. The differential diagnoses include aplastic anemia, systemic lupus erythematosus (SLE), and acute leukemias.

▶ Clinical Therapeutics

Although spontaneous remission often occurs, treatment is typically necessary and depends on the severity of the thrombocytopenia. Corticosteroids are the standard therapy, although other immunosuppressive drugs such as cyclophosphamide and danazol are sometimes used. IV gamma-globulin therapy is only transiently effective.

▶ Clinical Intervention

Splenectomy sometimes is required when medical management fails or when patients cannot be tapered off of steroids. Plasmapheresis, to reduce the circulating antibodies, may be required when other therapeutics fail.

## 2. Thrombotic Thrombocytopenic Purpura

▶ Scientific Concepts

Thrombotic thrombocytopenic purpura (TTP) is a microangiopathic, hemolytic anemia secondary to platelet aggregates or platelet fibrin thrombi in small blood vessels, intravascular aggregation, and endothelial injury. It is serious, progressive, and rapidly fatal unless intervention is taken. The etiology is unknown, with proposed mechanisms including inappropriate immune response, decrease prostaglandin formation, and stimulation by oral contraceptives. It may be initiated by endothelial injury, releasing procoagulant material into the circulation. The peak incidence is the third decade of life, with women affected more often than men.

▶ History & Physical

Fever, signs of hemorrhage including pallor and petechiae, neurologic signs due to vascular occlusions in brain (e.g., headache, delirium, altered state of consciousness, seizures), and renal dysfunction. However, neurologic symptoms are often remittent.

▶ Diagnostic Studies

CBC, peripheral smear, serum and urine chemistries, urinalysis, and coagulation profile should be obtained.

▶ Diagnosis

The CBC typically reveals a Hb that is <10 g/dL with significant thrombocytopenia and polymorphonuclear leukocytosis. The peripheral smear may reveal diffuse reticulocytosis, schistocytes (characteristic), and marked anisocytosis. An elevated bilirubin and LDH is seen, as in other types of hemolysis. Renal impairment can be found with an increased serum creatinine and blood urea nitrogen (BUN) secondary to decreased glomerular filtration rate.

Urine studies will reveal hemosiderinuria, hemoglobinuria, casts, and increased erythrocytes and leukocytes.

The differential diagnosis includes DIC. In contrast to DIC, there is typically normal fibrinogen, PT, and PTT, while the fibrin split products (FSP) may be slightly increased.

▶ **Clinical Therapeutics**

Plasmapheresis, whole-blood exchange transfusion, and plasma infusion are the primary therapies for this disorder. Platelet transfusions should be avoided as they will cause deterioration of the clinical condition. The LDH levels and platelet counts are used to monitor the response to therapy.

▶ **Clinical Intervention**

If the disease remains chronic, maintenance plasmapheresis or corticosteroids may be required.

### 3. Hemolytic Uremic Syndrome

▶ **Scientific Concepts**

Hemolytic uremia syndrome (HUS) results in acute intravascular hemolysis and renal failure with a variable amount of platelet destruction and thrombus formation (primarily affecting kidneys). Causes include mild febrile illnesses, certain immunizations, and GI disturbances. Those most frequently affected are infants and children (most < 8 years old), renal transplant patients, pregnant women, and particularly postpartum women.

▶ **History & Physical**

Vomiting and diarrhea usually precede anemia and renal failure. Signs include elevated blood pressure, pallor, fever, abdominal pain, bleeding from mucous membranes, and dark-colored urine. Progression to oliguria or anuria may result. Although hepatomegaly is typically present, splenomegaly is not. Neurological symptoms may be present but less frequently and severely than in TTP.

▶ **Diagnostic Studies**

CBC, peripheral smear, coagulation profile, chemistries, and urinalysis are indicated.

▶ **Diagnosis**

Severe anemia (Hb may be as low as 4 g/dL) in the presence of leukocytosis with predominance of neutrophils and severe thrombocytopenia indicates the possibility of HUS. Schistocytes and burr cells may be seen on the peripheral smear. Coagulation tests should be obtained to differentiate other causes of hemolysis, as they are usually normal in HUS. A decreased haptoglobin, increased bilirubin, hemoglobinuria and hemosiderinuria, extreme elevations in BUN and creatinine all point to this diagnosis. Urinalysis typically reveals proteinuria, increased erythrocytes and leukocytes, and casts.

▶ **Clinical Therapeutics**

Conservative management of fluids and electrolytes, monitoring of blood gases and blood pressure as indicated. Hemodialysis may be required for significant renal impairment. Mortality rates are less than with TTP. Long-term sequelae include chronic renal impairment.

## 4. Von Willebrand's disease

▶ **Scientific Concepts**

Von Willebrand's disease is an autosomal dominant trait with significant variability in the degree of clinical bleeding. It is the most common inherited bleeding disorder, occurring in 1 in every 800–1,000 individuals. There are three major types, with severity variable depending on penetrance and expression of the affected gene. Von Willebrand's factor (vWF) is a cofactor essential for platelet adhesion and is produced by endothelial cells. VWF has two functions: to facilitate platelet adhesion, and to act as a plasma carrier for factor VIII. The defect may be quantitative or functional. Normal plasma level is 10 mg/L.

▶ **History & Physical**

If mild, bleeding may occur only after surgery or trauma. If more severe disease, spontaneous epistaxis or oral mucosal, GI, or genitourinary bleeding may occur. Hemarthroses are not seen.

▶ **Diagnostic Studies**

Variable. The most diagnostic pattern is that of increased bleeding time, often prolonged PTT, normal PT, thrombin time, platelet count. Decreased vWF concentration in plasma, and often decreased factor VIII activity.

▶ **Diagnosis**

Requires high index of suspicion. All other drugs must be discontinued to accurately diagnose. Complete evaluation requires measurements of factor VIII:C activity, von Willebrand Factor antigen (vWF:Ag), von Willebrand factor activity (risocetin cofactor activity), and vWF multimer size. Acquired forms of von Willebrand's disease may develop in association with other autoimmune disorders and B cell lymphomas. Many (30%) have been associated with monoclonal gammopathy of unknown significance (MGUS).

▶ **Clinical Therapeutics**

Cryoprecipitate and factor VIII concentrates are used to correct moderate bleeding. DDAVP (desmopressin) increases the level of vWF in plasma in both normal individuals and in those with mild vWD, and should be given only to those with mild disease. Tachyphylaxis may occur if duration of therapy exceeds 48 hours in duration in some patients.

▶ **Clinical Intervention**

EACA may be useful to prevent bleeding from minor surgery and tooth extractions. Premarin may be useful to increase production of vWF by endothelial cells. IV gamma-globulin may provide a therapeutic effect on the bleeding in patients with acquired von Willebrand's disease.

# E. Disseminated Intravascular Coagulopathy (DIC)

▶ **Scientific Concepts**

This disorder results from the pathological activation of the clotting cascade with the generation of excess thrombin resulting in concomitant systemic thrombosis and hemorrhage. Precipitators include infection, with the most common microbes being gram-negative organisms (e.g., *Neisseria meningitidis*), intravascular hemolysis, obstetric accidents, burns, malignancies, crush injuries, and closed head injuries.

▶ **History & Physical**

Signs and symptom of abnormal bleeding and clotting may be present. These can include gross bleeding (e.g., bleeding surgical wounds, hematemesis, hemoptysis, hematuria), hematomas, petechiae, and purpura. Thrombosis may manifest with myocardial infarction, CVA, peripheral thrombosis, renal failure, and multisystem organ dysfunction.

▶ **Diagnostic Studies**

CBC, PT, PTT, and the DIC profile (FSP, d-dimer, fibrinogen) should be obtained immediately in patients suspected of having DIC.

▶ **Diagnosis**

The diagnosis is established in patients with a known precipitator and evidence of DIC on labs including elevated FSP and d-dimer. Fibrinogen may be elevated early in disease as acute-phase reactant but later becomes consumed. Thrombocytopenia may be present but not always in early stages of the disease.

▶ **Clinical Therapeutics**

No specific treatment is available for DIC. Blood products should be used as needed. Heparin has been used to treat complications from abnormal clotting, but this remains controversial in a disease that can also result in life-threatening bleeding.

▶ **Clinical Intervention**

Therapies should be directed at the underlying precipitating cause until the disease resolves. If the cause is unknown, empiric therapy for an infectious etiology should be initiated with broad-spectrum antibiotics. Treatment of the precipitator is the most important factor in outcome.

▶ **Health Maintenance Issues**

Early detection and treatment of precipitators may prevent or minimize DIC.

## III. MALIGNANT NEOPLASMS

### A. Acute Leukemias

▶ **Scientific Concepts**

The leukemias are a group of disorders characterized by the accumulation of abnormal white cells in the bone marrow. These defective cells may cause bone marrow failure, increased WBC, and ultimately infiltration of organs. Leukemias together comprise 2% of all adult cancers. Leukemias are divided into acute and chronic types, and are even further subclassified within these groups. It is essential to accurately diagnose leukemia, because treatment regimens are different and are highly successful in some types. In acute leukemias, the defective cells are unable to differentiate due to a maturation arrest. Rapid proliferation results in over 30% replacement of the normal hematopoietic precursors by the leukemic cells, which are also frequently found in the circulating blood. By definition, acute leukemia is diagnosed when the bone marrow has more than 30% blasts (< 5% is normal); further classification to acute myelocytic leukemia (AML) or acute lymphocytic leukemia (ALL) depends on morphology and which white cell line is most affected. AML is classified further into several subgroups depending on morphology, cytochemistry, immunophenotyping, and cytogenetics. The etiology of this malignant transformation is not known, but viral causes have been postulated. Also, alkylating agents, ionizing radiation, and benzene exposure have all been implicated as causative factors of leukemia, especially of AML and chronic myelocytic leukemia (CML).

## 1. Acute Myelocytic Leukemia (AML)

### ► Scientific Concepts

Acute myelogenous or myelocytic leukemia is a rare malignancy resulting from undifferentiated proliferation of granulocyte precursors, usually the myeloblast, in the bone marrow. This abnormality may disrupt normal production of other cell lines, such as platelets and erythrocytes. AML may be a primary malignancy, or may result as a consequence of prior chemotherapy or radiation exposure. Myelodysplastic syndromes often evolve to AML when the bone marrow blasts reach 30% of the bone marrow. In fact, 25% of adults diagnosed with AML have a history of myelodysplastic syndrome.

### ► History & Physical

Presenting complaints arise from failure of bone marrow to produce red cells, white cells, and platelets. Some patients may actually be asymptomatic, but most have complaints of fatigue, bleeding, persistent infections (including fungal and opportunistic infections), or fevers. Bleeding can be overt hemorrhage or minimal (bruising, petechiae, gingival, epistaxis). On exam, the patient may have pallor, fever, tachycardia, ecchymosis, petechiae, skin lesions (leukemia cutis), lymphadenopathy. Occasionally, splenomegaly is present; rarely one may have hepatomegaly.

### ► Diagnostic Studies

Anemia and thrombocytopenia may be profound; WBC may be elevated (> 100,000) or low, often extremely low. Usually, blasts are present in the periphery, with other immature forms sometimes present. Auer rods (cytoplasmic inclusion bodies) may be found in the blasts. The diagnosis is made by a bone marrow aspirate and biopsy; AML has > 30% blasts that are myeloperoxidase positive or esterase positive and terminal deoxynucleotidyl transferase (TdT) negative. Myeloid markers are positive on flow cytometry, and chromosomal abnormalities are often present on cytogenetic analysis.

### ► Clinical Therapeutics

The only treatment for AML is intensive induction combination chemotherapy, regardless of age or initial performance status. The other manifestations of bone marrow infiltration by leukemia (neutropenia, anemia, thrombocytopenia) will not improve unless the disease is treated. Success rates have improved due to a significant improvement in supportive care during chemotherapy. Patients are at risk of dying from complications of anemia, neutropenia, thrombocytopenia (heart failure, infections, bleeding), and occasionally organ infiltration. It is most important to diagnose acute promyelocytic leukemia (APL or M3) because great success can be achieved by early and proper treatment with idarubicin and a retinoid, all-*trans* retinoic acid (ATRA). Bone marrow or stem cell transplant should be considered in refractory, resistant, or relapsed cases.

▶ Clinical Intervention

A newly diagnosed AML patient with a WBC > 75,000 is at significant risk of leukostasis with pulmonary infiltration of the blasts, causing respiratory distress and possibly death. This is considered a medical emergency and leukapheresis should be started immediately prior to induction chemotherapy, which should also be initiated as soon as possible. Other emergencies include tumor lysis syndrome, which can occur when the WBC is high and during induction chemotherapy when the cells are killed. Hyperuricemia, renal failure, hyperkalemia, hypocalcemia, hyperphosphatemia, acidosis, and other metabolic disturbances may occur, leading to multiorgan failure. This syndrome can be prevented with aggressive hydration, alkalinization, and close observation. DIC is another emergency that can be caused by chemotherapy or the disease itself, especially in APL patients. Close observation and supportive care can prevent further complications, and ATRA has prevented this situation by pushing the progranulocytes into maturation prior to chemotherapy. Neutropenic fever in leukemia patients can be fatal, and close surveillance during and after chemotherapy administration is imperative to prevent adverse events. Broad-spectrum IV antibiotics should be started in any leukemia patient who is neutropenic and febrile, whether a source of infection is evident or not. Long-term follow-up is necessary, as late relapses have occurred; however, relapse is less likely after 2 years of remission.

## 2. Acute Lymphocytic Leukemia (ALL)

▶ Scientific Concepts

Eighty percent of all childhood leukemias are acute lymphocytic, and 25% of all adult acute leukemias are ALL. The physiology is similar to AML, but the defective cell is the lymphoblast rather than the myeloblast.

▶ History & Physical

Common complaints at presentation include fatigue, bleeding, fevers, lymphadenopathy, bruising, cough, and shortness of breath if a mediastinal mass (lymphoblastic T cell) is present. Findings may include pallor, bruising, petechiae, tachycardia, fever, lymphadenopathy, splenomegaly, hepatomegaly. Patients may present with central nervous system (CNS) disease with headaches, neck pain/stiffness, and other signs of increased intracranial pressure. Rarely a testicular mass is present.

▶ Diagnostic Studies

Usually the WBC is significantly elevated, often > 200,000, with a large percentage of blasts that stain TdT positive. Anemia and thrombocytopenia may be minimal or profound; LDH is often elevated. Bone marrow aspiration shows > 30% blasts that are TdT positive, myeloperoxidase negative, lymphoid markers are positive (CALLA, or CD10, and CD19) and may be T cell or B cell. Bone marrow biopsy is hypercellular, and cytogenetic abnormalities may be present. A chest radiograph may show a mediastinal mass (if T cell disease). A lumbar puncture should be done initially to rule out CNS disease. There are three subclassifications of ALL (L1, L2, L3); however, they are all treated the same in adults.

▶ **Clinical Therapeutics**

Induction chemotherapy should be started as soon as possible with combination chemotherapy, and supportive care should be similar to that of AML patients, avoiding complications of anemia, thrombocytopenia, and neutropenia that occur with treatment. Intrathecal chemotherapy has reduced the CNS relapse rate from >90% down to <5%.

▶ **Clinical Intervention**

Follow-up is important as late relapses have been seen. Bone marrow transplant (BMT) or stem cell transplant should be considered in patients with Philadelphia chromosome–positive disease, as this is a very poor prognostic indicator.

## B. Chronic Leukemias

### 1. Chronic Myelogenous Leukemia (CML)

▶ **Scientific Concepts**

Abnormal clonal proliferation of early progenitor stem cells resulting in an excess of cells of myeloid, erythroid, and megakaryocytic lineage. There are three phases (chronic, accelerated, blastic), and, in later phases, maturation arrest is a prominent feature. Associated with the tumor marker Philadelphia chromosome in 85–90% of cases, thus can be followed to monitor treatment success. The Philadelphia chromosome is a reciprocal translocation of genetic material between chromosomes 9 and 22 [t(9;22)]. Etiology is unknown, but increased incidence in atomic bomb survivors and those who received radiation as treatment for ankylosing spondylitis. CML is usually diagnosed in chronic phase, which is characterized by a high WBC and splenomegaly; usually well controlled with oral chemotherapy, alpha-interferon, or the signal transduction inhibitor imatinib mesylate (Gleevec). Currently, median survival, untreated, is 3.5 years but is expected to increase since the development and widespread use of imatinib mesylate. Accelerated-phase disease is less well defined and more difficult to control; median untreated survival is 6–12 months. Blast crisis is similar to an acute leukemia and is treated similarly; median untreated survival averages 3 to 6 months.

▶ **History & Physical**

Often, CML is diagnosed on a routine CBC. Some patients have complaints of fatigue, early satiety or left-sided abdominal pain (from splenomegaly), shortness of breath, or B symptoms (fever, drenching night sweats, fatigue, weight loss). Usually, the physical exam is normal other than splenomegaly and maybe some minor lymphadenopathy. Hepatomegaly may be present in some cases. In accelerated or blast phase, fever, weight loss, early satiety, and symptoms of worsening anemia and thrombocytopenia, or more commonly thrombocytosis, may be present.

▶ **Diagnostic Studies**

WBC is elevated, platelets are often elevated, anemia may be mild or absent. LDH is often elevated, and leukocyte alkaline phosphatase is low.

Hyperuricemia may be present due to the increased white cell mass. Bone marrow is hypercellular and has < 5% blasts in chronic phase. Chronic phase may also be defined as one where the granulocyte and platelet counts can be kept under control in an asymptomatic patient. Increased bone marrow blasts (> 30%) identify blast phase. Accelerated phase may contain blasts anywhere from 5 to 29% and may have increased numbers of basophils and megakaryocytes. The Philadelphia chromosome is present on cytogenetic analysis in ~ 90% of patients at diagnosis.

▶ Clinical Therapeutics

Control of WBC and decrease in splenomegaly can be obtained by using hydroxyurea, an oral chemotherapy; however, this treatment does not suppress the Philadelphia chromosome or prevent progression of the disease. Alpha-interferon has been used with success, often eliminates the disease and the Philadelphia chromosome, and prevents progression to more aggressive phases. The newest oral treatment imatinib mesylate shows incredible promise in those refractory or intolerant to interferon. To date, less success has been found in treating accelerated or blastic disease; however, some chemotherapeutic regimens are promising. A lymphoid blastic transformation can be treated as ALL, with the disease often returning to a second chronic phase.

▶ Clinical Intervention

Tumor lysis syndrome can occur on rare occasions but is easily prevented with the use of allopurinol and aggressive hydration. Interferon is poorly tolerated in some patients, especially those > age 60, so doses must be adjusted accordingly or other therapeutic regimens must be implemented. Some side effects of interferon are flulike symptoms that rarely last more than the initial 3 weeks of therapy, depression, disturbance in sleep cycle, fatigue, and, after longer periods of use, autoimmune complications. Follow-up is important; cytogenetics should be repeated during treatment and followed for presence of the Philadelphia chromosome.

## 2. Chronic Lymphocytic Leukemia (CLL)

▶ Scientific Concepts

Most common leukemia, usually in older age groups. Characterized by clonal proliferation and accumulation of mature-appearing lymphocytes of B lineage in blood and lymphoid tissues. Etiology is unknown, with no evidence of radiation or chemicals as causative agents.

▶ History & Physical

Twenty-five percent are asymptomatic at diagnosis; other complaints include B symptoms (fatigue, drenching night sweats, weight loss), frequent and/or persistent infections, lymphadenopathy. Less commonly, skin infections are present at diagnosis, and may include shingles.

▶ Diagnostic Studies

Clinical characteristics should be combined with lab results to determine Rai stage at diagnosis Table 14–1. Minimal criteria for diagnosis of chronic lymphocytic leukemia (CLL) are blood lymphocytes > $10 \times 10^9$/L and bone marrow lymphocytes >30%. If anemia and/or thrombocytopenia are present, the Rai stage is higher and more aggressive disease is present. Beta-2-microglobulin should be measured, and prognosis is better if

► table 14-1

**RAI STAGING SYSTEM**

| Stage | Clinical/Lab Features | Mean Survival (Months) |
|---|---|---|
| 0 | Lymphocytosis | >120 |
| 1 | Lymphadenopathy | 95 |
| 2 | Hepato/splenomegaly | 72 |
| 3 | Anemia (Hb < 11 g/dL) | 30 |
| 4 | Thrombocytopenia | 30 |
| Transformed | Richter's transformation (large cell lymphoma) | 6 |

it is <2.5. Immunophenotyping should be done on both the blood and marrow to determine B- or T-cell lineage. Cytogenetics are often normal, but the most common abnormalities involve chromosome 12. The pattern of infiltration on bone marrow biopsy is yet another prognostic indicator: nodular signifies a lower tumor burden and less aggressive disease than diffuse infiltration.

► Clinical Therapeutics

Usually, observation is recommended with early disease and/or favorable prognostic indicators. Rai stages 0, 1, and 2 are usually observed until signs of disease progression or bulky lymphadenopathy or symptoms of hepatosplenomegaly occur. Chemotherapy (fludarabine with or without cyclophosphamide) is recommended for more aggressive disease. Other agents such as cyclosporine A and monoclonal antibodies such as Rituxan and Campath are being investigated and have shown promising results.

► Clinical Intervention

Herpes zoster infections are more frequent in patients with CLL, so prophylaxis should be considered. CLL patients, for unknown reasons, have a higher incidence than the general population of additional malignancies and therefore should be followed closely, regardless of their CLL status.

### 3. Hairy Cell Leukemia

► Scientific Concepts

Prior to 1980, this was a universally fatal disease; now it is curable in most patients. B cell clonal malignancy; cells have characteristic cytoplasmic projections, thus looking "hairy." Patients present with anemia, neutropenia (rarely an elevated WBC), thrombocytopenia, and usually splenomegaly. They usually have an increased incidence of infections that persist longer than in their healthy cohorts.

► Diagnostic Studies

Neutropenia, anemia, thrombocytopenia. Bone marrow with hairy cells present, staining positive on tartrate-resistant acid phosphatase (TRAP) stain. Often a dry tap on bone marrow, thus making diagnosis more difficult.

► Clinical Therapeutics

Treatment formerly was interferon, now preferred treatment is one course of chemotherapy with a single agent, chlorodeoxyadenosine

(2-CdA) with excellent results. Pancytopenia should be supported with prophylactic antibiotics/antivirals/antifungals. Transfusion support may be necessary on rare occasions. In refractory cases or multiple relapsed cases, monoclonal antibody administration may prove to be beneficial.

## C. Lymphomas

### 1. Hodgkin's Disease

#### ▶ Scientific Concepts

Etiology of Hodgkin's disease (HD) is unknown, and the cell of origin is not yet completely defined. Current evidence shows that it evolves from the monocyte–macrophage cell line. Histologically, the cause of Hodgkin's disease was thought to be infectious, but that remains unproven. Epstein-Barr virus (EBV) may be important in the disease. Hodgkin's comprises 14% of all malignant lymphomas and has a bimodal age distribution, with the first peak in the 20s and the second in the 60s. Histologically, HD is unique in that a small proportion of cells are malignant; most are reactive cells. Sternberg-Reed cells (large polylobulated cells with large nucleoli) are the diagnostic malignant cells found in the background of reactive cells. There are four histologic subtypes; nodular sclerosing and mixed cellularity types make up 90%.

#### ▶ History & Physical

The most common complaint is that of painless lymphadenopathy in young adults, with or without B symptoms, malaise, or pruritus. Usually, the enlarged lymph node is supradiaphragmatic (90%) and is frequently (60–80%) in the cervical region. Mediastinal lymphadenopathy may manifest clinically with cough, wheezing, dyspnea, superior vena cava syndrome, and rarely pleural effusions. Affected lymph nodes are firm, mobile, rubbery. Tender nodes usually signify infectious or inflammatory processes. Splenomegaly may be present.

#### ▶ Diagnostic Studies

No specific laboratory findings. On CBC, may find mild neutrophilic leukocytosis, slightly increased platelets, and mild normochromic, normocytic anemia. Liver function tests may be slightly abnormal, and hyperuricemia may be present if there is bulky disease. Serum copper level is often elevated, and the patient is often anergic. Chest radiograph should be done, as well as computed tomographic (CT) scans of neck, chest, abdomen, pelvis. The largest and most central node should be biopsied with the capsule intact and Sternberg-Reed cells must be present in the proper reactive background for the diagnosis to be made.

#### ▶ Clinical Therapeutics

As Table 14–2 illustrates, staging is important for treatment.

### ▶ table 14-2

| Stage | Clinical Findings | Therapy |
|---|---|---|
| I, II | Local disease | Radiation alone |
| III | Nodal disease both above and below diaphragm | Radiation ± combination chemotherapy |
| IV | Extranodal disease | Combination chemotherapy |

HD has become a model of a curable neoplasm—almost 70% are long-term survivors.

▶ **Clinical Intervention**

Complications of radiotherapy include hypothyroidism, pericarditis, pneumonitis, sterility. Complications of chemotherapy are those associated with myelosuppression (bleeding, infections, anemia, vomiting, alopecia, paresthesias). Long-term complications include a 17% increased risk of secondary cancers and a 5–7% increased risk of acute leukemia.

## 2. Non-Hodgkin's Lymphomas

▶ **Scientific Concepts**

Lymphomas are the fifth most common cancer in the United States. Lymphomas are malignant tumors arising from lymphoreticular system and may occur at any site in the body. They are a group of heterogeneous tumors that vary greatly in response to treatment. There is progressive increase in incidence with age, but mortality rates are decreasing. Etiology unknown, but several causative relations: increased incidence in immunosuppressed patients and in those with hyperfunctioning immune systems (10% of patients with Sjögren's syndrome develop non-Hodgkin's lymphoma). Some seem to be caused by viruses (EBV, human T-lymphotropic virus-I [HTLV-I]). *Helicobacter pylori* has been implicated in mucosa-associated lymphoid tissue (MALT) lymphomas, but this association is not yet proven. Pathology is very important in classification and treatment. Histological subtypes are determined on the basis of architectural pattern, cellular atypia, and cell type. Progression often disseminates early and widely by hematogenous routes rather than by contiguous nodal extension.

▶ **History & Physical**

Most common reason for seeking medical attention is unexplained and/or persistent lymphadenopathy. Most patients are asymptomatic, but 20% have constitutional symptoms and waxing/waning lymphadenopathy months prior to diagnosis. Other complaints may be abdominal pain, vomiting, bleeding. Weight loss is common. Most common extranodal site at presentation is GI tract.

▶ **Diagnostic Studies**

No lab findings are specific for non-Hodgkin's lymphoma. At presentation, CBC is usually normal, but anemia, leukopenia, thrombopenia may occur. Occasionally, lymphoma cells are found in peripheral blood. Bulky disease may cause jaundice, azotemia, bowel obstruction. Studies necessary for staging include biopsy of lymph node, chest radiograph, CT scans of neck, chest, abdomen, pelvis; bilateral bone marrow biopsies; CBC, comprehensive metabolic panel, beta-2-microglobulin, HIV, HTLV serology.

▶ **Clinical Therapeutics**

Treatment is dependent on specific type of non-Hodgkin's lymphoma and usually involves combination chemotherapy with or without radiation therapy. In addition, monoclonal antibodies that specifically target the malignant cell line are currently being used with promising results. The currently available monoclonal antibodies include Rituxan and Campath.

## D. Multiple Myeloma

### ► Scientific Concepts

Multiple myeloma is a clonal malignancy of terminally differentiated B-lymphocytes, or plasma cells. It comprises approximately 1% of all malignancies, incidence increases with age, and it is currently incurable probably due to its innate resistance to chemotherapy. Myeloma often leads to organ dysfunction, susceptibility to infection, clotting abnormalities, neurological symptoms, and manifestations of hyperviscosity. Etiology is unknown, but there is an increased frequency in those exposed to radiation of nuclear warheads. Chemical exposure may increase the risk for myeloma. Increased frequency also exists in those who work with pesticides, paper, and leather tanners, and those with chronic immune stimulation.

### ► History & Physical

Most common symptom is bone pain, usually in the back/rib area, often precipitated by movement. Therefore, a careful physical exam should be done to search for tender bones and/or masses (plasmacytomas). Compression fractures may occur due to lytic bony lesions. Spinal cord compression is sometimes seen and requires emergent care. Recurrent infections signify a defect in immunity and may be the presenting complaint in one with myeloma. Most common infections are pneumonias and pyelonephritis. Signs and symptoms of anemia may be the presenting problems, and are present in approximately 80% at diagnosis. Symptoms of hypercalcemia may occur due to lysis of bone secondary to disease infiltration. These complaints may include lethargy, constipation, headache, fatigue, visual disturbances, even retinopathy. Renal failure or insufficiency occurs in 25%, with hypercalcemia the most common cause. Clotting abnormalities may occur.

### ► Diagnostic Studies

A complete skeletal survey should be done if myeloma is suspected. Plain films show lytic lesions, if present, better than any other diagnostic study. A CBC should be done and may show normocytic, normochromic anemia with rouleaux formation. Hypercalcemia may be present. Erythrocyte sedimentation rate (ESR) will be elevated. Serum and urine electrophoresis with immunofixation should be done and will show a monoclonal spike in 85%. A 24-hour urine will detect the presence of Bence–Jones proteins. Hypogammaglobulinemia may be present due to decreased production and increased destruction of normal antibodies. To date, lab tests most predictive of prognosis are beta-2-microglobulin and C-reactive protein, although they are not diagnostic of myeloma. A bone marrow aspirate and biopsy should be done for initial diagnosis and will show increased plasma cells and often an abnormal chromosome 13.

### ► Diagnosis

Multiple myeloma should be distinguished from MGUS and benign monoclonal gammopathies. The "classic triad" of plasmacytosis, lytic bone lesions, serum and/or urine M component, if present, is strongly suggested of myeloma. Current staging system is complicated and not predictive of outcome.

### ► Clinical Therapeutics

Myeloma, although treatable, is not yet curable. Glucocorticoids, alkylating agents, and local radiation therapy are the mainstays of therapy.

Melphalan and prednisone is a common combination; however, the use of melphalan can increase chances of developing myelodysplastic syndrome and/or acute myelogenous leukemia. Another is vincristine, coxorubicin, and dexamethasone in combination. Thalidomide appears to be an effective salvage therapy. Autologous stem cell transplants have shown superior disease-free and overall survival when compared to the above conventional therapy, with the median overall survival to date greater than 7 years.

► **Clinical Interventions**

Exogenous erythropoietin is often helpful for anemia related to the disease or therapy. Pamidronate (90 mg IV over 1–2 hours every 4 weeks) or Zoledronate (more potent and shorter infusion time) or other bisphosphonates are helpful for hypercalcemia. They also improve the quality of life by preventing lytic bone lesions. Palliative radiation therapy to painful bone lesions may also improve quality of life. Radiation therapy to any lesions contributing to cord compression should be done emergently in combination with dexamethasone.

## E. Others

### 1. Polycythemia Vera

► **Scientific Concepts**

Polycythemia vera is one of the myeloproliferative disorders characterized by erythrocytosis (hemoglobin > 17.5 g/dL in men, > 15.5 g/dL in women). It is a clonal disease, and leukocytosis, basophilia, and trilineage hyperplasia of bone marrow with clustering of megakaryocytes occurs. The endogenous myeloproliferation of increased red cells decreases the body's erythropoietin levels. Incidence is highest in those 60–70 years of age, with an equal male:female ratio.

► **History & Physical**

Clinically, patients may complain of problems related to hyperviscosity and hypervolemia, such as dyspnea, headaches, blurred vision; night sweats may result from the hypermetabolic state. Pruritus may also be present, probably due to increased levels of histamine or mast cells, and may worsen after a hot bath/shower. On examination, hypertension is found in 30%, splenomegaly in 60%, and the patient may appear plethoric. Peptic ulcers are present in 5–10%. Thrombotic and hemorrhagic complications are common as a result of high blood viscosity.

► **Diagnostic Studies**

Increased Hb, increased hematocrit and red cell count; neutrophils are increased in 50%, some with increased basophils. About half the patients have increased platelets, often three times the normal values. Serum $B_{12}$ and $B_{12}$ binding capacity are increased. Bone marrow is hypercellular with prominent megakaryocytes with or without clonal cytogenetic abnormalities. True red cell volume and erythropoietin levels are necessary for the diagnosis.

► **Diagnosis**

Primary polycythemia vera should be distinguished from secondary polycythemia, which can be due to hypoxia secondary to chronic obstructive pulmonary disease, cyanotic heart disease, renal causes, tumors, and cigarette smoking. Stress polycythemia is more common than polycythemia vera and may be associated with myocardial infarctions or transient ischemic attacks.

▶ **Clinical Therapeutics**

Median survival is 10–16 years; AML evolves in 10 to 15% of patients; 15–30% of cases evolve into myelofibrosis. If untreated, median survival is approximately 1.5 years. Treatment is therapeutic phlebotomy to keep hematocrit <44%; that is the point where thromboembolic events increase precipitously. All patients should be given aspirin and possibly dipyridamole. Older patients should also be treated with bone marrow suppressors such as hydroxyurea or busulfan. Platelet count should be maintained <400,000 to prevent further thrombotic events.

▶ **Clinical Intervention**

Thromboembolic events occur frequently in these patients; it is important to therapeutically phlebotomize and keep them on aspirin and other necessary medications long term.

## 2. Splenic Disorders

▶ **Scientific Concepts**

Splenomegaly occurs in a variety of disease states, including infections (e.g., mononucleosis, malaria, AIDS, viral hepatitis, splenic abscess), immunologic disorders (e.g., rheumatoid arthritis, SLE), congestive heart failure, some anemias (e.g., sickle cell, thalassemia, hemolytic), malignancies (e.g., leukemias, lymphomas, metastatic tumors), and chronic liver disease.

▶ **History & Physical**

Symptoms and signs associated with the underlying disorder.

▶ **Diagnostic Studies**

Evaluation should be guided based on history and physical.

▶ **Clinical Therapeutics**

Treatment of the underlying disorder.

▶ **Clinical Intervention**

Splenectomy may be required when hypersplenism accompanies splenomegaly and may provide important diagnostic information.

## BIBLIOGRAPHY

Beutler E, et al., eds. *Williams Hematology,* 6th ed. New York: McGraw-Hill; 2001.

Braunwald E, Fauci AS, Hauser SL, et al., eds. *Harrison's Principles of Internal Medicine,* 15th ed. New York: McGraw-Hill; 2001.

Hillman RS, Ault KA, eds. *Hematology in Clinical Practice, A Guide to Diagnosis and Management,* 3rd ed. New York: McGraw-Hill; 2002.

Hoffman R, Benz EJ Jr, Shattil SJ, et al., eds. *Hematology Basic Principles and Practice,* 3rd ed. New York: Churchill Livingstone; 2002.

Lotspeich-Steininger CA, Stiene-Martin EA, Koepke JA, Rosenthal DS, Eyre HJ. Hodgkin's disease and non-Hodgkin's lymphomas. pp. 456–469. In Murphy GP, Lawrence W, Lenhardt RE, eds. *American Cancer Society Textbook of Clinical Oncology,* 2nd ed. Atlanta: American Cancer Society; 1995.

Tierney LM Jr, McPhee SJ, Papadakis MA, eds. *Current Medical Diagnosis & Treatment,* 42nd ed. New York: Lange Medical Books/McGraw-Hill; 2003.

# Pediatrics 15

*Sarah A. Toth, MS, PA-C*

## I. EVALUATION OF THE NEWBORN

▶ History & Physical
See Table 15–1.

*General assessment:* TORCHS (toxoplasmosis, rubella, cytomegalovirus, herpes simplex, syphilis) screen if maternal history is positive or congenital infection apparent. Simian crease with trisomy 21 (Down syndrome).

*Skin:* Jaundice progresses from head to feet, occurs in 65% during first week of life; erythema toxicum common and self-limited; milia in 50% of newborns; lanugo is fine hair covering preterm infant's skin. Check for midline capillary hemangiomas (nap of neck, eyelids, forehead, occiput), mongolian spot (benign, bluish-black macule over back and buttocks), other "birthmarks."

*Head:* Check for caput succedaneum (edema that crosses over suture lines, indents with pressure); cephalohematoma (subperiosteal bleed contained within suture lines, fluctuant, may be associated with skull fractures). Limited mobility of sutures with craniosynostosis. Fontanels sunken with dehydration, bulging with increased intracranial pressure (ICP). Transilluminate if concerned about hydrocephalus.

*Eyes:* Pupils constricted for 21 days, then pupillary response; optical blink reflex; subconjunctival hemorrhages commonly due to birth process; red reflex should be visualized. If leukocoria present, can be caused by glaucoma (cloudy cornea), tumor (retinoblastoma), or cataract.

*Ears:* Low-set with Down syndrome, significant auricular anomaly often associated with renal disease; test hearing, especially if prenatal infection suspected.

*Nose/mouth/pharynx:* Check patency of nares (obligate nose breathers); cleft lip/palate; bifid uvula may indicate submucosal defect. Epstein pearls (retention cysts) at junction of hard/soft palate. Remove loose natal teeth to avoid aspiration. Prominent tongue with trisomy 21 and Beckwith–Wiedemann syndrome. High-pitched cry with increased ICP or drug withdrawal; hoarse cry with hypothyroidism or hypocalcemic tetany; absence of cry with vocal cord paralysis, severe illness, or profound mental retardation.

▶ table 15-1

### APGAR CHECKED AT 1 AND 5 MINUTES (BEST SCORE IS 10)

| Sign | 0 | 1 | 2 |
|------|---|---|---|
| Color | Blue, pale | Pink body, blue extremities | Completely pink |
| Heart rate | Absent | <100 | >100 |
| Reflex irritability | No response | Grimace | Sneeze/cough |
| Muscle tone | Flaccid | Some flexion of limbs | Good flexion of limbs |
| Respiratory effort | Absent | Weak/irregular | Good/crying |

*Adapted from: Rudolph C, Rudolph A, eds. Rudolph's Pediatrics, 21st ed. New York: McGraw-Hill; 2003, p. 99.*

***Neck:*** Check for masses: midline (commonly thyroglossal duct cyst or rarely congenital goiter); anterior to sternocleidomastoid (bronchial cleft cyst); within sternocleidomastoid (torticollis); posterior to sternocleidomastoid (cystic hygroma). Turner's syndrome with webbing of neck. Klippel–Feil syndrome with short, poorly mobile neck.

***Chest/lungs/heart:*** Check for fractured clavicle (crepitus, tenderness, asymmetric mass near neck); pectus excavatum or carinatum. Respiratory rate ~40–60 breaths/min; apnea and bradycardia with increased ICP or pulmonary disease; grunting, retractions, or nasal flaring with respiratory distress; plethora with increased hemoglobin; supernumerary nipples; breast discharge for ~ 2 weeks. Heart rate 120–140 beats/min, > 200 beats/min with congestive heart failure (CHF). Most common presentations of heart disease: cyanosis and CHF with abnormal pulses. Diminished pulses in all sites with hypoplastic left heart syndrome and aortic stenosis; diminished lower extremity pulses with coarctation of aorta. Murmurs are common (~ 60%), often benign.

***Abdomen:*** If scaphoid, suspect diaphragmatic hernia; marked distention with gastrointestinal/genitourinary (GI/GU) obstruction; umbilicus with three vessels should be two arteries and one vein, solitary artery may signify renal disease; check for anal agenesis; passage of meconium—if absent, cystic fibrosis or Hirschsprung's disease; more than just the lower poles of the kidneys may be palpable in congenital polycystic kidney disease.

***Genitalia:*** Check for ambiguity, edema common; testes descended in scrotum in 95% at birth; transilluminate hydroceles; hypospadias (ventral urethral orifice)/epispadias (dorsal urethral orifice). Labia majora should cover minora and clitoris; vaginal discharge with or without blood is normal response to maternal estrogen withdrawal; fecal urethral discharge indicates fistula; fingertip space between vagina and anus.

***Musculoskeletal:*** Clavicle fractures most common during delivery; multiple fractures with deformity associated with osteogenesis imperfecta; brachial palsy after delivery especially with shoulder dystocia; hip dislocation with positive Ortolani/Barlow maneuvers; flat feet normal.

***Neurological:*** Assess if newborn is hypotonic ("floppy infant") or hypertonic. Evaluate developmental milestones (Table 15–2) at initial and subsequent visits.

***Infantile automatisms:*** Rooting, sucking, traction, plantar and palmar grasp, Moro or startle reflex, tonic neck, placing and stepping responses, trunk incurvation or Galant's reflex are present at birth. Deep tendon reflexes: upgoing Babinski and ankle clonus are normal.

▶ Health Maintenance Issues

Every periodic visit for infants, children, and adolescents should include age-appropriate history and physical examination, immunizations, evaluation of growth and development, and patient education including anticipatory guidance (see Table 15–3).

► table 15-2

DEVELOPMENTAL MILESTONES DURING THE FIRST YEAR OF LIFE

| Age | Gross Motor | Fine Motor | Personal | Language |
|---|---|---|---|---|
| Newborn | Reflex head turn | — | Regards face | Alerts to bell |
| 1 month | Lifts head when prone | Eyes track horizontally | — | — |
| 2 months | Lifts shoulders when prone | Tracks past midline | Spontaneous smile | Coos; searches for sound |
| 3 months | Lifts up on elbows, head steady | Unfisted > 50%, tracks 180 degrees | — | — |
| 4 months | Lifts up on hands, rolls front to back | Reaches and brings object to mouth | Turns head to voice/noise | — |
| 5 months | Rolls back to front | "Rakes" at bright object | — | — |
| 6 months | Sits alone > 30 sec | Transfers hand to hand | Discriminates social smile | Babbles |
| 7–8 months | Crawls, sits well | Pincer grasp | Stranger anxiety | Mama, Dada |
| 9–10 months | Pulls to stand | Neat pincer grasp | Plays peek-a-boo | Understands "no" |
| 10–11 months | Cruises | — | — | — |
| 12 months | Walks | — | Drinks from cup | 3–5-word vocabulary |

*Adapted from: Rudolph C, Rudolph A, eds.* Rudolph's Pediatrics, *21st ed. New York: McGraw-Hill; 2003, p. 14, Table 1-9.*

► table 15-3

ANTICIPATORY GUIDANCE: TOPICS TO DISCUSS WITH PARENTS DURING THE FIRST YEAR OF LIFE

*Newborn:* Never leave child unattended; use car restraints; feeding topics; crying and sleeping patterns; stooling patterns; hiccups; sneezing and "wet burps"; startle reflexes; care of umbilical cord; circumcision; jaundice; how to take a temperature, when to call the office; fever, vomiting, and diarrhea; postpartum adjustment; sibling reactions

*2–4 Weeks:* Review above if needed; bath safety and sun exposure; feeding issues, fluoride supplementation; "colic"; bowel and bladder habits; when to call the office; time away from the child; giving time to siblings

*2 Months:* Review above; car restraints; do not leave unattended on bed/table; caution about hot liquids; do not use walkers; wait to introduce solids at 4–6 months; sleep, crying, and bowel patterns; immunizations; saline nose drops

*4 Months:* Review above; keep small objects out of reach; introduce solid foods, fruits, and vegetables; night awakening; teething/drooling; talking to baby; responds to vocalizations; immunizations

*6 Months:* Childproofing the house; syrup of ipecac; Poison Control Center; discourage walkers and encourage stair gates; bathtub safety; electrical outlets; introducing finger foods; discourage milk or juice as pacifier substitute; resistance to sleep; teething; shoes; separation and stranger anxiety; immunizations

*9 Months:* Toddler car restraint; ingestants such as peanuts, grapes; finger foods, self-feeding; weaning from bottle and introducing cup; sleep awakening; favorite toy; dental care; separation and stranger anxiety; imitation; social games; discipline, limit setting; distraction; child care support

*12 Months:* Reinforce above; kitchen, stairs, water, and car safety; fences, gates, and latches; table foods, decreased food intake; speech development; autonomy; limit setting, discipline

*Adapted from: Rudolph C, Rudolph A, eds.* Rudolph's Pediatrics, *21st ed. New York: McGraw-Hill; 2003, p. 28, Table 1-18.*

## II. IMMUNIZATIONS

*Note:* Because of dynamic changes occurring within field of immunizations, for most current information about immunizations and most recent updated immunization schedule, contact the Centers for Disease Control and Prevention (CDC) available via Internet (http://www.cdc.gov/mmwr) or the CDC National Immunization Hotline (1-800-232-2522).

### A. Diphtheria, Tetanus, and Pertussis

Preferred vaccine is diphtheria toxoid, tetanus toxoid, acellular pertussis (DTaP) in children followed by diphtheria toxoid and tetanus toxoid (dT) beginning after 7 years of age. It is one tenth the dose of pediatric DT. Given intramuscularly (IM) in anterolateral thigh or deltoid. Combination vaccine with *Haemophilus influenzae* type b may be used for fourth dose (booster). Contraindications include anaphylactic reaction to vaccine/vaccine constituent and encephalopathy within 7 days of administering vaccine. Precautions include acute febrile illness (temperature > 40.5°C) within 3 days; seizure, collapse, or shock-like state within 48 hours; inconsolable crying > 3 hours; and/or severe reaction to prior dose of DTaP. Reactions include local swelling and tenderness, slight fever, and irritability. Acetaminophen given beforehand may decrease symptoms. If schedule for DTaP is interrupted, it is resumed, not restarted.

### B. Polio

Recommended vaccine is inactivated poliovirus (IPV or Salk type). IPV contains neomycin and streptomycin and is contraindicated in patients with anaphylactic reactions to these drugs. Precautions should be taken when considering administering IPV to pregnant patients. Oral polio vaccine (OPV) is live attenuated (Sabin type) and is contraindicated with the exception of mass vaccination campaigns to control paralytic polio outbreak, unimmunized person traveling to endemic area within 4 weeks, and parental refusal to complete injection schedule.

### C. Measles, Mumps, and Rubella

Contraindications include pregnancy, as theoretically may injure developing fetus; anaphylactic reaction to neomycin; long-term therapeutic immunosuppression; severe human immunodeficiency virus (HIV). Precautions include recent (within 3–11 months) immune globulin administration, thrombocytopenia or thrombocytopenic purpura, personal or family history of convulsions. Measles and mumps components are derived from chick embryo fibroblast cultures, which do not contain significant amounts of egg proteins, thus may be administered to child with egg allergy and are no longer contraindicated. An intercurrent illness with low-grade fever is not a contraindication; however, if severe illness, vaccine should be delayed until child recovers. Adverse reactions include fever, rash, and transient arthralgia; encephalopathy rare with measles.

### D. *Haemophilus influenzae* Type B (Hib)

Combination vaccines are available for booster doses following primary vaccination. No known contraindications. Adverse reactions minimal with local reactions and fever.

### E. Hepatitis B

Recommended for all infants before hospital discharge or up to 2 months of age if born to hepatitis B surface antigen negative mother. Monovalent dose at birth, then subsequent doses with combination vaccine. Anaphylactic reaction to baker's yeast is only contraindication. There is no association between vaccine and multiple sclerosis, autoimmune disease, sudden infant death syndrome, or chronic fatigue syndrome.

## III. NUTRITION

### A. Growth Patterns

Average newborn weighs 3.5 kg, is 50 cm long, and has head circumference of 35 cm. Newborns lose 5–10% of body weight during first few days of life and regain weight by day 10; newborns gain about 30 g/day for first 3 months of life, then 10–20 g/day for remainder of first year; infants double birth weight by 6 months and triple birth weight at 1 year; average child weighs 10 kg at age 1, 20 kg at age 5, and 30 kg at age 10.

### B. Breastfeeding

Newborns nurse 8–12 times every 24 hours, with each feeding lasting around ½ hour; breastfed infants urinate ~ 8–10 times/day with colorless urine, stools seedy, yellow; postnatal bilirubin rises more in breastfed infant than formula-fed; human milk can be stored for 24 hours in refrigerator, 30 days in freezer; most medications and illicit drugs can be transmitted via breast milk; absolute contraindications to breastfeeding are rare and include tuberculosis in mother and galactosemia in infant; suspend breastfeeding if maternal group B streptococcal disease, herpes simplex or syphilitic lesions around nipple, pertussis, chickenpox, HIV, and non-B hepatitis. Colostrum, first milk produced, contains proteins, immunoglobulins, and secretory immunoglobulin A (IgA); mature milk produced at 7–10 days postpartum.

### C. Breast Milk Versus Formula

Both have 20 kcal/oz; casein-to-whey ratio is 40:60 in human milk and 80:20 in most formulas; polyunsaturated fat in human milk, saturated in cow milk; greater amount of lactose in human milk; breastfed infants may need supplements of vitamin K, vitamin D, iron, and fluoride (newborns should receive prophylactic dose of vitamin K); lesser amount of iron in breast milk but is more bioavailable; infections are less frequent in breastfed infants.

Most formulas attempt to reproduce human milk and are interchangeable; formula-fed infants do not require supplements. Bottle should not be propped as it causes pooling of feeds and secondary dental caries. Formulas do not have to be warmed and should never be microwaved. Infants should be burped every several ounces; stomach capacity at birth is 1–3 oz; therefore, newborn cannot take a 4-oz feeding. Formula intolerance includes diarrhea, vomiting, abdominal pain, asthma, eczema, failure to thrive, and shock.

### D. Addition of Other Foods

Risk of increasing food allergies may stem from too early introduction of solids as may childhood obesity; solid food added around 3–6 months; single-grain cereals first, then vegetables, followed by fruits, and later meats; add only one new food/week in case of allergies. "Baby food" is given as per label, and infant should not eat out of the jar as saliva may cause food to liquefy; open jars may be kept refrigerated for 2–3 days. Finger foods introduced at 9 months when child has pincer grasp; 1 year old should be able to eat same food as adults; avoid raw carrots, nuts, and hard candies as may be aspirated. Cow's milk, peanuts, egg whites, and citrus before age 1 year may be associated with allergies later on.

Honey is not recommended during first year of life as it may contain *Clostridium botulinum* and cause botulism. Infants (< 12 months of age) who drink cow's milk are at risk for hypocalcemia.

## IV. BEHAVIOR PROBLEMS

### A. Toilet Training

Initiate toilet training when child is physiologically and psychologically ready, usually around 2 years of age; takes 2 weeks to 2 months to learn; parental frustration from child's refusal to toilet train is second most common precipitant of fatal child abuse; occasional accidents months after training are not uncommon.

### B. Breath Holding

Most common between 12 and 18 months of age; apnea followed by color change prior to loss of consciousness and rhythmic clonic jerking of extremities mimicking seizure-like activity; cyanotic episodes occur with emotional provocation, pallid spells occur with injury or fear provocation; child may lose consciousness. Differential includes seizures, syncope, vertigo, cataplexy, central or obstructive apnea. Often associated with iron deficiency anemia; determine hemoglobin level and treat with iron if indicated. Treat with atropine sulfate for pallid episodes.

### C. Temper Tantrums

Occurs from 12 months to 5 years; ~ 20% of 2-year-old children have one daily; >5/d or harming others or destruction of property is abnormal; treatment is behavior modification.

### D. Crying

Average crying time at 2 weeks is 2 h/d; at 6 weeks 3 h/d, and at 12 weeks 1 h/d. If more frequent, consider colic, infections, intestinal gas, trauma, behavioral issues, drug or immunization reactions, child abuse, sickle cell crisis, CHF. Colic is inconsolable, excessive crying or fussiness > 3 h/d for > 3 d/week usually ~3:00 P.M. in an otherwise healthy < 3-month-old infant.

## E. Thumb Sucking

Occurs in 50–90% of all children; daily nonnutritive sucking occurs longer on average than nutritive sucking; intervention to stop thumb sucking should occur when child is > 4 years old as possible upper incisor protrusion may occur; risk for dental problems is lower with pacifiers.

## F. Enuresis

▶ Scientific Concepts
Involuntary or intentional urination in bed or clothing repeatedly (> 2 times/week for 3 consecutive months) in child whose age suggests achievement of bladder control. Occurrence in first-grade boys 10–20% and 8–17% of girls; epidemiologic factors: low birth weight, poverty, large family size, single-parent family, low intelligence quotient (IQ), poor speech and coordination, and encopresis. For nocturnal enuresis, majority (97%) are nonpathologic with remaining pathological causes including urinary tract infection (UTI), ectopic ureter, bladder calculus, neurogenic bladder, diabetes, obstructive sleep apnea.

▶ Diagnostic Studies
Urinalysis (UA), blood urea nitrogen (BUN), complete blood count (CBC), electrolytes. If abnormal UA, then renal ultrasound and voiding cystourethrogram (VCUG).

▶ Clinical Therapeutics
Conditioning alarms. Pharmacologic treatment: desmopressin and imipramine. Normal child bladder capacity in ounces is child's age + 2. (For example, a 2-year-old has a bladder capacity of 4 oz: 2-year-old + 2 = 4 oz; 3-year-old + 2 = 5 oz.)

▶ Health Maintenance Issues
Good prognosis; spontaneous cure rate 15%.

## G. Encopresis

▶ Scientific Concepts
Repeated passage of stool (monthly for > 3 months) in inappropriate places on an involuntary or voluntary basis by child who is developmental equivalent of 4 years. Occurs in 2% of 8-year-old boys and 0.7% of 8-year-old girls. Association may occur with enuresis, attention deficit hyperactivity disorder (ADHD), sexual abuse.

▶ History & Physical
Distended, stool-filled loops of bowel; tight sphincter tone; stool, pus, and mucus on undergarments.

▶ Diagnosis
Hirschsprung's disease, disorders of intestinal motility, lumbosacral spine, anal tone, and anatomy. Neurologic disorders, hypothyroidism, hypercalcemia, and lead poisoning are associated with constipation.

▶ Clinical Therapeutics
Rectal evacuation to include laxatives and enemas; dietary manipulation; behavior modification.

▶ Health Maintenance Issues
Prognosis is excellent, usually resolves by adolescence.

## V. ANEMIA, BLEEDING DISORDERS, LYMPHADENOPATHY

### A. Physiologic Anemia

▶ Scientific Concepts

Newborn has high hemoglobin (Hgb) and hematocrit (Hct); progressive decline from week 1 to 8 secondary to cessation of erythropoiesis with onset of respiration and expansion of blood volume. Full-term nadir at 8–12 weeks with Hgb level as low as 10 g/dL; premature nadir at 6–8 weeks with Hgb level as low as 7 g/dL.

▶ Diagnostic Studies

Hgb, Hct, and ferritin.

▶ Diagnosis

Vitamin E and folic acid deficiencies, failure to thrive.

▶ Clinical Therapeutics

Transfusion, but large transfusion may inhibit erythropoiesis.

### B. Iron Deficiency Anemia

▶ Scientific Concepts

Leading cause of anemia among infants and children; most common in ages 6–24 months; mainly due to dietary deficiency; need daily intake to counterbalance depletion of stores.

▶ History & Physical

Symptoms vary with severity; mild form is asymptomatic; more severe form: pallor, fatigue, irritability, delayed motor development, decreased exercise tolerance, anorexia, tachycardia, cardiomegaly, and pica.

▶ Diagnostic Studies

Hypochromic microcytic anemia with elevated red cell distribution width (RDW); ferritin < 10 mg/mL; serum iron < 30 g/dL; reticulocyte count > 600,000.

▶ Diagnosis

Associated with peptic ulcer disease, Meckel's diverticulum, menorrhagia, nasal bleeding, chronic intestinal blood loss by ingestion of cow's milk.

▶ Clinical Therapeutics

Supplementation with 4–6 mg/kg/d of elemental iron in three divided doses for at least 4–6 weeks; adequate response is reticulocytosis within 7 days and increase of Hgb > 1 g/dL in 1 month.

▶ Health Maintenance Issues

Children at increased risk for lead poisoning secondary to pica. Prophylactic iron supplementation (fortified formula or cereal or iron drops) for all infants > 4 months of age.

### C. Vitamin B$_{12}$ (Cobalamin) Deficiency Anemia

▶ Scientific Concepts

Uncommon, peaks at 4–7 months, secondary to deficient intake of vitamin B$_{12}$ (cobalamin) in infants breastfed by mothers who are strict vegetarians or who have pernicious anemia or may occur with intestinal malabsorption disorders.

▶ **History & Physical**

Pallor, mild jaundice, irritability, smooth and beefy red tongue, failure to thrive, chronic diarrhea, weakness, or paresthesias.

▶ **Diagnostic Studies**

Megaloblastic anemia; smear with macrocytic red blood cells (RBCs), increased indices, low reticulocyte count, low serum vitamin $B_{12}$ levels, elevated methylmaloninc acid and homocysteine levels. Schilling test identifies etiology.

▶ **Diagnosis**

Associated with thrombocytopenia, neutropenia, hypersegmentation.

▶ **Clinical Therapeutics**

Oral supplementation of cobalamin or if due to intestinal malabsorption then parenteral treatment.

▶ **Health Maintenance Issues**

May lead to neurological abnormalities.

## D. Folic Acid Deficiency Anemia

▶ **Scientific Concepts**

Uncommon; secondary to deficient intake of folic acid in diet of goat's milk; infants require 10 times more folate/body weight than adults; folic acid absorbed through small intestine. Etiologies include celiac disease, chronic infectious, enteritis, enteroenteric fistulas, and use of phenytoin or trimethoprim.

▶ **History & Physical**

Pallor, mild jaundice, smooth and beefy red tongue, failure to thrive, chronic diarrhea.

▶ **Diagnostic Studies**

Megaloblastic anemia; smear with macrocytic RBCs, increased indices, low serum folate levels of < 140 ng/mL, elevated homocysteine levels.

▶ **Clinical Therapeutics**

Folate 0.5–1.0 mg/d initially, then 0.05–0.10 mg/d as maintenance dose. Change to milk or soy-based formula.

▶ **Health Maintenance Issues**

Folate supplementation during first trimester of pregnancy decreases prevalence of neural tube defects in fetus, thus recommend routine supplementation for women of childbearing age.

## E. Sickle Cell Anemia

▶ **Scientific Concepts**

Countries associated—all of Africa, Italy, Greece, Middle East, and India; homozygosity for sickle gene have disease; heterozygosity for sickle gene have trait.

▶ **History & Physical**

Symptoms do not appear before 3–4 months; painful or vasoocclusive crises with painful swelling of hands and feet secondary to infarctions of small bones, severe abdominal pain, cerebrovascular accidents (CVAs), pulmonary consolidation, splenomegaly, aplastic crisis; pain precipitated by cold, dehydration, infection, stress but mostly indeterminate; about one third develop pneumococcal sepsis in first 5 years.

▶ Diagnostic Studies

Hgb electrophoresis conclusive study; markedly elevated reticulocyte count; sickle cells and target cells on peripheral smear.

▶ Clinical Therapeutics

Consider patient as compromised host; no antisickling drugs, narcotics for pain; correct dehydration and aggressive treatment of infections; prophylactic penicillin to prevent sepsis; bone marrow transplant; red cell transfusions for acute exacerbation.

## F. Coagulation Disorders

▶ Scientific Concepts

Platelet disorders, clotting factor abnormalities.

▶ History & Physical

Questions—bleeding with circumcision, immunizations, tooth eruption, after minor trauma; frequent epistaxis; drug intake such as aspirin, anticonvulsants, antibiotics; ingestion of warfarin; petechiae, mucosal bleeding with platelet disorders; soft-tissue bleeding, hemarthrosis with plasma clotting factors; hepatomegaly and splenomegaly.

▶ Diagnostic Studies

Screening tests: prothrombin time (PT), partial thromboplastin time (PTT), fibrinogen, bleeding time, CBC with platelet count, and examination of blood smear.

▶ Diagnosis

Consider hereditary deficiency: x-linked recessive inheritance hemophilia A (factor VIII) and Christmas disease (factor IX); autosomal dominant inheritance von Willebrand disease. Consider acquired deficiency: thrombocytopenia; disseminated intravascular coagulation (DIC); vitamin K deficiency.

▶ Clinical Therapeutics

Treat underlying abnormality, if possible.

## G. Lymphadenopathy

▶ Scientific Concepts

May be pathologic or nonpathologic; generalized adenopathy common in pediatric population and usually related to acute infection. *Staphylococcus aureus* and *Streptococcus pyogenes* most common infectious etiology; noninfectious inflammatory causes are collagen vascular disease, chronic granulomatous disease, and Kawasaki disease; noninflammatory congenital (thyroglossal duct cyst, cystic hygroma) and neoplasms.

▶ History & Physical

Prior illness; exposure to cats (cat scratch disease and toxoplasmosis); travel (histoplasmosis in southeastern United States and coccidioidomycosis in California); recent immigration (tuberculosis from Mexico,

Central America, Southeast Asia). Measure size of nodes at widest diameter; note redness, tenderness, warmth, mobility; hepatomegaly; splenomegaly; weight loss; lymph drainage in anatomical pattern; tender nodes with infection and fixed hard nodes with malignancy. Supraclavicular adenopathy associated with malignancy. Unilateral preauricular or submandibular adenopathy suggestive for nontuberculous mycobacterium. Pectoral nodes associated with cat scratch disease.

▶ Diagnostic Studies

CBC, erythrocyte sedimentation rate (ESR), liver function tests (LFTs), purified protein derivative (PPD), throat culture, viral studies, antinuclear antibody (ANA), rheumatoid factor (RF), biopsy to rule out lymphoma, chest x-ray (CXR) if suspect malignancy. Aspirate for culture and sensitivity if persistent.

▶ Clinical Therapeutics

Identify and treat cause. Antibiotics, antifungals, PPD, surgical removal/biopsy if present > 3 months.

▶ Health Maintenance Issues

Awareness of travel, presence of cats.

## H. Hodgkin's Versus Non-Hodgkin's Lymphoma

▶ Scientific Concepts

*Hodgkin's:* Peaks in adolescence, similar human lymphocyte antigen (HLA) typing in families; in developed countries more common in higher socioeconomic groups.

*Non-Hodgkin's lymphoma (NHL):* 1.5 times as common as Hodgkin's; peak age is 7 to 11 years but can occur in infants; seen with varied inherited disorders and chronic immunosuppressive therapy.

▶ History & Physical

*Hodgkin's:* Painless lymphadenopathy of cervical or supraclavicular nodes that are rubbery, firm, nontender and may be matted; noted incidentally; night sweats, fever, and 10% weight loss over 6 months.

*NHL:* 80% with GI involvement including abdominal mass (frequently right lower quadrant), abdominal pain and distension, vomiting diarrhea; 50–70% with mediastinal involvement including superior vena cava obstruction (plethora/edema of face, neck, and upper chest with dilated veins in these areas), trachea and main bronchi compression; 10% with Waldeyer ring (tonsil and adenoid) involvement; rapidly proliferating malignancy, thus brief (from days to a few weeks) duration of symptoms.

▶ Diagnostic Studies

*Hodgkin's:* Must obtain lymph node for pathology, histologically characterized by presence of Sternberg-Reed cells; CBC; ESR to follow success of treatment; CXR to ascertain mediastinal adenopathy; computed tomographic (CT) scan of chest, abdomen, and pelvis.

*NHL:* Must obtain lymph node or remove mass; lactate dehydrogenase (LDH) concentration serves as marker of disease activity; CBC; LFTs; renal function tests; electrolytes; uric acid; phosphorus; calcium; CXR and if abnormal then CT scan of chest; CT scan of pelvis and abdomen;

technetium or gallium bone scan; bone marrow aspirate; cerebral spinal fluid (CSF) examination.

▶ Diagnosis

*Hodgkin's:* Ann Arbor staging.

*NHL:* St. Jude's staging, similar but not the same.

▶ Clinical Therapeutics

*Hodgkin's:* Increasingly treated by multiagent chemotherapy or combined modality therapy (chemotherapy and radiation), if localized consider radiation therapy alone.

*NHL:* Chemotherapy is mainstay; surgery should not be performed for purpose of resection of lesions; radiation does not improve outcome; if relapse consider bone marrow transplantation.

# VI. CARDIOVASCULAR DISEASES

Epidemiology and prevalence of congenital heart disease (CHD): 10 per 1,000 live-born infants have congenital structural heart malformation. Division of classification: cyanotic (right-to-left shunt whether have recognizable cyanosis or not) versus noncyanotic (do not have right-to-left shunt even if cyanotic for other reasons). Frequency of common defects: ventricular septal defect (VSD), 32%; atrial septal defect (ASD), 7%; patent ductus arteriosus (PDA), 7%; pulmonary stenosis, 7%; coarctation of the aorta, 5%, tetralogy of Fallot, 5%.

## A. Ventricular Septal Defect (VSD)

▶ Scientific Concepts

Most common cardiac abnormality in children; hole in septum between right and left ventricle that may occur in either membranous or muscular part of septum. Increased incidence with genetic syndromes: trisomy 13, trisomy 18, and trisomy 21 (Down). Associated with maternal use of trimethadione during pregnancy.

▶ History & Physical

Harsh, high-pitched, holosystolic murmur heard best at left sternal border; first and second heart sounds normal; large defects may cause CHF without murmur.

▶ Diagnostic Studies

Electrocardiograph (ECG) with left ventricular hypertrophy (LVH) if large defect; echocardiograph (ECHO) diagnostic.

▶ Clinical Therapeutics

Medical management of CHF.

▶ Clinical Intervention

Surgical repair if medical treatment for CHF and failure to thrive or pulmonary hypertension fails; small defects close spontaneously.

## B. Atrial Septal Defect (ASD)

► **Scientific Concepts**

Third most common congenital heart defect; hole in septum between right and left ventricle; small defects of no hemodynamic significance, larger defects with shunting of blood; common cardiac defect associated with Noonan syndrome and CHARGE syndrome (coloboma of eye, heart defects, choanal atresia, retardation, genital, and ear anomalies).

► **History & Physical**

Symptoms range from asymptomatic to exercise intolerance; CHF; atrial arrhythmia may present in mid to late adulthood; heart sounds: pulmonary systolic murmur that peaks in early systole; crescendo–decrescendo murmurs, fixed wide splitting of the second heart sound at left upper sternal border; may have rumbling, mid-diastolic murmur at left lower sternal border.

► **Diagnostic Studies**

ECG with left axis deviation (rSR′ pattern in lead V1), sinus rhythm usually, atrial arrhythmia after second decade; CXR with cardiac enlargement and increased pulmonary vascularity; ECHO diagnostic.

► **Clinical Intervention**
Large defect surgically closed.

## C. Patent Ductus Arteriosus (PDA)

► **Scientific Concepts**

Persistence of normal fetal blood vessel that connects main pulmonary artery with descending aorta; spontaneous closure in term infant at 3–5 days of life; second most common heart defect.

► **History & Physical**

Increased incidence: preterm infants weighing < 1,500 g, birth at high altitude (hypoxia), pulmonary disease, and maternal rubella during first trimester; heart sounds: continuous, rumbling, "machinery like" murmur, maximal at second left intercostal space at left upper sternal border or left infraclavicular area, bounding pulses.

► **Diagnostic Studies**

CXR with cardiomegaly, prominent main artery segment, dilated ascending aorta and increased pulmonary vasculature markings; ECG normal or LVH; ECHO diagnostic.

► **Clinical Intervention**

Spontaneous closure usually within several weeks of birth. If symptomatic in preterm infant, pharmacological closure with indomethacin (high success rate 80–90%); closure by transcatheter coil embolization or surgical ligation by age 2 years if above not effective. Potential complications if not closed include infective endocarditis, pulmonary hypertension, and CHF.

## D. Coarctation of the Aorta

► **Scientific Concepts**

Common, leading cause of CHF in first month of life; coarctation usually occurs in thoracic region of descending aorta distal to left subclavian artery in juxtaductal region. Increased in males and Turner's syndrome.

▶ **History & Physical**

Classic physical finding is diminution or absence of femoral pulses and delayed relative to brachial pulses; blood pressure lower in lower extremities; may be asymptomatic or present with CHF, hypertension, or murmur; heart sounds: generally normal, however, systolic ejection murmur, radiates to left-sided interscapular area with associated apical ejection click in right upper sternal border. Scoliosis common in teenagers.

▶ **Diagnostic Studies**

ECG normal at birth or if severe shows RVH, later with LVH; CXR with normal heart size, with evidence of left ventricular enlargement; reverse "3" sign (dilatation of ascending aorta, coarctation, poststenotic dilatation); rib notching secondary to enlargement of intercostal collaterals after 1 year of age. Two-dimensional ECHO and Doppler flow mapping valuable in assessing anatomy; magnetic resonant imaging (MRI) necessary if ECHO unclear.

▶ **Clinical Intervention**

Anticongestive measures until surgical intervention (treatment of choice in infants and young children) or balloon angioplasty (older children, adolescents, or adults).

## E. Transposition of the Great Arteries

▶ **Scientific Concepts**

Failure of rotation of great vessels so aorta originates from right ventricle, pulmonary artery from left ventricle; principal problem is severe hypoxia. Male predominance.

▶ **History & Physical**

Extreme cyanosis, unresponsive to increasing oxygen, lack of respiratory distress, no characteristic murmur or have murmur associated with ventricular septal defect or pulmonic stenosis, loud single second heart sound in left upper sternal border and prominent right ventricular impulse.

▶ **Diagnostic Studies**

CXR nonspecific or classic finding "egg on a string" with cardiomegaly; ECG with right axis deviation (RAD) and RVH (normal in newborn); ECHO important for diagnosis.

▶ **Clinical Intervention**

Surgical with arterial switch operation (ASO), including transplantation of both coronary arteries into reconnected aorta.

## F. Tetralogy of Fallot

▶ **Scientific Concepts**

Spectrum of abnormalities including: large unrestrictive VSD, aorta overriding ventricular septum, pulmonary stenosis, and RVH. Most common cyanotic heart lesion. Associated with DiGeorge syndrome, velocardiofacial syndrome, Klippel–Feil syndrome (congenital cervical vertebral body anomalies), and genetic abnormalities of chromosome 22.

▶ History & Physical

Asymptomatic to severely hypoxic; hallmark sign: "Tet spells" sudden onset or worsening cyanosis secondary to increase in right-to-left shunting; paroxysmal hypoxemia (self-limited, last <30 min, occur mostly in morning, precipitated by fright), sudden onset of dyspnea, alterations in consciousness and decrease in intensity of murmur; decreased exercise intolerance; squatting is position of comfort after exertion; heart sounds: rough systolic ejection murmur heard best over left sternal border in third intercostal space radiating to back, palpable right ventricular heave.

▶ Diagnostic Studies

CXR with characteristic "boot-shaped" heart, enlargement of right ventricle with concavity of upper left heart border secondary to absence of main pulmonary artery segment, right-sided aortic arch (25%); ECG with right axis deviation and RVH; ECHO with increased blood flow in main pulmonary artery.

▶ Clinical Intervention

Pulmonary stenosis worsens with age; definitive treatment surgical with modified Blalock–Taussig shunt; treatment for acute hypercyanotic episode is placement in knee–chest or squatting position; medical management for secondary polycythemia.

## G. Hypoplastic Left Heart Syndrome

▶ Scientific Concepts

Group of malformations, usually with underdeveloped left ventricle and atrium, marked hypoplasia of ascending aorta, mitral stenosis, mitral hypoplasia, aortic atresia, or mitral atresia; male preponderance; accounts for 25% of cardiac deaths in first year of life.

▶ History & Physical

Stable at birth, deteriorate rapidly with closure of ductus arteriosus as symptoms develop by day 2–3 with cyanosis, tachypnea, tachycardia, diminished then absent peripheral pulses, occasional rales, soft grade I/VI systolic murmur at left sternal border.

▶ Diagnostic Studies

ECG with right axis deviation, right atrial hypertrophy, RVH, absence of Q wave in lead V6 and qR pattern in V1; CXR with increased vascular markings and cardiac enlargement; ECHO definitive.

▶ Clinical Intervention

Surgical: orthotopic cardiac transplantation or reconstruction with Norwood procedure, followed by Glenn anastomosis and Fontan procedure.

## H. Rheumatic Fever

▶ Scientific Concepts

Sequela to upper respiratory infection (URI) with group A beta-hemolytic *streptococcus,* diffuse inflammatory disease that involves heart, joints, central nervous system (CNS), and subcutaneous tissues; peak risk in school-age children (5–15 years) during fall, winter, and spring as does pharyngitis.

► History & Physical

Antecedent streptococcal pharyngitis 1–5 weeks prior to symptoms. Jones criteria major: polyarthritis of large joints often migratory; carditis frequently with new onset murmur of mitral regurgitation followed by Carey Coombs murmur (soft, mid-diastolic murmur at apex); Sydenham's chorea; subcutaneous nodules movable, nontender over extensor surfaces and bony prominences of arms, legs, scalp, and vertebrae; erythema marginatum over trunk and proximal extremities. Jones criteria minor: polyarthralgia; fever; ECG with prolonged P-R interval; and acute-phase reaction (elevated ESR and C-reactive protein, leukocytosis). Other associated findings: epistaxis, vomiting, abdominal pain, anorexia, weight loss.

► Diagnostic Studies

Increased ESR, C-reactive protein, and antistreptolysin-O titer (ASO). May see anemia and leukocytosis. ECG with prolongation of P-R interval (first degree), second degree, or complete block.

► Diagnosis

Use Jones criteria—two major or one major and two minor criteria plus evidence of preceding streptococcal infection documented by positive throat culture for group A beta-hemolytic *streptococcus* (gold standard), scarlet fever, elevated ASO.

► Clinical Therapeutics

Treat streptococcal pharyngitis with antibiotics (benzathine penicillin G is drug of choice); aspirin for clinical manifestations; corticosteroids if moderate to severe carditis.

► Health Maintenance Issues

Must treat and follow-up group A beta-hemolytic streptococcal pharyngitis. Prophylaxis necessary with controversial duration.

## VII. GASTROINTESTINAL DISORDERS

### A. Vomiting

► Scientific Concepts

Vomiting is forceful expulsion of stomach contents through mouth, regurgitation is effortless, rumination is voluntary induction of regurgitation; three phases of vomiting: nausea (response to noxious stimuli coordinated by CNS), retching, and emesis; input to vomiting center in medulla arises from pharynx (gagging), brain (ICP and dizziness), and GI tract (distension and noxious substances); 50% of infants have spitting up or vomiting as isolated complaint, less frequent in older children.

► History & Physical

Morning vomiting without nausea may be secondary to increased ICP; bilious vomiting indicative of intestinal obstruction; projectile vomiting and peristaltic waves associated with pyloric stenosis; nonbloody and nonbilious vomiting consider infectious, metabolic, neurologic, and endocrine etiologies. Evaluate for dehydration; assess growth pattern (weight) to determine chronicity; neurologic exam; examine fundi for papilledema or retinal hemorrhages; check for signs of abdominal obstruction (mass or distension).

▶ **Diagnosis**

*Infants:* Structural abnormalities—"the higher the lesion, the earlier the symptoms"; esophageal atresia; overfeeding in bottle-fed infants; food allergies especially cow's milk; gastroesophageal reflux (GER); metabolic disorders; infectious associated with UTI, otitis media, meningitis; non-accidental trauma (intracranial hemorrhage); pyloric stenosis; intussusception (classic triad: colicky pain, vomiting, bloody and mucoid stools).

*Children:* Usually gastroenteritis; UTI; otitis media; streptococcal pharyngitis; sinusitis; delayed gastric emptying secondary to diabetes mellitus; CNS-related problems to include migraine headaches, tumor, Reye's syndrome; medications, especially theophylline, erythromycin, and digitalis; appendicitis and other surgical lesions.

*Adolescents:* Ingestion of illicit drugs/alcohol, pregnancy, eating disorders, sinusitis, migraine headaches.

▶ **Diagnostic Studies**

Stool for leukocytes, occult blood, and cultures (viral and bacterial); CBC with differential, electrolytes, urinalysis, pregnancy test, metabolic workup last; abdominal x-ray, ultrasound or contrast-enhanced CT scan to rule out obstructive lesions.

▶ **Clinical Therapeutics**

Hydrate, oral better than intravenous (IV), clear liquids, discourage antiemetics; further management dependent on diagnosis.

## B. Diarrhea

▶ **Scientific Concepts**

Characterized by increased volume of stool with looser consistency and increased frequency; average child with one episode yearly (if in day care center, increases to 4.5 episodes per annum); may be associated with abdominal pain, bloating, dehydration, fever, vomiting, and weight loss; infants excrete 5–10 g/kg of stool daily; children excrete 10 g/kg/d and adults excrete 200 g/d. *Osmotic diarrhea (malabsorptive)*—stooling decreases with fasting; *secretory diarrhea*—bowel continues to secrete water and electrolytes with absence of leukocytes, stooling continues despite cessation of eating, elevated sodium content in stool, associated with malignancies (neuroblastoma, ganglioneuroma); *motility diarrhea*—occurs without malabsorption (irritable colon syndrome); *inflammatory diarrhea*—acute or chronic (Crohn's disease or ulcerative colitis). Steatorrhea is fat in stools—occurs with problems in small intestine (giardiasis), liver, and pancreas.

▶ **History & Physical**

Look for signs of dehydration (altered vital signs, delayed capillary refill, sunken fontanel, dry mucous membranes, absent tearing, decreased skin turgor, and anuria) and growth retardation.

▶ **Diagnosis**

Acute diarrhea: most common cause is acute gastroenteritis, predominantly viral, primarily with *rotavirus*, occurs in winter months, preceded by URI, followed by fever and vomiting with voluminous watery, diarrhea without leukocytes or blood, hypernatremia, and 10% with otitis media. Second most common viral pathogen is enteric *adenovirus,* which occurs in summertime. Bacterial causes include mainly *Shigella, Salmonella, Campylobacter; Shigella/Campylobacter* with blood/mucus in stools; *Shigella* with high fever and are seizure prone; *Salmonella* often with headache and meningismus; *Giardia lamblia, Entamoeba histolytica,* and *Cryptosporidium parvum* are parasitic infections requiring to be cultured separately; *Escherichia coli* in newborns, with epidemic outbreaks of large, explosive watery, green stools without blood; toxigenic *E. coli* is most common pathogen for traveler's diarrhea. Necrotizing enterocolitis (NEC) with blood and watery stools often affects preterm infants with respiratory distress syndrome; consider food intolerance/allergies, overfeeding of fruit juices high in fructose or sorbitol-containing products (osmotic diarrhea), cow's milk intolerance with associated steatorrhea, growth retardation, anemia, hypoproteinemia, edema, eczema, eosinophilia, and elevated immunoglobulin E (IgE).

Chronic diarrhea: defined as lasting > 2 weeks; inflammatory bowel disease; Crohn's disease; irritable bowel disease; use of antibiotics most commonly pseudomembranous colitis due to toxin-producing *Clostridium difficile;* heavy metals such as iron; cystic fibrosis with large, bulky, foul-smelling stools and failure to thrive; celiac disease with mushy, bulky, foul-smelling stools; related to allergy or wheat protein (gluten).

▶ **Diagnostic Studies**

Evaluate stools for quantity; gross appearance (undigested food secondary to poor chewing); chemical and microscopic analysis for unabsorbed nutrients such as carbohydrates, fats (Carmine red stain), blood, leukocytes (methylene blue stain for white blood cells); culture for bacteria/ova/parasites, immunoassay for rotavirus; levels of sodium, potassium; and stool osmolality. Sigmoidoscopy or barium enema last.

▶ **Clinical Therapeutics**

Hydrate and correct electrolyte imbalances; if severe dehydration: IV hydration as inpatient; if moderate dehydration: oral rehydration solutions as outpatient; dietary manipulation with BRAT diet (bananas, rice, applesauce, toast). Antimicrobial agents for pathogens such as *Shigella, G. lamblia, E. histolytica,* and *Campylobacter.* DO NOT use antidiarrheal agents as this retains toxins. Usually self-limited, may lead to malnutrition if chronic.

## C. Constipation

▶ **Scientific Concepts**
About 3% of outpatient visits.

▶ **History & Physical**

Hard, dry stools, with painful defecation; often exhibit withholding patterns or behavioral changes; abdominal or rectal pain, hematochezia; anorexia; fecal soiling. Examination usually normal but may palpate feces in left lower quadrant. Relaxed anal tone with spinal cord disease, tight sphincter with loose stools after exam with Hirschsprung's disease.

▶ **Diagnostic Studies**

Flat plate of abdomen, barium enema, thyroid function studies, stool culture for botulism, and rectal biopsy.

▶ Diagnosis

Hirschsprung's disease if meconium delayed > 24 hours, may not be diagnosed until age 5–6 years, associated with syndromes (Down, Smith–Lemli–Opitz, Waardenburg). Barium enema: narrow distal segment with proximal megacolon; rectal biopsy if absence of ganglion cells. Hypothyroidism—if secondary to hypopituitarism, not diagnosed through newborn screening process due to normal thyroid-stimulating hormone (TSH). Imperforate anus with perineal fistula may not be recognized early. Botulism—constipation between 6 weeks to 6 months of age; history of breastfed or exposure to honey, corn syrup, homegrown herbal teas; often febrile, lethargic, and hypotonic with flattened facies; inability to gaze away from light shone directly in eye. Gentamicin administration may potentiate neuromuscular blockade and precipitate respiratory arrest. Other considerations—medications (aspirin, codeine, vincristine, iron, bismuth [Pepto-Bismol], imipramine); dehydration; neurologic disorders.

▶ Clinical Therapeutics

Dietary manipulation: discontinue iron, add fruit and vegetables. Medications to soften and increase bulk to stool: Maltsupex, **no** corn syrup. In older children, dietary manipulation: add fruit (papaya, cantaloupe), add stool softener (mineral oil) and laxatives (Milk of Magnesia, lactulose). For chronic problems, use enemas.

▶ Clinical Intervention

Surgical intervention for Hirschsprung's disease and imperforate anus.

## D. Congenital Diaphragmatic Hernia

▶ Scientific Concepts

Varied presentations, 80% left-sided.

▶ History & Physical

If severe, immediate postnatal respiratory distress, scaphoid abdomen, absent breath sounds on affected side, pulmonary hypertension, displacement of cardiac impulse to contralateral side.

▶ Diagnostic Studies

CXR positive.

▶ Clinical Therapeutics

High-frequency mechanical ventilation is mainstay of respiratory support pre- and postsurgery. Role of extracorporeal membrane oxygenation (ECMO) is controversial, and role of inhaled nitric oxide has not proven useful.

▶ Clinical Intervention

Stabilization of respiratory system. Surgical repair.

▶ Health Maintenance Issues

Lung on affected side hypoplastic, mediastinal shift, pulmonary infections, associated with cardiac, GI, CNS, GU malformations.

## E. Hirschsprung's Disease

▶ Scientific Concepts

Congenital aganglionic megacolon. Absence of ganglion cells in mucosal and muscular layers of colon; rectum and rectosigmoid usually affected; increased in males and Down, Smith–Lemli–Opitz, and Waardenburg syndromes.

▶ **History & Physical**

In newborn, failure to pass meconium, then vomiting, abdominal distention, anorexia, bouts of enterocolitis. In older children, constipation with foul-smelling, ribbon-like stools. Examination with enlarged abdomen, prominent veins, peristaltic pattern visible, rectal exam without solid feces in anal canal, usually with gush of liquid stool as finger is withdrawn.

▶ **Diagnostic Studies**

Biopsy of bowel to detect ganglion cells; x-ray of abdomen with dilated proximal colon/absence of gas in pelvic colon; barium enema with narrowed segment distal to dilated portion.

▶ **Clinical Intervention**

Surgical with colostomy and resection of aganglionic segment at 6 months of age.

▶ **Health Maintenance Issues**

Chronic constipation, fecal incontinence, strictures.

## F. Acute Appendicitis

▶ **Scientific Concepts**

Most common childhood emergency abdominal surgery, obstruction of appendix by fecaliths.

▶ **History & Physical**

Classically, with anorexia, low-grade fever followed by periumbilical pain localizing to right lower quadrant, nausea, and vomiting. Present with peritoneal signs of guarding, rebound tenderness, localized mass, tenderness on rectal exam, positive psoas/obturator signs on some.

▶ **Diagnostic Studies**

Mild leukocytosis; ultrasound with noncompressible, thickened appendix with localized fluid collection; limited CT with rectal contrast (CTRC) is emerging as powerful tool to visualize abnormal appendix with or without presence of fecalith; abdominal x-ray shows radiopaque fecalith on two thirds with ruptured appendix. Rule out pregnancy with negative human chorionic gonadotropin (hCG) in females of childbearing age; negative UA; and negative CXR (symptoms mimic pneumonia).

▶ **Diagnosis**

Differential includes: pneumonia, UTI, ectopic pregnancy, mechanical obstructions, and inflammatory diseases.

▶ **Clinical Intervention**

Appendectomy.

▶ **Health Maintenance Issues**

Appropriate postoperative antibiotics.

## G. Intussusception

▶ **Scientific Concepts**

Most frequent intestinal obstruction in first 2 years of life; commonly ileocolic; increased in males; etiology unknown but common lead points for obstruction include polyps, lymphoma, Meckel's diverticulum, parasites, foreign bodies, and adenovirus or rotavirus infections with hypertrophied Peyer patches; associated with celiac disease and cystic fibrosis.

▶ **History & Physical**

Paroxysmal abdominal pain with drawing up of knees; followed by vomiting, diarrhea afterward, then bloody, mucous bowel movement or "currant jelly stools"; fever; tender, distended abdomen with palpable sausage-shaped mass in upper midabdomen. May last several days and be recurrent.

▶ **Clinical Therapeutics**

Conservative with diagnostic and therapeutic barium enema.

▶ **Clinical Intervention**

If barium enema not effective, surgical correction.

▶ **Health Maintenance Issues**

Rotavirus vaccine (Rotashield) was suspended due to increased risk of intussusception among young infants within weeks following its use.

## H. Pyloric Stenosis

▶ **Scientific Concepts**

Hypertrophy of circular muscle of pylorus, increased in full-term males; positive family history (13%); incidence increased in infants (< 30 days old) treated with erythromycin therapy.

▶ **History & Physical**

Progressive nonbilious projectile vomiting during first few weeks of life; infants take feedings; dehydration with hypochloremic, hypokalemic metabolic alkalosis; abdominal exam may yield palpation of "olive" and visualizing prominent peristaltic waves.

▶ **Diagnostic Studies**

Upper GI contrast series with absence of air distal to pylorus with characteristic "string sign" and enlarged "shoulders" bordering elongated and obstructed pyloric channel; ultrasound with hypertrophic pyloric musculature.

▶ **Clinical Therapeutics**

Correction of dehydration/electrolyte imbalance.

▶ **Clinical Intervention**

Pylorotomy.

## I. Neonatal Jaundice

▶ **Scientific Concepts**

Bilirubin is byproduct of hemoglobin metabolism with two forms: direct (conjugated) and indirect (unconjugated); defective bilirubin conjugation; metabolism of heme is incomplete in newborn.

▶ **History & Physical**

Vomiting, lethargy, acholic (white stools), dark urine; poor feeding with metabolic disorders; check jaundice, yellow discoloration in skin/mucous membranes/sclerae progresses from head to feet; hepatomegaly; with metabolic disorders unusual facies; other masses.

► Diagnosis

Physiologic jaundice peaks at 3–5 days postpartum, breast-milk jaundice at 2 to 3 weeks; hemolytic diseases, ABO or Rh incompatibility; erythrocyte defects, glucose-6-phosphate dehydrogenase (G6PD); polycythemia; vitamin K; varied syndromes; antibiotics. Intestinal obstruction for unconjugated hyperbilirubinemia enterohepatic disorders. For conjugated hyperbilirubinemia intrahepatic disorders: sepsis; metabolic: alpha-1-antitrypsin deficiency, cystic fibrosis; infectious: hepatitis, TORCHS.

► Diagnostic Studies

Need to differentiate unconjugated from conjugated hyperbilirubinemia; serum total and fractionated bilirubin, Coombs' test, infant and maternal blood types, Hct, CBC with reticulocyte count, peripheral blood smear to rule out hemolysis, blood and urine cultures, viral titers, thyroid function tests, LFTs, sweat chloride, alpha-1-antitrypsin phenotype, urine Clinitest to rule out galactosemia, scintigraphy to rule out hepatitis, ultrasound for choledochal cyst/cholelithiasis, biopsy.

► Clinical Therapeutics

Phototherapy for unconjugated hyperbilirubinemia; exchange transfusion if continued elevation. Surgical correction with biliary atresia.

► Health Maintenance Issues

Kernicterus, due to toxic hyperbilirubinemia, results in encephalopathy with subsequent neurologic problems.

# VIII. RESPIRATORY DISORDERS

## A. Sinusitis

► Scientific Concepts

Five to 10% of URIs complicated by sinusitis; predominant organisms are *Streptococcus pneumoniae, H. influenzae*-nontypeable, and *Moraxella caterallis,* along with *Staphylococcus aureus* and anaerobes less frequently; *Pseudomonas aeruginosa* is common with cystic fibrosis. Virus' isolated, but role is unclear; ethmoid and maxillary sinus' most commonly affected, present at birth and developed by 3 years of age; frontal and sphenoid sinus' not developed until 12 years of age.

► History & Physical

Mucopurulent discharge in nose or posterior pharynx, prolonged nasal drainage, cough at night, malodorous breath, painless periorbital swelling, headache, sense of facial fullness or pain, erythematous nasal mucosa, possible tenderness over sinuses; transillumination of sinus' of limited value. If chronic (symptoms > 30 days), consider complicating factors of GER, allergic rhinitis, decreased host immunity, nasal foreign body, or anatomic variations (enlarged adenoids, septal deviation, nasal polyp), exacerbation of reactive airway disease.

► Diagnostic Studies

X-ray with mucosal thickening (> 4 mm) or air–fluid level (rare in children < 5 years) or opacification of sinus cavities. Preferred views: Caldwell (anteroposterior) and Water's (occipitomental), but lack sensitivity and specificity. CT (maxillofacial) is preferred diagnostic test if lack of resolution of symptoms with adequate antibiotics or suspect complications. Sinus aspirate yields precise organism; nasal or pharyngeal cultures do not reflect bacteria in sinuses.

▶ Clinical Therapeutics

Antimicrobials such as amoxicillin, high dose amoxicillin-clavulanate (Augmentin ES-600), cefidinir, cefuroxime, clindamycin; treat initially for 10–14 days; if prompt relapse of symptoms, then 21-day course.

▶ Clinical Intervention

Antral lavage, surgical enlargement of natural meatus.

▶ Health Maintenance Issues

Complications include orbital cellulitis/abscess, frontal sinus abscess (Pott's puffy tumor), meningitis, epidural abscess, subdural empyema, brain abscess, sagittal sinus thrombosis.

## B. Pharyngitis

▶ Scientific Concepts

Etiologic agents are predominantly viral (90%), most commonly adenovirus, coxsackievirus, herpes simplex virus (HSV), Epstein–Barr virus (EBV), influenza, parainfluenza; bacterial etiologies are most often group A beta-hemolytic *streptococcus,* followed by *Mycoplasma pneumoniae, Chlamydia pneumoniae,* groups B, C, and G beta-hemolytic streptococci, *Arcanobacterium haemolyticum, Neisseria gonorrhoeae* (in sexually active teens or sexual abuse in prepubertal child), *Corynebacterium diphtheriae* (nonimmunized child).

▶ History & Physical

Pain in throat, fever, may be associated with headache, nausea, vomiting, and occasionally abdominal pain; suspect viral if concurrent rhinorrhea or cough or conjunctivitis; history of exposure to contact. Examination with pharyngeal erythema, tonsillar enlargement and/or exudate, cervical adenitis; follicular, ulcerative, and petechial lesions more common with viruses. Cannot make etiologic diagnosis by visualization, only an educated guess.

▶ Diagnostic Studies

Throat culture is gold standard for diagnosis of streptococcal infection, must confirm diagnosis because of sequelae; rapid antigen tests specific but may lack sensitivity; Thayer–Martin culture if suspect gonorrhea.

▶ Clinical Therapeutics

Supportive, treat suspected (pending cultures) or proven bacterial pharyngitis; penicillin VK is drug of choice for group A streptococcal pharyngitis, except if penicillin-allergic then erythromycin estolate. Return to school or day care 24 hours after treatment initiated.

▶ Health Maintenance Issues

Untreated may lead to rheumatic fever, peritonsillar abscess (Quinsy), glomerulonephritis.

## C. Otitis Externa

▶ **Scientific Concepts**

"Swimmer's ear"; etiologies include primarily trauma and water exposure, followed by excessive cleaning; secondary infection due to drainage from perforated tympanic membrane or patent ventilating tubes; most common bacterial etiologies *S. aureus* and *P. aeruginosa;* frequent underlying fungal infection with *Candida albicans.*

▶ **History & Physical**

Severe ear pain, especially with movement of pinna or tragus; itching and fullness; edema/erythema of external ear canal with possible debris or purulent discharge; cervical adenitis.

▶ **Clinical Therapeutics**

Remove moist cerumen, foreign body, or debris. Keep canal dry. Topical antibiotic and steroid combination ear drops (e.g., ciprofloxacin + hydrocortisone otic suspension) are usually sufficient for most infections; if surrounding cellulitis, then add oral antibiotics. Adequate analgesia, if severe narcotics justifiable. Otowick if severe canal edema.

▶ **Health Maintenance Issues**

Pain and conductive hearing loss are temporary complications. If predisposed, combination of white vinegar and alcohol into ear canals prior to swimming.

## D. Otitis Media

▶ **Scientific Concepts**

One third of all pediatric visits, most common from 6 to 36 months, increased in boys, greater prevalence in Alaskan natives and Native Americans. Predisposing factors include cleft palate or other craniofacial anomaly, genetic susceptibility (twins/triplets), low socioeconomic status, bottle feeding in horizontal position, secondhand smoke exposure, day care attendance, winter months. Increased risk associated with Down, Goldenhar's, and Treacher Collins syndromes. Breastfeeding reduces incidence. Organisms predominantly are *S. pneumoniae, H. influenzae*-nontypeable, *Moraxella catarrhalis.*

▶ **History & Physical**

Fever, otalgia, irritability, anorexia, pulling on ears, vomiting, hearing loss. Examination reveals hyperemic opaque tympanic membrane (TM) with distorted or absent light reflex with impaired visibility of ossicular landmarks, pneumatic otoscopy with decreased or absence of movement of TM; erythema alone may be secondary to crying.

▶ **Clinical Therapeutics**

Acetaminophen or ibuprofen for pain. Antibiotics for treatment, with amoxicillin (90 mg/kg/d) remaining first-line drug of choice, cefuroxime, cefdinir, amoxicillin/clavulanate (Augmentin ES-600), azithromycin, ceftriaxone. Antihistamines, decongestants, or steroids have no documented role in therapy. Chemoprophylaxis is controversial, but used if > three episodes in past 6 months or four in past 12 months.

▶ **Clinical Intervention**

Surgical placement of tympanostomy tubes and/or adenoidectomy. Pneumococcal vaccine with limited reduction.

▶ **Health Maintenance Issues**

Complications include cholesteatoma, mastoiditis, osteomyelitis of temporal bone, facial nerve (CN VII) paralysis, epidural/subdural abscesses, meningitis, lateral venous sinus thrombosis, brain abscess, bacterial labyrinthitis, conductive and/or sensorineural hearing loss, delayed speech and language development; educate to encourage breastfeeding, avoid passive smoke, minimize or cease day care, avoid pacifier.

## E. Epiglottitis

▶ **Scientific Concepts**

True medical emergency. Infection of supraglottic larynx. Predominately (>90%) by *H. influenzae* type b, infrequently by *S. pneumoniae, Streptococcus pyogenes, S. aureus;* usually 3–7 years of age; year-round. Incidence dramatically decreased due to *H. influenzae* type b (Hib) vaccine.

▶ **History & Physical**

Abrupt onset of high fever (> 39°C), dysphagia, muffled voice, throat pain; shortly thereafter, toxic appearance, sits upright with chin extended to maximize airway ("sniffing dog position"), followed by rapid onset (within 12 hours) of low-pitched inspiratory stridor progressing to severe airway obstruction in < 24 hours.

▶ **Diagnosis**

Laryngotracheobronchitis (croup) with secondary bacterial infection, diphtheria.

▶ **Diagnostic Studies**

Lateral neck x-ray with "thumb sign"; diagnosis confirmed in operating room under direct visualization.

▶ **Clinical Therapeutics**

Secure airway by endotracheal tube or tracheostomy; IV antibiotics.

▶ **Health Maintenance Issues**

Rifampin prophylaxis for certain contacts; complications include death, pulmonary edema; recurrence is unusual.

## F. Croup (Laryngotracheobronchitis)

▶ **Scientific Concepts**

Most common 3 to 36 months of age; potentially life-threatening, peaks in late fall to early winter; boys > girls; etiologies include most often parainfluenza virus, followed by other viruses—respiratory syncytial virus (RSV), influenza virus, adenoviruses.

▶ **History & Physical**

Prodromal URI with nasal congestion, sore throat, typical high-pitched barking cough, hoarseness, inspiratory stridor and fever, gradual development (24–72 hours); disturbing the child increases likelihood of crying and further laryngeal swelling. As laryngeal inflammation increases, respiratory distress develops.

▶ **Diagnosis**

Epiglottitis, bacterial tracheitis, spasmodic croup, laryngeal or esophageal foreign body, angioneurotic edema, or retropharyngeal abscess should be considered in differential.

► Diagnostic Studies

Lateral neck x-ray with subglottic narrowing ("steeple sign").

► Clinical Therapeutics

Humidified oxygen or cool mist, racemic epinephrine, corticosteroids (dexamethasone is drug of choice or budesonide) may be helpful, IV hydration. Minimize agitation and crying, which increases respiratory distress and oxygen demand. If severe, may need hospitalization.

## G. Sudden Infant Death Syndrome (SIDS)

► Scientific Concepts

Second leading cause of death in infancy, but declining; incidence < 12 months of age, peaks at 2–4 months of age; unexplained death after thorough investigation; occurs mostly at night; increased during winter; male predominance; history of low birth weight, maternal drug addiction, and maternal smoking especially prenatally; association with prone sleeping position; etiology remains unknown.

► History & Physical

Present in early morning hours in cardiopulmonary arrest with history of preceding good health or antecedent URI. Symptoms of apnea, bradycardia, hypotonia, cyanosis, pallor, or altered level of consciousness. Look for signs of external trauma (e.g., bruises, long bone fractures), injury to genitalia; ophthalmologic exam for retinal hemorrhages.

► Diagnosis

Diagnosis of exclusion in any unexplained death, consider apparent life-threatening event (ALTE); Munchausen's syndrome by proxy (MSBP); child abuse; RSV; inborn errors of metabolism; cardiac anomalies/arrhythmias; infantile botulism.

► Diagnostic Studies

Comprehensive autopsy. Laboratory workup guided by history and physical.

► Health Maintenance Issues

"Back to sleep" campaign—supine sleeping position is recommended.

## H. Foreign Body Aspiration

► Scientific Concepts

Peaks at 6 months to 4 years; principally small objects such as peanuts, seeds, popcorn, hard candy, coins, toys.

► History & Physical
History of choking.

*Upper:* Respiratory distress, laryngospasm, stridor, sudden onset; if partial, child may be able to vocalize and cough, drooling; if complete, aphonia and cyanosis.

*Lower:* Large airway obstruction with respiratory distress; cough and wheeze may resolve only to recur then have chronic cough or persistent wheezing or recurrent pneumonia; asymmetric breath sounds.

► Diagnostic Studies
*Upper and Lower:* Lateral neck x-ray focus on esophageal area, possible radiopaque object; inspiratory and expiratory CXRs, with former show-

ing hyperinflation of a segment and possibly radiopaque object itself, with latter showing mediastinal shift away from affected side. If clinical suspicion persists despite negative imaging, bronchoscopy is indicated.

▶ Clinical Intervention

***Upper:*** Allow child to cough; as per basic life support, if < 1 year, deliver five measured back blows with heel of hand with child face down, then five rapid chest compressions; if > 1 year, perform abdominal thrusts; do not probe blindly; possible emergency intubation, tracheostomy, needle cricothyrotomy; if not treated, progressive cyanosis, loss of consciousness, seizures, bradycardia, and cardiac arrest.

***Lower:*** If acute, hospitalize for evaluation; bronchoscopy followed by beta-adrenergic nebulizer treatment and chest physiotherapy; if long-standing, may develop bronchiectasis and lung abscess.

▶ Health Maintenance Issues

Monitoring small objects, toys, and food.

## I. Bronchiolitis

▶ Scientific Concepts

Most common outbreaks in winter and spring in children < 2 years of age; RSV most common, followed by parainfluenza, influenza, adenovirus, *M. pneumoniae, Chlamydia trachomatis, C. pneumoniae, Ureaplasma,* and *Pneumocystis* which is least common.

▶ History & Physical

With RSV, 1–2 days of fever, rhinorrhea, cough then wheezing, tachypnea, respiratory distress with shallow breathing, nasal flaring, cyanosis, retractions, rales/rhonchi.

▶ Diagnostic Studies

Mild lymphocytosis, CXR with hyperinflation, diffuse interstitial infiltrates.

▶ Clinical Therapeutics

Most managed as outpatients by supportive therapy; oxygen guided by results of pulse oximetry; hydration; hospitalization required for < 2 months of age or hypoxemia on room air, apnea, underlying chronic cardiopulmonary disorders; beta-adrenergics and corticosteroids are controversial; rapid diagnostic testing for RSV permits early intervention; antiviral, ribavirin, used in severe cases; Palivizumab (monoclonal anti-RSV antibody) or RSV-IVIG (RSV intravenous immune globulin) are used for prophylaxis for high-risk children, but are expensive and do not treat active infection.

## J. Cystic Fibrosis

▶ Scientific Concepts

Most common lethal genetic disease in United States; incidence 1:3,000 to 1:2,500 among Caucasians; inherited in autosomal recessive manner; median survival ~ 29 years; disorder of exocrine glandular dysfunction characterized by chronic pulmonary disease, pancreatic insufficiency, and intestinal malabsorption.

▶ History & Physical

At birth, 17% with meconium ileus and 50% with failure to thrive and/or respiratory compromise; frequent respiratory infections with *S. aureus,* later with *P. aeruginosa* and *Burkholderia cepacia,* productive cough, wheezing, tachypnea, rales, digital clubbing, decreased exercise tolerance, pulmonary function abnormalities, nasal polyps. Other system involvement includes GI with abdominal distention; bulky, greasy stools; flatulence; hypoalbuminemia; edema; hepatomegaly; intestinal blockage from inspissated stools; rarely portal hypertension; cor pulmonale (late complication with poor prognosis).

► **Diagnostic Studies**

Gold standard is quantitative pilocarpine iontophoretic sweat test with sweat chloride > 60 meq/L; identified presence of cystic fibrosis transmembrane conductance regulator (CFTR) gene on long arm of chromosome 7 that codes for CFTR protein; elevated immunoreactive trypsinogen; pulmonary function tests.

► **Clinical Therapeutics**

Pancreatic enzyme supplementations for GI, no dietary restrictions. For respiratory, chest physical therapy, antibiotics, bronchodilators, anti-inflammatory agents, recombinant human DNAase inhalations. Gene therapy trials underway for agents to restore CFTR function.

► **Health Maintenance Issues**

Improvement of prognosis with specialized treatment centers and comprehensive, progressive treatment programs. Lung transplant for end-stage treatment is acceptable. Gene therapy trials being developed. Prenatal genetic testing for families with known genotype. Immunizations are critical including annual influenza vaccine.

## K. Pneumonia

► **Scientific Concepts**

*Viral:* RSV, parainfluenza, and influenza for > 75% of infections; few varicella-zoster virus.

*Mycoplasmal:* Two- to 3-week incubation; onset of symptoms is slow; mainly *M. pneumoniae* ("walking pneumonia"); most common in school children and adolescents.

*Hypersensitivity:* Exposure to birds/bird droppings or organic dusts such as moldy hay, compost, tree bark, aerosols.

*Bacterial:* *S. pneumoniae, H. influenzae*-nontypeable, *S. aureus.*

► **History & Physical**

*Viral:* Preceded by URI, wheezing, stridor; cough, retractions, grunting, nasal flaring, rales, decreased breath sounds may not distinguish from bacterial pneumonia.

*Mycoplasmal:* Classic prodrome of fever, headache, malaise, sore throat followed by dyspnea and cough (sputum production later); associated with otitis media, bullous myringitis. Upon exam: rales, decreased breath sounds, dullness to percussion. Complications include autoimmune hemolytic anemia, coagulation defects, thrombocytopenia, cerebral infarction, Guillain–Barré syndrome, cranial nerve involvement, psychosis, erythema multiforme, Stevens–Johnson syndrome.

*Hypersensitivity:* Episodic cough/fever; chronic exposure with weight loss, fatigue, dyspnea, cyanosis, death.

*S. pneumoniae:* Abrupt onset of fever, chills, chest pain, and dyspnea; restlessness; respiratory distress with diminished breath sounds, crackles, dullness on affected side, and possible pleural friction rubs; most common in child with sickle cell disease due to impaired splenic function.

*H. influenzae:* No unique findings.

*S. aureus:* High fever, rapid progression of respiratory distress with toxic-appearing child, possible abdominal distension; formation of pneumatoceles and empyema.

▶ Diagnostic Studies

*Viral:* Mild leukocytosis, rapid viral diagnostic tests, CXR with perihilar streaking, increased interstitial markings, patchy bronchopneumonia, lobar consolidation, hyperinflation, pneumatoceles with adenovirus.

*Mycoplasmal:* CBC and differential normal, cold hemagglutinin titer > 1:64 supports diagnosis; CXR with interstitial or bronchopneumonic infiltrates in middle or lower lobes.

*Hypersensitivity:* Eosinophilia, obstruction on pulmonary function test acutely, restrictive chronically.

*S. pneumoniae:* Leukocytosis, positive blood cultures, CXR with lobar consolidation.

*H. influenzae:* CXR with lobar consolidation; positive tracheal, blood, urine, or pleural fluid cultures.

*S. aureus:* CXR with pneumatoceles, empyema, and pyopneumothorax; often unilateral (right) lung involvement; positive blood, pleural fluid, or bronchial washings.

▶ Diagnosis

*Viral:* Asthma, airway obstruction by foreign-body aspiration, viral/bacterial tracheitis or parasitic disease.

*Hypersensitivity:* Asthma, collagen-vascular or immunologic or interstitial disease.

▶ Clinical Therapeutics

*Viral:* Supportive care, respiratory isolation; high-risk infants with severe RSV disease treat with ribavirin; varicella-zoster virus susceptible administer varicella-zoster immune globulin on exposure and treat with acyclovir.

*Mycoplasmal:* Treat dehydration; antipyretics; erythromycin is treatment of choice, clarithromycin or azithromycin are alternatives.

*Hypersensitivity:* Elimination of precipitant, corticosteroids.

*S. pneumoniae:* Oral (PO) penicillin or erythromycin or clindamycin is effective but second-generation cephalosporin is standard of care; IV cefuroxime or ceftriaxone or cefotaxime plus PO/IV macrolide in child > 4 years.

*H. influenzae:* IV cefuroxime or cefotaxime.

*S. aureus:* Hospitalize, obtain cultures then treat with penicillinase-resistant penicillin; drainage of empyema or pyopneumothorax; contact isolation.

▶ Health Maintenance Issues

*Viral:* Most recover, but death possible if underlying cardiorespiratory disease or immunodeficiency disease or superimposed bacterial pneumonia.

*Mycoplasmal:* Excellent recovery if no extrapulmonary complications.

## L. Asthma

▶ Scientific Concepts

Most common chronic childhood illness, affects 5–15% of population; increased in boys until onset of puberty then equalizes; airflow obstruction is partially reversible; triggers include URI, allergic reactivity (mold, dust mites, animal dander, cockroaches), cigarette smoke, air pollutants, exercise, rapid change in barometric pressure, psychologic factors; aspirin and food are uncommon precipitators; "atopic triad" is eczema, seasonal rhinitis, and asthma; atopy is strongest predisposing factor.

▶ History & Physical

Wheezing is most characteristic sign but may occur in absence with "cough variant," shortness of breath, prolonged cough, dyspnea, excessive secretions, "noisy" breathing. Examination with prolongation of expiration; wheezes: higher pitched with increasing obstruction and silence with poor air exchange; rhonchi; intercostal and suprasternal retractions; nasal flaring; restlessness and apprehension; cyanosis of lips and nail beds with underlying hypoxia; tachycardia and pulsus paradoxus.

▶ Diagnostic Studies

Decreased peak expiratory flow rates (PEFR) on pulmonary function test, leukocytosis, elevated Hct, eosinophils accumulate in sputum, respiratory acidosis and metabolic acidosis signify imminent respiratory failure; CXR with bilateral hyperinflation, flattening of diaphragm, patchy atelectasis.

▶ Diagnosis

Bronchiolitis, foreign body aspiration, congenital structural anomalies, bronchopneumonia, croup, pertussis, cystic fibrosis. Chronic sinusitis, GER, and rhinitis may increase severity.

▶ Clinical Therapeutics

Choice of therapy based on clinical features prior to treatment: mild intermittent, mild persistent, moderate persistent, and severe persistent; low-dose inhaled corticosteroids for mild persistent asthma; low-to-medium dose inhaled corticosteroids and long-acting beta-2-agonists for moderate persistent asthma; preferred strategy: initiate at high level to gain control then step down; medications classified as quick-relief (short-acting inhaled beta-2-agonist, albuterol, or levalbuterol) and long-term control (cromolyn sodium, nedocromil sodium, inhaled corticosteroids, and leukotriene modifiers); if not controlled, then add long-acting inhaled beta-2-agonist (salmeterol, formoterol) or alternative, but not preferred, sustained-release theophylline; maintain oxygen saturation > 95%; allergan immunotherapy. If admitted to hospital: IV hydration, moisturized oxygen, monitor potassium, inhaled beta-2-agonist, ipratropium bromide and systemic corticosteroids (prednisone, prednisolone, methylprednisolone), antibiotics if co-existing bacterial infection; intubation if impending respiratory arrest.

► Health Maintenance Issues

Avoid allergens (mold, dust mites, animal dander, cockroaches, tobacco smoke) and aggravating factors (exertion outdoors with high levels of air pollution); environment control measures (encase mattress/ pillow, cleanse bed linens frequently, low indoor humidity, remove carpet/upholstered furniture); educate patient/family/school personnel about triggers, gaging disease activity and step-wise care plan; peak flow meters at home; close follow-up as significant morbidity and mortality if lack of appropriate care; exercise encouraged; annual influenza vaccine; referral to asthma specialist if severe disease or multiple hospital visits.

# IX. MUSCULOSKELETAL AND RHEUMATOLOGIC DISORDERS

## A. Scoliosis

► Scientific Concepts

Lateral curvature of spine, coronal plane deformity ($> 15°$ coronal curve); right thoracic curve is most common; usually discovered on routine exam.

► History & Physical

Idiopathic: most common (75–80%) are structural; five times more common in females; occurs during growth spurt; curve may progress if onset before menarche; classically painless, but if painful, consider other causes (e.g., bone tumor, spondylolisthesis, spondylolysis); usually asymptomatic, but if severe, curvature may lead to impaired pulmonary function. Upon examination, asymmetry of shoulder heights, scapular prominence or position, uneven waistline or pelvic levelness, flexion at waist to angle of $90°$ accentuates curvature and rotational deformity of spine, characteristic rib hump is apparent on convex side of curve in thoracic scoliosis, fully expose back to include observation for café-au-lait spots or midline skin defects associated with underlying spinal lesions, complete neurologic exam.

► Diagnostic Studies

X-ray using erect thoracoabdominal spinal view to determine Cobb angle (geometric measurement of severity of curve).

► Diagnosis

Congenital associated cardiac and renal anomalies. Neuromuscular associated with cerebral palsy, poliomyelitis, muscular dystrophy, Friedreich's ataxia.

► Clinical Intervention

Idiopathic with $< 20°$ curve, monitor progression (serial exams every 4–6 months); $> 20°$ curve requires bracing in growing child to prevent progression; if $> 40°$ curve, surgical correction (Harrington rod or posterior spinal fusion). Congenital not braceable; if progressive, needs surgery. Paralytic is progressive and not braceable; surgery may be indicated.

► Health Maintenance Issues

Routine screening at health maintenance exam to detect early curvature allowing for bracing to cease progression of curvature. If severe and left untreated, may result in cardiopulmonary impairment or cosmetic deformity.

## B. Osgood–Schlatter Disease

► Scientific Concepts

Related to adolescent growth spurt and/or repetitive microtrauma, usually sports related.

► History & Physical

More common in boys, typically 10–15 years of age; painful swelling over tibial tubercle with occasional avulsion of patellar tendon at insertion of tibia; > 50% bilateral; activity worsens symptoms.

► Diagnostic Studies

X-ray normal or may show fragmentation of tibial tubercle, soft-tissue swelling.

► Diagnosis

Other fractures, arthritis, infections, neoplasms.

► Clinical Therapeutics

Rest, restrict activity, nonsteroidal anti-inflammatory drugs (NSAIDs), quadriceps stretching and strengthening.

► Health Maintenance Issues

Self-limited, symptoms resolve with skeletal maturity.

## C. Legg–Calvé–Perthes Disease (LCPD)

► Scientific Concepts

Idiopathic juvenile avascular necrosis of femoral head; idiopathic with capital femoral epiphysis becomes avascular, then is reabsorbed, then later revascularized. Most common in males (ratio 5:1) ages 4–8 years; associated with low birth weight, delayed bone age, short stature.

► History & Physical

Acutely, slowly progressive limp with hip pain referred to groin, inner thigh, or knee, which is aggravated by internal rotation/abduction and relieved by rest. Later in disease, painless limp more common.

► Diagnostic Studies

X-ray (anteroposterior and frog-leg views). Early stage: negative or widening of joint space; later stage: increased density of femoral head, radiolucency near epiphysis, flattening of femoral head. Radionucleotide bone scans useful if early x-rays are negative. Joint aspirates are normal.

► Diagnosis

Transient synovitis of the hip, osteomyelitis, septic arthritis, juvenile rheumatoid arthritis.

► Clinical Intervention

Supportive care, goal of treatment is to maintain full joint mobility and prevent deformity of femoral head. Bracing is not beneficial; surgery in severe cases.

▶ Health Maintenance Issues

Better prognosis with less femoral head involvement and younger age (< 6 years) at onset.

## D. Slipped Capital Femoral Epiphysis (SCFE)

▶ Scientific Concepts

Capital femoral epiphysis slips off metaphysis through growth plate; most common in obese, adolescent males; etiology unknown; may be related to hormonal factors that lessen bone's ability to resist shearing forces; associated with irradiation for malignancy, endocrine, and metabolic disorders.

▶ History & Physical

Insidious limp often occurring following trauma to hip; intermittent or constant pain referred into thigh or medial side of knee; examination with limitation of internal rotation of hip with localized tenderness and hip flexion contracture.

▶ Diagnostic Studies

Anteroposterior and frog-leg lateral views of hip show widening of physis (growth plate) and increased density (blush sign) over proximal metaphysis, epiphysis slipping posteriorly and inferiorly with respect to neck of femur ("like ice cream falling off a cone").

▶ Clinical Intervention

Surgical and emergency surgery if abrupt slippage of proximal femur.

▶ Health Maintenance Issues

Long-term prognosis is guarded due to overstress of hip from being overweight. Monitor limb lengths. Complications are leading cause of degenerative hip joint disease in adults.

## E. In-Toeing and Out-Toeing

▶ Scientific Concepts

Rotational problems of lower extremities.

***In-toeing:*** Infants commonly have metatarsus adductus and metatarsus varus (rotation of foot), toddlers (12–24 months of age) have medial tibial torsion (tibia), young children (3–5 years) have medial femoral torsion/femoral anteverison (femur).

***Out-toeing:*** Physiologic in infants arises from rotation of hip; lateral tibial torsion in childhood arises from rotation of tibia; may be from intrauterine positioning except for femoral origin.

▶ History & Physical

Often positive family medical history; determine age of onset, developmental milestones as may be sign of underlying neuromuscular/neurologic disorder; upon exam assess gait, rotational profile: foot progression angle (with foot, curved lateral border of foot, may be flexible or rigid); with tibia inward, foot/thigh angle; with femur, increased inward hip rotation. Lab tests unnecessary.

▶ Clinical Intervention

Most metatarsus adductus resolve spontaneously; for metatarsus varus, refer to orthopedist for serial casting followed by corrective shoes or inserts, rarely surgery; medial tibial torsion corrects with time unless > 10 years of age, then possible surgery; medial femoral torsion/femoral anteversion usually no treatment, if > 10 years of age with severe gait disturbance refer to orthopedist for surgery; physiologic out-toeing spontaneous resolution by 18 months of age; severe lateral tibial torsion requires surgery.

## F. Developmental Dysplasia of Hip (DDH)

▶ Scientific Concepts

More common in first-born, Caucasian, female (ratio of 8:1), via breech presentation, with left hip (60%); associated with congenital torticollis, metatarsus adductus, clubfoot, skull or facial abnormalities; mechanical, physiologic, genetic, hormonal, environmental factors as etiology.

▶ History & Physical

Classic signs: positive Ortolani (hip clunk) and Barlow tests (examiner attempts to dislocate femur) in a newborn; positive Galeazzi's sign (compares level of knees when patient flat on bed with legs flexed), asymmetric gluteal/thigh folds, and limitation of hip abduction in a child; once child walking, obvious signs are limping, toe-walking, waddling gait.

▶ Diagnostic Studies

Ultrasound (preferred) confirms diagnosis revealing flat, shallow acetabulum and delayed ossification of femoral head. In infants < 6 months of age, cartilaginous joint not visible on x-ray.

▶ Clinical Intervention

Pavlik harness in newborn; closed or open reduction with spica cast if > 6 months of age.

▶ Health Maintenance Issues

Prognosis dependent upon age of diagnosis, "the earlier the better"; if missed or delayed diagnosis, possible severe degenerative hip disease.

## G. Foot Abnormalities

*Talipes equinovarus (clubfoot):* Not rotational deformity, but pathologic with deformity and hypoplasia of talus and tarsal bones; may be from intrauterine positioning or molding; isolated deformity or associated with neuromuscular anomalies; requires intervention at birth with manipulation, serial casting, and surgery within first year of life.

*Calcaneovalgus foot:* Common, due to intrauterine position; dorsum of foot lies on tibia; resolves with stretching.

*Congenital vertical talus:* Rare, associated with trisomy 18, "rocker-bottom" deformity, serial castings and surgery to treat.

*Pes planus (flat feet):* Flexible flat foot is usually benign; rigid may be associated with neurological disease, arthritis, trauma, infection, congenital vertical talus, tumors; orthotics not necessary unless leg pain present.

## H. Fracture Facts

▶ Scientific Concepts

Four developmental regions of bone: diaphysis (shaft of bone), metaphysis (flared region of bone at end of diaphysis), physis (region of growth cartilage), epiphysis (end of bone that was initially cartilaginous). Physeal (growth plate) and metaphyseal fractures are most common in children. Clavicle, distal radius, distal ulna are most frequent sites. Growth plate fractures are classified by Salter–Harris method: Type I, epiphysis and metaphysis separate without displacement; Type II, fragment of metaphysis splits with epiphysis; Type III, partial plate fracture of physis and epiphysis to joint surface when growth plate partially fused; Type IV, extensive fracture of epiphysis, physis, metaphysis and joint surface; Type V, crush injury to physis. Pathologic fractures often secondary to bone cysts. Colles' fracture, distal radius fracture, seen in young child from fall on outstretched arms. Boxer's fracture, distal fifth metacarpal fracture, typically seen after teenager punches object in anger. In adolescent with wrist trauma, scaphoid is commonly fractured leading to "snuffbox" tenderness with high risk for nonunion or avascular necrosis. Visibility of posterior fat pad on elbow x-ray is indicative of bleeding, inflammation, or fracture.

## I. Juvenile Rheumatoid Arthritis (JRA)

► **Scientific Concepts**

Defined as onset < 16 years of age with persistent synovitis in one or more joints for > 6 weeks excluding other forms of juvenile arthritis; cardinal feature of synovitis is morning stiffness for > 15 minutes; varied presentation secondary to immunologic, genetic, and environmental factors.

► **History & Physical**

Three major patterns based upon presentation in first 6 months of disease. *Pauciarticular* (oligoarticular): most common accounting for 40–60%, female predominance, characterized by chronic arthritis in ≤ four joints, insidious onset, asymptomatic iridocyclitis. *Polyarticular:* chronic pain and swelling of ≥ five joints in scattered or symmetric fashion that commonly involves cervical spine, hips, shoulders, and temporomandibular joints; insidious onset with fatigue; perhaps low-grade fever, rheumatoid nodules, weight loss; female predominance; subtype division with positive rheumatoid factor (RF) seen in adolescents without iridocyclitis or with negative RF seen in children (3–9 years of age) with iridocyclitis; arthritis waxes and wanes. *Systemic onset* (Still's disease): affects 10–20% of either gender of children; hallmark of spiking fever daily or twice daily, accompanied by salmon-pink macular rash, preceding arthritis of variable joint involvement; other manifestations are hepatosplenomegaly, leukocytosis, polyserositis; do not develop iridocyclitis; remission within a year.

► **Diagnostic Studies**

No diagnostic test for JRA; RF-positive in ~ 15%; ANA positive with pauciarticular, ESR nonspecific; joint fluid aspirate with 5,000–60,000 white blood cells (WBCs), mostly neutrophils, distinguishes from infectious; x-ray not diagnostic, may have soft-tissue swelling, regional osteoporosis; MRI with early joint damage.

► **Diagnosis**

Orthopedic condition (avascular necrosis, slipped capital femoral epiphysis, Osgood–Schlatter disease), reactive arthritis (rheumatic fever), infections (osteomyelitis, Lyme disease, parvovirus), collagen-vascular disease, malignancy (leukemia, neuroblastoma, bone tumor), psychological.

► Clinical Therapeutics

NSAIDs are drugs of choice; second-line agent is methotrexate; injectable gold salts, corticosteroid injections, joint replacement are options in selected patients; combinations of drugs may be necessary; physical therapy (range of motion and muscle strengthening); joint casting is never indicated; iridocyclitis should be treated by ophthalmologist.

► Health Maintenance Issues

Worse prognosis with progression from pauciarticular to polyarticular, presence of positive RF or ANA, persistent synovitis, hip involvement; mortality is rare.

## J. Kawasaki Disease

► Scientific Concepts

Leading cause of acquired heart disease in children in developed countries; affects children < 5 years, boys > girls; greater in Asians.

► History & Physical

Well-established clinical criteria: fever > 40°C for 5 days, unresponsive to antibiotics, *and* four of the following: extremity changes—palmar/plantar erythema, indurative edema, or desquamation of hands/feet; nonvesicular polymorphous exanthem—primarily on trunk and perineum; lymphadenopathy—cervical, unilateral, > 1.5 cm, firm, nonfluctuant; mucosal changes—injected or dry fissured lips, "strawberry tongue," erythema of oropharyngeal mucosa; conjunctival injection—bilateral bulbar, nonexudative. Other symptoms include extreme irritability, abdominal pain, diarrhea, vomiting, anterior uveitis, arthralgias/arthritis, aseptic meningitis, hepatic dysfunction.

► Diagnostic Studies

Elevation of platelet count, ESR, C-reactive protein (CRP), alpha-1-antitrypsin, IgE; normocytic/normochromic anemia; sterile pyuria. Evaluate with ECHO for coronary artery aneurysm, with ECG for arrhythmias, with ultrasound for gallbladder hydrops.

► Diagnosis

Scarletina, measles, toxic shock syndrome, Rocky Mountain spotted fever, erythema multiforme.

► Clinical Therapeutics

IVIG 2 gm/kg over 10–12 hours in single dose and high-dose salicylates (100 mg/kg/d divided every 6 hours) for 14 days, then reduce dose (3–5 mg/kg/d) for 3 months if normal ECHO or indefinitely if coronary abnormalities.

► Clinical Intervention

Cardiac catheterization and bypass surgery may be required if evidence of myocardial ischemia or infarction.

► Health Maintenance Issues

Coronary artery dilatation and aneurysms are major complications (20%); serial ECHO is recommended.

## X. GENITOURINARY DISORDERS

### A. Hematuria

▶ Scientific Concepts

Microscopic: defined as three or more positive consecutive urine dipsticks for blood and five or more RBCs per high-power field (hpf) on centrifuged urine; common in school-aged child; twice as common in girls; majority of cases benign. Gross: large number of RBCs in urine resulting in red or brown colored urine; less common than microscopic.

▶ History & Physical

Determine positive family history for hematuria, renal disease, bleeding diathesis, hemolytic anemia, inborn errors of metabolism; question about trauma, recent skin infection, pharyngitis, dysuria, abdominal or flank pain. If microscopic hematuria present with dysuria or if gross hematuria with appearance of red or brown urine associated with flank/urethral pain, examine for rashes/petechiae/peripheral edema; check joints for arthritis; palpate for renal masses; check genitalia for trauma, mass, or rash; funduscopic for hypertensive changes; obtain blood pressure.

▶ Diagnostic Studies

First morning urine to differentiate upper/lower; if RBC casts, then ASO titer, ANA, C3 complement, CBC with differential and platelet count, BUN/creatinine, albumin; if no casts/bacteriuria, then CBC with differential and platelet count, urine culture and sensitivity, PT/PTT; sickle cell prep; renal ultrasound to rule out structural abnormalities and tumors; abdominal CT scan if history of trauma; CXR to evaluate for CHF; if family history significant for renal disease, obtain hearing screen; renal biopsy on selected cases for definitive etiology.

▶ Diagnosis

UTI, cystitis, urethritis, vaginitis, prostatitis, perineal irritation, meatal stenosis, trauma including insertion of foreign object into urethra/bladder, passage of renal stones, following vigorous exercise, glomerulonephritis, (acute poststreptococcal glomerulonephritis, IgA nephropathy, anaphylactoid purpura, hemolytic–uremic syndrome), hypercalciuria, hemolytic anemias, drug-induced hemolysis, mismatched blood transfusions, myoglobinuria secondary to rhabdomyolysis, varied drugs/dyes/pigments, sickle cell hemoglobinopathies and hemophilia. Rare causes include renal artery or vein thrombosis coagulopathies, tumors, and congenital obstructive uropathy.

▶ Clinical Intervention

Treat underlying disease.

### B. Proteinuria

▶ Scientific Concepts

Defined as random urine total protein-creatinine (Upr:Ucr) ratio > 0.25 or 24-hour urine protein > 4 mg/m$^2$/h or presence of > 1+ protein on dipstick on three occasions; small amount normally present; levels may increase with vigorous exercise, fever, heat/cold stress, trauma, or CHF.

► **History & Physical**

Question for recent fever, vigorous exercise, heat/cold stress, trauma. Morning periorbital edema, check height/weight for gain/loss, orthostatic blood pressure, impetigo to rule out strep infections, joints for swelling, ascites, organomegaly.

► **Diagnostic Studies**

If detected in asymptomatic patient, should be repeated. Gold standard is timed (24-hour) urine collection, orthostatic proteinuria with A.M./P.M. dipstick (A.M. negative/P.M. positive), Upr:Ucr ratio, electrolytes, BUN/creatinine, serum total protein and albumin, ANA, C3, C4, ASO titer, hepatitis B surface antigen (in populations at risk). Possible renal imaging and renal biopsy.

► **Diagnosis**

Four categories: physiologic or transient; orthostatic; glomerular (glomerulonephritis, IgA nephropathy, Alport syndrome, Henoch–Schonlein purpura, systemic lupus erythematosus, poststreptococcal); and tubular (Fanconi's syndrome, drug/heavy metals).

► **Health Maintenance Issues**

If abnormal 24-hour collection, refer to nephrologist. If physiologic/orthostatic, evaluate annually; no restrictions on physical activity, excellent long-term prognosis.

## C. Posterior Urethral Valves (PUV)

► **Scientific Concepts**

Rare, male only, congenital, prostatic urethra, bilateral hydronephrosis, and long-term renal insufficiency.

► **History & Physical**

Detected prenatally with ultrasound; at birth with distended bladder, palpable kidneys, UTI, renal insufficiency, poor stream; later with failure to thrive, vomiting, hematuria, enuresis, hesitancy.

► **Diagnostic Studies**

Ultrasound, VCUG is best.

► **Clinical Intervention**

Transurethral catheter, correction of underlying medical problems, transurethral ablation of valves, temporary vesicostomy.

► **Health Maintenance Issues**

Best predictor is decline of serum creatinine after treatment, renal failure and dialysis in those whose creatinine stays > 1.0, vesicoureteral reflux, voiding problems.

## D. Hypospadias

► **Scientific Concepts**

Most common congenital penile abnormality. Consider virilization disorder, familial tendency.

► **History & Physical**

Displacement of urethral meatus along ventral surface of glans, shaft (distal or proximal), or perineum; often with chordee (ventral band of fibrous tissue causing ventral curvature of penis); prepuce incompletely formed with thin or absent ventral skin and abundance of dorsal skin (dorsal hood).

▶ **Clinical Intervention**
Surgical at 6–18 months; usually one-step procedure; two-stage surgeries if severe form.

▶ **Health Maintenance Issues**
Delay neonatal circumcision.

## E. Vesicoureteral Reflux (VUR)

▶ **Scientific Concepts**
Retrograde flow of urine from bladder into ureters; graded on scale of I to V with stage V most severe; increases incidence of UTI.

▶ **Diagnostic Studies**
VCUG.

▶ **Clinical Intervention**
Low-dose prophylactic antibiotics (amoxicillin if < 2 months of age, otherwise trimethoprim and sulfamethoxazole [TMP-SMZ] or nitrofurantoin); urine cultures every 4 months and when febrile, repeat VCUG every 12–18 months until resolved; surgical (reimplantation of ureter) if severe grade of reflux (grade V) when ≥ 12 years of age.

▶ **Health Maintenance Issues**
Lower grades of reflux spontaneously resolve; increased incidence in siblings.

## F. Cryptorchidism

▶ **Scientific Concepts**
Undescended testes; 3–4% of full-term and 30% of preterm male newborns; 50% descended by 3 months of life and 80% by 12 months of age; most common genital problem in pediatric urology; predisposition with abnormalities in hypothalamic-pituitary-gonadal axis.

▶ **History & Physical**
Examination in warm environment, repetitive exams in multiple positions, palpable/nonpalpable.

▶ **Diagnostic Studies**
Plasma testosterone concentrations after hCG stimulation to confirm presence or absence of abdominal testes.

▶ **Diagnosis**
Retractile testes secondary to hyperactive cremasteric. Associated with recessive x-linked ichthyosis and Prader–Willi syndrome. If bilateral, evaluate for sex chromosome abnormalities such as fully virilized female with congenital adrenal hyperplasia.

▶ **Clinical Therapeutics**
Intramuscular hCG therapy is controversial.

▶ **Clinical Intervention**
Surgery at 6–18 months is treatment of choice.

▶ Health Maintenance Issues

At risk for infertility and testicular malignancy (seminoma is most common).

## G.  Urinary Tract Infections

▶ Scientific Concepts

One of most common pediatric infections; twice as frequent in females except during neonatal period when more common in males; incidence 10 times higher in uncircumcised than circumcised males; most common pathogens: *E. coli.* (80 to 90%), *Klebsiella pneumoniae, Enterobacter, Proteus mirabilis* (increased in males), *Pseudomonas,* group B *streptococcus* (neonates), and *Staphylococcus saprophyticus* (sexually active adolescents).

▶ History & Physical

In neonates: often nonspecific, fever or hypothermia, poor feeding, failure to thrive, jaundice, or sepsis. In infants: fever, irritability, or foul-smelling urine. In preschool children: fever, vomiting, abdominal pain, foul-smelling urine, incontinence, or dysuria. In school-aged children: classic signs of enuresis, frequency, urgency, dysuria, and often afebrile. Upper tract infections with constitutional symptoms of high fever, flank and back tenderness. Examine abdomen for masses/tenderness, genitalia for lesions. Measure blood pressure.

▶ Diagnostic Studies

Gold standard is urine culture; suprapubic aspirate or catheterized specimen for infants; clean-catch, midstream urine collection in older children who can void upon request; clean-bagged specimen is not reliable except to exclude if negative. After first diagnosis, VCUG and renal ultrasound to determine structural anomalies and VUR. Intravenous pyelogram (IVP) replaced by ultrasound. Routine use of nuclear scan is not recommended due to expense and radiation exposure.

▶ Clinical Therapeutics

Seven- to 10-day course of antibiotics with follow-up urine culture, prophylactic antibiotics if needed.

▶ Health Maintenance Issues

Refer to urologist if VCUG demonstrates VUR or obstructive anomalies.

## H.  Acute Poststreptococcal Glomerulonephritis

▶ Scientific Concepts

Most common postinfectious nephritis, possible genetic susceptibility, always preceded by group A beta-hemolytic streptococcal throat or skin infection with clinical glomerulonephritis 7 to 14 days later, primarily in school-aged children (5–15 years of age).

▶ History & Physical

Asymptomatic to renal failure; typical presenting symptoms are gross/microscopic hematuria, proteinuria with periorbital or peripheral edema, and hypertension. Other symptoms are oliguria and headache. Rarely CHF and encephalopathy are associated. Fever is not expected.

▶ **Diagnostic Studies**

Urinalysis with RBCs or RBC casts; elevated serum ASO titers or anti-deoxyribonuclease-B (anti-DNAase B) titers or anti-hyaluronidase titers (AHT), positive throat and/or skin cultures; depressed serum C3; BUN elevated disproportionately to creatinine; renal biopsy if progressively deteriorating renal function.

▶ **Diagnosis**

Benign hematuria, IgA nephropathy, hereditary nephritis, membranoproliferative glomerulonephritis, Henoch–Schonlein purpura, systemic lupus erythematosus.

▶ **Clinical Therapeutics**

Supportive, treat hypertension, reduce sodium intake, treatment with diuretics, antistreptococcal antibiotics for throat/skin infections, corticosteroids not beneficial.

▶ **Health Maintenance Issues**

Full recovery in > 95%; some with chronic renal failure; hematuria/proteinuria for up to 3 months or longer. If C3 elevated after 8 weeks, question diagnosis; suggestive of membranoproliferative glomerulonephritis.

## I. Ambiguous Genitalia

▶ **Scientific Concepts**

Intersex abnormality; classified as male/female pseudohermaphroditism or true hermaphroditism or gonadal dysgenesis; 1/4,000 live births.

▶ **History & Physical**

Question use of virilizing drugs during pregnancy, consanguinity, sterility, female hirsutism. Upon exam: variable, enlarged phallus, labioscrotal fusion, hyperpigmented labia, labial rugae, perineal hypospadias, inguinal hernia; look for nongenital dysmorphic features, palpate testes; hypospadias and cryptorchidism together associated with intersex disorder 50% of time.

▶ **Diagnostic Studies**

Karyotype, serum 17-hydroxyprogesterone, urine 17-ketosteroids and pregnanetriol, sex steroids, electrolytes if suspect congenital adrenal hyperplasia (CAH), pelvic ultrasound for müllerian structures, pelvic CT/MRI for gonads, genitography to visualize duct structures.

▶ **Diagnosis**

CAH, adrenogenital syndrome, chromosomal mosaicism, maternal androgen ingestion, biochemical defects.

▶ **Clinical Therapeutics**

Hormonal supplementation to include cortisol for CAH, testosterone or estrogen at puberty; surgical procedures after medical treatment.

▶ **Health Maintenance Issues**

Excellent prognosis; undiagnosed and untreated CAH may lead to neonatal shock and death; interdisciplinary team approach; discuss gender assignment; females with amenorrhea/sterility.

## XI. PSYCHOLOGICAL AND DEVELOPMENTAL PROBLEMS

### A. Mental Retardation

▶ Scientific Concepts

Onset < 18 years of age; IQ < 70 on Wechsler Intelligence Scale; most common preventable cause is iodine deficiency; etiologies include chromosomal, CNS abnormalities, multiple congenital anomaly syndromes, inborn errors of metabolism, idiopathic.

▶ History & Physical

Cardinal symptom is delayed developmental milestones; syndromic appearance including craniofacial malformations; seizures; behavioral difficulty adapting; early personality changes.

▶ Diagnostic Studies

Developmental assessment, screen hearing and vision, full psychological evaluation, three-generation pedigrees, chromosome or DNA testing, metabolic screen, neuroimaging if neurologic symptoms, electroencephalogram (EEG).

▶ Diagnosis

Autism, progressive neurologic disorder.

▶ Health Maintenance Issues

Treat associated problems, impact on families (refer to parent support groups), education (vocational training), rehabilitation, protection.

### B. Attention Deficit Hyperactivity Disorder (ADHD)

▶ Scientific Concepts

Most common neurobehavioral disorder characterized by inattention, impulsivity, hyperactivity; 3–5% of school-aged children; increased in males; genetic link with high rate of heritability.

▶ History & Physical

Symptoms persist > 6 months without associated psychosis, onset prior to age 7 years, evident in more than two settings, especially at school, clinical diagnosis based on parent/child interviews, neurological exam may be normal.

▶ Diagnostic Studies

Conners' Parent and Teacher Rating Scales or ADHD Rating Scale IV or Child Behavior Checklist by Achenbach are used to measure baseline symptoms and monitor progress.

▶ Diagnosis

Parents or teachers who are inexperienced or overly critical may provide ADHD history for child. Other disorders that may mimic include specific developmental disorders, anxiety, affective disorder, hyperthyroidism, drugs, or obstructive sleep apnea.

▶ Clinical Therapeutics

Therapy prior to or concurrent with first-line psychostimulants—methylphenidate (Ritalin or Concerta), dextroamphetamine (Dexedrine), dextroamphetamine in combo with amphetamine (Adderall). Pemoline (Cylert) is no longer recommended due to associated liver failure. Secondary medications are tricyclic antidepressants (bupropion and venlafaxine), alpha-2 adrenergic agonists (clonidine and guanfacine).

▶ **Clinical Intervention**
Multimodal approach: behavior modification, family education/ counseling, educational interventions (preferential front-row seating, small teacher–student ratio).

▶ **Health Maintenance Issues**
Prognosis better with higher intellect.

## C. Autism

▶ **Scientific Concepts**
Rare, increased in males, onset before age 3 years, 75% function at mental retardation level, strong familial component, possible genetic association.

▶ **History & Physical**
Qualitative impairment in social interaction and communication and repetitive stereotypical patterns of behavior, rituals, or mannerisms; infants fail to make eye contact or delayed social smile; impaired imitation; language delay or echolalic/nonsensical speech; self-injurious behavior.

▶ **Diagnostic Studies**
Checklist for Autism in Toddlers (CHAT) administered at 18 months of age, reliable specificity; vision and hearing screen.

▶ **Diagnosis**
Mental retardation, metabolic disorders, fragile X syndrome, Rett syndrome.

▶ **Health Maintenance Issues**
Incurable, behavior modification, sensory integration intervention, limited success with medication, most require lifelong support/ supervision.

## D. Child Abuse and Neglect

▶ **Scientific Concepts**
Nonaccidental physical/psychological/sexual harm and/or physical/ emotional neglect; wide spectrum from obvious trauma to failure to thrive; increasing frequency; social risk factors in abusive families include poverty, violence, psychiatric illness, substance abuse.

▶ **History & Physical**
Family stress, unrealistic expectations of child by caregiver, discrepant history of injury or unknown injury, delay in seeking care, previous inadequate medical care, interview child alone if possible; note growth and state of hygiene; retinal hemorrhages and full fontanel with shaken baby syndrome; burns, especially cigarette or immersion-type without splash marks on perineum/buttocks; patterned bruises (bites, belt, looped cord) or over soft tissue instead of boney prominences; withdrawn or

explosive personality; long bone fractures in preambulatory infants; genital trauma or sexually transmitted disease; child disclosure of sexually assault.

▶ Diagnostic Studies

Funduscopic; x-rays—extremities, skull, sternum, scapula, and posterior/anterior ribs (side-to-side thorax compression); spiral fractures or metaphyseal chip fractures (forceful jerking of extremity); skeletal survey shows multiple fractures in different stages of healing; CT scan and MRI if head injury; CBC with differential and platelets, PT/PTT; pregnancy test if postmenarchal; evidence kit for sexual assault; often negative exam for sexual assault.

▶ Diagnosis

Platelet disorders, leukemia with bruising, rickets, osteogenesis imperfecta with fractures, SIDS, neuroblastoma, Crohn's disease mistaken for sexual abuse.

▶ Clinical Intervention

Protection of child is priority; stabilize existing and immediate environment. Medical stabilization and psychosocial investigation. Mandatory reporting of suspected maltreatment to child protective services.

▶ Health Maintenance Issues

Variable prognosis; psychological counseling.

## XII. NEUROLOGICAL PROBLEMS

### A. Febrile Seizures

▶ Scientific Concepts

Criteria: fever > 38.8°C, 3 months to 5 years of age, and non-CNS infection; 2–5% of children; familial preponderance.

*Simple:* Brief (< 15 minutes), solitary event, generalized, tonic–clonic seizure associated with febrile illness without CNS infection or neurologic etiology.

*Complex:* Lengthy (> 15 minutes), focal, extended, or multiple attacks within 24 hours, abnormal neurologic exam; fever may cause solitary seizure in patient without seizure disorder or may provoke seizure in patient with seizure disorder.

▶ History & Physical

Rapid onset of fever, tonic–clonic posturing, normal neurological exam if simple febrile seizure or abnormal if complex febrile seizure.

▶ Diagnostic Studies

EEG not indicated for simple febrile seizure; strongly consider lumbar puncture (LP) if < 12 months of age; MRI and CT scan low yield if simple febrile seizure but if complex febrile seizure shows possible structural lesion.

▶ Diagnosis

CNS infection, structural or metabolic disease, epilepsy.

► Clinical Therapeutics

Prophylactic antipyretics and/or anticonvulsants not given for solitary febrile seizure; if > 5-minute duration, manage as status epilepticus: secure airway, draw blood, start IV, administer lorazepam.

► Health Maintenance Issues

Treating febrile seizures does not decrease risk of afebrile seizures; educate about benign nature of seizure; 30% recurrence rate.

## B. Weakness

► Scientific Concepts

Paresis or impaired strength, static versus evolving weakness, central (produces hemiplegia) versus peripheral (weakness of extension), proximal (muscle disorder or myopathy) versus distal (peripheral nerve disorder or polyneuropathy), upper versus lower motor neuron.

► History & Physical

In older children, upper motor neuron lesions with spasticity, hyperreflexia, Babinski and lower motor neuron lesions with hypotonia, hyporeflexia, but in infancy may have overlap of symptoms; also cortical thumb, persistent primitive reflexes; Gower maneuver (hip-girdle).

► Diagnosis

Cerebral palsy, myelitis, spina bifida, polio, spinal muscle atrophy, inflammatory, myasthenia gravis, hereditary polyneuropathies, infantile botulism, muscular dystrophy.

► Diagnostic Studies

Electromyography/nerve conduction velocity (EMG/NCV), biopsy.

► Clinical Therapeutics

Treat underlying cause.

## C. Abnormal Head Size

► Scientific Concepts

Brain growth drives skull growth, head size is two or more standard deviations below (microcephaly) or above (macrocephaly) the norm for age; premature closure of cranial sutures with microcephaly, bulging fontanels seen with hydrocephalus, intracranial tumors, or arachnoid cysts.

► History & Physical

Serial measurements with tape measure over occipital, parietal, and frontal prominences, plot on growth charts; transillumination for macrocephaly; measure head circumference of parents.

► Diagnosis

**Microcephaly:** Chromosomal abnormalities, infections (intrauterine-TORCH or perinatal), radiation, toxemia, familial, perinatal hypoxia, metabolic, Tay–Sachs disease, craniosynostosis.

**Macrocephaly:** Increased ICP caused by hydrocephalus, subdural hematomas, tumors or may be benign. Megalencephaly (large brain) may cause benign familial, neurofibromatosis, achondroplasia, Soto's syndrome, or fibrous dysplasia (thickened skull).

► Diagnostic Studies

TORCH screen, IgM, urine culture, serum and urine amino and organic acids, MRI or CT scan for microcephaly. MRI or CT scan or cranial ultrasound (if anterior fontanel open) for macrocephaly.

► Clinical Intervention

Surgical for some macrocephaly and microcephaly, treat underlying disorder, supportive for microcephaly.

► Health Maintenance Issues

Advise genetic counseling, mental retardation often with microcephaly.

## D. Bacterial Meningitis

► Scientific Concepts

Most common pathogens: group B streptococci, *E. coli*, *Listeria monocytogenes*, *H. influenzae* type b, coagulase-negative staphylococci, Enterobacteriaceae for 0–1 month; *S. pneumoniae*, *N. meningitidis*, *H. influenzae* type b, group B streptococci, Enterobacteriaceae for 1–23 months; *N. meningitidis*, *S. pneumoniae*, *H. influenzae* type b for > 2 years.

► History & Physical

Headache; meningeal irritation: nuchal rigidity (stiff neck) and positive Kernig and Brudzinski signs, fever or hypothermia, hyperirritability, seizures, focal sensory/motor changes indicative of infarct; papilledema and cranial nerve abnormalities (especially sixth cranial nerve) in older children; bulging fontanel or increasing head circumference in infants.

► Diagnostic Studies

CBC with differential; blood culture; chemistry panel; obtain CSF for chemistry/cell count/Gram stain/culture (after intracranial mass is ruled out), expect increased polymorphonuclear leukocytes, elevated protein, decreased glucose (with viral, expect no or mild leukocytosis, elevated protein, and normal glucose); CT or MRI to rule out intracranial masses and show meningeal inflammation; EEG nonspecific.

► Clinical Therapeutics

Early aggressive, supportive therapy; hydrate at two thirds maintenance; correct electrolytes, acidosis, nothing by mouth. Empiric broad-spectrum antibiotics until Gram stain/culture returned: cefotaxime, ampicillin if < 3 months; ceftriaxone, cefotaxime, or ampicillin plus chloramphenicol for > 3 months, add vancomycin or rifampin if *S. pneumoniae* not ruled out; duration of therapy is 7 days for meningococcal, 10 days for *H. influenzae* type b or pneumococcal, and 14–21 days for neonatal meningitis with group B streptococci and *L. monocytogenes*. With *H. influenzae* type b, early addition of dexamethasone may decrease sensorineural hearing loss.

► Health Maintenance Issues

Seizures, brain abscess, subdural effusions, cerebral edema are complications; long-term effects include blindness, hearing loss, seizures, hydrocephalus, cranial nerve deficits, mental retardation, behavioral problems. Prevention with chemoprophylaxis of susceptible individuals exposed to index patient, active immunization (*H. influenzae* type b and *S. pneumoniae*), and patient isolation. Dramatic reduction of *H. influenzae* type b due to conjugate vaccine.

## E. Cerebral Palsy

▶ **Scientific Concepts**

Static, nonprogressive motor and postural disorder of cerebral or cerebellar origin; increased in small-for-gestational-age infants; causes included intrauterine hypoxia/bleeding, infections (intrauterine/extrauterine), toxins, congenital malformations, kernicterus, stroke, trauma, genetic.

▶ **History & Physical**

Impaired function of voluntary muscles—75% spastic or pyramidal (upper motor neuron lesion), 15% ataxic (cerebellar lesion), 5% dyskinetic or extrapyramidal (basal ganglia lesion), rarely hypotonic, any combination of limbs affected. Associated with mental retardation, seizures, behavioral/emotional problems, speech/language/sensory perception/vision/hearing deficits. Examination with variable findings, "clasp knife" rigidity (spastic), hyperreflexia, ataxia, decreased fine motor voluntary responses, clonus, extensor/plantar responses, possible contractures, "floppy infant," microcephaly, smaller hand/foot.

▶ **Diagnostic Studies**

No routine studies, EEG, urine screening for amino and organic acidurias, serum amino acids, IgG and IgM antibodies, cranial ultrasound (most useful in premature), MRI (most useful in full term), CT scan to understand cerebral injury.

▶ **Diagnosis**

Progressive neurological change is *not* cerebral palsy; consider other neurological/metabolic disorders.

▶ **Clinical Intervention**

Physical, occupational, speech therapy, special education, family support, diazepam/dantrolene sodium/baclofen for spasticity, recently use of botulinum toxin to disrupt release of acetylcholine from motor nerve terminals, selective dorsal rhizotomy.

▶ **Health Maintenance Issues**

Ranges from resolution for mild to death for severe.

## F. Amblyopia and Strabismus

▶ **Scientific Concepts**

Amblyopia is reduction in central visual acuity. Strabismus is misalignment of visual axes of two eyes.

▶ **History & Physical**

Amblyopia occurs only in critical period of visual development during first decade of life, may occur in strabismic patient, with untreated refractive errors, with cataracts, media opacities, or complete ptosis. Strabismus with esotropia (excessively convergent) or exotropia (excessively divergent).

▶ Clinical Intervention

*Amblyopia:* Correct refractive errors, cataracts, opacities, visual rehabilitation, patching good eye.

*Strabismus:* Surgical correction, patching, glasses.

## XIII. COMMON CHILDHOOD DISEASES

### A. Respiratory Syncytial Virus (RSV)

▶ Scientific Concepts

Accounts for most hospitalizations for pulmonary reasons of children < 2 years, midwinter and spring outbreaks, transmitted by nasal secretions.

▶ History & Physical

Four- to 7-day incubation, rhinorrhea, progressive cough, tachypnea, retractions, diffuse wheezing, variable fever, irritability, poor feeding, cyanosis in severe cases; younger infants may present with apnea; associated with otitis media, pharyngeal hyperemia, conjunctivitis.

▶ Diagnostic Studies

CXR with hyperinflation of lungs, increased peribronchial thickening, flat diaphragm, horizontal ribs; nasal secretions positive via enzyme immunoassay (EIA).

▶ Diagnosis

Bronchiolitis, asthma, foreign body, pertussis, cystic fibrosis. SIDS not associated with RSV.

▶ Clinical Therapeutics

Humidified oxygen, supportive, corticosteroids are ineffective, variable relief with beta-adrenergic agonists, possible hospitalization, ribavirin in children with underlying compromising conditions or < 6 weeks of age or prematurity if severe disease process.

▶ Health Maintenance Issues

One percent morbidity, respiratory isolation, strict handwashing techniques, prophylaxis initiated at beginning of RSV season for infants at high risk with either intramuscular palivizumab (Synagis), a monoclonal antibody directed against RSV, or RSV intravenous immune globulin (IVIG) (RespiGam), a polyclonal antibody.

### B. Infectious Mononucleosis

▶ Scientific Concepts

Epstein–Barr virus (EBV) is etiologic agent.

▶ History & Physical

Prodrome of headache, malaise, nausea, abdominal pain; followed by classic triad of fever, nontender cervical lymphadenitis, tonsillopharyngitis (often exudative); other findings of palatal petechiae, hepatosplenomegaly, rhinitis, eyelid edema, rash and/or possible rash with penicillin/ampicillin administration; failure to thrive and otitis media are commonly found in young children.

▶ **Diagnostic Studies**
Atypical lymphocytes, relative neutropenia, mildly elevated serum transaminase levels; heterophil antibodies, EBV-specific serologic testing.

▶ **Diagnosis**
Bacterial/viral tonsillopharyngitis, cytomegalovirus infection, rubella, hepatitis A and B, HIV infection.

▶ **Clinical Therapeutics**
Symptomatic relief, avoid penicillin/ampicillin, artificial airway if respiratory compromise, steroids for swollen pharyngeal lymphoid tissue with secondary respiratory compromise.

▶ **Health Maintenance Issues**
Potential complications are pneumonia, seizures, Guillain–Barré syndrome, meningitis, thrombocytopenia, bacteremia, myocarditis, jaundice; no contact sports for 6–8 weeks if patient has splenomegaly.

## C. Roseola

▶ **Scientific Concepts**
Roseola infantum or exanthema subitum, etiologic agent is human herpesvirus-6 (HHV-6) or human herpesvirus-7 (HHV-7), benign illness, incidence 6–36 months, peaks 6–7 months of age.

▶ **History & Physical**
Characterized by abrupt onset of fever to 40°C for 4–8 days, accompanied by febrile seizures (10%) then defervesces with rose-pink macular or maculopapular rash on face, neck, and/or trunk. Examination shows characteristic rash, eyelid edema, suboccipital lymphadenopathy, pharyngeal erythema, erythematous papules on soft palate/uvula (Nagayama spots), frequently bulging anterior fontanel in infants.

▶ **Diagnostic Studies**
Leukopenia and lymphocytopenia, CSF positive for HHV-6 DNA.

▶ **Diagnosis**
Erythema infectiosum, measles, rubella, infectious mononucleosis, bacterial meningitis.

▶ **Clinical Therapeutics**
Supportive, acetaminophen.

▶ **Health Maintenance Issues**
If antibiotics prescribed at beginning of illness, often rash incorrectly attributed to drug allergy.

## D. Varicella (Chickenpox)

▶ **Scientific Concepts**
Chickenpox; most common vesicular exanthem in childhood; lifelong immunity; most cases in late winter and early spring; virus lies in dorsal root ganglion and may reappear as "shingles"; contagious 1–4 days prior to rash and until lesions scabbed over.

▶ **History & Physical**
Known exposure 11–20 days prior to vesicular eruption; prodrome with malaise and low-grade fever; rash progresses in stages, macule to

papule to vesicle ("dew drop on a rose petal") to crusted vesicle mainly on trunk and extremities, intensely pruritic rash.

▶ **Diagnostic Studies**
Rarely need antigen detection studies.

▶ **Diagnosis**
Poison ivy/oak, scabies.

▶ **Clinical Therapeutics**
Supportive, acetaminophen, calamine lotion, diphenhydramine. If immunosuppressed or high-risk infected neonates varicella-zoster immune globulin (VZIG) and acyclovir early.

▶ **Health Maintenance Issues**
Prevention with live attenuated vaccination; avoid aspirin-containing medications because of association with Reye's syndrome; neonates born to mother who develop varicella from 5 days prior to 2 days after delivery are at high risk for severe or fatal (5%) disease; complications include secondary bacterial skin infections, pneumonia, neurologic syndromes (encephalitis, meningitis, myelitis, Guillain–Barré syndrome); less commonly hepatitis, arthritis, glomerulonephritis, Reye's syndrome; rarely myocarditis, pericarditis, pancreatitis, orchitis.

## E. Rubella (German Measles)

▶ **Scientific Concepts**
German measles occurs rarely with sporadic outbreaks usually in springtime, infectious 5 days before and 5 days after rash; congenital rubella syndrome (CRS) follows maternal infection in first trimester.

▶ **History & Physical**
Prodrome in older children with low-grade fever, coryza, lymphadenopathy (postauricular and suboccipital), erythematous, discrete, maculopapular, noncoalescing rash that starts on face and spreads to entire body after it disappears from face and is gone by fourth day; characteristic Forschheimer sign of red spots on buccal mucosa and palate; congenital defects include growth retardation, deafness, chronic encephalitis, congenital heart disease (PDA, pulmonary artery stenosis, ASD), cataracts, retinitis, jaundice, thrombocytopenia, purpuric "blueberry muffin" rash at birth.

▶ **Diagnostic studies**
Mild leukopenia with relative lymphocytosis, viral isolates from nasopharyngeal secretions, rubella-specific IgM, EIA, latex agglutinations, hemagglutination-inhibition antibody determination.

▶ **Clinical Therapeutics**
Supportive, acetaminophen, aspirin for rubella arthritis only, prognosis is excellent in children but poor in congenitally infected infants.

▶ **Health Maintenance Issues**
Prevention with vaccination.

## F. Rubeola (Measles)

▶ **Scientific Concepts**
Highly contagious, transmitted via respiratory secretions, winter/spring disease.

► History & Physical

Incubation ~ 10 days, 3- to 5-day prodrome of fever and malaise, then cough, conjunctivitis, coryza, then 2 days prior to rash develop Koplik's spots (pathognomonic white papules on diffusely red base of buccal mucosa) followed by discrete, erythematous maculopapular rash that descends from head behind ears spreading to trunk coalescing to a bright red rash over 3 days, fine desquamation may occur, fever falls when rash appears, lymphadenopathy (posterior cervical), splenomegaly, headache, diarrhea, vomiting, abdominal pain.

► Diagnostic Studies

Lymphopenia is characteristic, leukopenia, elevated measles IgM antibody 3 days after rash appears, EIA that peaks 2–6 weeks after rash, multinucleate giant cells in nasal secretions during prodromal period.

► Diagnosis

Kawasaki disease, rubella, infectious mononucleosis, roseola, scarlet fever, enterovirus.

► Clinical Therapeutics

Supportive therapy, encourage fluid intake, acetaminophen, cough suppressants, consider ribavirin in immunocompromised patients, vitamin A supplementation for malnourished child.

► Health Maintenance Issues

Prevention with attenuated vaccination; immune globulin (IG) prevents or modifies disease if given within 6 days of exposure; complications include pneumonia, encephalitis, secondary bacterial infections, arthritis, bronchiolitis, croup, encephalitis, seizures, myocarditis, pericarditis, appendicitis, corneal ulcerations; reportable disease.

## G. Mumps

► Scientific Concepts

Contagious; transmitted by direct contact/infected respiratory droplets; uncommon disease with widespread use of vaccine; single attack confers lifelong immunity.

► History & Physical

Parotid gland swelling and tenderness, Hatchcock sign—tenderness with upward pressure applied to angle of mandible, increased parotid discomfort following eating/drinking acidic foods (e.g., orange juice), Stensen duct red and swollen may express yellow secretions, fever, facial lymphedema, presternal edema is a classic sign, ear displaced upward/outward, headache, anorexia, abdominal pain. Associated with meningocephalitis, pancreatitis, oophoritis or orchitis (postpubertal males), mastitis (adolescent females).

► Diagnostic Studies

Viral cultures from Stensen duct, urine, or CSF; serologic with paired sera 2–4 weeks apart; elevated serum amylase; mumps-specific IgM antibody.

► Diagnosis

Other viral parotitis, cervical adenitis, Stensen duct calculus, parotid gland tumors, leukemia, tooth infections.

► Clinical Therapeutics

Supportive, acetaminophen, respiratory isolation for 9 days after swelling begins if hospitalized and when able to return to school.

► Health Maintenance Issues

Orchitis is most serious complication and results in sterility if bilateral, auditory nerve neuritis with unilateral deafness, facial nerve paralysis, diabetes mellitus, myocarditis; prevention with vaccination.

## H. Rotavirus

► Scientific Concepts

"Winter gastroenteritis," 6 months to 2 years; nosocomial in pediatric wards, transmitted by contact with infected feces, respiratory, or waterborne (swimming pools).

► History & Physical

Fever; URI; vomiting, then 3 to 5 days of voluminous watery diarrhea without leukocytes or blood.

► Diagnostic Studies

Rotavirus in feces seen with electron microscopy, enzyme-linked immunoabsorbent assay (ELISA).

► Diagnosis

Other viral gastroenteritis (Norwalk virus, adenovirus).

► Clinical Therapeutics

Supportive care, hydrate, correct electrolytes; possible hospitalization; antibiotics and antidiarrheals not indicated.

► Health Maintenance Issues

Complications include hypernatremic dehydration, metabolic acidosis from bicarbonate loss in stool, ketosis from poor intake and lactic acidemia from hypotension and hypoperfusion; good hand-washing techniques to prevent spread. Rotavirus vaccine (Rotashield) suspended due to association with increased risk for intussusception within 3 weeks of vaccination.

## XIV. ENDOCRINE DISORDERS

### A. Diabetes Mellitus-Type IA

► Scientific Concepts

Immune-mediated diabetes, formerly juvenile onset or insulin dependent; most common type in < 40-year-olds; ketosis prone; immunologic damage to beta cells of pancreas; genetic predisposition and affected by environmental factors; associated with carrier of HLA-DR3 or HLA-DR4.

► History & Physical

Classic triad polyuria, polydypsia, polyphagia; weight loss; hyperglycemia and glucosuria with or without ketonuria; if presenting in ketoacidosis then vomiting dehydration, Kussmaul respirations, altered mental status; if presenting < 1 year of age, nonspecific symptoms (irritability, tachypnea, poor weight gain, vomiting).

► Diagnostic Studies

Fasting glucose ≥ 126 mg/dL, random glucose ≥ 200 mg/dL oral glucose tolerance test (OGTT) with 2-hour postprandial glucose ≥ 200 mg/dL.

► Clinical Therapeutics

Insulin, dietary, exercise, stress management, frequent blood glucose and urine ketone monitoring.

► Health Maintenance Issues

Somogyi phenomenon: elevated morning glucose as a physiologic response to nighttime hypoglycemia; close clinical follow-up: glycosylated hemoglobin (HbA$_{1C}$) every 3 months, cholesterol yearly, TSH yearly, 24-hour urine for microalbumin if patient diabetic > 5 years, ophthalmology yearly for retinal photographs. Ketoacidosis is major cause of morbidity and mortality. Acute complications are ketoacidosis/ketonuria, hypoglycemia; long-term complications include renal failure, retinopathy, early onset of cardiovascular disease, peripheral and autonomic neurologic impairment.

## B. Short Stature

► Scientific Concepts

Defined as height ≥ 3 standard deviations below mean for age. Differentiate between constitutional growth delay (CGD), familial short stature (FSS) and pathologic etiologies. CGD characterized by slow growth rate in first 3 years of life followed by low-normal growth velocity, positive family history, and delayed puberty. FSS is characterized by short target height and normal linear growth velocity. Deceleration of linear growth after 6 months of age is typical of growth hormone deficiency, hypothyroidism, or glucocorticoid excess. Initial decrease in weight is followed by decreased height velocity suggestive of malnutrition or systemic illness (chronic renal failure, inflammatory bowel disease, liver disease, CHF, asthma, cystic fibrosis, hemoglobinopathies). Dysmorphic features suggest chromosomal abnormalities (Turner's syndrome, Down syndrome, Prader–Willi syndrome). Skeletal abnormalities are associated with rickets, osteogenesis imperfecta, achondroplasia.

► History & Physical

Height velocity is critical factor; detailed family history; intrauterine growth retardation; height, weight, head circumference for growth patterns.

► Diagnostic Studies

CBC, ESR, thyroid function tests, BUN/creatinine, LFTs, electrolytes, calcium, phosphorous, urinalysis, x-ray of left hand/wrist for bone age, karyotype (females only), insulin-like growth factor-1 (IGF-1), insulin-like growth factor binding protein-3 (IGFBP-3), growth hormone levels (random and with clonidine challenge) highly variable results thus not diagnostic.

► Clinical Therapeutics

Directed toward cause of growth failure.

▶ Health Maintenance Issues

Growth hormone therapy is approved for GHD, growth retardation with chronic renal failure, Turner's and Prader–Willi syndromes, and small-for-gestational-age children. Side-effects include benign hypertension and slipped capital femoral epiphysis.

## C. Abnormalities of Puberty

▶ Scientific Concepts

Pubertal delay defined as lack of increase in testicular size above prepubertal size by age 14 in boys and lack of initiation of breast development by age 13 in girls. Etiologies include trauma, infection, auto-immune, chemotherapy, radiation therapy, hypopituitarism, chronic diseases, Prader–Willi syndrome, Turner's syndrome, Kleinfelter's syndrome. Precocious puberty is defined as development of secondary sexual characteristics before age of 8 years in girls or 9 years in boys; more common in girls.

▶ History & Physical

*Pubertal delay:* No signs of puberty as listed above.

*Precocious puberty:* Advanced Tanner Stage, when and rate of change; palpate thyroid; check for abdominal mass; measure size of penis and testes (diameter > 2.5 cm or volume > 4 mL); examine clitoris, labia, and vagina; examine optic fundus; check for acne, facial and axillary hair.

▶ Diagnostic Studies

*Pubertal delay:* Follicle-stimulating hormone (FSH) and luteinizing hormone (LH) response to gonadotropin-releasing hormone (GnRH), testosterone in males, karyotype, bone age, cranial MRI or CT to identify abnormalities of CNS.

*Precocious puberty:* FSH, LH, GnRH, estradiol in females, testosterone in males, dehydroepiandrosterone (DHEA), adrenocorticotropic hormone (ACTH) stimulation test, urinary 17-ketosteroids, bone age, ultrasound of pelvis/abdomen to rule out adrenal or ovarian mass/cysts, cranial MRI or CT to identify abnormalities of CNS.

▶ Clinical Therapeutics

*Pubertal delay:* Replacement of sex steroids, if hypogonadism then calcium supplements.

*Precocious puberty:* GnRH analogs, calcium supplements, thyroid replacement if indicated.

▶ Health Maintenance Issues

*Pubertal delay and precocious puberty:* Psychological support.

## XV. POISONINGS

## A. Acetaminophen

▶ Scientific Concepts

Acetaminophen is a frequently used antipyretic/analgesic metabolized in liver; most common drug overdose. Hepatotoxic dose is 150 mg/kg in children, which is extrapolated from adult data. In some children (< 10 years), this same dose may have little effect. Death can occur from fulminant hepatic failure.

▶ **History & Physical**

If spontaneous vomiting after ingestion, unlikely to have toxic level. With acute overdose, initially either asymptomatic or mild GI disturbance, diaphoresis 6–12 hours after ingestion, asymptomatic period from 12 to 48 hours after which hepatic enzymes rise, followed by signs (clinically and laboratory) of hepatotoxicity 24–48 hours after ingestion. Hepatic failure with encephalopathy, then coma and death.

▶ **Diagnostic Studies**

Acetaminophen level > 4 hours after ingestion then plot on nomogram, LFTs, and glucose.

▶ **Diagnosis**

Acute gastroenteritis, encephalopathy, and chemical hepatitis.

▶ **Clinical Therapeutics**

Stabilize patient, gastric lavage and activated charcoal. If acetaminophen level within toxic range per nomogram, treat with *N*-acetylcysteine (NAC) (Mucomyst) diluted to 5% solution in sweet fruit juice or carbonated soft drink within first 8 hours of ingestion. Loading dose is 140 mg/kg orally followed by 70 mg/kg orally every 4 hours for 17 doses. If levels not available, may start then withdraw treatment

▶ **Health Maintenance Issues**

All patients requiring Mucomyst must be hospitalized and follow daily aspartate aminotransferase (AST), alanine aminotransferase (ALT), bilirubin, and PT.

## B. Anticholinergics

▶ **Scientific Concepts**

Multiple drugs including antihistamines, atropine, cyclic antidepressants (amitriptyline, imipramine, doxepin, nortriptyline), scopolamine. Varied plants such as jimsonweed, horse nettle, night shade (black, climbing, deadly), potato leaves, and some mushrooms.

▶ **History & Physical**

"Mad as a hatter, red as a beet, blind as a bat, hot as a hare, and dry as a bone." Tachycardia; hyperthermia; hypertension; flushed skin and dry mucous membranes; dilated pupils; urinary retention; dysrhythmias; delirium with disorientation; uncontrollable agitation; hallucinations; impaired speech and swallowing; movement disorders such as myoclonus; seizures; coma; respiratory failure and cardiovascular collapse.

▶ **Diagnostic Studies**

Must notify lab; glucose, ECG, arterial blood gases, cyclic antidepresants radiopaque on abdominal x-ray.

▶ **Clinical Therapeutics**

Supportive care: cardiac monitoring, IV access; gastric lavage and administer activated charcoal. Physostigmine is used to treat antihistamine overdose with dose of 0.02 mg/kg/dose up to 0.5 mg IV every 5 minutes until therapeutic effect seen. Contraindications: abnormal ECG and concurrent tricyclic antidepressant overdose. Use is controversial due to side effects: seizures, bradycardia, asystole, and death. Phenytoin may be used to treat seizures/dysrhythmias.

► **Health Maintenance Issues**
Hospitalize/monitor.

## C. Carbon Monoxide

► **Scientific Concepts**
Odorless/colorless. Seen after fires, automobile exhaust with propane or gasoline engines operating in enclosed space, faulty furnaces or gas stoves, and with methylene chloride (paint strippers). Binds to hemoglobin 240 times more avidly than oxygen.

► **History & Physical**
Mild to moderate exposure includes headache, dizziness, nausea, confusion, chest pain, dyspnea, weakness, syncope. Severe exposure causes dysrhythmias, seizures, coma, myocardial ischemia, pulmonary edema, myoglobinuria, renal failure, encephalopathy with agitation.

► **Diagnostic Studies**
Carboxyhemoglobin (COHgb) levels elevated. Pulse oximetry *not* reliable. Arterial blood gas with measured, not calculated, oxygen saturation. ECG. CXR normal in first 24 hours and may show pulmonary edema after 1–4 days.

► **Diagnosis**
Flu-like illness, tension or migraine headache, food poisoning.

► **Clinical Therapeutics**
Administer 100% oxygen. Hyperbaric oxygen chamber if possible, indications include COHgb level 30–40%, coma, neurological or neuropsychiatric impairment, pulmonary edema, acidosis, abnormal ECG, pregnant patient with COHgb level >15%. Half-life of COHgb on room air is ~ 4 hours, 60–90 minutes on 100% oxygen, 30 minutes on hyperbaric oxygen therapy.

► **Health Maintenance Issues**
Possible permanent liver, renal, or CNS damage. Long-term neuropsychiatric changes and memory loss.

## D. Cocaine

► **Scientific Concepts**
May be teratogenic. Absorbed intranasally or via ingestion or inhalation. Intentional ingestion by "body packers" or "stuffers."

► **History & Physical**
Euphoria, agitation, paranoia, insomnia, dilated pupils, tachycardia, hypertension, cardiac arrhythmia, seizures, respiratory stimulation. Complications include myocardial infarction, tachyarrhythmias, stroke, rhabdomyolysis with acute renal failure, hyperthermia, intestinal ischemia.

▶ Diagnostic Studies

Serial ECGs, cardiac isoenzymes/tropin levels. Cocaine metabolites in urine for up to 3 days after acute exposure and up to 2 weeks in habitual use.

▶ Clinical Therapeutics

Stabilize; administer activated charcoal; treat seizures with IV diazepam, agitation with benzodiazepines, and dysrhythmias with phenytoin.

▶ Health Maintenance Issues

Hospitalize.

## E. Iron

▶ Scientific Concepts

Ingestion of > 40 mg/kg is dangerous. Easily accessible in multivitamins.

▶ History & Physical

Pattern of progression.

**Stage I:** 30 minutes to 6 hours. GI toxicity causing vomiting, hematemesis, diarrhea, hematochezia, and abdominal pain.

**Stage II:** 6–24 hours. Patient improves.

**Stage III:** 6–48 hours. Systemic toxicity with hepatic injury and/or renal failure, hyperglycemia, metabolic acidosis, bleeding, fever, convulsions, shock, coma, death.

**Stage IV:** 4 to 8 weeks. Late complications. Pyloric or antral stenosis.

▶ Diagnostic Studies

Serum iron > 350 µg/dL is associated with mild toxicity, > 500 µg/dL with serious toxicity, > 1,000 µg/dL with death. Obtain serum iron and total iron binding capacity (TIBC), CBC (leukocytosis), electrolytes, total protein, glucose, LFTs, blood type/cross match. Radiopaque tablets on abdominal x-ray.

▶ Diagnosis

Acute gastroenteritis, GI bleed, shock.

▶ Clinical Therapeutics

Supportive care. Gastric lavage. Whole bowel irrigation (WBI) is method of choice. Fluid and acid–base corrections. Deferoxamine IV at 15 mg/kg/h via continuous infusion for minimum of 8 hours; 100 mg can chelate 8.5 mg of elemental iron; rapid administration can cause hypotension, facial flushing, urticaria, tachycardia, shock. Transfusion.

▶ Health Maintenance Issues

If level > 500 µg/dL, admit. Follow-up visit 2–4 weeks after discharge to assess possible obstruction.

## F. Aspirin (Salicylates)

▶ Scientific Concepts

In over-the-counter medications such as Alka-Seltzer. Methyl salicylate is in oil of wintergreen. Becoming uncommon as replaced by acetaminophen or NSAIDs. Acute toxic overdose is > 150 mg/kg.

▶ **History & Physical**

Acute ingestion: tachypnea, vomiting, tinnitus, hyperthermia, lethargy or excitability, seizures, coma. Chronic ingestion: confusion, altered mental status, dehydration, metabolic acidosis, respiratory alkalosis, cerebral edema, pulmonary edema, cardiovascular collapse.

▶ **Diagnostic Studies**

Salicylate level > 6 hours after ingestion, electrolytes, glucose, arterial blood gas (respiratory alkalosis and metabolic acidosis), PT/PTT, LFTs, ECG. To 1 mL of urine, add a few drops of 10% ferric chloride—urine will turn purple if salicylates present.

▶ **Diagnosis**

Reye's syndrome, uremia, diabetes mellitus, meningitis.

▶ **Clinical Therapeutics**

Stabilize; administer activated charcoal; consider WBI if ingested enteric-coated preparations; IVs to correct fluid–electrolyte and acid–base disturbances; cooling blanket for hyperpyrexia, diazepam for seizures, vitamin K for bleeding problems. Consider hemodialysis: acute ingestion > 100 mg/dL, acute renal failure, CNS deterioration, unresolving acid–base disturbances, pulmonary edema.

▶ **Health Maintenance Issues**

Admit if > 60 mg/dL. Complications include metabolic acidosis, respiratory alkalosis, hypokalemia, hyponatremia, hypoglycemia, pulmonary edema, seizures secondary to lab abnormalities, coma, bleeding secondary to hypothrombinemia and platelet dysfunction, chemical hepatitis, allergic manifestations.

## BIBLIOGRAPHY

Barkin R, Rosen P. *Emergency Pediatrics: A Guide to Ambulatory Care,* 5th ed. St. Louis, MO: Mosby-Year Book; 1999.

Barness L. *Handbook of Pediatric Physical Diagnosis.* Philadelphia, PA: Lippincott-Raven; 1998.

Bickley L, Szilagyi P. *Bates' Guide to Physical Examination and History Taking,* 8th ed. Philadelphia, PA: Lippincott Williams and Wilkins; 2003.

Berkowitz C. *Pediatrics: A Primary Care Approach,* 2nd ed. Philadelphia, PA: W.B. Saunders; 2000.

Gunn V, Nechyba C, eds. *The Harriet Lane Handbook: A Manual for Pediatric House Officers,* 16th ed. Philadelphia, PA: Mosby; 2002.

Hay W, Hayward A, Levin M, Sondheimer J, eds. *Current Pediatric Diagnosis and Treatment,* 16th ed. New York: Lange Medical Books/McGraw-Hill; 2003.

Johnson K, Oski F. *Oski's Essential Pediatrics.* Philadelphia, PA: Lippincott-Raven; 1997.

Polin R, Ditmar M. *Pediatric Secrets,* 3rd ed. Philadelphia, PA: Hanley and Belfus; 2001.

Rudolph C, Rudolph A, eds. *Rudolph's Pediatrics,* 21st ed. New York: McGraw-Hill; 2003.

# Infectious Disease 16

*William R. Duryea, PhD, PA-C*

## I. CANDIDIASIS

► Scientific Concepts

*Candida* is a commensal, dimorphic fungus that exists primarily in the yeast form. It is part of the normal body flora and does not cause disease unless host defenses are altered. Over 150 species are known, but the majority of human infections are caused by *C. albicans*. Human candidiasis ranges from superficial infections of the skin and mucous membranes to highly invasive, life-threatening disease. Vaginal candidiasis is among the most common superficial infections, affecting over 75% of women at some time in their lives. Oral thrush is also a frequent manifestation of superficial candidiasis.

► History & Physical

Increased incidence of candidiasis is seen in those with risk factors that include diabetes, pregnancy, recent antibiotic and/or contraceptive use, and immunodeficiency states (e.g., resulting from human immunodeficiency virus [HIV] infection, cancer chemotherapy, etc.). Such risk factors, especially immunodeficiency disorders, predispose patients to more severe, potentially life-threatening, systemic candidiasis. Nosocomial candidiasis has markedly increased in recent years, with *Candida* now the fourth most frequently reported organism in hospital blood cultures.

Candidal skin infections may be found in warm, moist areas in the axillae, under the breast, or in the groin. Diabetics and those who frequently immerse their hands in water are predisposed to candidal paronychia; and HIV patients have a high incidence of onychomycosis. Oral thrush presents with multiple white patches on oral mucosa, including the tongue and palate. *Candida* vulvovaginitis is manifested by cottage cheese-like discharge in the vaginal vault, and discrete papular or pustular lesions on the vulva along with erythema and swelling of the vulva and labia.

► Diagnostic Studies

Potassium hydroxide (KOH) preparations of scrapings of candidal lesions will reveal the characteristic budding yeast and hyphae morphology of the organism. In cases of systemic candidiasis, recognition of candidemia is made by blood culture.

► Diagnosis

Diagnosis is based on knowledge of patient risk factors, recognition of the clinical pattern of infection, KOH studies, and/or blood culture.

► Clinical Therapeutics

*Candida* skin infections respond to application of topical nystatin, azoles, and amphotericin B. Topical cream should be applied 2–3 times daily. Effective treatment of onychomycosis requires several months of treatment with oral azoles (e.g., terbenifine). Troublesome chronic mucocutaneous candidiasis (CMC) requires months to years of treatment with oral ketoconazole or fluconazole.

Oral thrush is treated with nystatin suspension or clotrimazole troches 4–5 times daily for 7–10 days. Nystatin suspension is also effective in the treatment of uncomplicated esophageal candidiasis. Topical azoles (e.g., clotrimazole, miconazole, etc.) and oral agents (e.g., fluconazole) are available for treatment of *Candida* vulvovaginitis. Both approaches are equally effective, but oral agents are more expensive. Ketoconazole has demonstrated efficacy in prophylaxis. The first choice for treatment of disseminated candidiasis/candidemia is oral or intravenous (IV) fluconazole.

▶ Clinical Intervention

Patients with recurring candidal infection or infection at multiple sites should be further investigated for immune system deficits or evidence of other underlying disease, such as diabetes.

▶ Health Maintenance Issues

See above regarding prophylaxis.

## II. CRYPTOCOCCOSIS

▶ Scientific Concepts

*Cryptococcus* infection (cryptococcosis) is caused by an encapsulated yeast, *C. neoformans*. Most infections are acquired through inhalation of infected particles from concentrations of pigeon droppings in barns or old buildings, or from airborne organisms released from windblown contaminated soil. Another variety of *C. neoformans* (var. *gatti*) is acquired from flowering *Eucalyptus* trees in southern California.

Cryptococcosis is most commonly manifested as meningoencephalitis, with or without pulmonary involvement. Immunodeficiency states (e.g., acquired immunodeficiency syndrome [AIDS]) predispose to more serious, often life-threatening, disease.

▶ History & Physical

Occupational exposure through farming or working in old buildings may be known, but often there is no clear history of exposure to the organism. Underlying immunodeficiency portends more serious, multisystem manifestations of cryptococcosis. For most patients, however, the disease is usually subclinical, and many remain asymptomatic. The most common symptoms of pulmonary infection are dry cough, low-grade fever, sputum production, and pleuritic chest pain. Headache is the most frequent presenting symptom of central nervous system (CNS) involvement. Meningeal inflammation is marked by stiff neck and photophobia. Progressive CNS disease may produce altered mental status, visual loss, cranial nerve palsies, ataxia, seizures, coma, and death.

▶ Diagnostic Studies

Cryptococcal CNS infection is identified by a positive culture of CSF. Also, CSF will be positive for cryptococcal antigen in 95% of patients. The gold standard for identification of pulmonary infection by *C. neoformans* is culture of sputum or bronchoalveolar lavage. Lab diagnosis of disseminated cryptococcosis (cryptococcemia) is made by the presence of cryptococcal antigen in the patient's serum.

▶ Diagnosis

Diagnosis is based on the clinical presentation, and appropriate studies cited above.

► Clinical Therapeutics

The choice of therapy for cryptococcosis is based on the HIV status of the patient, and whether they have localized pulmonary, CNS, or disseminated disease. Mild to moderate disease responds to fluconazole in both HIV-positive and -negative patients, except that HIV-positive patients must take the drug for life. Amphotericin B and fluconazole should be used to treat CNS, severe pulmonary, or disseminated disease.

► Health Maintenance Issues

AIDS patients with CD4 counts < 200 should receive daily fluconazole prophylaxis.

## III. HISTOPLASMOSIS

► Scientific Concepts

Histoplasmosis is a fungal infection endemic within the Mississippi and Ohio River valleys of the United States. The infection is caused by *Histoplasma capsulatum,* a dimorphic fungus. Outside the human host it grows as a mycelial form; but when it invades human tissue, it becomes a pathogenic yeast. Disease usually arises from inhalation of mycelial fragments, after which the organism converts to a thin-walled, oval yeast form. In the immunocompetent host, T cell immunity develops within 2–4 weeks, and stops further spread of the disease. Subsequent formation of calcified granulomas containing *H. capsulatum* allows the organism to persist in a dormant state in body tissues for long periods. Histoplasmosis is considered one of the AIDS–defining infections, which may be manifested as severe pulmonary disease, meningitis, encephalitis, disseminated intravascular coagulation, organ failure, and/or septic shock.

► History & Physical

Low-inoculum exposure to mycelia of *H. capsulatum* in immunocompetent persons results in mild, asymptomatic disease, with no conclusive findings on the history and physical exam. Immunodeficient patients and those exposed to a high inoculum of the fungus may develop pulmonary symptoms of dyspnea and hypoxemia, or more severe signs of chronic or disseminated disease (e.g., cough, malaise, weight loss, fatigue, focal consolidation, hepatosplenomegaly, CNS manifestations, etc.)

► Diagnostic Studies

In symptomatic patients with acute disease, chest X-ray may show focal infiltrates, hilar, and/or mediastinal lymphadenopathy. If the patient has developed chronic histoplasmosis, chest radiographs may reveal necrosis, cavitation, and fibrosis. In AIDS patients, the blood count may be diminished (e.g., anemia, leukopenia, thrombocytopenia). When possible, one should try to recover the organism from culture of blood, sputum, biopsied tissue, or other sources. In some cases, histopathologic examination of presumptively infected tissue can establish the diagnosis earlier than culture. Complement fixation titers ≥1:32 or the presence of antibodies to H antigens are indicative of active infection.

► Differential Diagnosis

In the workup of histoplasmosis, tuberculosis and pneumonia caused by other fungi or bacteria must be ruled out. Definitive diagnosis is made by identification of *H. capsulatum* in culture, or in specially stained tissue samples. Positive serology, as describe above, indicates active infection.

▶ Clinical Therapeutics

For most immunocompetent patients, the disease is mild and uncomplicated, requiring no antifungal treatment. Those with persistent pulmonary and constitutional symptoms, should receive a 6- to 12-month course of itraconazole. For AIDS patients and others who have severe, life-threatening disease, amphotericin B is the drug of choice.

▶ Clinical Intervention

HIV-positive persons with diagnosed histoplasmosis should receive itraconazole for life to prevent recurrent infection.

▶ Health Maintenance Issues

Persons at increased risk for acquiring serious *H. capsulatum* infection should be advised to avoid situations or activities that will bring them into contact with possible histoplasma-contaminated dust or soil.

## IV. PNEUMOCYSTIS

▶ Scientific Concepts

*Pneumocystis carinii* is a protozoan-like fungus that is the agent of severe, life-threatening pneumonia in AIDS patients with CD4 counts of < 200. Infection is acquired via inhalation between human hosts. Since 1983, *Pneumocystis carinii* pneumonia (PCP) has been considered an AIDS-defining illness.

▶ History & Physical

PCP in AIDS patients typically presents with the triad of fever, dyspnea on exertion, and nonproductive cough. Severe hypoxia late in the course of the disease will produce resting shortness of breath. The pulmonary exam may reveal fine rales in cases of severe disease, but is likely to be negative in early stages.

▶ Diagnosis

While chest radiography and serum lactic dehydrogenase (LDH) are important tools in the assessment of PCP, the gold standard is identification of *P. carinii* in stained bronchoalveolar lavage and/or transbronchial biopsy specimens obtained via bronchoscopy. The typical appearance of PCP on chest x-ray is one of diffuse bilateral infiltrates. The serum LDH is usually elevated, but the test lacks diagnostic specificity. A persistently elevated LDH is of greater prognostic value, portending a poorer outcome.

▶ Clinical Therapeutics

The combination of trimethoprim (TMP) and sulfamethoxazole (SMX), oral (PO) or IV, continues to be the primary treatment for moderate to severe PCP. However, adverse effects of treatment with TMP-SMX are common, with morbilliform rashes most frequently observed. Survival of patients with moderate to severe disease appears to be enhanced by the concomitant administration of corticosteroids.

A relatively new drug in the treatment of PCP, trimetrexate, appears to be as effective as TMP-SMX with fewer side effects in patients with moderate to severe disease. Two other combinational regimens have proven efficacy in the treatment of mild to moderate PCP: clindamycin/primaquine, and dapsone/TMP. The incidence of side effects with dapsone/TMP is much lower than that of TMP-SMX. Pentamidine isethionate continues to be a suitable alternative in the treatment of mild to moderate PCP.

▶ **Health Maintenance Issues**

Prevention of PCP in AIDS and other immunocompromised patients is best achieved with TMP-SMX, three times weekly, for life.

## V. BOTULISM

▶ **Scientific Concepts**

Ingestion of the neurotoxin of *Clostridium botulinum* causes the syndrome of botulism, a paralytic disease that begins with cranial nerve impairment progressing to the extremities and terminating with respiratory failure. In some cases, the illness is mild and no medical intervention is necessary. *C. botulinum* synthesizes seven types of neurotoxins (A–G), all of which affect peripheral neuromuscular junction by inhibiting the release of acetylcholine. Ingestion of the preformed toxin in home-canned meats, fish, fruits, and vegetables occurs in the majority of cases. Toxin types A, B, and E are most commonly associated with human botulism. In the United States, type A predominates west of the Rocky Mountains; type B is more common in the East; and type E outbreaks occur most frequently in Alaska, the Pacific Northwest, and the Great Lakes region where it is often associated with consumption of contaminated fish. Among the other forms of botulism (e.g., wound botulism, infant botulism, adult infectious botulism), food-borne botulism is most common worldwide. Infant botulism, produced from ingestion of spores in contaminated food and production of toxin in the intestine, is the most frequently encountered form of botulism in the United States. This type of botulism has been linked to sudden infant death syndrome (SIDS).

▶ **History & Physical**

Following ingestion of food containing neurotoxin, patients present with acute onset of symmetrical facial muscle paralysis with bilateral involvement of the cranial nerves, marked by diplopia, dysarthria, and/or dysphagia. Dizziness, blurred vision, and dry mouth are common. Other eye signs may include fixed or dilated pupils, depressed pupillary reflexes, and ptosis. Symmetric descending paralysis progressively involves the neck, arms, thorax, and legs. Although patients may be anxious, drowsy, or agitated, they remain alert and oriented. There is usually no fever.

▶ **Diagnosis**

The clinical presentation, physical exam findings, and assays of stool and serum toxins will establish the diagnosis.

▶ **Differential Diagnosis**

The differential diagnosis includes myasthenia gravis, poliomyelitis, mushroom intoxication, Guillain–Barré and Lambert–Eaton syndromes.

► Clinical Therapeutics

Hospitalization and supportive measures, including intubation and mechanical ventilation, must be considered if signs of respiratory failure accompany paralysis. Trivalent (types A, B, and E) antitoxin should be administered in cases of food-borne illness.

# VI. CHLAMYDIA

► Scientific Concepts

Chlamydia are obligate intracellular bacteria that cause a variety of human diseases. Three pathogenic species of chlamydia are recognized: *Chlamydia trachomatis, C. psittaci,* and *C. pneumoniae.* A number of serotypes of *C. trachomatis* exist, with types D to K most frequently responsible for sexually transmitted disease (STD) in adolescents and young adults. Genital infection by *C. trachomatis* is currently the most common notifiable infectious disease in the United States. Serotypes A–C of *C. trachomatis* cause trachoma, the predominant infectious cause of blindness worldwide.

*C. pneumoniae* is linked to upper respiratory infection and pneumonia mainly in children and young adults. *C. psittaci* causes zoonotic illness (psitticosis) transmitted to humans from birds. The illness may range from pneumonia to systemic disease.

► History & Physical

Nongonococcal urethritis (NGU) caused by chlamydia will usually present with history of dysuria and frequency, along with urethral discharge (in men). Many infected women are asymptomatic. Complaints of vaginal bleeding and/or discharge, abdominal pain, and dysuria may signal mucopurulent cervicitis (MPC). Pelvic inflammatory disease (PID) should be ruled out in sexually active women who have abdominal pain/tenderness and associated adnexal and/or cervical motion tenderness.

In men who have sex with men, the combination of rectal pain/exudates tenderness, and hematochezia suggests proctitis (which may also occur in heterosexual women). Suspect chlamydial epididymitis in anyone under 35 years of age presenting with unilateral testicular pain/tenderness or swelling. The combination of urethritis, uveitis, arthritis, and mucocutaneous lesions is seen in Reiter's syndrome. Lymphogranuloma venereum (LGV) should be considered in those who present with tender unilateral inguinal or femoral lymphadenopathy. The presentation of trachoma is similar to herpes simplex conjunctivitis.

► Diagnostic Studies

Gram stain of discharge should be followed by confirmatory studies: culture and/or microimmunofluorescent (micro-IF) antibody or nucleic acid probe testing. Seek evidence of HLA-B27 in suspected Reiter's syndrome.

► Diagnosis

The absence of gonococci on Gram's stain combined with a positive culture confirms the diagnosis of chlamydial infection. In the absence of a positive culture, a positive micro-IF or DNA probe study is also confirmatory.

► Clinical Therapeutics

For adults with NGU, a single 1-g dose of azithromycin is effective. For other types of chlamydial infections (LGV, NPC, PID, etc.), doxycycline, erythromycin, and tetracycline (for *C. psittaci*) also have proven effectiveness.

► Clinical Intervention

Obtain sexual history from all sexually active patients as first step in identifying those at risk for STDs. Educate patients on preventive strategies for avoiding STDs. Utilize screening programs to detect those with asymptomatic chlamydial infection. Prevalence of trachoma can be reduced by improving living standards and practicing basic hygiene, such as hand washing. Prevention of human psitticosis is achieved by quarantining, and treating imported birds with tetracycline.

## VII.  CHOLERA

► Scientific Concepts

Cholera is an acute diarrheal illness caused by *Vibrio cholerae,* a curved, gram-negative rod. Once ingested, the organism's enterotoxin acts on intestinal epithelium, raising intracellular cyclic adenosine monophosphate (AMP) levels, resulting in massive fluid and electrolyte transport into the bowel lumen. Devastating outbreaks of cholera have occurred since ancient times, when epidemics were first chronicled by early physicians.

Cholera is endemic to the Ganges River delta from which most of the major pandemics have originated in recent centuries. The disease continues to be a public health problem in underdeveloped areas where water treatment facilities and adequate sewage disposal systems are lacking. Overcrowded refugee camps in war-torn areas are breeding grounds for new epidemics.

► History & Physical

Rapid clustering of cases in endemic areas underscores cholera's epidemic potential. Within a few hours after ingestion of the organism, patients present with profuse, watery diarrhea. Fever and abdominal pain are often minimal. Decreased skin turgor, sunken eyes, weak pulses, and postural hypotension accompany rapid fluid loss and portend development of hypovolemic shock. Patients should be checked for altered mental status, muscle weakness, and cardiac manifestations of electrolyte depletion.

► Diagnostic Studies

Gross exam of the stool shows typical "rice water" appearance. No blood or pus is present. Stool microscopic exam may reveal rapidly motile, curved bacilli, suggestive of *V. cholerae.* Serotype can be determined by immobilization of organisms with specific antiserum (e.g., Ogawa). Latex agglutination and enzyme-linked immunosorbent assay (ELISA) methods have proved useful for rapid diagnosis in early stages of the disease. Culture of the organism yields flat yellow colonies on TCBS medium. Excessive fluid accumulation due to development of ileus may occur and can be identified via abdominal ultrasound.

▶ **Differential Diagnosis**

Diarrheal disease caused by other enteric pathogens includes *Shigella*, *Salmonella*, and *Campylobacter* species, enteropathogenic *Escherichia coli*, *Yersinia enterocolitica*, rotavirus, Norwalk agent; and various protozoan parasites, including *Giardia lamblia*, *Cryptosporidium*, and *Cyclospora* species.

▶ **Clinical Therapeutics**

IV fluid and electrolyte replacement is critical to reversal of severe dehydration. Include IV glucose when mental status changes. Oral fluid replacement (e.g., WHO Oral Rehydration Solution) is as effective as IV treatment, if no vomiting. Tetracycline administration may shorten the duration of illness.

▶ **Health Maintenance Issues**

Epidemic cholera can be prevented by effective public health programs that include clean water supplies, and adequate sewage treatment and disposal. New cholera vaccines are undergoing field trials.

## VIII. DIPHTHERIA

▶ **Scientific Concepts**

Diphtheria is an acute tonsillopharyngitis caused by *Corynebacterium diphtheriae*, a gram-positive rod with club-shaped swellings at each end. The organism chiefly infects the respiratory tract; however, toxigenic strains of *C. diphtheriae* are capable of producing both local, respiratory, and systemic disease, particularly affecting the heart, kidneys, and nerves.

Pseudomembrane development in the pharynx is a characteristic feature of the disease, resulting from tissue necrosis caused by the organism's exotoxin. Nontoxigenic diphtheria involves only the respiratory tract, and is typically local, mild disease.

▶ **History & Physical**

After an incubation period of several days to a week, patients develop a low-grade fever and present with nasopharyngeal symptoms and signs, including sore throat, nasal discharge, pharyngeal erythema, white tonsillar exudates, and/or grayish adherent pseudomembrane. Dislodging the membrane causes bleeding. Cervical adenopathy may confer a "bull neck" appearance. Laryngeal involvement is marked by hoarseness, stridor, and dyspnea. Some patients develop cutaneous diphtheria manifested by pustules that later ulcerate, forming a gray-brown membrane at the base. Toxic patients need to be carefully checked for cardiac and/or neurologic involvement.

▶ **Diagnostic Studies**

Gram-stained smears from pseudomembrane swabs, or from cutaneous lesions, will demonstrate the characteristic club-shaped, gram-positive rod. Cultures are best isolated on selective media. A presumptive diagnosis can be made on the basis of a positive smear and culture. Polymerase chain reaction (PCR) testing enables both detection of the organism and determination of toxigenicity.

▶ Differential Diagnosis

Tonsillopharyngitis caused by other bacteria (e.g., streptococci), viruses (e.g., infectious mononucleosis), or fungi (e.g., candidiasis) must be ruled out. Acute epiglottitis and Vincent's angina should also be considered.

▶ Clinical Therapeutics

Hospitalize and provide supportive care, including airway management, cardiac monitoring, and prevention of neurologic complications. The mainstay of therapy is diphtheria antitoxin, dose-adjusted to the severity of disease. Also, add a 2-week course of erythromycin. Keep patients in strict isolation until culture-negative.

▶ Health Maintenance Issues

Notify local health authorities of positive diagnosis of diphtheria, culture close contacts, and begin prophylactic antibiotics. Droplet precaution isolation should be observed until two negative nasopharyngeal cultures are returned. The only effective means of prevention is inoculation with diphtheria toxoid. Administer booster every 10 years.

## IX. GONOCOCCAL INFECTIONS

▶ Scientific Concepts

Gonococcal infection (gonorrhea) is caused by the sexual transmission of *Neisseria gonorrhoeae*, a gram-negative, intracellular diplococcus. Infections range from genital involvement in men and women to disseminated spread of gonococci, usually manifested as an arthritis–dermatitis syndrome. Death from endotoxic shock may occur with disseminated gonorrhea. Neonatal gonococcal conjunctivits may be transmitted from an infected mother during delivery or postpartum. Anorectal gonorrhea is seen in men who have sex with men and in women who have receptive anal intercourse.

▶ History & Physical

Gonococcal infections should be suspected in sexually active persons who present with urethritis (men, predominantly) or cervicitis. The male genital exam reveals a creamy yellow discharge. Symptomatic women have a mucopurulent vaginal discharge, and complain of dyspareunia, intermenstrual bleeding, and/or dysuria. Exam of the cervix will reveal the discharge along with cervical edema and friable mucosa. Suspect PID in women with genital gonorrhea who complain of bilateral lower abdominal pain and exhibit cervical motion tenderness. Anorectal gonorrhea is manifested by purulent rectal discharge, rectal bleeding, and tenesmus. Disseminated disease is marked by predominantly unilateral arthritis affecting the wrists, knees, and/or ankles. There may be accompanying skin lesions (e.g., pustules and hemorrhagic papules).

▶ Diagnostic Studies

Gram stain and culture of discharge are the mainstays of diagnosis. Gram stain of urethral discharge in men has high sensitivity and specificity, making cultures unnecessary. Blood cultures are required in cases of systemic infections. PCR or ligase chain reaction (LCR) studies have high sensitivity and specificity, and offer a diagnostic alternative when smears or cultures are problematical.

### ▶ Clinical Therapeutics

The treatment of choice for uncomplicated gonorrhea is single-dose ceftriaxone. Increased incidence of concurrent chlamydial infection warrants the addition of doxycycline or azithromycin. A higher dose and longer duration of ceftriaxone treatment is required for complicated infections, including septic arthritis, endocarditis, and/or meningitis.

### ▶ Health Maintenance Issues

Gonorrhea and other STDs are primarily prevented by sexual abstinence or condom use during sexual intercourse. Effective treatment of cases and sexual partners is essential to disease control.

## X. SALMONELLOSIS

### ▶ Scientific Concepts

Diseases caused by *Salmonella* species range from mild gastroenteritis to life-threatening enteric fever (e.g., typhoid). In contrast to *Salmonella* enteritis, enteric fever produces systemic manifestations resulting from dissemination of the organism throughout the host. *Salmonella typhi* and *S. paratyphi* are the predominant causes of enteric fevers. *Salmonella* gastroenteritis commonly results from eating contaminated, undercooked food; whereas enteric fever is associated with drinking water contaminated with human feces. Ingestion of undercooked chicken contaminated with *S. enteritidis* is a frequent cause of gastroenteritis. Salmonellae are gram-negative bacilli that are easily identified from stools cultured on selective media, such as bismuth-sulfite agar.

### ▶ History & Physical

Patients with *Salmonella* gastroenteritis typically experience fever, abdominal cramps, nausea, vomiting, and diarrhea 6–48 hours after eating contaminated food. The diarrhea usually consists of loose, nonbloody stools. One should have a high index of suspicion of enteric (typhoid) fever when a patient presents with fever/chills and recent history of foreign travel. Along with fever and chills, the prodrome of enteric fever may be manifested by a variety of other nonspecific symptoms, including malaise, cough, weakness, and/or myalgia. Patients may also experience diarrhea or constipation. Physical findings such as hepatosplenomegaly, rose spots (on trunk), epistaxis, paroxysmal bradycardia, and profound mental status changes ("typhoid psychosis") are important clues to the diagnosis.

### ▶ Diagnostic Studies

*Salmonella* gastroenteritis is diagnosed by positive stool culture. In cases of enteric fever, *S. typhi* is more likely to be found in blood than in stool culture during early to mid stages of the disease. In the late phase, stool and urine cultures will become more strongly positive. A presumptive diagnosis of typhoid fever can be made with the Widal serological test, but final diagnosis requires finding the organism in culture.

▶ Differential Diagnosis

Other bacterial and parasitic causes of infectious diarrhea must be considered, particularly *Escherichia, Shigella,* and *Giardia.* Noninfectious causes include colitis and neoplasia.

▶ Clinical Therapeutics

Rehydrate with fluids and electrolytes, and give antimicrobials (drugs of choice are TMP-SMZ for children, and quinolones for adults).

▶ Health Maintenance Issues

Person-to-person transmission is prevented by education in proper food handling, personal hygiene, and washing of hands. Enteric fever is effectively controlled by supplying potable water and adequately treating and disposing of sewage. Travelers to endemic typhoid fever areas should be vaccinated.

## XI. SHIGELLOSIS

▶ Scientific Concepts

*Shigella* enteritis (shigellosis) ranges from mild, watery diarrhea to severe dysentery. Shigellae are gram-negative bacilli encompassing four species: *S. boydii, S. dysenteriae, S. flexneri,* and *S. sonnei* (most prevalent in the United States). Shigellosis largely affects infants and children in the United States via person-to-person transmission, commonly in schools and day care centers. Bacillary dysentery, caused by *S. dysenteriae* and *S. flexneri,* is predominantly a disease of underdeveloped areas where transmission through ingestion of contaminated water is a major public health problem.

▶ History & Physical

A history of travel to endemic areas or clustering of cases of acute, watery diarrhea from schools or day care centers may indicate an outbreak of shigellosis. Fever and abdominal pain accompany diarrhea. In cases of severe dysentery, diarrheic stools contain blood, pus, and mucous. Dysentery patients may become toxemic and develop high fevers. Pain with digital rectal exam is common.

▶ Diagnosis

The presence of leukocytes in diarrheic stool suggests shigellosis; however, definitive diagnosis requires identification of the organism in culture.

▶ Differential Diagnosis

In cases of watery diarrhea, consider a variety of other bacterial, parasitic, or viral agents (e.g., *Salmonella, Giardia,* rotavirus, etc.). When dysentery predominates, *Entamoeba histolytica* and enteroinvasive *E. coli* must be ruled out.

▶ Clinical Therapeutics

Fluid and electrolyte rehydration must be accompanied by antibiotic treatment. The drug of choice for children is TMP-SMX; adults should be given a quinolone. Antimotility drugs are contraindicated.

▶ Health Maintenance Issues

In developing countries, dysentery can be effectively controlled by installation of effective drinking water treatment and sewage disposal systems. Personal hygiene and clean living conditions are important preventive measures in both developed and underdeveloped areas.

## XII. TETANUS

▶ Scientific Concepts

Tetanus is a toxin-mediated neurologic syndrome caused by *Clostridium tetani,* an anaerobic gram-negative bacillus. The disease is manifested by severe muscle spasms due to blocking of inhibitory neuron transmission by *C. tetani* toxin (tetanospasmin).

▶ History & Physical

Patients often present with irritability, restlessness, diaphoresis, and drooling, due to dysphagia and hydrophobia, and have a history of a recent contaminated wound infection. Trismus (lockjaw) is also a frequent early sign, associated with risus sardonicus, the classic tetanus facial expression. Waves of opisthotonos progress to painful extremity spasms and generalized convulsions. The patient remains lucid in the midst of pain and spasmodic contractions.

▶ Diagnosis

In most cases, the diagnosis of tetanus is made clinically; the organism is difficult to recover from wound cultures.

▶ Differential Diagnosis

Meningitis, seizure disorders, alcohol withdrawal, hypocalcemic tetany, and strychnine poisoning all have some tetanus-like features and must be ruled out.

▶ Clinical Therapeutics

Inpatient supportive care must be provided, with special attention to airway maintenance and administration of IV diazepam (to relieve muscle rigidity). Also, give human tetanus immunoglobulin (TIG) and IV penicillin G.

▶ Health Maintenance Issues

Tetanus prevention is achieved by active immunization of infants and children with DTaP (combined diphtheria, tetanus toxoid, and absorbed pertussis vaccine), and booster every 10 years for life with Td vaccine (consisting of tetanus and diphtheria toxoids for adult use).

## XIII. TUBERCULOSIS

▶ Scientific Concepts

Tuberculosis (TB) is primarily a pulmonary infection caused by the acid-fast bacillus, *Mycobacterium tuberculosis.* The infectious agent is transmitted from person to person via inhaled aerosol droplets, and then bacilli implant and multiply in bronchioles. The infection may remain localized at the primary pulmonary site (in 80% of cases) or disseminate and infect multiple organs (miliary TB). Most infected immunocompetent persons do not develop active disease (with clinical signs and symptoms). Active pulmonary tuberculosis may be the presenting infection in HIV patients and is considered an AIDS-defining illness. Infection by *M. tuberculosis* results in a positive TB (purified protein derivative [PPD]) test.

▶ **History & Physical**

Patients typically complain of fever, fatigue, productive cough (including hemoptysis), and weight loss. Physical findings may include adenopathy and apical rales.

▶ **Diagnostic Studies**

Chest radiograms may show apical pulmonary infiltrates, but occasionally are normal. Sputum may be positive for acid-fast bacilli. Culture of *M. tuberculosis* takes from 2 to 6 weeks for colony development. Other lab findings are typically normal for uncomplicated pulmonary TB; but miliary TB can exhibit lab evidence of anemia and metabolic abnormalities due to adrenal insufficiency, liver and/or kidney failure, and gastrointestinal involvement.

▶ **Diagnosis**

A positive PPD test establishes the diagnosis of both pulmonary and miliary TB infection. The interpretation of a positive test is dependent on the at-risk status of the patient (e.g., AIDS patients and others at high risk for TB infection are considered positive if the PPD test exhibits ≥ 5 mm of induration; whereas ≥ 15 mm is considered positive for low-risk patients). The TB diagnosis is supported by findings of pulmonary infiltrates on chest x-ray and identification of acid-fast bacilli in sputum or in other body fluids or tissues.

▶ **Clinical Therapeutics**

Drug therapy for TB is based on the guiding principle that multiple drugs should be administered on schedule for several months via directly observed therapy. The CDC recommends directly observed therapy to increase compliance with treatment and to avoid the development of resistant strains. Isoniazid (INH), rifampin (RIF), pyrazinamide (PZA), streptomycin (SM), and ethambutol are first-line drugs for treatment of both pulmonary and extrapulmonary TB. Immunocompetent patients can be effectively treated with a combination of three or four of the above drugs for 6 months. Immunocompromised and/or those exposed to multidrug resistant TB (MDR-TB) should have several other drugs added to their primary regimens (e.g., amikacin, ciprofloxacine, cycloserine, ethionamide, etc.). Antibiotic therapy should be accompanied by rest, oxygen, and respiratory therapy.

▶ **Clinical Intervention**

Before treatment is begun, a baseline blood count and lab studies of liver and kidney function should be obtained. Follow-up with monthly checks for symptoms and signs of drug toxicity.

▶ **Health Maintenance Issues**

Prophylactic INH therapy should be given to those who convert to a positive PPD to prevent the development of active TB infection. Isolation of patients with active infection will prevent exposure to the general population.

# XIV. ATYPICAL MYCOBACTERIAL INFECTIONS

► **Scientific Concepts**

Atypical TB-like infections occur most often in immunocompromised hosts and comprise up to 30% of all infections caused by mycobacteria. The most common of these infections, caused by *M. avium* complex (MAC), usually produces pulmonary disease, but disseminated infection may also occur. Disseminated MAC is a particular problem in AIDS patients and may be manifested as osteomyelitis, hepatitis, lymphadenitis, meningitis, or multi-organ/system disease. MAC are acid-fast bacilli, morphologically and culturally similar to *M. tuberculosis*.

► **History & Physical**

An immunodeficiency history along with a TB/pneumonia-like presentation may signal MAC infection. Pulmonary MAC manifests itself with fever, productive cough (perhaps, hemoptysis), and weight loss. Prolonged fever, night sweats, weight loss, generalized lymphadenopathy, jaundice, and hepatosplenomegaly may occur with disseminated disease. AIDS patients can present with a history of chronic diarrhea, jaundice, and abdominal pain suggestive of gastrointestinal MAC disease.

► **Diagnostic Studies**

Chest radiograms often mimic reactivation TB, showing upper lobe infiltrates and cavitation. An acid-fast positive smear provides a presumptive diagnosis of mycobacterial infection. A definitive diagnosis is made by isolation and molecular-probe identification of MAC in sputum, blood, or tissue-biopsy cultures grown on special media (e.g., Bactec).

► **Differential Diagnosis**

*M. tuberculosis* must be ruled out, as well as other atypical *Mycobacterium* species (e.g., *M. kansasii, M. scrofulaceum, M. bovis,* etc.)

Nonmycobacterial infection, such as viral, bacterial, or fungal pneumonia, should also be considered.

► **Clinical Therapeutics**

Multidrug treatment of MAC infection for 12–24 months is recommended. Combinations of the following drugs have proven effective for treatment of MAC in both immunodeficient and immunocompetent patients: clarithromycin, ethambutol, rifabutin, clofazimine, amikacin, azithromycin, and ciprofloxacin. The combination of choice for adult AIDS patients is clarithromycin + ethambutol + rifabutin. Treatment protocols for pediatric AIDS patients are not well established.

► **Clinical Intervention**

Baseline blood counts (including CD4 levels) and liver and kidney function tests should be obtained before beginning therapy. Continue with monthly monitoring during treatment period.

► **Health Maintenance Issues**

AIDS patients with CD4 counts < 100 require life-long prophylaxis with antibiotics (clarithromycin, azithromycin, or rifabutin daily). The same regimen is effective in posttreatment suppression of MAC in AIDS patients. (For treatment of less common atypical mycobacterial infections, see *The Sanford Guide® to Antimicrobial Therapy*.)

## XV.  AMEBIASIS

▶ Scientific Concepts

Infection with *E. histolytica* causes amebiasis, a syndrome ranging from asymptomatic gastrointestinal (GI) infection to chronic colitis. The majority of infections are subclinical. Infection results from ingestion of *E. histolytica* cysts via fecal–oral transmission. Trophozoites emerge from cysts, colonize the large bowel, and may disseminate via the portal circulation. Extraintestinal amebiasis is most commonly manifested as liver abscess, which may be complicated by pleuropulmonary or peritoneal involvement. During active infection, both trophozoites and cysts may be shed in the stool.

▶ History & Physical

Note history of travel to areas of endemic amebiasis. Homosexual males and institutionalized persons are also at higher risk for infection. Intestinal amebiasis presents with symptoms of acute or chronic colitis manifested by lower abdominal pain and diarrhea. With acute disease, patients will complain of frequent watery stools, containing blood and mucous. Chronic amebic colitis is more likely to present with a prolonged (months to years) history of intermittent bloody diarrhea and abdominal pain. Amebic liver abscess produces fever, right upper quadrant pain, and/or hepatomegaly. There may be cough and crackles at the right lung base.

▶ Diagnostic Studies

Obtain stool for ova and parasites. Check for eosinophilia and leukocytosis on the complete blood count (CBC). Colonoscopy may be necessary to directly visualize the intestinal mucosa and to obtain a mucosal biopsy. In cases of suspected liver abscess, check for lesions with hepatic ultrasound. Chest x-ray may reveal lower lobe consolidation adjacent to area of liver abscess (pleuropulmonary amebiasis).

▶ Diagnosis

The definitive diagnosis of amebiasis if made by identification of cysts and/or trophozoites in stool or biopsy material.

▶ Clinical Therapeutics

Asymptomatic infection (with evidence of cyst-passage in stool) should be treated with a luminal agent, such as paromomycin. Patients with active amebic infection (dysentery, hepatic abscess, etc.) require treatment with metronidazole and paromomycin. Dysentery patients will also need rehydration and electrolyte replacement.

▶ Health Maintenance Issues

Persons traveling in endemic areas should take precautions against ingestion of contaminated food and water.

## XVI.  HOOKWORM

▶ Scientific Concepts

Hookworm is a roundworm infection caused by *Ancylostoma duodenale* or *Necator americanus* (predominant in North America). Hookworm larvae in soil initiate human infection by directly penetrating the host's skin, then migrating hematogenously to the lungs. Larvae are coughed up, swallowed, and travel to the small intestine, where they mature into adult worms. Adult hookworms then attach to intestinal mucosa and feed on host nutrients. Eggs are released with feces; when deposited in soil, they hatch into larvae, thus completing the worm's life cycle. Humans are the only hosts, with children most often affected.

### ▶ History & Physical

Rural children, especially those from warmer climates, are more likely to present with hookworm symptoms. Patients frequently complain of itching at the site of larval penetration (often the feet), and there may be evidence of larval subcutaneous migration tracts. Cough, wheezing, and fever may indicate pulmonary migration of larvae. In the intestinal phase of infection, patients complain of abdominal pain often accompanied by diarrhea. Severe worm infestation may produce signs of malnutrition.

### ▶ Diagnosis

The diagnosis is made by finding hookworm eggs in feces. *A. duodenale* and *N. americanus* eggs have identical morphology. Eosinophilia supports the diagnosis.

### ▶ Clinical Therapeutics

Mebendazole will effectively eradicate hookworm. Correct iron and/or protein deficiency when necessary.

### ▶ Health Maintenance Issues

Patients with asymptomatic infections may not require antihelminthic drug therapy and can be maintained with regular monitoring of serum iron levels and iron supplementation.

## XVII. MALARIA

### ▶ Scientific Concepts

Malaria is a parasitic disease of human erythrocytes caused by four species of *Plasmodium*: *P. falciparum*, *P. malariae*, *P. ovale*, and *P. vivax*. The parasite is transmitted to humans via bite of the female *Anopheles* mosquito. On a global scale, malaria impacts the human population more than any other parasitic disease, affecting over 1 billion people. The highest incidence of disease is seen in sub-Saharan Africa. Cases of malaria in the United States are predominantly seen in persons who have emigrated from endemic areas. Severity of infection is directly related to the species of *Plasmodium* involved. The most severe form, caused by *P. falciparum*, produces widespread microvascular complications; whereas *P. malariae*, *P. ovale*, and *P. vivax* tend to produce milder disease and no microvascular damage. Complications of falciparum malaria are myriad, including severe anemia, pulmonary edema, renal failure, CNS manifestations (delirium, seizures, coma), and death.

### ▶ History & Physical

Note history of emigrating from, or travel to, endemic areas. Patients will complain of regular fevers and may indicate that they occur every

2 to 3 days. The periodicity of fever depends on the infecting species—every 48 hours for *P. ovalex* and *P. vivax* infection, and every 72 hours for *P. malariae.* Patients with falciparum malaria will be more likely to have a history of continuous fever. Shaking chills characteristically accompany fever. Nonfalciparum malaria presents with many nonspecific symptoms, which may include headache, weakness, muscle aches, and fatigue. Pale conjunctiva, hepatosplenomegaly, and repeated fevers followed by exhaustion occur in patients with more advanced disease. Progressive falciparum malaria is manifested by nausea/vomiting, CNS changes (described above), signs of respiratory distress, hypotension, and shock.

▶ **Diagnosis**

Diagnosis is established by identifying the parasite on Giemsa-stained blood smears.

▶ **Clinical Therapeutics**

Chloroquine or mefloquine are effective for the treatment of "benign" malaria (*P. malariae, P. ovale, P. vivax*). The development of chloroquine-resistance in the treatment of falciparum malaria has made quinidine gluconate the new drug of choice for falciparum malaria in the United States. Severe falciparum malaria often requires inpatient management of complications (e.g., enterocolitis, hypoglycemia, renal failure, pulmonary edema, disseminated intravascular coagulation [DIC], adult respiratory distress syndrome [ARDS], etc.).

▶ **Clinical Intervention**

Severe falciparum malaria is a medical emergency and requires prompt and aggressive intervention to prevent serious microvascular complications.

▶ **Health Maintenance Issues**

Persons planning travel to malaria-prone areas should begin chloroquine or mefloquine prophylaxis 1–2 weeks before travel, and should continue taking the drug during and after the trip (for 1 month post travel).

## XVIII.  PINWORMS

▶ **Scientific Concepts**

Pinworm infection (Enterobiasis) is caused by the roundworm, *Enterobius vermicularis,* and is the most common worm infection in the United States, affecting mostly school-aged children. Enterobiasis is spread among family members and young school children via hand-to-mouth transmission of infective eggs. The eggs hatch in the intestine, and mature into adult worms within a month. During active infection, adult females nocturnally migrate to the host's perianal area and deposit eggs. The presence of eggs provokes perianal scratching and transfer of eggs to the host's hands, from which self-reinfection and/or passage of eggs to others may occur. Most cases of enterobiasis are benign.

▶ **History & Physical**

Enterobiasis is usually asymptomatic. When symptomology develops, it is generally limited to perianal pruritis. Since the pruritic episodes occur at night, hosts will often exhibit altered sleep patterns.

▶ Diagnosis

Diagnosis is established by identifying *E. vermicularis* eggs obtained from the host's perianal area. Eggs may be obtained by applying "Scotch" tape to the perianal area in the early morning, and then examining the tape microscopically.

▶ Clinical Therapeutics

*Enterobius* can be eradicated with a single dose of mebendazole or pyrantel pamoate, which should be repeated in 2 weeks.

▶ Clinical Intervention

In a setting of potential reinfection, treat household members to eliminate the worm from asymptomatic carriers.

▶ Health Maintenance Issues

Household members and those working with young children should practice frequent hand washing and give attention to thorough house-cleaning and laundering to eliminate eggs on bedding and clothing.

## XIX. TOXOPLASMOSIS

▶ Scientific Concepts

Toxoplasmosis is a zoonotic infection caused by *Toxoplasma gondii,* an obligate intracellular protozoan. Humans acquire the disease from cats (the definitive host) by ingestion of food, water, or soil contaminated with *Toxoplasma* cysts, or by transplacental transmission of the parasite to the fetus. Fetal toxoplasmosis can lead to a variety of congenital disorders including chorioretinitis and blindness, hydrocephalus, hearing loss, psychomotor retardation, epilepsy, and hematologic abnormalities.

▶ History & Physical

Toxoplasmosis in immunocompetent persons generally produces no symptoms or results in mild disease manifested by fatigue and regional lymphadenopathy. Occasionally, it develops an infectious mononucleosis-like syndrome with fever, sore throat, lymphadenopathy, muscle aches, and hepatosplenomegaly. Immunocompromised persons infected with *T. gondii* are likely to develop encephalitis, with a myriad of possible neurologic deficits, the most common of which are dysphasia and hemiparesis.

▶ Diagnostic Studies

Acute *T. gondii* infection can be established by serologic (ELISA) testing for the presence of specific IgG and IgM antibodies to the parasite. A positive IgA-ELISA test for toxoplasmosis in a newborn confirms the presence of congenital infection. In immunocompromised persons, serologic methods may not be productive and will require the isolation and identification of the parasite from tissue or the use of PCR studies on body fluids. Ocular toxoplasmosis is usually diagnosed on clinical grounds.

▶ Differential Diagnosis

Toxoplasmosis in an immunocompetent person may present like infectious mononucleosis, cat-scratch disease, cytomegalovirus (CMV) infection, lymphoma (including metastatic carcinoma), or tuberculosis. Immunodeficient persons with toxoplasmosis encephalitis may have symptoms and signs suggesting brain abscess, brain tumor, CNS tuberculosis, CMV meningoencephalitis, cryptococcoma, or progressive multifocal leukoencephalopathy.

▶ Clinical Therapeutics

Children and adults with uncomplicated *Toxoplasma* lymphadenitis do not require treatment. Acute toxoplasmosis acquired during pregnancy should be treated with spiramycin. Add pyrimethamine, sulfadiazine, and folinic acid to the maternal drug regimen if amniotic fluid tests positive for *T. gondii* at ≥ 18 weeks gestation. Toxoplasmosis in immunodeficient patients should be treated with the same drug regimen as that for fetal toxoplasmosis. Toxoplasmosis prophylaxis in immunodeficient persons is accomplished with TMP-SMX.

▶ Health Maintenance Issues

See prophylaxis measures described above. Also, acquisition of cysts can be prevented by avoiding contact with cat feces; thorough hand washing after gardening or disposing of cat litter; washing fruits and vegetables before eating; and thoroughly cooking meat before consumption.

## XX. LYME BORRELIOSIS

▶ Scientific Concepts

The most common manifestation of Lyme borreliosis in the United States is Lyme disease, caused by *Borrelia burgdorferi*, a spirochete transmitted to humans via tick bite. Lyme disease occurs most commonly in areas endemic to its principal vector, the deer tick (*Ixodes* species): the northeastern, upper midwestern, and western states. After transmission to a human host, the spirochete replicates in the dermis (manifested as erythema chronicum migrans [ECM]), and then spreads via the bloodstream to other organs/systems. Besides the skin, the disease principally affects the joints, heart, and nervous system.

▶ History & Physical

Those who engage in outdoor activities in tick-infested areas are at higher risk for contracting Lyme disease. Early symptoms and signs of infection include ECM, headache, fever/chills, fatigue, lymphadenopathy, myalgias, and arthralgias. Later in the illness, neurologic, cardiac, and/or increased musculoskeletal involvement are likely, with arthritis being the most common occurrence. Lyme arthritis is typically asymmetric and migratory, involving the large joints, one or two at a time. The knee is most frequently affected, followed by the shoulder and elbow. Patients often complain of recurrent attacks of arthritis, at varying intervals, involving several joints at a time. The most common CNS manifestations of Lyme disease are headaches, photophobia, stiff neck, bilateral facial nerve palsy, and peripheral radiculoneuropathy. Various degrees of heart block occur in some patients after 1–2 months of infection.

▶ Diagnosis

The characteristic clinical picture coupled to positive serologic testing establishes the diagnosis. A positive antibody response to *B. burgdorferi* may not develop until 1–4 weeks into the infection. Two-step serologic testing is recommended—positive ELISA confirmed by Western blot. Positive serologic tests do not distinguish between active and inactive infection.

### ▶ Differential Diagnosis

The presenting features of Lyme disease can mimic a number of bacterial, fungal, or allergic diseases affecting the skin, including cellulitis, ringworm, and eczema. The clinical picture of disseminated Lyme disease can be confused with rheumatic fever, rheumatoid arthritis, psoriatic arthritis, septic arthritis, viral or bacterial meningitis, CNS malignancy, collagen vascular disease, and a host of less common autoimmune disorders.

### ▶ Clinical Therapeutics

Doxycycline or amoxicillin are recommended for the treatment of uncomplicated Lyme disease in children and adults. Do not use doxycycline in pregnant persons. IV ceftriaxone is effective for treating severe Lyme disease associated with cardiac, CNS, and/or musculoskeletal complications. Nonsteroidal anti-inflammatory drugs (NSAIDs) can be given for symptomatic arthritis.

### ▶ Health Maintenance Issues

Persons involved in outdoor activities in endemic areas should protect against tick bites by wearing protective clothing, applying tick repellants, inspecting skin areas regularly during outdoor activity, and immediately removing attached and unattached ticks. Lyme vaccine (recombinant OSP-A) is available and is recommended for those who live and/or work in tick-infested areas.

## XXI. ROCKY MOUNTAIN SPOTTED FEVER

### ▶ Scientific Concepts

Rocky Mountain Spotted Fever (RMSF) is a tick-borne rickettsial disease, manifested by fever, headache, and rash. The etiologic agent, *Rickettsia rickettsii,* is a gram-negative coccobacillus and an obligate intracellular parasite of eukaryotic cells. *Dermacentor* ticks, the vectors of RMSF, are found only in the western hemisphere. Virtually every state reports cases of RMSF, but the highest incidence is in the mid-Atlantic region.

### ▶ History & Physical

Patients may report a prior tick bite (< 5% of cases). The presentation may be flu-like in the early stages of illness, with headache, fever, malaise, and myalgias. With disease progression, nausea, vomiting, anorexia, abdominal pain, high fever, and chills are usually accompanied by a maculopapular rash, spreading from the distal extremities to the trunk and face. The rash characteristically evolves into petechial and hemorrhagic lesions, if antibiotics are not given early in the illness.

Be alert to signs of encephalitis, renal and/or liver failure in severe cases of RMSF.

### ▶ Diagnosis

Suspicion of RMSF may be made on clinical grounds, with diagnosis by positive serologic immunofluorescent antibody (IFA) testing. Seropositivity does not develop in most cases until 7–10 days after onset, making definitive diagnosis difficult in the early, acute stage of illness. Immuno-histochemical identification of the organism from punch biopsy of skin lesions may be required for diagnosis in some cases.

▶ Differential Diagnosis

The nonspecific, early manifestations of RMSF can mimic influenza, infectious mononucleosis, or viral hepatitis. As RMSF progresses and the rash develops, one must consider other rickettsial diseases, such as rickettsial pox, murine typhus, and epidemic typhus, and a host of other possible rash-associated illnesses (e.g., rubella, rubeola, idiopathic thrombocytopenic purpura [ITP], thrombotic thrombocytopenic purpura [TTP], meningococcemia, Kawasaki syndrome). Abdominal symptoms may suggest enterocolitis. Pulmonary findings can be confused with bronchitis or pneumonia.

▶ Clinical Therapeutics

The drug of choice for treatment of RMSF is doxycycline. Severe cases with pulmonary, renal, or liver complications may require hospitalization and appropriate supportive therapy.

▶ Health Maintenance Issues

See recommendations for prevention of tick bites in Lyme Borreliosis section.

## XXII. SYPHILIS

▶ Scientific Concepts

Syphilis is a chronic infection caused by the spirochete, *Treponema pallidum*. It is primarily an STD, characterized by active infection interrupted by periods of latency. Syphilis is less commonly transmitted in utero or via blood transfusion. Three stages of syphilis are recognized: primary infection, manifested by a single, painless genital ulcer; secondary syphilis, in which the development of generalized mucocutaneous lesions occurs; and tertiary infection (5–20 years after initial infection), characterized by progressive, destructive disease affecting the cardiovascular, musculoskeletal, and central nervous systems. Latent periods of variable duration may occur between each stage.

▶ History & Physical

At high risk for syphilis are those with a history of unprotected sexual activity with multiple partners. Primary syphilis classically presents with a solitary (sometimes multiple) painless genital ulcer (chancre). The patient with primary disease is also likely to exhibit local and regional lymphadenopathy.

Secondary syphilis patients may complain of fever, headache, sore throat, and malaise. Such patients are likely to exhibit a generalized nonpruritic macropapular rash, seen on the bilateral distal extremities and/or trunk and mucous membranes. As the secondary lesions erode, they may fuse into flat, highly infectious patches, termed *condylomata lata*. Look for condylomata lata in moist, intertriginous body areas, such as beneath pendulous breasts, perianal area, etc. Also, there may be patchy alopecia affecting the scalp, eyebrows, and/or beard. Physical findings suggestive of CNS, GI, renal and/or musculoskeletal involvement in secondary syphilis are less common.

Patients who progress to tertiary syphilis may not be aware that they ever had primary or secondary disease, and therefore were not treated for syphilis. At this stage of the disease, patients may present with an array of signs and symptoms ranging from minor musculoskeletal complaints to signs of serious cardiovascular damage (e.g., endarteritis obliterans), advanced CNS involvement (e.g., meningeal syphilis), and/or destructive musculoskeletal changes. Widespread neural damage may produce changes in personality, affect, sensorium, speech, and intellect ("general paresis"). Further deterioration leads to tabes dorsalis, manifested by ataxic gait, areflexia, and loss of sensation (which may result in Charcot's joints).

A maternal history of syphilis during pregnancy raises the index of suspicion for congenital syphilis. Such infants may present with fever, low birth weight, maculopapular rash, and CNS signs.

### ▶ Diagnosis

The diagnosis of syphilis is established by direct microscopic visualization of the spirochete from infectious lesions or by positive serologic testing. Direct visualization by fluorescent antibody staining is preferable to dark-field examination. A positive screening test (e.g., rapid plasma reagin [RPR] or Venereal Disease Research Laboratory [VDRL]) should be confirmed by a more sensitive and specific treponemal antibody test (e.g., fluorescent treponemal antibody [FTA] test).

### ▶ Differential Diagnosis

Syphilis is known as "the great impersonator," making the differentiation of the disease based on its presentation and physical findings a daunting task. The syphilis-like conditions in this section constitute a partial list, limited to the most obvious and/or common diseases. The lesion of primary syphilis should be differentiated from chancroid, herpes simplex, lichen planus, granuloma inguinale, and malignancy. The rash of secondary syphilis may suggest a host of other conditions, including viral exanthems, drug eruption, pityriasis rosea, and scabies. The possibilities to be ruled out in tertiary syphilis include miliary tuberculosis, malignancy, brain abscess, Alzheimer's dementia, cerebrovascular accident, and trauma.

### ▶ Clinical Therapeutics

Penicillin is the drug of choice for all stages of syphilis, including congenital syphilis. In cases of penicillin allergy, doxycycline, tetracycline, or erythromycin can be used. For complications of tertiary syphilis, hospitalization and appropriate supportive therapy may be required.

### ▶ Health Maintenance Issues

Patient education and community health programs directed at the high risks associated with sexual promiscuity and the importance of seeking prompt treatment for syphilis are important to an effective syphilis prevention and control effort.

## XXIII. CYTOMEGALOVIRUS INFECTIONS

### ▶ Scientific Concepts

Cytomegalovirus (CMV) is a double-stranded DNA virus related to herpes. CMV infection can be acquired congenitally, perinatally, and via sexual transmission. CMV, like herpes, becomes latent after primary infection and may reactivate many years later. Reactivation CMV is common in AIDS patients with low CD4 counts and may lead to life-threatening, multiorgan disease. CMV retinitis is an important cause of blindness in immunocompromised patients. Most CMV infections in immunocompetent persons are asymptomatic.

▶ History & Physical

Immunocompetent persons seldom present with signs and symptoms of CMV infection. If symptoms develop, the patient usually exhibits a mild mononucleosis-like syndrome. Aside from congenital CMV infection (in which < 1% of newborns are symptomatic), clinical CMV is seen mostly in immunodeficient children and adults. Such persons may be organ transplant recipients, AIDS patients, or persons undergoing radiation therapy for cancer. CMV in the immunodeficient patient can present with signs of localized or disseminated disease. For example, CMV pneumonitis patients will complain of fever, cough, dyspnea, and night sweats. There may be associated retinitis. Gastrointestinal CMV may produce ulceration and bleeding, leading to complaints of nausea/vomiting, abdominal pain/tenderness, and bloody stools. Also, be alert to signs of CMV meningoencephalitis in AIDS patients.

Infants born with symptomatic CMV generally are premature and have undergone retarded intrauterine growth. At birth, they present with petechiae, jaundice, microcephaly, and hepatosplenomegaly.

▶ Diagnostic Studies

The diagnosis of CMV infection is made by cytopathological studies, by isolating and identifying the virus in tissue cultures, or by demonstrating seroconversion. Positive cytopathology is the finding of characteristic CMV nuclear inclusions ("owl eye" cells) in tissue biopsy specimens.

▶ Clinical Therapeutics

Ganciclovir is the drug of choice for the treatment of all CMV syndromes, including retinitis. Its effectiveness can be enhanced by the addition of CMV hyperimmune globulin to the regimen.

▶ Health Maintenance Issues

Prophylactic ganciclovir has been shown to reduce the frequency of CMV disease in immunocompromised persons.

## XXIV. EPSTEIN–BARR VIRUS INFECTIONS

▶ Scientific Concepts

Epstein–Barr virus (EBV) is a double-stranded DNA virus associated with several human disorders, the most common of which is heterophil-positive infectious mononucleosis. The infection is transmitted by contact with infected human secretions, principally saliva. The classic manifestation of EBV infectious mononucleosis is the presence of atypical lymphocytes in the peripheral blood smear. Most EBV infections in healthy persons are asymptomatic. EBV is also connected with the development of several lymphoproliferative diseases, including Burkitt's lymphoma, B-cell lymphoma, Hodgkin's disease, and nasopharyngeal carcinoma.

► History & Physical

The clinical syndrome of infectious mononucleosis is typically seen in healthy, young adults who present with fever, sore throat, tender lymphadenopathy (usually posterior cervical), and splenomegaly. The patient may have a history of intimate contact with other infected persons and frequently note a prodrome of malaise, fatigue, and persistent headache. A rash or jaundice with hepatic involvement will occur in some cases. Persons with lymphoma typically present with painless lymph node enlargement (e.g., Hodgkin's patients often note a painless mass in the neck). AIDS patients who develop multiple painless nodes should be further investigated for B-cell lymphoma.

► Diagnostic Studies

In patients with EBV infectious mononucleosis, the CBC will exhibit leukocytosis (commonly, 12,000–20,000), with predominantly lymphocytosis and > 10% atypical lymphocytes. Liver enzymes are often moderately increased. Confirmation of EBV infection is made by demonstration of heterophil antibodies (positive monospot test) or a positive test for antibodies to EBV-specific antigen. The diagnosis of lymphoma is made by cytopathological examination of biopsied lymph node tissue.

► Differential Diagnosis

EBV infectious mononucleosis may be confused with other bacterial, fungal, and viral causes of pharyngitis (e.g., *Candida, Streptococci*, diphtheria, adenoviral infection); with other causes of lymphadenopathy (e.g., HIV, CMV, toxoplasmosis); and with the manifestations of carbamazepine hypersensitivity. Differentiation among various types of lymphomas is impossible without cytological identification.

► Clinical Therapeutics

EBV infectious mononucleosis is a self-limited disease for most immunocompetent persons, and therapy is mainly supportive. The treatment of lymphoma, depending on the stage of disease and the status of the patient, ranges from no therapy to irradiation, chemotherapy, and stem-cell transplantation.

► Clinical Intervention

For complications of infectious mononucleosis (e.g., EBV hepatitis), corticosteroids may lessen the extent and duration of illness. Secondary bacterial pharyngitis should be treated with appropriate antibiotics.

► Health Maintenance Issues

Patients in the acute stage of infectious mononucleosis should be advised to avoid contact sports and heavy lifting because of the risk of splenic rupture.

## XXV. ERYTHEMA INFECTIOSUM

► Scientific Concepts

Erythema infectiosum is an exanthematous illness of childhood caused by parvovirus B19 (P-B19), a single-stranded DNA virus. The virus is presumably transmitted via respiratory droplets. P-B19 is the only known human pathogen among the more than 50 types of parvoviruses, causing a diverse range of syndromes, from fifth disease in children to arthritis in adults. The term *fifth disease* evolved from the early classification of diseases of children in which erythema infectiosum was fifth on the list of the six exanthems of childhood. The classic feature of fifth disease is a fiery red "slapped cheek" rash. In immunocompromised patients, P-B19 attacks erythroid precursor cells, producing anemia or aplastic crisis. Nosocomial outbreaks of erythema infectiosum have been traced to patients in P-B19 aplastic crisis, who are highly infectious during that period. P-B19 infection during pregnancy has been associated with hydrops and fetal death.

### ► History & Physical

Children usually develop fifth disease during the winter or spring months. Many have a mild subclinical infection, but others present with the characteristic "slapped cheek" rash. The rash often spreads to the arms and legs, becomes pruritic and erythematous, with a lacy, reticular pattern. A mild fever may precede the development of the rash. In adults, P-B19 infection often presents with arthritic symptoms referred to the knees, ankles, hands and/or wrists, in symmetrical distribution. Adults usually do not develop a rash. Patients note diminishing arthritic symptoms with time, and no residual joint damage occurs. The presence of pallor in adults with P-B19 infection may denote accompanying anemia.

### ► Diagnosis

The diagnosis of P-B19 infection is based on clinical findings, and is confirmed by a positive test for IgM anti-P-B19 antibodies in the patient's serum.

### ► Differential Diagnosis

In cases of fifth disease, the principal rule-out is scarlet fever. P-B19 arthritis in adults may mimic a number of arthritic disorders including rheumatoid arthritis, lupus erythematosis, and Lyme disease.

### ► Clinical Therapeutics

Treatment is supportive for those with normal immune systems. Give NSAIDs for arthritis/arthralgia in adults. Aplastic crisis requires whole blood transfusion. Immunodeficient patients should receive hyperimmune antiP-B19 globulin.

### ► Clinical Intervention

Chronic anemia associated with persistent P-B19 infection in immunodeficient persons can be controlled with administration of immune globulin.

### ► Health Maintenance Issues

Hospitalized immunodeficient patients who develop P-B19–associated aplastic crisis should be isolated to prevent nosocomial spread of infection. Hyperimmune antiP-B19 globulin is recommended for pregnant persons.

## XXVI.  HERPES SIMPLEX

### ► Scientific Concepts

Herpes simplex is a double-stranded DNA virus that causes painful infections, most often in the oral and genital areas. Two antigenic types of the virus persist in the human population: HSV1 and HSV2, both of which are transmitted by direct intimate contact with infected secretions. Herpes infections affecting the oral area (herpes labialis) result in single or multiple mucocutaneous lesions, largely caused by HSV1. Oral herpes infections are commonly referred to as *cold sores*. Genital herpes is mainly an HSV2 infection; however, both types of herpes can infect the oral and genital areas.

Herpes simplex virus also infects the eye, often producing corneal damage that may lead to blindness. Painful HSV infections of the finger and nail (herpetic Whitlow) may occur, especially among health care workers. Both types of HSV cause neonatal and congenital infections that may produce congenital abnormalities. Erythema multiforme and Stevens–Johnson syndrome have an HSV etiology, in some cases.

Immunocompromised persons are at particular risk for the development of serious HSV infections that may disseminate to multiple organs and systems, with tropism for the neurologic system.

### ► History & Physical

Patients with oral HSV often have a prior history of similar lesions and note that they develop during an illness or when under psychological stress. In cases of oral and/or genital HSV, there may be a history of sexual contact with an HSV-infected partner. Patients typically present with either a single lesion or a cluster of small, clear vesicles in the circumoral and/or genital area. In a few days, the vesicles break and ulcerate, becoming more painful; after 1–2 weeks, the lesions crust over and begin to heal. Vulvovaginal HSV may be accompanied by vaginal discharge. Patients with HSV keratitis complain of eye pain (generally unilateral) and diminished visual acuity. Fluorescein eye exam reveals branching corneal ulceration.

HSV in immunocompromised patients can present without external lesions, but may exhibit symptoms and signs relative to the organ/system(s) involved. Be especially alert to CNS herpes (e.g., note signs of meningitis or encephalitis). Neonatal herpes may present with widespread skin lesions or signs of disseminated infection.

### ► Diagnostic Studies

Oral or genital HSV is diagnosed on clinical findings and a positive Tzanck smear on scrapings from a lesion or a positive test for HSV antigen in lesion material. PCR testing should be done on CSF in cases of suspected HSV encephalitis.

### ► Differential Diagnosis

Mucocutaneous HSV must be distinguished from herpangina., impetigo, aphthous stomatitis, Stephens–Johnson syndrome, primary syphilitic chancre, and common viral exanthems. Disseminated HSV with multiple organ/system involvement broadens the differential considerably, with special attention to other viral or bacterial causes of meningoencephalitis.

### ► Clinical Therapeutics

Mucocutaneous HSV is effectively treated with oral or topical acyclovir. Use ophthalmic acyclovir or tirfluridine for HSV keratitis. (*Note:* HSV keratitis can progress to corneal scarring and should be afforded prompt emergent care with topical antiviral agents.) Congenital and disseminated HSV requires parenteral acyclovir. Acyclovir-resistant HSV can be treated with foscarnet.

► Health Maintenance Issues

Acyclovir is effective in the primary and secondary prevention of HSV infections (recommended for immunodeficient patients). Patients should be educated about avoidance of high-risk sexual practices that increase the likelihood of contracting HSV infection. Maternal transmission of HSV to the child at delivery can be prevented by cesarean section.

## XXVII.  HIV INFECTION

► Scientific Concepts

HIV infection was first encountered in the United States in 1981, when homosexual men began developing severe opportunistic infections and peculiar neoplasms associated with a syndrome, later named AIDS. It is now known that HIV infection targets CD4 lymphocytes, components of the T cell immune system. The virus is transmitted sexually and perinatally and via contact with HIV-contaminated blood and blood products. There is no evidence that the disease is transmitted by casual (nonsexual) contact with HIV-positive persons or by insect vectors.

After primary, acute infection, many years may elapse before development of full-blown AIDS. The severity of HIV infection increases as CD4 lymphocyte counts decline. A CD4 count of less than 200 signals the onset of full-blown AIDS, making the patient at very high risk for a variety of potentially life-threatening opportunistic infections. Such infections include *Pneumocystis carinii* pneumonia, tuberculosis, *Herpes* and *Toxoplasma* encephalitis, cryptococcal meningitis, and disseminated *Mycobacterium avium* complex (MAC). Other AIDS-defining conditions include AIDS dementia complex and Kaposi's sarcoma.

Over the past 5 years, the increasing incidence of HIV infection in the United States has shifted from homosexual men to heterosexual females, particularly African American women. The heterosexual shift in the epidemic has resulted from increasing HIV transmission among IV drug abusers engaging in heterosexual practices with multiple partners. Current estimates are that approximately 1 million persons are living with HIV/AIDS in the United States. From a global perspective, HIV infection/AIDS is a pandemic, with disease occurrence in virtually every country, totaling over 40 million cases. Since the first reported cases in 1981, over 3 million persons have died from AIDS and AIDS-related illnesses.

► History & Physical

Patients at risk for HIV infection will usually have a history of promiscuous sexual practices, IV drug abuse, blood transfusion, occupational accident (e.g., needle stick), or perinatal exposure. Primary HIV infection may be asymptomatic, or patients may present with a mononucleosis-like syndrome, consisting of fever, headache, sore throat, lymphadenopathy, and general malaise. Following primary acute infection, patients may experience a decline in symptoms and enter a latent period before further signs of disease progression are noted.

As the CD4 count declines and the disease progresses, a variety of clinical presentations are likely to occur. These include signs and symptoms of pneumonia (e.g., *P. carinii*), meningitis (e.g., *Cryptococcus*), TB, GI disease (esophageal candidiasis, shigellosis, giardiasis), toxoplasmosis, malignancy (e.g., lymphoma, Kaposi's sarcoma), disseminated viral infections (e.g., HSV, CMV, Varicella-zoster virus [VZV]), fungal infections (e.g., histoplasmosis, cryptococcosis, candidiasis, etc.), disseminated MAC, and AIDS dementia complex.

Dermatologic conditions are very common in AIDS patients and include STD lesions (e.g., HSV, all stages of syphilis, disseminated gonorrhea), malignancy (e.g., Kaposi's sarcoma), staphylococcal/streptococcal conditions (e.g., folliculitis, impetigo, cellulites), fungal lesions (e.g., mucocutaneous candidiasis, cryptococcosis), and viral rashes (e.g., VZV, HSV).

### ▶ Diagnostic Studies

ELISA is the standard screening test for HIV infection. A positive screening test must be confirmed by the Western blot (WB) method. A positive test for antibodies to all three HIV antigens (*env, gag, pol*) on the WB is conclusive evidence of infection with HIV. An indeterminate WB may indicate an evolving antibody response, and should be repeated in 1 month. HIV-infected patients may remain WB-negative for up to several months after primary infection. Definitive diagnosis of HIV infection should be followed by a baseline CD4 count to stage the disease. In early HIV disease, the CD4 level is greater than 500. At midstage, the CD4 ranges between 200 and 500. Late-stage HIV disease is marked by CD4 levels that drop below 200. At this stage of the infection, patients usually develop full-blown AIDS, and other diagnostic testing appropriate to onset of AIDS-related illnesses will be necessary.

### ▶ Differential Diagnosis

The constitutional symptoms in primary HIV infection may suggest a number of common disorders, including EBV-infectious mononucleosis, viral influenza, tuberculosis, or malignancy. HIV/AIDS, by itself, has no defining set of signs and symptoms. The differential diagnosis in cases presenting with advanced HIV disease and full-blown AIDS becomes very broad due to the wide variety of opportunistic infections, malignancies, and other AIDS-related disorders that occur (often concurrently) in such patients.

### ▶ Clinical Therapeutics

HIV/AIDS patients must receive therapy directed at: (1) reduction of their HIV load, (2) treatment of opportunistic infections and malignancies, (3) hematopoietic stimulation, and (4) prophylaxis against further development of opportunistic infections. HIV load is reduced with antiretroviral drugs used in combination: nucleoside analogs (e.g., zidovudine), protease inhibitors (e.g., indinavir), and nonnucleoside reverse transcriptase inhibitors (e.g., nevirapine). Opportunistic infections and malignancies should be treated with appropriate antibiotics and chemotherapeutic agents (e.g., *P. carinii* pneumonia [PCP] is effectively treated with TMP-SMX; Kaposi's sarcoma responds to vinblastine). Appropriate hematopoietic-stimulating agents should be given (e.g., erythropoietin for anemia). Multiple prophylactic antibiotic regimens will be required to prevent recurrent PCP, MAC, TB, CMV, toxoplasmosis, cryptococcosis, and candidiasis (e.g., clarithromycin and azithromycin for prevention of MAC).

► Clinical Intervention

Some of the above-described therapeutic interventions must be initiated before CD4 levels drop below 200 (e.g., treatment of opportunistic infections); but all available interventions must be employed in advanced disease, including reduction of HIV load, hematopoietic stimulation, and prophylaxis against opportunistic infections.

► Health Maintenance Issues

Young persons must be educated on the dangers of unprotected and promiscuous sexual activity. Sexual abstinence or the use of condoms is the best means for preventing HIV infection. Once HIV infection begins, prophylaxis against opportunistic infections should be used as described above.

## XXVIII. HUMAN PAPILLOMAVIRUS INFECTIONS

► Scientific Concepts

Human papillomavirus (HPV) infections are generally manifested as benign skin or genital warts. Skin warts are typically superficial or deep (plantar). Genital warts (condyloma acuminata) are sexually transmitted infections occurring on the external genitalia and perianal areas. HPV infection of the female genital tract increases the risk of cervical cancer.

► History & Physical

Children and young adults frequently present with warts (verruca vulgaris) on the hands or feet and sometimes the face. Common warts on the hands will appear as one or more flat, generally painless, superficial growths. The lesions are variably sized (1 mm to 1 cm), hyperkeratotic, flesh-colored papules. Plantar warts are painful, single, multiple, or coalesced lesions typically found on the plantar pressure points (metatarsal heads and heel).

Persons presenting with anogenital warts (condyloma acuminata) may indicate a history of sexual activity with infected partner(s). Perianal warts have a higher incidence among homosexual men. In women, the presence of warts on the labia warrants a search for additional lesions in the vagina and cervix. Conversely, vaginal and cervical warts may occur without external warts. Penile warts usually develop around the urethral meatus and may extend proximally on the shaft.

► Diagnosis

The diagnosis is usually based on clinical findings. Suspicious lesions should be biopsied for cytopathological examination (e.g., colposcopy with biopsy in cases of cervical epithelial changes).

► Differential Diagnosis

Other wart-like lesions that must be considered are skin tags, plantar corns, nevi, and seborrheic keratosis. In cases of anogenital warts, other dysplastic/malignant conditions must be ruled out, including actinic keratoses and squamous cell carcinoma.

► Clinical Therapeutics

The approach to treatment depends on location, cosmetic considerations, and premalignant potential of the lesion. Therapeutic options range from watch and wait to chemical or surgical removal. Spontaneous disappearance commonly occurs. Chemical destruction can be accomplished with topical salicylic acid, podophylline, and formalin. Electrocautery, cryotherapy, or laser surgery are additional options.

▶ **Health Maintenance Issues**

Anogenital warts can be prevented by avoidance of sexual activity with HPV-infected partners. Sexual partners should be examined and treated. Females with a history of genital warts should be advised to receive periodic screening for malignancy via Pap smears.

## XXIX.  INFLUENZA

▶ **Scientific Concepts**

Influenza is an acute, febrile illness caused by influenza A and B viruses. The infection is highly contagious and epidemic, beginning each year in the late fall and winter, and continuing into spring. The viruses affect all age groups, predominantly targeting the respiratory system. Most cases are uncomplicated and resolve in 1–2 weeks; however, serious infections and secondary bacterial involvement (e.g., pneumococcal pneumonia) may complicate influenza in the very young and very old. New influenza vaccine is produced each year, formulated from the predominant antigenic types involved in that year's outbreak (e.g., the 2003–04 trivalent influenza vaccine is designated by three antigenic types: H1N1, A/New Caledonia/20/99; H3N2, A/Moscow/10/99; and B/Hong Kong/330/2001). Each year's new vaccine significantly reduces the risk of serious influenza infections and complications.

▶ **History & Physical**

In the late fall and early winter months, clusters of cases presenting with acute onset of febrile respiratory illness often signal the beginning of "flu season." Patients typically complain of sudden onset of chills, fever, headache, sore throat, nonproductive cough, muscle aches, and general malaise. Physical exam findings are nonspecific, but may include cervical lymphadenopathy, rhinorrhea, hyperemic pharynx, substernal and/or abdominal tenderness. In neonates, the only presenting sign may be fever.

▶ **Diagnosis**

Rapid diagnostic tests are now available to detect the presence of influenza viral antigens. However, the diagnosis is often made clinically within the context of the seasonal outbreak pattern.

▶ **Differential Diagnosis**

*Mycoplasma* pneumonia and other viral pneumonias, such as parainfluenza, adenovirus, and respiratory syncytial virus, must be considered in the context of influenza.

▶ **Clinical Therapeutics**

Most cases of influenza are uncomplicated and can be treated supportively with bed rest, adequate hydration, and antipyretics. (*Note:* avoid salicylates in children because of the risk of Reye's syndrome.) M2 inhibitors or neuraminidase inhibitors can be given to shorten the course of illness.

▶ Clinical Intervention

Primary influenza pneumonia may require hospitalization and appropriate supportive care.

▶ Health Maintenance Issues

Influenza vaccine should be administered yearly to those at risk for complications of influenza (e.g., persons ≥ 65 years of age) and to those who can transmit influenza to others at high risk (e.g., physician assistants, nurses, physicians). Since the most common, serious complication of influenza is pneumococcal pneumonia, it is also advisable that persons at high risk receive polyvalent pneumococcal vaccine. For further information on influenza and pneumococcal vaccination, consult the Centers of Disease Control and Prevention (CDC) National Immunization Program website: www.cdc.gov/nip/

## XXX.  MUMPS

▶ Scientific Concepts

Mumps is a paramyxovirus infection of childhood that is largely controlled in the United States by vaccination. The virus is transmitted via respiratory droplets. The distinctive feature of the infection is painful swelling of the parotid glands. Humans are the only natural reservoir for the virus. Preschool children who receive combined measles-mumps-rubella (MMR) vaccine are protected against infection.

▶ History & Physical

In this country, most new cases of mumps lack a vaccination history, and clusters of infections are occasionally seen in religious communities opposed to vaccination. Patients may present with a prodrome of fever, headache, muscle aches, and anorexia; but more often, parotid pain and swelling are the initial complaints. Be alert to stiff neck, headache, and drowsiness that may signal complicating aseptic meningitis. Unilateral testicular pain, swelling, and tenderness may indicate orchitis, an uncommon complication of mumps.

▶ Diagnosis

A presumptive diagnosis of mumps can be made on clinical grounds, and can be confirmed by ELISA testing for specific IgM antibodies to mumps virus.

▶ Differential Diagnosis

Parotid swelling may be associated with a variety of conditions, including parainfluenza virus type 3, coxsackie virus, and influenza A infections; cervical lymphadenitis; supportive parotitis; and salivary calculi. Testicular torsion may be confused with mumps orchitis. Signs of aseptic meningitis may occur with a myriad of viral syndromes.

▶ Clinical Therapeutics

Treatment of mumps is symptomatic, including analgesics, warm or cold compresses to painful glands and/or testicles, and adequate hydration.

► Health Maintenance Issues

The disease can be prevented by administering MMR vaccine to children 12–15 months of age and again between ages 4–6.

## XXXI. RUBELLA

► Scientific Concepts

Rubella (German measles) is an acute exanthematous viral infection of children and adults. The disease is spread by respiratory droplets and by direct contact. The illness is usually mild and accompanied by a rash. However, rubella infection during pregnancy places the fetus at risk for development of congenital rubella syndrome (CRS). A fetus with CRS may be spontaneously aborted or develop a variety of abnormalities, including sensorineural deafness, retinopathy, cataracts, fetal growth retardation, and heart defects (e.g., patent ductus arteriosus). CRS may lead to postnatal mental retardation and developmental delays. The widespread use of MMR vaccine (see the section on Mumps) has dramatically reduced the incidence of rubella in the United States.

► History & Physical

Rubella is highly contagious, and patients may have a history of family exposure or institutional contact with other infected persons 1–2 weeks prior to onset of symptoms. A prodrome of fever, cough, anorexia, lymphadenopathy, muscle aches, and malaise is often seen in adults; soon followed by the development of a erythematous maculopapular rash. Children typically develop the rash without a prodrome. The rash initially erupts on the face, spreads to the distal extremities within 24–48 hours, and usually disappears in 3–5 days. Forschheimer spots (soft palate petechiae) may occur in some cases. Adults may complain of concurrent arthritic pain, a complication most often seen in women.

► Diagnosis

Rubella can be provisionally diagnosed by history of exposure and clinical presentation. Confirmation of rubella infection is made by the finding of a positive ELISA test for rubella-specific IgG and/or IgM antibodies. The finding of active infection in a pregnant person before 20 weeks of gestation poses a highest risk for the development of CRS.

► Differential Diagnosis

The presentation of rubella mimics other viral exanthems, including fifth disease, measles, roseola, and scarletina. One should also consider toxoplasmosis, scarlet fever, and infectious mononucleosis.

► Clinical Therapeutics

There is no specific treatment for rubella, other than symptomatic therapy.

► Clinical Intervention

Children born with congenital rubella syndrome will require intervention to treat or correct specific defects. For example, sensorineural hearing deficits warrant early audiologic evaluation. Early assessment and intervention for developmental delays and mental retardation should be done.

► **Health Maintenance Issues**

Rubella is prevented by the administration of MMR vaccine. Prenatal screening of reproductive-aged women's immune status is important for the prevention of CRS.

## XXXII. ROSEOLA

► **Scientific Concepts**

Roseola is an acute febrile illness in infants caused by a human herpesvirus. The illness is characterized by a relatively high fever followed by a rose-pink maculopapular rash. Seizures may be precipitated by the high fever. The infection predominantly affects children aged 6 months to 3 years and is the most common cause of exanthematous fever in this age group.

► **History & Physical**

Be alert to roseola in any mildly ill young child who presents with a continuously high fever (up to 8 days) and/or rash. A fever > 40°C is not uncommon. There may be associated vomiting and diarrhea. A rose-pink, nonpruritic, maculopapular rash first appears on the trunk, and later spreads to the neck, face, and extremities. Various degrees of coalescence of the rash usually occur before it disappears in 1–2 days. Febrile seizures may be followed by signs of meningitis or meningoencephalitis. Some infants will exhibit a bulging anterior fontanelle.

► **Diagnosis**

There is no specific test for roseola. A presumptive diagnosis can be made on clinical findings.

► **Differential Diagnosis**

Other common viral exanthems must be considered. The high fever may also suggest bacterial sepsis.

► **Clinical Therapeutics**

Roseola is generally a benign viral infection and can be managed with symptomatic therapy, with particular attention to antipyretics to prevent febrile seizures.

► **Clinical Intervention**

Particular attention should be given to control of fever with antipyretics and sponge baths in children with a history of febrile seizures.

## XXXIII. MEASLES

► **Scientific Concepts**

Measles (rubeola) is an exanthematous viral infection that has been largely controlled in the United States by preschool immunization. The disease is transmitted via respiratory droplets or direct contact, and outbreaks occur in winter and spring months. Nonimmune persons are highly susceptible. Children and young adults are primarily affected, but the disease can occur at any age.

► **History & Physical**

Clustering of cases can be expected during seasonal outbreaks, but for some, there may be no known history of exposure. Persons in the prodromal phase may complain of fever, sneezing, cough, tearing, lethargy, and photophobia. Examination of the buccal mucosa during this phase is likely to reveal small white or light blue plaques (Koplik's spots). Within a few days, a maculopapular rash develops around the hairline and face, and coalesces to bright red patches as it spreads to the trunk. The rash generally appears as the fever peaks. Spreading of the rash to the extremities occurs while it fades from the face and trunk. Desquamation may accompany clearing of the rash. Atypical measles commonly presents with signs and symptoms of pneumonia, but CNS or GI complications may also occur. Adult measles often is accompanied by hepatitis and/or asthmatic symptoms.

► **Diagnosis**

A presumptive diagnosis can be made on clinical findings and confirmed by positive test for IgG or IgM antibodies.

► **Differential Diagnosis**

Other viral exanthems must be ruled out, as well as staphylococcal and streptococcal infections (e.g., scalded skin syndrome), Kawasaki's disease, Stevens–Johnson syndrome, and drug allergy.

► **Clinical Therapeutics**

Treatment is largely supportive directed principally at cough relief and fever reduction. Full recovery can be expected within 2 weeks.

► **Clinical Intervention**

Prolonged fever suggests secondary bacterial infection. Otitis, sinusitis, and/or bacterial pneumonia are the most common complications and require appropriate antibiotic therapy.

► **Health Maintenance Issues**

The current two-dose schedule of MMR vaccination is recommended for prevention of measles. Nonimmune persons can be protected from infection if given the vaccine within 72 hours after exposure.

## XXXIV. VARICELLA-ZOSTER VIRUS INFECTIONS

► **Scientific Concepts**

Primary infection with varicella-zoster virus (VZV) commonly occurs in infants and children, resulting in varicella (chickenpox). Primary infection confers life-long immunity; however, the virus continues to reside in the sensory ganglia in a dormant condition. Later in life, often under conditions of stress, the virus reactivates causing secondary infection (herpes zoster = shingles). Immunodeficient persons have a higher incidence of herpes zoster.

Chickenpox is highly contagious and is spread via respiratory droplets and direct contact with infectious lesions. After a 2- to 3-week incubation period, the infection manifests itself with fever and a generalized vesiculopustular rash. Vaccination with live varicella virus is now recommended for all susceptible children and adults.

Although not as contagious as the primary infection, herpes zoster is capable of being transmitted from cases of shingles to susceptible persons, causing primary chickenpox. Herpes zoster characteristically produces a painful eruption of grouped vesicles along a single dermatome, stopping at the midline. Ophthalmic zoster may result in serious corneal damage and visual impairment.

### ► History & Physical

There is often a history of prior exposure to chickenpox or shingles. Chickenpox develops in those with no prior history of varicella. Minor constitutional symptoms are followed by the eruption of clusters of red macules on the trunk and face that rapidly evolve into tiny vesicles on an erythematous base. The vesicles become pustular and very itchy, then encrust and scab over. Transition stages vary among lesions, producing a variety of forms at any one time. After about a week, new lesions stop forming.

The rash of shingles presents as clusters of vesicles on an erythematous base, found unilaterally along a single dermatome, often on the trunk or face. Pain or pruritis may occur prior to the appearance of the rash, in the area of eventual eruption, continue during the active rash, and then may recur for a variable period after the rash disappears (postherpetic neuralgia).

### ► Diagnosis

The diagnosis is based on the characteristic clinical picture, and the finding of multinucleated giant cells with inclusions in stained tissue from lesions (Tzanck test). The diagnosis is supported by detection of VZV antigen in skin lesions.

### ► Differential Diagnosis

Other conditions with rashes similar to varicella include impetigo, scabies, coxsackievirus infection, and rickettsialpox. Shingles may be confused with contact dermatitis, herpes simplex, and linear impetigo lesions.

### ► Clinical Therapeutics

Acyclovir is the drug of choice for varicella and herpes zoster infections. Supportive treatment is directed at pain/itching control, maintenance of hydration, and good general hygiene. Chicken pox and zoster lesions are infective until they begin to crust over and heal. Therefore, children should not return to school until all lesions show evidence of healing.

### ► Clinical Intervention

Secondary bacterial infection is the most common complication of VZV infection, requiring treatment with topical or systemic antibiotics.

► Health Maintenance Issues

VZV infections can be prevented by administration of live attenuated vaccine.

## XXXV. RABIES

► Scientific Concepts

Rabies is a life-threatening viral infection of the CNS transmitted to humans predominantly from infected (rabid) animals. The disease manifests itself as an acute, fulminant encephalitis that is invariably fatal without early and aggressive postexposure prophylaxis. Average survival time after onset of symptoms is 4 days. Human infection usually occurs via animal bite. Infected dogs, cats, bats, raccoons, skunks, wolves, and foxes are the most common vectors of human rabies. Domestic animal immunization is widely practiced in the United States; however, rabies transmission from infected wild animals remains a serious public health threat. The availability of human diploid cell vaccine provides for safe and effective rabies prophylaxis.

► History & Physical

A history of a bite from a suspected rabid animal is important. Also, contamination of a wound by infected animal saliva may be reported. The patient is likely to note numbness and tingling in the bite area, along with nonspecific symptoms, such as headache, fever, nausea, and vomiting. Also, there may be various degrees of limb and facial weakness. Combat-iveness, agitation, hallucinations, signs of meningeal irritation, muscle spasms, and seizures signal the onset of encephalitis. As the encephalitis progresses, the patient enters the "hydrophobic period" of the disease, manifested by dysphagic drooling, confusion, double vision, decreased lucidity, and violent involuntary muscle contractions. Finally, respiratory paralysis occurs, resulting in death.

► Diagnosis

The diagnosis is based on the history of rabid animal bite, and the finding of viral antigen in infected tissue. Anti-rabies antibody levels increase too late to be of diagnostic value in saving the patient's life. Definitive diagnosis is made by postmortem finding of Negri bodies in the brain tissue of the presumed rabid animal and/or the patient; by isolation of the virus from infected tissue; or detection of rabies virus DNA by PCR studies.

► Clinical Therapeutics

Once symptomatic rabies is evident, patients very rarely survive. Aggressive intensive care is required but offers little chance for recovery.

► Clinical Intervention

Postexposure prophylaxis should be initiated in any instance of known or suspected rabies in an animal involved in human exposure (to infected saliva or bite). The prophylactic regime consists of thorough wound cleansing and debridement and administration of human antirabies immune globulin and human diploid cell vaccine. If reference lab findings are negative for rabies virus in the suspected animal, the prophylaxis regime may be discontinued.

### ► Health Maintenance Issues

Preexposure prophylaxis with human diploid cell vaccine should be considered in any person at high risk for contact with rabies, such as laboratory personnel, veterinarians, cave explorers, and humane service workers.

## BIBLIOGRAPHY

Braunwald E, Faud AS, et al., eds. *Harrison's Online.* New York: McGraw-Hill; 2002. www.harrisonsonline.com

Bryan CS. *Infectious Diseases in Primary Care.* Philadelphia, PA: WB Saunders; 2002.

Gilbert DN, Moellering RC, Sande MA. *The Sanford Guide to Antimicrobial Therapy;* 32nd ed. Hyde Park, VT: Antimicrobial Therapy; 2002.

Holmes HN, ed. *Handbook of Infectious Diseases.* Springhouse, PA: Springhouse Corp.; 2001.

Rakel RE, Bope ET, eds. *Conn's Current Therapy: 2002.* Philadelphia, PA: WB Saunders; 2002.

Wilson WR, Sande MA, eds. *Current Diagnosis & Treatment in Infectious Disease.* New York: Lange Medical Books/McGraw-Hill; 2001.

# Surgery 17

*Steve B. Fisher, MHA, PA-C*

## I. GENERAL SURGERY

### A. Cholecystitis/Cholelithiasis

▶ Scientific Concepts

An inflamed gallbladder lining can be due to infection, "sludge," or obstructive stone in the cystic or common bile duct. Predisposing factors include genetics, oral contraceptives, female gender, and multiparity. Most stones are cholesterol; others are bilirubin pigmented. Greatest incidence is adults 30–80 years old.

▶ History & Physical

Intolerance of fatty foods; moderate, intermittent abdominal pain in epigastric and right upper quadrant; nausea; and vomiting. Possible radiation to right scapula or posterior thorax.

▶ Diagnostic Studies

Ultrasound of the gallbladder is the study of choice, followed by hepato-iminodiacetic acid (HIDA) scan for clarification if necessary. Oral cholecystogram is rarely used today. Endoscopic retrograde cholangiopancreatography (ERCP) can be both diagnostic and therapeutic. White blood cell (WBC) count and serum liver enzymes and amylase are helpful, but nonspecific.

▶ Diagnosis

Lab tests will be elevated. The ultrasound will show stones or sludge or a thickened gallbladder wall.

▶ Clinical Therapeutics

Cholecystitis should be treated with cholecystectomy, either immediately (within 72 hours of initial onset) or 6 weeks after IV fluids and antibiotics to treat a longer acute attack.

▶ Clinical Intervention

Laparoscopic cholecystectomy is the technique of choice. Urgent surgery is required for emphysematous, gangrenous, or perforated cholecystitis.

▶ Health Maintenance Issues

Individuals demonstrating early signs of fatty food intolerance may delay or avoid progression of disease with low-fat diet.

### B. Pancreatic Tumors

▶ Scientific Concepts

Pancreatic adenocarcinoma occurs most often between ages 50 and 70 with increased incidence among males, African Americans, and persons of Jewish descent. Risk factors include diabetes, chronic pancreatitis, familial cancer, polyposis, tobacco use, and dietary and occupational exposures.

▶ History & Physical

Weight loss, jaundice, and pain are the most common symptoms. Back pain and depression may also occur. Courvoisier's sign (palpable nontender gallbladder with jaundice) is more indicative of pancreatic malignancy than cholecystitis. Signs and symptoms are related to the location of the tumor, the most common being the head and, less commonly, the body or tail of the pancreas.

### ▶ Diagnostic Studies

Ultrasound of the upper abdomen including gallbladder, liver, and pancreas is the study of choice for patients with jaundice. Computed tomography (CT) of the abdomen can be the initial study when pancreatic carcinoma is suggested by history and physical findings. ERCP may be helpful to find small tumors, but requires a highly skilled endoscopist. For patients with obstructive jaundice, percutaneous transhepatic cholangiography is useful.

### ▶ Diagnosis

Percutaneous fine-needle aspiration is reliable for diagnosing a malignancy, but should not be used when ultrasound or other studies demonstrate a lesion that is potentially resectable.

### ▶ Clinical Therapeutics

Palliative procedures are more frequent than curative ones. Procedures to relieve biliary obstruction or gastric outlet obstruction, chemotherapy, or combination therapy including intraoperative radiotherapy are alternatives.

### ▶ Clinical Intervention

Patients without preoperative evidence of metastatic disease may be treated with resection. Pancreaticoduodenectomy (Whipple procedure) is standard for tumor of the pancreatic head, when not involving the portal vein or superior mesenteric artery region. Prior laparoscopy can be used to rule out peritoneal seeding, which would be a contraindication to radical surgery. Distal pancreatectomy including splenectomy and lymphadenectomy is performed for carcinoma of the midbody and tail location. Laparoscopy should be included for staging of the condition. Total pancreatectomy has potential advantages, but survival rates are not significantly better and it results in a brittle type of diabetes requiring careful management postoperatively.

### ▶ Health Maintenance Issues

Sobriety to halt progress of chronic pancreatitis, avoidance of tobacco and other environmental exposures may decrease incidence in high-risk populations. In general, measures are supportive and palliative, since most pancreatic tumors are characterized as being fast growing, aggressive, and eventually fatal.

## C. Malignant Breast Masses

### ▶ Scientific Concepts

During her lifetime, a woman has a 12% chance of developing breast cancer. Of new cases each year, less than 1% is in men. The overall mortality rate for breast cancer has not changed in several decades. Primary risk factors include first-degree relatives, carrying the hereditary breast cancer gene, atypical hyperplasia, prior contralateral breast cancer, and nulliparity. The role of unopposed estrogen use is again under question at the time of this writing. Noninvasive breast cancers include ductal carcinoma in situ (DCIS), lobular carcinoma in situ (LCIS), and Paget's disease. Invasive breast cancer has favorable histologic types of tubular (grade 1 intraductal), colloid or mucinous, and papillary. Less favorable outcomes are seen with medullary cancer, invasive lobular, invasive ductal, and inflammatory breast cancer. Staging and prognosis is based on the T (tumor size) N (axillary node status) M (distant disease/metastasis) table.

### ▶ History & Physical

Sixty percent of patients present having discovered a lump on self-examination. Twenty-five percent of masses are discovered by examiners. Another presenting symptom is evidence of metastatic disease, particularly axillary nodes or distant organs (especially lung, liver, bone, brain, adrenal). Physical exam includes inspection and palpation of both breasts and axillae.

### ▶ Diagnostic Studies

Mammography should begin with a baseline study at age 40 or immediately at any age with symptomatology. Ultrasound, though not a good screening tool, is useful to evaluate a particular mass. Magnetic resonance imaging (MRI) may be used to clarify a questionable lesion on mammogram. Fine-needle aspiration is for any palpable mass to determine if it is cystic or solid as well as for cytology. Large, locally advanced lesions should receive a core-needle biopsy.

### ▶ Diagnosis

Biopsies will differentiate between benign and cancerous lesions. Staging using the TNM method assists in determining prognosis and selection of treatment.

### ▶ Clinical Therapeutics

Radiation, chemotherapy, and hormonal therapy are considered in addition to excision of the mass, based on biopsy typing and staging.

### ▶ Clinical Intervention

Surgical procedures are based on staging. Breast conservation surgery is done for stage 1 and 2 and some stage 3 patients. Procedures include lumpectomy, axillary lymphadenectomy, sentinel node biopsy, and postoperative radiation. Modified radical mastectomy (entire breast and axillary contents are removed), Halstead radical mastectomy, and simple mastectomy (all breast tissue removed) are other procedures used as indicated. Haagensen criteria are used to determine inoperability. Postoperative care should focus on mobilization of the ipsilateral arm, psychological support, and a breast prosthesis. Surveillance for recurrent disease is essential.

### ▶ Health Maintenance Issues

Breast-self exam should be taught to all females beginning in puberty, and yearly clinical exam should begin at age 18. Screening mammography should begin at age 40 and continue every 2 years until age 50, when it should become an annual event.

## D. Thyroid Masses

### ▶ Scientific Concepts

Most commonly, a thyroid nodule is found on physical exam of an asymptomatic patient. Although most solitary nodules are benign, the concern is for malignancy. In children, 85–90% are benign. During childbearing years most nodules are nonmalignant. Malignant incidence in a nodule increases about 10% per decade after age 40. Women have a greater likelihood of thyroid cancer than men, but benign nodules are more common in women. Tumors in males are more likely to be malignant. Head or neck radiation exposure increases the incidence of thyroid cancer.

### ► History & Physical

Physical exam on an otherwise healthy patient may reveal a thyroid nodule. Nodules that are firm suggest malignancy, but may soften through cystic degeneration. Benign nodules are characteristically soft. Sudden appearance or rapid growth point toward malignant character.

### ► Diagnostic Studies

Thyroid function tests, antithyroid antibody levels, thyrocalcitonin assay, and radioisotope scanning are all laboratory studies to evaluate the general thyroid function. Ultrasonography can determine whether a mass is solid or cystic, or may reveal a nonpalpable lesion. Needle biopsy obtains cells for histo- or cytopathologic examination to aid in diagnosis.

### ► Diagnosis

Biopsies will differentiate between benign and cancerous lesions.

### ► Clinical Therapeutics

Thyroid hormone supplement is necessary after partial or complete thyroidectomy. If a postoperative scan reveals any radioiodine uptake, then further use of radioiodine for ablation is necessary to complete the treatment.

### ► Clinical Intervention

Surgical excision for thyroid cancer is the mainstay of treatment. The extent of tissue removal is based on aggressiveness of the tumor, extent of the tumor, and histological type. The range includes simple lobectomy and isthmus excision for a solidary nodule to gland excision and lymph node excision.

### ► Health Maintenance Issues

Monitor for evidence of recurrent or metastatic disease. Most common sites are bone, brain, and lung.

## E. Splenectomy

### ► Scientific Concepts

There are multiple functions of the spleen, some of which continue to be poorly understood. Blood filtration and immunologic processes are the most important functions. Indications for splenectomy can be classified as absolute or relative based on the type of pathology. Absolute indications include massive splenic trauma or spontaneous rupture, primary splenic tumors, splenic abscess or echinococcal cyst, hereditary spherocytosis, and bleeding esophagogastric varices associated with splenic vein thrombosis. Relative indications include chronic lymphocytic or myelogenous leukemia, staging for Hodgkin's disease or non-Hodgkin's lymphoma, immune and infliltrative disorders, hematopoietic disorders other than spherocytosis, and primary splenic disorders.

▶ History & Physical

Symptoms of conditions that might indicate splenectomy vary based on the etiology. Conditions may present as chronic, slowly progressive with generalized symptoms (the leukemias, systemic lupus erythematosus [SLE], etc.) to acute, fulminating, specific symptoms (massive trauma or thrombotic thrombocytopenic purpura) requiring immediate action.

▶ Diagnostic Studies

Various blood tests (complete blood count [CBC] with peripheral smear, serum protein electrophoresis, bone marrow samples) and visualization studies (CT, MRI) aid in establishing the diagnosis and then indicating the course of treatment.

▶ Diagnosis

Diagnoses vary widely as indicated in the Scientific Concepts section.

▶ Clinical Therapeutics

In some of the splenic conditions, medical treatment in itself is sufficient, or is at least the front-line approach. Steroids for thrombocytopenic purpura is an example. Chemotherapy and radiation therapy are used in Hodgkin's disease.

▶ Clinical Intervention

Surgical excision of the spleen is absolutely indicated in some medical conditions and some traumatic conditions, as noted above. Traditionally, splenectomy is accomplished through a laparotomy incision by either first ligating the ligaments or approaching the vessels first. With the greater sophistication of laparoscopic techniques, some surgeons use this approach.

▶ Health Maintenance Issues

Postoperative complications may include hemorrhage, abscess, or thrombocytosis. Because of the role the spleen plays in the immune system, caution to avoid sepsis, particularly use of polyvalent pneumococcal vaccine, should be used in all patients who have had the spleen removed.

## F. Aortic Aneurysm

▶ Scientific Concepts

A pseudoaneurysm is covered only by a thickened fibrous capsule after trauma or infection. A true aneurysm involves all three layers of the arterial wall and is usually associated with atherosclerosis. It is defined as a focal dilation of an artery to 1.5–2 times or more greater than its normal diameter. Aneurysms are most common in the infrarenal aorta, iliac arteries, and popliteal arteries, and it is estimated that 2–3% of men over 70 years old have an aortic aneurysm. High-risk factors (smoking, hypertension, positive family history) may increase the incidence to 10%, and gender ratio is 4:1 male to female. The risk of rupture is diameter dependent.

A 4-cm abdominal aortic aneurysm (AAA) has an annual risk of rupture of less than 5%, but this increases to 15% when the diameter reaches 6 cm. Because surgical mortality rate for elective repair of AAA is reported at 2–4%, and patients with an aneurysm greater than 5 cm are encouraged to undergo repair.

### ▶ History & Physical

Aneurysms often are discovered on routine physical exam as an asymptomatic mass. Of the 20% that are symptomatic, localized pain or tenderness, thrombosis, or distal embolization with secondary peripheral ischemia are the findings. A bruit may be heard by auscultation over the upper midline abdomen. Severe acute back pain, hypotension, and hemodynamic collapse indicate the clinical catastrophe of rupture.

### ▶ Diagnostic Studies

The "eggshell sign" of aortic calcification is seen in 60% of patients. If an abdominal aortic aneurysm is suspected by history or exam, the best screening test is ultrasonography, which can assess the size and location with >95% accuracy. CT or MRI can then evaluate the full extent of the aneurysm.

### ▶ Diagnosis

Defined as diameter of ≥4 cm confirmed by examination and diagnostic studies.

### ▶ Clinical Therapeutics

Patients with serious surgical risk factors such as pulmonary disease, renal insufficiency, or coronary artery disease are managed with conservative measures of monitoring symptoms and follow-up ultrasonography every 3–12 months.

### ▶ Clinical Intervention

An abdominal incision is usually the approach of choice. Proximal dissection of the aorta to the aneurysm and heparinization are accomplished before the aorta is clamped and the aneurysm incised. The residual aneurysm sac is used as a cover once a prosthetic graft is sewn in place. Sophisticated catheter techniques and devices have led to an alternative repair of the endovascular graft. Success rate for patients who have an aneurysm rupture is less than 25–50%, even with immediate surgical care.

### ▶ Health Maintenance Issues

Complications after surgery include myocardial infarction (MI), renal failure, ischemia of the colon, and distal emboli. A pseudoaneurysm may develop at the graft/vessel junction. All patients should be encouraged to follow guidelines to reduce occurrence of atherosclerotic disease.

## G. Inguinal Hernias

### ▶ Scientific Concepts

Indirect inguinal hernias are congenital but cannot develop if the processus vaginalis does not remain patent. It is related functionally to the communicating hydrocele that has serous fluid, not bowel, protruding into the groin. Direct inguinal hernias are not associated with the processus vaginalis and proceed directly through the posterior inguinal wall, medial to the inferior epigastric vessels. They are thought to be acquired lesions and not to protrude into the scrotum. The femoral hernia is like the direct hernia in that it is acquired and has no hernia sac. Indirect hernias are the most common type in both sexes and in all age groups. A hernia may be reducible (contents pushed back into the abdomen), incarcerated (contents cannot be pushed back), obstructing (kinked loop of bowel obstructs gastrointestinal [GI] tract), strangulated (ischemic tissue contained in the hernia will necrose), sliding (the wall is partly formed by the colon or bladder not just the peritoneum), or Richter's type (one side of bowel wall is trapped allowing necrosis without obstructive symptoms). Once discovered, it is usually wise to repair hernias electively rather than after signs of major complications ensue such as obstruction, strangulation, or perforation.

### ▶ History & Physical

Inguinal hernias usually cause a bulge in the groin that typically increases with increased abdominal pressure. The mass may be tender. The examiner's finger should be placed along the spermatic cord at the scrotum and passed into the external ring along the canal. A direct hernia causes a forward bulge low in the canal. An indirect hernia touches the tip of the finger. The femoral hernia bulges lateral to the inguinal ligament.

### ▶ Diagnostic Studies

History and physical exam suffice.

### ▶ Diagnosis

While differentiation of hernia type is based on history and examination, surgical repair technique is essentially the same. Differential diagnosis from other conditions includes hydrocele, thrombosed varix, lymphadenopathy, undescended testicle, or abscess or tumor.

### ▶ Clinical Therapeutics

If necessary, pain management until repair is warranted. In patients of older age with high surgical risk, mechanical "truss" support is palliative and not curative.

### ▶ Clinical Intervention

Surgical repair is the mainstay of treatment for all groin hernias. Several techniques exist (Marcy, Bassini, McVay, Shouldice, Lichtenstein), but the principle of returning hernia contents to the place of origin and securing the defect is the foundation of repair. More frequently, prosthetic mesh is the repair material of choice as opposed to layer reconstruction and reinforcement. Laparoscopic techniques are now commonly used, but are contraindicated for intestinal infarction within the hernia.

### ▶ Health Maintenance Issues

Hernias that are discovered in infants should be repaired as early as possible. This is also true of patients at any age. The recurrence rate is approximately 1 in 7 over a 15-year postoperative period. Proper body mechanics for lifting and weight control can reduce the incidence.

## H. Appendicitis

### ▶ Scientific Concepts

Appendicitis is the most common cause of acute surgical abdomen, and 80% are in the 5- to 35-year age range. Increased incidence is also found in patients over age 60. The appendix mucosa has a high concentration of lymph follicles, and obstruction of the appendiceal lumen from lymphoid hyperplasia associated with an acute viral or bacterial illness may account for 60% of acute appendicitis cases. Another 35% are caused by blockage of the lumen by fecal material that hardens. When the lumen is blocked, the appendix distends and ischemia and then necrosis may occur. Perforation may occur if all layers of the appendix are involved, resulting in an abscess or diffuse peritonitis.

### ▶ History & Physical

Loss of appetite, nausea, or vomiting may accompany the initial symptoms of upper abdominal or periumbilical pain. Generalized pain becomes more focused in the right lower quadrant as inflammation progresses; fever and leukocytosis develop. Rebound tenderness at McBurney's point (two thirds distance from the anterior iliac spine to the umbilicus) often develops. Bowel sounds decrease or become absent. Pressure applied to the left lower quadrant causing pain in the right lower quadrant (Rovsing's sign), pain on extension of the right hip (positive psoas sign), and pain with passive rotation of the flexed right thigh in the supine position (positive obturator sign) all aid in determining this diagnosis and the possible position of the appendix. Rupture may occur that temporarily lessens the pain and other symptoms, only to have them return more severely.

### ▶ Diagnostic Studies

The most important diagnostic tool is the history and physical exam. A WBC with a left shift is helpful. Radiographic studies including flat plate of the abdomen, CT, or ultrasound may be useful in cases that present atypically, but usually are not necessary.

### ▶ Diagnosis

Multiple organs from several systems can cause right lower abdominal symptoms. Gastroenteritis, colitis, pyelitis, salpingitis, tuboovarian abscess, and ruptured ovarian cyst should be included in the differential. Other possibilities are Meckel's diverticulum, acute ileitis, obstructing tumors of the ascending colon, sigmoid or cecal diverticulitis, or perforated gastric or duodenal ulcer. Some nonsurgical conditions such as right lower lobe pneumonia, acute hepatitis, acute pyelonephritis, cystitis, and epididymitis must be eliminated also. Testicular torsion is another condition to consider. Younger children may have an intussusception. Rarely an appendiceal carcinoid tumor is found and only 3% of those are malignant.

### ▶ Clinical Therapeutics

Fluid and electrolyte replacement should be instituted before surgical intervention as well as antibiotics (second- or third-generation cephalosporin).

### ▶ Clinical Intervention

Surgery should be done promptly. Laparoscopic technique is favored for reduced postoperative pain and quicker return to work, although studies have shown no reduced hospital stay. A greater incidence of recurrent abscess is thought to occur in ruptured appendix cases that are removed laparoscopically. A localized abscess identified by CT may be drained through radiologic visualization, antibiotics instituted, and appendectomy performed 6 to 12 weeks later.

### ▶ Health Maintenance Issues

Wound infection is the most common postoperative complication, or an abscess. Abdominal or pelvic adhesions may present problems of abdominal pain or reduced fertility, particularly in females.

## I. Small Bowel Tumors

▶ **Scientific Concepts**

Benign neoplasms are 10 times more common than malignant tumors according to autopsy data and are usually asymptomatic. However, malignant tumors constitute 75% of *symptomatic* small bowel tumors. Surgery is indicated for the benign lesions of polyps, leiomyomas, lipomas, adenomas, hemangiomas, fibromas, and neurofibromas only if associated with bleeding, obstruction, or intussusception. The most common malignant neoplasms are adenocarcinoma, carcinoid, lymphoma, and sarcoma. Metastases from other intra-abdominal sites are common, but from extra-abdominal sites are rare. Because symptoms are often subtle and slow in onset, diagnosis is often late in the course of the disease. Although not classified as tumor disease entities, ulcerative colitis and Crohn's disease may also reach a point where surgical intervention is the treatment of choice. These entities are described in greater detail in another chapter.

▶ **History & Physical**

For adenocarcinomas, obstruction is the most common finding; it is associated with weight loss, and sometimes occult bleeding can occur. In carcinoid tumors, presenting symptoms include anorexia, weight loss, and fatigue. These are the same symptoms, in addition to vague abdominal pain, that are found with primary small bowel lymphoma. Ulceration and bleeding occur in more than half of patients with leiomyosarcoma. On examination, if the condition has progressed to obstruction, bowel sounds are decreased and high-pitched. The abdomen may be distended, tympanic, and varying levels of tenderness may be found.

▶ **Diagnostic Studies**

An abdominal series that includes supine and upright views of the abdomen and an anteroposterior (AP) view of the chest will help ascertain mechanical obstruction. Although not specific for diagnostic purposes, a CBC and basic chemistry panel with urinalysis will indicate the patient's overall condition.

▶ **Diagnosis**

Nearly half of all small intestinal adenocarcinomas are diagnosed at operation by histological exam.

▶ **Clinical Therapeutics**

For adenocarcinomas, chemotherapy has little role in treatment. Lymphomas can be treated postsurgically with chemoradiation.

▶ **Clinical Intervention**

Treatment includes segmental resection of the intestine with adequate margins and removal of as much mesentery as possible without compromising blood supply to the remaining intestine.

▶ **Health Maintenance Issues**

Supportive treatment for nutrition is important.

## J. Large Bowel Tumors

▶ **Scientific Concepts**

Polyps are important because those with certain physical characteristics have a greater incidence of malignant potential (villous type have

33% propensity). Familial polyposis syndrome is characterized by extensive polyposis, and nearly all persons develop colon cancer if not treated.

Cancer of the colon and rectum is a major cause of death in the United States. It is the most common malignancy of the GI tract and is the third most lethal cancer in both men and women. Most detection is after the age of 50. Historically, the most common location has been the left colon and rectum, but there has been a shift to the right colon. Neither pathogenesis nor cause is well understood, but the polyp–cancer sequence is a factor and patients with ulcerative colitis have an increased risk as do patients with Crohn's disease. Genetics (familial adenomatous polyposis) and dietary factors have all been implicated in pathogenesis. Peak incidence is at approximately 70 years of age, but the incidence begins to increase in the 30s.

► History & Physical

Clinical presentation depends on the location, size, and extent of the tumor. Right-sided cancers are associated with melanotic stools, iron deficiency anemia, and right-side mass. Left-sided tumors produce a change in bowel habits, red blood per rectum, and cramping abdominal pain from partial obstruction. History findings include change of appetite, malaise, and possible change in stool caliber, as well. Physical exam should always include digital rectal exam with stool guiac.

► Diagnostic Studies

Colonoscopy is the evaluation tool of choice to exclude or confirm synchronous lesions. A barium enema can be avoided if the colonoscopy exam reaches the cecum and visualization is satisfactory. Labs should include carcinoembryonic antigen (CEA), liver enzymes, and CBC. CT scan is used to evaluate the abdomen and especially the liver for metastases.

► Clinical Therapeutics

Surgical resection is the preferred treatment for most cases of colorectal cancer. Chemotherapy and radiation therapy are palliative for recurrent nonresectable tumors.

► Clinical Intervention

Important aspects of surgery include proper bowel preparation, thorough exploration of the abdomen for metastases, segmental excision with node excision, and anastomosis without tension. A temporary colostomy is used for all "pull-through" operations. The TNM staging system is useful in predicting survival rates, as is the Dukes' classification.

► Health Maintenance Issues

Since most recurrences are in the first 18–24 months postoperatively, reevaluation as often as monthly with CEA and 6-month intervals for barium enema or colonoscopy is recommended.

## K. Gastrointestinal Diverticula

► Scientific Concepts

A diverticulum is an abnormal sac or pouch protruding from the wall of a hollow organ, and by age 80 about 70% of persons have it. True diverticula are composed of all layers of the bowel wall, whereas false diverticula lack a portion of the bowel wall. Diverticulosis appears related to low-fiber diet, which is typical of Western cultures. The sigmoid colon is the most common site. Diverticulitis results from perforation of a diverticulum after blockage by a fecalith and can be as benign as localized cellulitis or as fulminant as fistula formation and an acute abdomen condition.

▶ History & Physical

Hallmark symptoms are left lower quadrant abdominal pain, alteration of bowel habits, fever, and occasionally a palpable mass. All are dependent on the progression of the infection after perforation.

▶ Diagnostic Studies

CT scan is the study of choice. Abdominal x-rays are appropriate if acute diverticulitis is suspected. A barium enema is contraindicated in the acute phase, and should be deferred 2 to 3 weeks. If fistula or obstruction are of concern, a contrast enema is indicated.

▶ Diagnosis

Diagnosis is based on the radiograph findings and history and physical.

▶ Clinical Therapeutics

Treatment is directed at the specific complication. Eighty-five percent of acute cases are treated medically with intravenous (IV) antibiotics and no oral intake. More than two acute episodes is a good indication that surgery will be needed.

▶ Clinical Intervention

Elective sigmoid colectomy should be scheduled for any one with two or more hospitalizations for acute diverticulitis. If the condition is serious enough, immediate resection with temporary colostomy may be needed. For fistula conditions, sigmoid colectomy after adequate bowel preparation is recommended.

▶ Health Maintenance Issues

Proper diet, avoiding seeds and nuts, is important to reduce incidence of diverticular blockage.

## L. Ulcerative Colitis and Crohn's Disease

▶ Scientific Concepts

Ulcerative colitis is an idiopathic inflammatory disorder of the large bowel and rectum that involves the mucosa and submucosa. It is most often seen in persons age 15–30, but also may have an onset at about age 55. Twenty percent of patients have a family history, suggesting a predisposition genetically. The etiology is unknown and the male:female ratio is nearly 1:1. Ethnically, Jews have an increased incidence and African Americans and Native Americans are essentially spared. Microabscesses are a part of the disease progression and may lead to pseudopolyp formation. Crohn's disease, if limited to the colorectal area, can be confused with ulcerative colitis. Crohn's more commonly occurs in the terminal ileum region and is transmural. The overall distinguishing features of Crohn's from ulcerative colitis include involvement of any portion of the alimentary canal, "skip lesions" where normal segments alternate with diseased segments, linear ulcerations, aphthous sores, and extraintestinal manifestations. Like ulcerative colitis, Crohn's has two parts of the life span when it most commonly occurs: during the teens and early 20s and again in the 5th and 6th decades.

### ► History & Physical

In ulcerative colitis, bloody diarrhea is the most common symptom, with mucus and pus. Cramping abdominal pain, malaise, fever, weight loss, and anemia are common. A condition of "toxic megacolon" may result from a fulminant course that includes dilatation of the transverse colon and risk of perforation. Physical exam for ulcerative colitis is consistent with the severity of the symptoms and may be essentially negative or consistent with findings of an acute abdomen. In Crohn's, most patients have the triad of abdominal pain, diarrhea, and weight loss, of which abdominal pain is the most common presenting symptom. The diarrhea rarely is bloody, assisting the clinician in differentiating from ulcerative colitis. Perianal involvement can be seen with Crohn's but rarely with ulcerative colitis. Extraintestinal manifestations involving the skin, eyes, joints, and liver are commonly found with Crohn's, and patients often appear chronically ill.

### ► Diagnostic Studies

Proctoscopy is the most valuable test to establish the diagnosis of ulcerative colitis. Radiographic evaluation is useful for both of these disease entities to determine extent if severity of condition (acute abdomen) does not contraindicate barium studies. The aforementioned skip lesions are characteristic of Crohn's as well as a cobblestone appearance from granulomas; the loss of haustral markings may be noted in ulcerative colitis. The order of studies is important to be effective: barium studies should be done after nuclear scans, ultrasonography, plain films, and IV contrast because expulsion of barium from the GI tract is slow and it interferes with the other tests. Additionally, the barium studies should be done in the following order so as not to complicate the interpretation of results: enema, upper GI, small bowel, and enteroclysis (small bowel enema).

### ► Diagnosis

Diagnosis is made by a combination of typical radiographic patterns and histology evaluation of biopsies. Radiologic studies should confirm location and pattern of lesions in the alimentary canal that will distinguish between ulcerative colitis and Crohn's. This is necessary because it is difficult to differentiate Crohn's from ulcerative colitis when specimens are examined microscopically.

### ► Clinical Therapeutics

For ulcerative colitis, medical therapy is the usual initial treatment and is successful in about 80% of cases. This includes initial steroid therapy that must be used only short term and is then changed to sulfasalazine. Crohn's also responds to steroids, but immunosuppressive agents are the agent of choice thereafter. Broad-spectrum antibiotics are beneficial to decrease luminal bacterial concentrations.

### ► Clinical Intervention

Surgical treatment in ulcerative colitis is indicated for hemorrhage, toxic megacolon not responding to intensive medical treatment, colonic stricture, dysplasia or cancer, and debilitating disease not responding to medical treatment. Procedures may include total proctocolectomy with permanent ileostomy, proctocolectomy with anal preservation and ileal–anal anastomosis, abdominal colectomy with closure of the rectal stump, or other less often used procedures. Surgical indications for Crohn's include intestinal obstruction, fistulas or abscesses, debilitating disease, fulminant colitis, or cancer. It should be noted that the propensity for cancer is much less with Crohn's than with ulcerative colitis. The goal of surgery is to conserve bowel; it is palliative, not curative. Abdominal exploration is performed and sites of transection are chosen conservatively, based on obvious gross involvement. Microscopic confirmation of the absence of disease at the margins does not determine future recurrence and is not necessary for a safe anastomosis, thus eliminating the need for frozen-section evaluation. It is likely that Crohn's patients will require surgery in the future because recurrence is the rule rather than the exception, especially in patients with small bowel involvement. Since multiple segment resection may result in "short-bowel syndrome," management of strictures with stricturoplasty as opposed to further resection is preferred. Unfortunately, the efficacy of prophylactic pharmacotherapy after resection in preventing recurrence is not convincing.

### ► Health Maintenance Issues

Particularly for Crohn's patients, psychosocial support long term is important. Yearly colonoscopy has been recommended because of predisposition to cancer, particularly for ulcerative colitis patients.

## M. Volvulus

### ► Scientific Concepts

Volvulus is the twisting or torsion of an organ on a pedicle. Although rare in the United States overall, more than 80% of volvulus in the colon are in the sigmoid portion. The most typical patient is male, average age of 60, who has been in long-term care or mental institutions. Cecal volvulus is more rare and is found most commonly in women under age 40. Sigmoid volvulus is predisposed when there is a long, freely movable sigmoid portion, sufficient mobile mesentery, and a fixed point about which the colon can twist. A congenital anatomic anomaly wherein there is incomplete peritoneal fixation of the right colon is necessary for cecal volvulus to develop. Competence of the ileocecal valve aids in distinguishing findings between small and large bowel sites of obstruction. An incompetent valve allows large bowel findings to mimic small bowel findings.

### ► History & Physical

History reveals abdominal distention, discomfort, and obstipation in both types of volvulus. The cecal type may have some initial diarrhea. Exam demonstrates distention and tympany, and rebound tenderness suggests gangrenous bowel.

### ► Diagnostic Studies

Abdominal x-rays assist in differentiation: in sigmoid type, there is a massively distended loop of bowel with both ends in the pelvis and the "bow" near the diaphragm (known as bent inner tube sign). A large distended cecum in the left upper quadrant associated with the "bird's beak" deformity or "ace of spades" on barium enema indicates cecal volvulus.

### ► Diagnosis

It is extremely important to distinguish between complete and partial obstruction because of the need for immediate surgery in the former with its inherent risks, particularly adequate bowel prep.

► Clinical Therapeutics

All patients with large bowel obstruction should be treated with IV fluids, nasogastric (NG) suction, and continuous observation until the diagnosis is established and specific therapy is instituted. If the volvulus involves the sigmoid, then sigmoidoscopy with rectal tube insertion for decompression is the initial step.

► Clinical Intervention

Cecal volvulus is always treated surgically, either by suturing the cecum to the parietal peritoneum (cecopexy) or, if there is gangrene, by right hemicolectomy with ileotransverse colonic anastomosis. Colonoscopic decompression may provide temporary resolution to allow adequate surgical prep. Prompt sigmoid resection with temporary colostomy is required if strangulation or perforation is suspected in that portion of the colon or if decompression does not succeed. Elective sigmoidectomy with colorectal anastomosis is recommended even in the case of successful decompression to prevent future episodes.

► Health Maintenance Issues

No specific recommendations are indicated.

## N. Hemorrhoids

► Scientific Concepts

Hemorrhoids are the expansion of the vessels in the anal cushions, usually caused by increased abdominal pressure from straining with defecation, pregnancy, obesity, or increased pressure of the portal vasculature. Vessel anatomy predisposes hemorrhoid location to left lateral, right anterior, and right posterior. Typification is commonly internal, above the dentate line, or external, below the dentate line. Because of innervation, external hemorrhoids are the type that are painful and have no further subclassification; they are either present or absent. Internal hemorrhoids are not painful and are classified from first to fourth degree based on prolapse magnitude, fourth being the most serious and unable to be manually reduced.

► History & Physical

Protrusion and bleeding are the primary presenting symptoms. Bleeding may be minimal after anal wiping or severe enough to cause anemia. It is painless, bright red in color, and coats the stool rather than being mixed in. First degree internal hemorrhoids can be visualized only with an anoscope. Thrombosis is indicated by purplish color, and erosion may be present. Digital rectal exam may not be tolerated in fourth degree or tender thrombosed conditions.

► Diagnosis

History and physical exam are the diagnostic methods of choice.

► Clinical Therapeutics

First and second degree conditions can be treated by sclerotherapy with phenol in oil or infrared photocoagulation. Rubber band ligation of internal lesions above the dentate line are satisfactory for first, second, and selected third and fourth degree cases. Most thromboses resolve within 2 weeks without specific therapy, the most severe pain subsiding rapidly after the first 48 hours.

► Clinical Intervention

Sometimes excision is necessary in thrombosed cases. Excision of all hemorrhoidal tissue may be required in some third and fourth degree cases.

► Health Maintenance Issues

Patient education to avoid prolonged straining and addition of dietary fiber and stool softeners is foundational.

## II. CARDIOVASCULAR AND THORACIC SURGERY

### A. Coronary Artery Disease

► Scientific Concepts

Obstruction of the coronary arteries is predominantly caused by atherosclerosis and is the most common cause of death in the United States and other developed countries. Other coronary artery disease (CAD) causes are vasculitis, radiation injury, and trauma. The male to female ratio is 4:1, but the female rate is increasing rapidly. Documented risk factors include hypertension, smoking, hyperlipidemia, positive family history, diabetes, obesity, and stress.

► History & Physical

Ischemic heart disease may present as angina pectoris, which is substernal chest pain lasting 5 to 10 minutes, precipitated by physical or emotional exertion and relieved by rest. Some patients have heart failure with pulmonary edema or hypotension. Others may present with acute MI. The clinician should also be aware of the "silent" MI in diabetics. Physical examination should include a thorough cardiac exam to assess for associated symptoms of atherosclerotic disease such as bruits, diminished peripheral pulses, cardiac enlargement, or signs of heart failure (rales, edema, hepatic enlargement).

► Diagnostic Studies

Baseline electrocardiogram may be normal at rest, so exercise stress testing with or without radionuclide is of value. Cardiac catheterization remains the gold standard.

► Diagnosis

History of chest pain type and pattern as related by the patient is essential. Additional studies of electrocardiogram (ECG), stress test, and ultimately catheterization are most useful. An obstruction of 50% of the lumen is considered physiologically significant.

► Clinical Therapeutics

Elimination of negative lifestyle habits is foundational. Treatment of stable angina without congestive heart failure is initiated with use of nitrates, beta-blockers, digitalis, and calcium channel blockers. Percutaneous transluminal coronary angioplasty is the next option, the purpose of which is to widen the lumen while leaving the vessel intact, sometimes placing a stent to lengthen the time of patency.

### ▶ Clinical Intervention

The decision to use coronary artery bypass grafting is based on anatomy, symptoms, and the potential risks and benefits. Stable angina that is unresponsive to medication, unstable angina, and multivessel blockage with decreased left ventricular function are indications for bypass. Bypass may also be done on patients concomitantly if vessel occlusions are noted when a patient is having heart surgery for other reasons such as elective valve replacement or complications of MI. Not all patients are good surgical candidates, and some may be better served by percutaneous procedures. Bypass vessels are created most often from the greater saphenous vein, but when arteries (mammary and others) are used, the residual patency over time is improved. Minimally invasive bypass utilizing the internal mammary artery can be performed through limited incisions without cardiopulmonary bypass, but is limited to bypassing the left anterior descending or right coronary artery.

### ▶ Health Maintenance Issues

Continued preventive measures through modified lifestyle changes can prolong the effectiveness of coronary artery bypass. Low-fat diet, smoking cessation, and aerobic exercise are all helpful parameters.

## B. Cardiac Valve Disease

### ▶ Scientific Concepts

Cardiac valvular disease can be either acquired or congenital. Mitral and aortic valves are most commonly affected. Stenosis or regurgitation are the most common functional problems of the valves. Rheumatic fever, Marfan's syndrome, and bacterial endocarditis are the leading causes. Mitral stenosis causes distention of the left atrium (sparing the left ventricle) and subsequent right heart failure and arrhythmias, especially atrial fibrillation, leading to thrombosis and systemic embolization. Mitral regurgitation can lead to signs of pulmonary hypertension, atrial arrhythmia, and left and right heart failure with severe left ventricle injury. Aortic stenosis is progressive and silent until cardiac enlargement, especially left ventricular hypertrophy, and congestive failure develop. Aortic regurgitation can be even more insidious until left ventricular overload can lead to fulminant failure without emergent treatment. Tricuspid disease is usually regurgitation secondary to pulmonary hypertension associated with mitral valve disease.

### ▶ History & Physical

For mitral stenosis, dyspnea is the most significant symptom, indicating pulmonary congestion due to increased left atrial pressure. Chronic cough, hemoptysis, pulmonary edema, and systemic arterial embolization may also be present. The typical patient is cachectic with apical diastolic rumble, opening snap, and loud first heart sound found on auscultation. In mitral insufficiency, there may be many years between the first evidence and development of symptoms. Dyspnea on exertion, fatigue, and palpitations occur late during cardiac decompensation. A holosystolic blowing murmur at the apex radiating to the axilla and accentuated apical impulse are findings on physical exam. The classic symptoms of aortic stenosis are angina, syncope, and dyspnea. Average life expectancy after onset of symptoms is 4 years because symptoms occur late in the disease process and represent myocardial decompensation. Sudden death may occur at this stage. A crescendo–decrescendo murmur at the second right intercostal space is the classic finding, often with radiation to the carotid arteries. An associated thrill and narrowed pulse pressure may also be present. Aortic insufficiency may have early symptoms of palpitations and dyspnea on exertion, while severe congestive failure is seen later. A diastolic murmur along the left sternal border is heard, radiating to the left axilla. The pulse pressure is widened. Tricuspid insufficiency produces a systolic murmur, and stenosis of this valve produces a diastolic murmur, both best heard at the lower end of the sternum. Pulmonic valve acquired lesions are uncommon. Multiple valvular disease is usually reflected as signs and symptoms of the most severely affected valve.

### ► Diagnostic Studies

Chest x-ray, ECG, and echocardiography are appropriate to evaluate any of the valvular conditions. Cardiac catheterization gives additional important information for all of the conditions. Each specific diagnosis has its own findings on all of these studies.

### ► Diagnosis

Mitral stenosis shows prominent pulmonary vasculature in upper lung fields on x-ray, whereas an enlarged left ventricle and atrium are found with insufficiency. ECG may be normal in stenosis or show abnormal P waves; left ventricular hypertrophy is found in 50% of ECGs in mitral insufficiency. Cardiac catheterization procedure calculates valve cross-sectional area, end-diastolic pressure gradient, pulmonary artery pressure in stenosis and additionally determines left ventricular function in mitral insufficiency. To diagnose aortic stenosis, the chest x-ray shows a heart of normal size, possibly with calcification of the valve. Insufficiency in this valve is revealed by a chest x-ray with enlarged left ventricular dilatation. Cardiac catheterization with aortography will quantitate the degree of insufficiency and estimate the cross-sectional area. Important parameters in stenosis from the cardiac catheterization are pressure gradient across the valve and assessment of mitral or coronary artery disease, which is found in 25% of patients.

### ► Clinical Therapeutics

Mitral insufficiency and tricuspid disease are the only entities that significantly benefit from medical treatment of digitalis, diuretics, and vasodilators. For all others, surgery is the treatment of choice when symptoms progress.

### ► Clinical Intervention

For mitral stenosis, closed or open mitral valve commissurotomy for simple fusion of the commissures and minimal calcification. Valve replacement is required for severe disease of the chordae tendineae and papillary muscles, along with permanent anticoagulant therapy to prevent thromboembolization. Surgical intervention for mitral insufficiency is indicated for progressive congestive heart failure or cardiac enlargement, acute onset from ruptured chordae tendineae, or multi-valve disease. Valve repair and annuloplasty are performed when possible, or the valve is replaced if necessary. Aortic stenosis requires surgical correction if there are symptoms of syncope, angina, or dyspnea, or if the peak systolic gradient is greater than 50 mmHg or with valve area less than $0.7$ cm$^2$. Excision and replacement are required. Aortic insufficiency requires valve replacement when ventricular decompensation is demonstrated, with or without significant symptoms. Tricuspid valve disease that does not respond to medical treatment is remedied with surgery (commissurotomy or valve replacement for stenosis, valve excision alone for insufficiency).

### ► Health Maintenance Issues

Patients that are treated with valve replacement require permanent anticoagulation, especially in mitral stenosis.

## C. Septal Defects

### ► Scientific Concepts

Incidence of congenital heart disease is approximately 3 in 1,000 births, and in most cases the etiology is unknown. Ventricular and atrial septal defects are among the five most common types. Atrial septal defect ratio is 2:1, female to male. If there is a large defect, atrial pressures are equal on both sides, and the flow is left to right across the defect because of ventricular compliance when the atriums empty during diastole. If atrial defect is left uncorrected, pulmonary vascular obstructive disease may develop.

Ventricular septal defects are the most common congenital heart defect, and the most common ventricular septal defect is conoventricular (70–80%). Muscular defects may be single or multiple and may be of an inlet or an outlet type. Like atrial dynamics, ventricular pressures are equal on either side of a large defect and flow is left to right, but the determining factor is pulmonary vascular resistance being less than the systemic resistance. This causes increased pulmonary flow with left ventricular overload and early congestive failure.

### ► History & Physical

In atrial defects, mild dyspnea and easy fatigability present in infancy and early childhood. Untreated symptoms may progress to congestive failure during adulthood. Initial presentation may be neurologic, including cerebrovascular accident (CVA) or transient ischemic attack (TIA), from atrial thrombus embolic event. Systolic murmur and fixed, split second heart sound in left second or third intercostal space are revealed on exam.

In ventricular defects, infancy and early childhood symptoms are rarely seen in small defects, which may close spontaneously. Symptomatology is most often noted in defects equal to or larger than the aortic root diameter, and children have dyspnea on exertion, easy fatigability, and increased frequency of respiratory infections. Severe cardiac failure is seen more often in infants than children. A harsh pansystolic murmur is found on exam.

### ► Diagnostic Studies

Chest x-ray in patients with significant atrial septal defect reveals enlargement of right ventricle and prominent pulmonary vasculature. ECG demonstrates right ventricular hypertrophy and echocardiogram demonstrates the direction of blood flow shunting and definition of the defect.

In ventricular defects, biventricular hypertrophy is evident by x-ray and ECG in large defects. Catheterization is essential for documenting severity of left-to-right flow shunting, vascular resistance in the pulmonary system, and location of the defects.

▶ Diagnosis

Diagnosis is made by exam and study findings.

▶ Clinical Therapeutics

Some atrial defects close spontaneously. Medical treatment of heart failure symptoms is appropriate until control is no longer adequate in either atrial or ventricular defects. Then surgical intervention is required.

▶ Clinical Intervention

In atrial septal defects, surgical closure is indicated if the blood flow of the pulmonary system is 1.5–2 times greater than the corporal system or if a neurologic event occurs due to atrial embolism source. The ideal timing for closure is age 3–5 years. A percutaneous approach in the catheterization lab may be attempted. Otherwise, sternotomy with polyester textile fiber patch is required. Mortality risk of surgery is less than 1%.

Ventricular septal defect should be closed when infants have significant cardiac failure or increased pulmonary vascular resistance. Surgery should still be initiated in asymptomatic patients if spontaneous closure is not complete by age 2 years in patients with significant flow shunts, and if pulmonary flow is 1.5–2 times greater than systemic blood flow. Operative mortality risk is related to the degree of preoperative pulmonary vascular disease, but is less than 5%.

▶ Health Maintenance Issues

Complications of atrial repair may be sick sinus syndrome or patch leak. For ventricular repair, low-output syndrome and complete heart block are the major complications.

## D. Peripheral Occlusive Disease

▶ Scientific Concepts

Atherosclerosis is the most common cause of arterial occlusive disease, the most predisposed locations being iliac, superficial femoral, and tibial arteries. Predisposing factors are family history, tobacco abuse, diabetes, hypertension, and hyperlipidemia. Aortoiliac occlusion is more common in adults between ages 40 and 60. Occlusion may be acute or chronic, but the critical common factor is that distal pressure becomes insufficient to adequately perfuse tissues. In chronic situations, collateral circulation may develop as multiple pathways around a stenosis, but collateral vessels have higher resistance and symptoms will ensue if it is poorly developed or compromised by further atherosclerotic occlusion. When an artery occludes acutely by embolism or local thrombus from an ulcerated plaque, collateral circulation does not have time to develop and leads to acute ischemia and distal tissue loss.

▶ History & Physical

Frequently atherosclerosis is asymptomatic until pressure is low enough to limit adequate perfusion of tissues. Then claudication (cramping pain) develops in large muscle groups distal to the occlusion after exercise because of the demand for greater perfusion. Vascular claudication is reproducible by exercise and is promptly relieved by rest. Ischemic rest pain is considered limb-threatening if revascularization is not done. The same is true for gangrene or tissue necrosis. A thorough review of systems, particularly cardiac and pulmonary, is important. Assessment of neurologic, cardiac, and pulmonary systems on exam, including bruits, pulses, and skin integrity is essential.

### ▶ Diagnostic Studies

The ankle-brachial index that compares the systolic pressure of the ankle with that of the arm is a general indicator of lower extremity occlusion. A ratio of ankle to arm pressure of 0.8 correlates with claudication and 0.4 correlates with resting pain. Arterial duplex scanning allows calculation of blood flow velocity, correlating high flow with areas of stenosis. Ultimately, arteriography is done in cases of rest pain or gangrene. Magnetic resonance arteriography is becoming more accurate and common, with an advantage of being noninvasive.

### ▶ Diagnosis

Claudication is differentiated from neurogenic or musculoskeletal pain by history, physical exam, and noninvasive studies. Exercise is not usually an exacerbating factor for neurogenic pain, nor in major muscle groups. Musculoskeletal pain often remains at rest. Spinal stenosis is sometimes the finding for neurogenic claudication.

### ▶ Clinical Therapeutics

Up to 50% of patients with claudication have significant relief with cessation of tobacco usage and regimented exercise. Medical treatment with agents to provide easier passage of blood cells through the vessels is beneficial to some.

### ▶ Clinical Intervention

Percutaneous transluminal angioplasty by accessing the stenotic area with balloon inflation to fracture the plaque produces variable results, usually better in larger vessels. This may be supplemented with stent placement. Complications with this approach include atheroembolism, intimal hyperplasia, thrombosis, and rupture. Open operative procedures include bypass and local endarterectomy with patch angioplasty, which is for less common focal lesions in the femoral system. Bypass procedures are done either with autogenous veins, especially the greater saphenous, or prosthetic conduits usually of Dacron. The most common site for proximal anastomosis is the common femoral artery. If disease is isolated to the tibial vessels, such as in diabetics, the popliteal artery may be suitable. Distal anastomosis is determined by the vessel with the unobstructed distal outflow. When an autologous vein is used, it is usually placed in reversed position and the internal valves are left in place. If there is a large discrepancy in diameter between the vessel being bypassed and the reversed graft, then the vein is used *in situ* and the valves are lysed and branches are ligated. Limb amputation is used as a last resort in patients with rest pain or tissue loss. Consideration is given to the fact that the more distal the amputation, the more functional gait the patient will retain. This must be balanced, however, with the fact that the more proximal the amputation, the better opportunity for healing without significant complications.

► Health Maintenance Issues

Primary patency of a bypass ranges 65 to 89% at 5 years for most greater saphenous veins, with limb salvage rates at 90%. Assisted primary patency and secondary patency refer to grafts that have required some type procedure to maintain patency after original placement. Major limb amputation (below or above knee) has a perioperative mortality rate up to 10% for coronary vessel disease. Up to 50% will have contralateral amputation within 3 years.

## E. Lung Neoplasms

► Scientific Concepts

Cancer of the lung is the most common cause of nondermatologic cancer in North America. It is the leading cause of cancer death in both men and women. More than 85% are related to smoking greater than one pack per day for 20 years. Other causes may be exposure to radioactive materials, asbestos dust and fluorspar, nickel, arsenic, and petroleum products. Lung cancer may be primary or secondary, the former progressing from dysplastic changes to in situ changes to invasive carcinoma, and develops from two distinct cell lines of large cell or small cell types. Identification of cell lines is important in determining treatment. Small cell lines (oat cell, intermediate cell, and mixed cell) metastasize earlier and are treated systemically with chemotherapy and radiation therapy. Large cell types (squamous cell, adenocarcinoma, and mixed cell type) are evaluated with surgical removal in mind, the best chance for cure. Secondary lung cancers are cause by metastasis of tumors that start elsewhere in the body, usually from the breast, GI system, genitourinary tract, or soft tissues. Surgical option for single metastatic lesions is justified by improvement in the survival rate, but any metastasis to the lung generally has a poor prognosis.

► History & Physical

Pulmonary symptoms of lung cancer include cough, dyspnea, chest pain, fever, sputum production, and wheezing. Asymptomatic patients may discover there is tumor only by evidence on routine chest x-ray. Systemic manifestations include weight loss, malaise, bone pain, and symptoms referable to the central nervous system (CNS). Nonmetastatic manifestations are secondary to hormone-like substances with signs of Cushing's syndrome, hypercalcemia, myasthenic neuropathies, hypertrophic osteoarthropathies, and gynecomastia. Pancoast's tumor involves the superior sulcus and may produce symptoms of brachial plexus involvement, vertebral collapse, pain or weakness of the arm, edema, or Horner's syndrome. Physical exam, including auscultatory findings, will be consistent with extent of disease and location of tumor.

► Diagnostic Studies

Abnormal chest x-ray is the most common finding and tumor may present as a nodule, infiltrate, or as atelectasis. CT scan of the chest reveals extent of the tumor and possibility of mediastinal metastasis. Bronchoscopy for visualization, tissue biopsy, and/or bronchial washings for cytology evaluation will specify the histologic type of tumor and assist in treatment planning.

► Diagnosis

Diagnosis must be confirmed by histologic typing to determine treatment. Tumor must be distinguished from tubercular lesions.

► Clinical Therapeutics

The stage of tumor, of which size and spread are the key factors, determines the treatment. The TNM (Tumor, Nodal involvement, and Metastasis) system is used to provide a basis for prognostication. One half of patients are not candidates for thoracotomy with pulmonary resection at the time of diagnosis. For these patients, radiotherapy, chemotherapy, or a combination of both may be indicated.

► Clinical Intervention

Pulmonary resection is the only potential cure for bronchogenic carcinoma. It is the best treatment for patients with localized non–small cell primary lung lesions. Resection for any surgical candidate is accomplished through a thoracotomy incision. Depending on extent of involvement, the excision may require pulmonary segmentectomy, lobectomy, or pneumonectomy. For more peripheral lesions, a lesser wedge resection may be possible. More complex operations are becoming possible with the advent of bronchoplastic procedures and reconstruction of the tracheobronchial tree. Thoracoscopic surgery techniques are being developed, but their application is dependent on tumor location and size.

► Health Maintenance Issues

Common postoperative complications include bleeding, pneumonia, wound infection, and cardiac events, but these are rarely seen. Early mobilization and full expansion of the lungs appear to influence recovery favorably.

## F. Laryngeal Cancer

► Scientific Concepts

Squamous cell carcinoma is the most common laryngeal malignancy, making up about 95%. Verrucous carcinoma is a squamous variant limited to local invasion and is rarely metastatic. Alcohol and tobacco (smoking and smokeless) use are risk factors. Men are more often affected than women, most commonly ages 50 to 69. The larynx is divided into three regions, the supraglottis (drained by nodes that cross the midline, deep to the jugular nodes), the glottis (poorly developed lymphatics), and the subglottis (drained through cricothyroid membrane to the prelaryngeal and pretracheal nodes).

► History & Physical

The most common symptom is hoarseness, but stridor, cough, hemoptysis, dysphagia, and aspiration may also occur.

► Diagnostic Studies

All patients suspected of having laryngeal carcinoma must have direct laryngoscopy and biopsy. CT and MRI can determine depth and node involvement. Laryngograms, barium swallow, and stroboscopic laryngoscopy may be helpful.

► Diagnosis

Biopsy is required. Staging then determines the course of treatment.

► Clinical Therapeutics

Radiation is used for stage T1 when the tumor is confined to the site of origin to preserve voice quality, but surgery is still often indicated.

► Clinical Intervention

Extent of surgery depends on the extent of tumor spread. Large supraglottic tumors are treated with horizontal procedure to spare the true vocal folds. Transglottic tumors that spread to a true vocal fold may require a suprahemilaryngectomy with radical neck dissection and radiation if nodal metastases are found. Tumor that is confined to the larynx with fixation of the hemilarynx that has destroyed cartilage or extends beyond the larynx requires a total laryngectomy with total neck dissection. Radiation therapy is indicated both pre- and postoperatively. Verrucous carcinoma is treated with conservation laryngectomy without need for radical neck dissection.

► Health Maintenance Issues

If total laryngectomy is performed, intelligible speech can be produced by using an electrolarynx or by learning to vibrate the esophagus and neopharynx. Sometimes prosthetic valves are placed into the tracheostoma. Avoidance of tobacco and alcohol are important.

## III. NEUROSURGERY

### A. Brain Masses

► Scientific Concepts

Each factor of brain tumor categorization is important in determining diagnosis and management. These categories are relation to brain tissue (intrinsic or extrinsic), site (supratentorial or posterior fossa), and age at presentation (pediatric or adult). Extrinsic tumors more often are benign and can be excised totally; infratentorial tumors are accompanied by increased intracranial pressure and hydrocephalus than supratentorial. Pediatric tumors are more often infratentorial and adult tumors are supratentorial. The distribution regarding age is bimodal: the first is ages 3–10, and the second is in the 50s. Most brain tumors are more common in males than females. Classification of tumors is broadly based on cell origin, either astrocyte cell lines or nonglial cell tumors.

► History & Physical

Tumors become apparent by the symptoms they produce. This may be from mass effect when normal brain tissue is exposed to excessive pressure from a large tumor expanding within the closed intracranial space. "Eloquent" areas of the brain will be affected more quickly by a small tumor than a "silent" area. CNS dysfunction may occur because of blood flow impairment due to compression of normal blood vessels, a "steal" phenomenon as blood flow is diverted from normal areas of the brain to the growing tumor, or by production of substances that cause metabolic impairment. Headaches and seizures may result. A neurologic evaluation will elicit acute onset or progressive neurologic deficits. Asymmetry of motor strength, sensation, or reflexes on examination may be present. Papilledema on fundoscopic exam may indicate increased intracranial pressure.

▶ **Diagnostic Studies**

Skull films, CT scan, and MRI are appropriate initial studies. The CT and MRI should be done with contrast to demonstrate any disruption of the blood–brain barrier, which is often manifested in the tumor area. Angiography and positron emission tomography (PET) scan may also be useful.

▶ **Diagnosis**

Relation to brain tissue, site, and age of presentation assist in diagnosis of what type of tumor, but tissue evaluation histologically is essential. Supratentorial tumors include the following: Astrocytomas of the cerebrum are usually slow growing. Ependymomas are well-circumscribed and occur in the vicinity of the ventricles. Oligodendrogliomas are slow growing and are calcified. Meningiomas are most common in females and are usually adjacent to the dura. Metastatic tumors most often are from lung, breast, prostate, kidney, and melanoma. Infratentorial tumors include acoustic neuromas, epidermoid cysts, meningiomas, and hemangioblastomas. Medulloblastomas are malignant, ependimomas usually present with obstruction of cerebral spinal fluid (CSF) pathways, and brain stem gliomas present with cranial palsies of the brain stem in the first 10 years of life. Cerebellar astrocytomas have much more benign effects than astrocytomas in other locations.

▶ **Clinical Therapeutics**

Usually pharmaceutical regimens are not employed to treat this disease entity.

▶ **Clinical Intervention**

Surgery is necessary to establish a diagnosis, but is also important and even essential in treatment for many intrinsic type tumors. Surgical excision's goal is gross total removal of the tumor while minimizing iatrogenic neurologic deficits. Often the tumor must be entered and aspirated. Gross margins around metastatic tumors are more clearly defined than benign glioma margins. There is benefit demonstrated from the combination of surgical excision and postoperative radiation of single metastatic lesions. Vascular tumors are excised without biopsy because of the risk of bleeding. Chemotherapy is of limited efficacy. Extrinsic tumors can often be totally excised because they invaginate into the brain rather than arise from within it. A variety of surgical approaches are used, depending on the location of the tumor.

▶ **Health Maintenance Issues**

Supportive therapy is necessary in patients with poor prognosis and short-term survival rates. Functional losses (motor weakness, speech and cognitive impairments, and activities of daily living restrictions) may benefit from various therapy programs.

## B. Spinal Cord and Nerve Root Impingement

▶ **Scientific Concepts**

The spinal cord begins at the base of the cerebellum and proceeds through the spinal canal, floating in the dural sac, which is filled with cerebrospinal fluid. At each level between the vertebrae (7 cervical, 12 thoracic, and 5 lumbar), nerve roots depart to specific symmetrical areas of the body to transmit neuronal messages. In adults, at about the level of lumbar vertebrae 1 or 2, the tip of the cord ends and only the nerve roots remain. Injury to the cord itself or the nerve roots will produce specific symptoms and signs depending on the level of injury. Cord and nerve root injury can be differentiated by the dermatomal/myotomal patterns as well as the pattern of reflexia (hypo for individual nerve roots and hyper for cord injury above T8), muscle tone (hyper for cord injury above T8 and hypo for cord injury below T8 and any nerve root). The most common cause of cord or nerve root impingement (pressure) is intervertebral disc protrusion. Less frequent impingement sources are trauma, spondylolisthesis (slippage of one vertebra on another), or stenosis (narrowing of the canal or intervertebral foramen due to bone thickening of arthritis). Discs contain a soft fibrous center (nucleus pulposus) encased by a tough fibrous covering (anulus fibrosis). Herniation (slipped disc) occurs when the pulposus pushes through a weakness or tear in the anulus. If the fragment does not maintain its continuity with remnants of pulposis inside the disc space, it is called a *free fragment*. Depending on its position (typically underneath or through the posterior longitudinal ligament), the fragment may apply pressure to the thecal sac, spinal cord, or most commonly the nerve root, producing the classic "radicular" symptoms. The most common levels of disc herniation are C6/C7 and C5/C6 in the cervical region and L5/S1 in the lumbar region. The thoracic region rarely has disc herniation.

### ▶ History & Physical

Disc herniation typically presents as neck or low back pain; if a nerve root is involved, symptoms radiate to the limb of innervation. Muscle spasm often will be part of the symptomatology and range of motion of the spine is often limited, especially extension for cervical and flexion for lumbar discs. The nerve root affected in the cervical spine is usually the one above the disc level involved, and in the lumbar spine it is usually the nerve root below the involved level. Physical examination will demonstrate appropriate dermatomal changes in reflexes, motor strength, and sensation. For lumbar radiculopathy, the classic straight-leg raising sign is often positive. The longitudinal organization of the spinal cord dictates that a lesion at any given level can cause functional loss at all levels below that level. Bladder, bowel, and sexual function can be affected by pressure on the sacral nerves and can present a neurologic emergency.

### ▶ Diagnostic Studies

In the case of trauma, immobilization is necessary and plain x-ray films must confirm proper alignment and lack of impinging fracture. The most useful studies for disc disease are CT scan or MRI. Contrast is not necessary unless tumor is suspected or to distinguish scar tissue from new pathology if previous surgery has been done. Myelography is often used for specific surgical technique planning, especially in cases of stenosis or when fusion is required.

### ▶ Diagnosis

Mechanical stability must be established in trauma and spondylolisthesis. Tumor will require consideration of adjuvant therapy. Extent of functional loss is a better indicator of need for surgical intervention than size of herniation found on studies.

▶ Clinical Therapeutics

Approximately half of all patients with disc herniations will respond sufficiently to conservative treatment including limited activities, but not bed rest. Methylprednisolone in the acute phase of radicular symptoms followed by nonsteroidal anti-inflammatory drugs (NSAIDs) and muscle relaxers are a useful medical regimen. Narcotic analgesia is often required short term, but should be dispensed with caution. Physical therapy or chiropractic modalities of ultrasound, heat, massage, and electrical stimulation can be beneficial, and, in appropriate cases, a trial of traction is useful. If adequate relief of symptoms is not attained in 6–8 weeks after onset of symptoms, surgery must be considered.

▶ Clinical Intervention

Surgery is a last resort and is reserved for conditions where a clear need for decompression is found. Because of the structure of the cervical spine, disc excision is accomplished from an anterior approach, and fusion is required. Use of bone bank donor bone and placement of a metal plate, usually titanium, is usually selected over the option of autologous bone graft from a pelvic donor site. Lumbar microdiskectomy is a posterior procedure and no fusion is required. Lumbar fusion for mechanical instability is a more extensive procedure often utilizing disc space preservation in the form of metal or carbon cylinders and fixation between the adjacent vertebrae. For the occasional thoracic disc repair, an anterior approach involving thoracotomy and lung decompression is required, making this procedure one that is utilized with great caution. For canal stenosis, posterior laminectomy in any of the spinal regions is the procedure of choice.

▶ Health Maintenance Issues

Most patients who require microdiskectomy are able to return to normal daily activities with minimal restrictions in 6 to 8 weeks. No specific therapy is necessary, but reminders about proper body mechanics, weight control, and cessation of tobacco products is helpful. Patients requiring lumbar fusion wear a stabilizing brace for about 4 months and then progress to therapy with goals of lumbar stabilization and mobilization. The same reminders apply as above. Active lifestyles may be resumed, but restrictions on lifting and bending and twisting must be considered. Pain management may become an issue and such patients should be referred to a specialist.

# IV. UROLOGIC SURGERY

## A. Renal Masses

▶ Scientific Concepts

Renal masses are classified as benign or malignant, with malignant masses further classified as primary or metastatic. The most common renal mass is a simple cyst (70%). Renal cell carcinoma is the most common primary renal tumor and is more common in men than women, being most frequently found from age 40 to 69. This type of tumor usually arises from the proximal convoluted tubules. Renal cell tumors are usually unilateral and are spherical with a pseudocapsule of parenchyma and fibrosis. Transitional cell carcinoma of the renal pelvis may present as a renal mass or a filling defect in IV pyelogram. Upper tract lesions may seed the lower urinary tract, thus making upper tract evaluation mandatory when lower tract findings are of transitional cell type.

▶ History & Physical

Painless hematuria is often a presenting symptom, but more tumors are being found on CT and ultrasound as an incidental finding. Patients may have flank pain, abdominal mass, and hematuria, but rarely have all three to form the complex of Charcot's triad. Masses are rarely palpable.

▶ Diagnostic Studies

Ultrasonography is useful for differentiating a simple from a complex cyst or solid tumor. CT scan is the most cost-effective diagnostic and staging modality; it evaluates local tumor, venous extension, regional lymph nodes, and liver metastases. MRI may be better at defining venous extension. Renal arteriography is best for determining renal-sparing surgery, but its diagnostic role has been replaced by CT scan. Percutaneous aspiration and biopsy is usually unnecessary, but may be a reasonable method of diagnosis for patients with metastatic disease.

▶ Diagnosis

Simple cysts require no treatment. Complex cysts are regarded as malignant tumors until diagnosed otherwise by biopsy. Renal adenoma, historically thought to be benign, is now classified the same as small renal cell carcinoma.

▶ Clinical Therapeutics

Chemotherapy is essentially ineffective, as is hormonal therapy. Immunotherapy using interferon, interleukin, lymphokine-activated killer cells, and tumor-infiltrating lymphocytes have shown some objective responses.

▶ Clinical Intervention

Radical nephrectomy (surgical removal of ipsilateral adrenal gland, kidney, and adipose tissue and fascia) with regional lymphadenectomy is performed for tumor within or without the renal capsule but still within Gerota's fascia. Excision of the renal vein is required if involvement is found.

▶ Health Maintenance Issues

Postoperative complications include bleeding, retroperitoneal abscess, ileus, and wound infection, as well as other complications of abdominal surgery such as pulmonary embolism.

## B. Ureteral Obstruction

▶ Scientific Concepts

Ureteral obstruction is caused primarily by stone disease, extrinsic masses, gynecologic malignancy, vascular aneurysm, inflammatory disease of the colon, and retroperitoneal fibrosis. Urinary calculi have a variety of compositions, but the most common are calcium oxalate calculi, which are radiopaque.

▶ History & Physical

The most frequent symptom is colicky pain from ureteral obstruction. Other symptoms include gross or microscopic hematuria, nausea and vomiting, and irritative bladder symptoms. Costovertebral angle tenderness is found on physical exam and paralytic ileus may be associated. Hematuria is usually present.

### ► Diagnostic Studies

Urinalysis usually reveals hematuria. A stone composed of uric acid is rarely found with urine pH of 6.5 or higher. Excretory urography (intravenous pyelogram [IVP]) is the diagnostic test of choice and can define stone size, location, and degree of obstruction. Renal function should be assessed before IVP to avoid contrast nephrotoxicity. In patients where IVP is contraindicated, ultrasound in conjunction with plain abdominal radiograph provides useful information. Cystourethroscopy and retrograde pyelography can reveal calculi not identified on other imaging studies.

### ► Diagnosis

Retrieved calculi or fragments should be evaluated to determine their composition. The type may reveal some systemic pathologic process that can be treated (hyperparathyroidism, renal tubular acidosis, *Proteus* urinary tract infection, or hyperuricemia).

### ► Clinical Therapeutics

Metabolic evaluation should be conducted on patients younger than age 40 with their initial event, patients with multiple calculi, and patients with recurrent stone formation. Generally, a medically treatable metabolic abnormality will be found. Observation for spontaneous stone passage is allowable for patients who have adequate orally administered pain control, the ability to take fluids by mouth, and a stone less than 5 mm in diameter.

### ► Clinical Intervention

Almost any calculus can be removed by open surgical procedure, which would be indicated by severe pain, nonprogression of calculus passage, and emergent infection or prolonged obstruction. Percutaneous nephrostomy procedure is best suited for large calculi that cannot be fragmented and removed using ultrasonic, electrohydraulic, or laser lithotriptors. Ureteroscopic procedures are most efficacious for stones in the distal half of the ureter and may be caught intact by a wire basket or fragmented with various lithotriptors. Fever and renal insufficiency are indications for emergency surgery.

### ► Health Maintenance Issues

If possible, determination of predisposing metabolic conditions and appropriate treatment may prevent recurrences.

## V. TRAUMA REPAIR

### ► Scientific Concepts

Plastic and reconstructive surgery is concerned with the reconstruction or improvement of the form and function of areas of the body. Three properties of skin are essential for understanding reconstruction—elasticity (constant tension due to underlying collagen fibers), extensibility (ability to stretch), and resilience (resistance to infection and puncture). Healing of wounds has three phases: the inflammatory phase, the proliferative phase, and the maturation phase. It is classified as healing by primary (simple repair of recent clean wounds), secondary (left open to heal without surgical intervention), and tertiary (delayed primary closure). Abnormal healing may take the form of keloids, which are hypertrophic scars. Different types of wounds require varying treatment guidelines. These types are lacerations, abrasions, contusions, avulsions, bites, contaminated wounds, and contaminated chronic wounds. A general principle is to use the least complicated form of closure of a wound that provides sufficient approximation of skin edges and other tissues.

▶ History & Physical

Mechanism of injury is an important aspect of the history to determine potential tissue injury depth and extent. Injury to vital structures (nerves, blood vessels) below the surface must be considered. The ABCs of emergency medicine (airway, breathing, circulation) must always be considered in head and neck trauma. Careful inspection of breadth, depth, preciseness of laceration margins, and contamination with foreign bodies must be considered. Function of the tissue at the site of injury, such as bending at a joint or stretching across the trunk, will influence repair technique.

▶ Diagnostic Studies

X-ray may be useful to rule out underlying fracture or to identify radiopaque foreign bodies.

▶ Diagnosis

Careful physical exam leads to an appropriate assessment of injury and repair planning.

▶ Clinical Therapeutics

Abrasions usually do not require surgical closure, but should be kept clean and moist after thorough cleansing. Contusions have external skin surfaces intact, but must be assessed for deeper tissue injury such as hematomas. Contaminated wounds must be thoroughly cleansed and debrided and usually heal best by secondary intention. Antibiotic use is reserved for severely contaminated wounds or in immunocompromised patients, or in injuries that involve deeper structures (fractures). Lacerations and open injuries older than 24 hours require debridement and irrigation. Topical antibiotic creams can help partial-thickness wounds, but care must be taken so that toxic solutions do not adversely affect wound healing by destroying normal tissue or inhibiting epithelialization. Patients must be assessed for tetanus-prone parameters and appropriate measures should be taken.

▶ Clinical Intervention

The goal of surgical repair is repair of interrupted structures and approximation of tissues. Appropriate debridement is important and preparation of wound edges for close approximation. Even approximation of skin edges is essential to avoid the casting of a shadow in lighting, which is the mechanism that makes a scar more noticeable. The principle of surgical repair is to use the technique of least complexity and tissue involvement. This order is primary closure, skin graft, local flap, distant flap, and free tissue transfer. A particular laceration may actually have a more satisfactory closure if it is extended in a Z-shaped fashion to create less tension on the suture line.

▶ Health Maintenance Issues

Keeping the site of injury clean is important for all healing wounds. Closed lacerations should be kept dry and abrasions should be kept moist to enhance best healing conditions.

# VI. PRINCIPLES OF PERIOPERATIVE CARE

There are many factors that influence operative risk. These include baseline general medical status of the patient, natural history of the disease process, and changes of the patient's baseline medical status by the surgical process. When emergency conditions do not preempt available time, a thorough medical history including current medications and allergies is important as well as a careful review of systems. Key systems to evaluate are cardiac, pulmonary, hematologic (coagulation), renal, and metabolic (diabetes, hepatic, adrenal cortex, nutritional). Specialized testing is reserved for patients who have significant risk factors. Pulmonary complications are the most common cause of postoperative morbidity. In general, patients who have an obstruction to expiration flow are in greatest jeopardy. Goldman and associates attempted to quantitate the perioperative hazards of myocardial infarction based on the history, physical findings, and laboratory data of patients, establishing the Goldman cardiac risk scale. The most cost-effective and best screening test for hemostatic abnormality is a careful history, not laboratory determinations of coagulation profiles. Metabolic and nutritional consequences of chronic renal disease frequently require special preparation of the patient. Meticulous fluid management is necessary. Diabetes presents increased risks in the area of hyper- or hypoglycemia, cardiovascular events, or infectious susceptibility.

Postoperative risks include blood loss; inadequate pulmonary function that influences perfusion of brain, heart, and kidney; cardiac dysfunction; and fluid imbalance. Central venous pressure and pulmonary capillary wedge pressure assist in evaluation of right and left heart function, respectively. Shock is traditionally described as systolic hypotension of 90 mmHg or less, but a broader definition is a condition in which total body cellular metabolism is malfunctional. Inadequate oxygen delivery and toxic cellular insult from systemic inflammation are now thought to be a dual mechanism with additive effects that are the prime factors in shock. Endpoints for resuscitation of the circulation depend on variables such as the primary etiology of the circulatory deficit, the underlying state of the patient's circulation, and the magnitude of cellular and organ malfunction during the hypoperfusion episode. Usually bedside assessment of normal circulation is adequate to predict the outcome of resuscitation.

## BIBLIOGRAPHY

Cohn SL, Goldman L. Preoperative risk evaluation and perioperative management of patients with coronary artery disease. *Med Clin North Am* 2003; 87(1):111–136.

Jarrell BE, Carabasi RA, eds. *National Medical Series for Independent Study: Surgery*, 4th ed. Philadelphia, PA: Lippincott Williams & Wilkins; 2000.

Lawrence PF, Bell RM, Dayton MT, eds. *Essentials of General Surgery*, 3rd ed. Philadelphia, PA: Lippincott Williams & Wilkins; 2000.

Lawrence PF, Bell RM, Dayton MT, eds. *Essentials of Surgical Specialties*, 2nd ed. Philadelphia, PA: Lippincott Williams & Wilkins; 2000.

# Index